The Doctors Book
OF
Home Remedies for
MEN

The Doctors Book
OF
Home Remedies® for
MEN

FROM HEART DISEASE AND HEADACHES
TO FLABBY ABS AND ROAD RAGE,
OVER 2,000 SIMPLE SOLUTIONS

EDITED BY JACK CROFT

Men'sHealth.
BOOKS

RODALE

© 1999 by Rodale Inc.
Illustrations © 1999 by Michael Gellatly

All rights reserved. No part of this publication may be reproduced or transmitted in any form or by any means, electronic or mechanical, including photocopying, recording or any other information storage and retrieval system, without the written permission of the publisher.

The Doctors Book of Home Remedies, Men's Health, and *Men's Health Books* are registered trademarks of Rodale Inc.

Printed in the United States of America on acid-free ∞, recycled paper ♻

The six-step strategy for controlling anger, on page 53, was adapted from *When Anger Hurts: Quieting the Storm Within,* by Matthew McKay, Peter D. Rogers, and Judith McKay. © 1989 by New Harbinger Publications, Inc., Oakland, California. Reprinted by permission of New Harbinger Publications.

Library of Congress Cataloging-in-Publication Data

The doctors book of home remedies for men : from heart disease and
    headaches to flabby abs and road rage, over 2,000 simple solutions /
    edited by Jack Croft.
        p.   cm.
    "Men's health books."
    Includes index.
    ISBN 0–87596–529–6 hardcover
    ISBN 1–57954–261–1 paperback
    1. Men—Diseases.   2. Men—Health and hygiene.   3. Medicine,
Popular.   4. Self-care, Health.   I. Croft, Jack.
RC48.5.D63   1999
616'.0081—dc21   98–46311

Distributed to the book trade by St. Martin's Press

2   4   6   8   10   9   7   5   3   1   hardcover
2   4   6   8   10   9   7   5   3   1   paperback

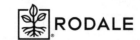

RODALE

WE **INSPIRE** AND **ENABLE** PEOPLE TO IMPROVE
THEIR LIVES AND THE WORLD AROUND THEM

The Doctors Book of Home Remedies for Men Staff

Managing Editor: Jack Croft

Contributing Editor: Stephen C. George

Principal Writers: Alisa Bauman, Bridget Doherty, Larry Keller, James McCommons, Donna Raskin, Julia VanTine

Contributing Writers: Dave Caruso, Abel Delgado, Doug Hill, Christian Millman, Linda Mooney, Judith Springer Riddle, Carla Thomas

Associate Research Manager: Jane Unger Hahn

Book Project Researcher: Jan Eickmeier

Editorial Researchers: Jennifer Abel, Tanya H. Bartlett, Jennifer Fiske, Grete Haentjens, Lois Guarino Hazel, Jennifer L. Kaas, Mary Kittel, Mary S. Mesaros, Deanna Moyer, Deborah Pedron, Paula Rasich, Staci Ann Sander, Lorna S. Sapp, Lucille Uhlman, Nancy Zelko

Copy Editor: David R. Umla

Associate Art Director: Charles Beasley

Cover and Interior Designer: Richard Kershner

Cover Photographer: Mitch Mandel

Illustrator: Michael Gellatly

Layout Designer: Donna G. Rossi

Manufacturing Coordinators: Brenda Miller, Jodi Schaffer, Patrick T. Smith

Office Manager: Roberta Mulliner

Office Staff: Julie Kehs, Mary Lou Stephen

RODALE HEALTH AND FITNESS BOOKS

Vice President and Editorial Director: Debora T. Yost

Executive Editor: Neil Wertheimer

Design and Production Director: Michael Ward

Marketing Manager: Kris Siessmayer

Research Manager: Ann Gossy Yermish

Copy Manager: Lisa D. Andruscavage

Production Manager: Robert V. Anderson Jr.

Associate Studio Manager: Thomas P. Aczel

Manufacturing Managers: Eileen F. Bauder, Mark Krahforst

Introduction

Scientists have yet to isolate it, but there can be little doubt that a home-repair gene is embedded deep within the Y chromosome. If you're looking for empirical evidence, head down to your local hardware store on any Saturday morning. Clearly, there has to be some powerful, biological imperative at work to drive men to own a full set of crescent wrenches *and* a 100-piece ratchet set *and* a toolbox full of adjustable wrenches.

There's just something about a man and his tools. The natural urge to fix things, to do it yourself, is one of the most celebrated traits among men. And rightly so. That makes it all the more perplexing that men don't bring the same can-do attitude to their health. It's the same basic principle at work. With the right tools and knowledge, you can build a body that will stand the test of time. And when minor things go wrong with your health, you can fix them. You just need to know how. That's where *The Doctors Book of Home Remedies for Men* comes in. Think of this as the ultimate repair manual for your body.

On the pages that follow, you'll find the know-how and the tools you need to do the job right. Healing from Home, the opening section of the book, offers an overview for men who want to manage their health wisely. There, you'll find specific strategies to help you choose the right doctor and make him (or her) your health-care partner because when it comes to health, there are certain things a man just can't do himself. You'll discover clear, no-nonsense explanations of the various alternative health disciplines that you'll encounter throughout the book and learn the simple, basic steps that every man can take to dramatically decrease his odds of dying before his time. You'll also find a handy list of the most common, effective, and versatile items you'll need in your home remedies toolbox.

To get the latest and best self-care tips and techniques for the Remedies section, we talked to hundreds of doctors and other experts about all the problems men face. And we came up with more than 2,000 ways to get fast relief for common ailments such as, well, the common cold, back pain, headaches, heartburn, jet lag, jock itch, muscle cramps, sore throat, and toothaches. We also collected scores of smart strategies to avoid such serious health concerns as diabetes, heart disease, high blood pressure, impotence, and stress.

But that's not all. Because we at *Men's Health* understand that virtually everything a man does can affect his health, we've included a lot of topics that you won't find in any other medical manual. Things that can cause stress and deny you your constitutionally guaranteed right to the pursuit of happiness. Things like being henpecked, Internet addiction, low self-esteem, midlife crisis, pessimism, road rage, and sports addiction. Even how to ogle other women without getting the evil eye from them or, worse, from the woman you're with.

Each Remedies chapter spotlights a "Do This Now" tip, which is your best bet for fast relief from the problem at hand. You'll find a brief description in plain English of the problem, its cause, and how serious it is. And you'll find a variety of home remedies, ranging from tried-and-true cures to the latest options culled from the fascinating world of alternative medicine. Then you'll learn what you can do to avoid ever having the problem again.

The last section of the book, In Case of Emergency, features an illustrated guide to essential lifesaving techniques that can help you be the man who keeps his cool while everyone around you loses theirs. From cardiopulmonary resuscitation to the Heimlich maneuver to saving someone from drowning, these techniques are required learning for the man who wants to always be prepared. They may help you save a life someday—maybe even your own.

Like any great repair manual, you'll find this one comprehensive yet straightforward and easy-to-use. The job of building a stronger, leaner, healthier body is a big one—no doubt about it. But I'm confident that you're just the man to do it.

Michael Lafavore
Editor-in-Chief, *Men's Health* Magazine

Contents

PART THREE: IN CASE OF EMERGENCY

Part One

HEALING FROM HOME

Who Needs a Doctor?

The book you hold in your hands will help you take care of scores of health problems by yourself. Use it well, and you'll gain as much personal control over your health and healing as you could possibly ask for. So does that mean that you'll never have to see the inside of a doctor's office again? Absolutely not.

Every man needs a doctor. And the savvy medical consumer puts at least as much effort into choosing a doctor he can trust and developing a professional relationship with his physician as he does picking an auto mechanic, accountant, lawyer, or investment broker. The idea is essentially the same: When problems come up that you can easily and safely handle, you take care of them. But when problems emerge that require a trained professional, you have a trusted expert ready and waiting to help.

This book is primarily for dealing with those problems for which a doctor might not be needed. But just so there is no confusion, we'll reiterate our point: *Every* man needs a good doctor, no matter how much he disdains the probing and questioning and undressing and waiting and paying. And to show you we mean it, we're offering right here at the beginning—before we get to the hundreds of tips and techniques that can help you feel better fast—our best wisdom on finding the perfect doctor for your particular needs.

MEN AND DOCTORS

Between the ages of 25 and 44, 63 percent of all office visits to doctors are made by women. And they have twice as much contact during the year with their doctors as men. Overall, about 7 out of 11 adults visiting a doctor are women—despite the fact that men die younger than women.

"It's a paradox," says Mack Lipkin, M.D., director of primary care at New York University in New York City. Why is it that for so many of us, a visit to a doctor is as rare as a physician making a house call? Here are a few reasons.

- We're bulletproof. "We think we're invincible," says Kenneth Goldberg, M.D., a urologist who is the founder and director of the Male Health Institute in Irving, Texas, and author of *How Men Can Live As Long As Women.*

- We're busy. Men are still in the workforce in greater numbers than women, says Dr. Lipkin. It's simply very difficult for guys to make the time for a visit to a doctor, he says.
- We're tough. "There's a cultural attitude that men share that they should tough it out," says Dr. Lipkin. "I think that because men engage in harder labor and more active and violent sports as they're growing up, they are used to pain and pain going away as just kind of a natural thing. You just take your lumps. There are many men from macho cultures where that is even more the case."
- We're frightened. Being poked, probed, and touched in embarrassing places is unnerving. "We're scared out of our wits," says Dr. Goldberg.
- We're skeptical. "Men may be skeptical because of their fears and past experiences with doctors," says Dr. Goldberg.
- And some men also have the attitude that if they can't fix it themselves, then it can't be helped, adds Dr. Lipkin.

Still, there are times when it is foolish and potentially deadly not to see a physician. "Any time you have a symptom that persists, you should see a doctor," Dr. Goldberg says. "It doesn't matter if it's a headache or abdominal pain. If it's there and it doesn't go away or it significantly intensifies, it's worth pursuing."

And there are some symptoms that should send you immediately to your doctor's office, say Dr. Goldberg and Dr. Lipkin. They are:

- Sudden pain at any location in your body, especially in the chest or abdomen.
- Sudden dizziness, change in vision, or headache.
- A change in bowel or urinary habits.
- Blood in urine, semen, stool, or mucus.
- Bleeding that is persistent from the rectum, chest, nose, or ears.
- Difficulty breathing or shortness of breath. "Young men frequently have asthma and don't know it and can really get in trouble," says Dr. Lipkin.
- Weakness or faintness. It could signal depression, a hormonal problem, chronic fatigue syndrome, or HIV infection.
- Severe or persistent diarrhea or vomiting.
- Any suicidal, homicidal, or persistent depressive feelings.

GIVING YOUR DOCTOR A CHECKUP

Even if you decide to ask a doc what's up, there remains the dilemma of choosing a good one. Most of us give more thought to what shirt to wear today than selecting a doctor. Chances are that you pick your doctor out of the Yellow Pages, along with the plumber and lawn mower repairman. Those guys, however, are unlikely to physically harm you if they make a mistake. A doctor might. So how do you pick a good one?

Go when you're well. If you wait until you're sick to call a doctor, you probably won't have the time or desire to check out his credentials. And if he's not a good doctor, this is a bad time to find out. Instead, schedule an appointment for a routine checkup or some other mundane medical matter. "It's the same thing as when you have a car," Dr. Lipkin says. "When your car breaks down, if the mechanic knows you and you have a history together, you're going to get much better attention when you need him—especially if you need the car fixed the same day—than if you've never met him before and you drive in cold."

Check the doctor's affiliations. Your odds of getting a good doctor improve if he is associated with a medical center or a teaching institution, says Dr. Lipkin. That's because they have a rigorous screening process whereby only the physicians most respected by their peers are added to the staff. And a doctor who also teaches is asked many questions by bright students, requiring him to keep informed of new developments in medicine, Dr. Lipkin says.

Ask friends and colleagues. Word of mouth can be an effective means of locating a doctor that you will like if you respect the judgment of the people recommending him, says Dr. Lipkin. Or if you know somebody who was seriously ill, ask if he was treated by any physicians that he particularly admired.

Tune in to *Dr. Quinn, Medicine Woman*. We know that some of you might find the idea of dropping your drawers for a lady doctor about as soothing as the cold metal of a stethoscope on your skin. But there is some evidence that female doctors conduct longer visits with patients, ask more questions, and make more positive statements. Other studies have found that the amount of time female physicians spend with patients hardly differs from that of their male colleagues, yet patients are often happier with a woman doctor.

In case you're wondering, about one doctor in five in America is a woman. As recently as 1980, the ratio was only about one in nine.

Check your doctor's birth certificate. One of the keys to a good doctor-patient relationship is communication. One study concluded that doctors are more receptive to patient input when the patient is not the same age as they. If true, a 25-year-old patient may find that a 60-year-old doctor listens more attentively to him, or a 60-year-old patient may do best with, say, a 35-year-old doctor.

Ask other doctors. If you know a doctor, ask him for the names of colleagues he considers to be especially competent, or ask him who his doctor is, Dr. Lipkin suggests.

Practice complimentary medicine. Researchers found that when internists were given a small bag of candy, they were more likely to diagnose a hypothetical illness quickly, and they were perceived as more humane and understanding. A compliment when your doctor provides quality care presumably would have the same effect.

Here are some other qualities to look for in a primary care physician:

A good listener. "Active listening is a key to being an effective doctor," says Dr. Lipkin.

A good talker. Your doctor should explain matters in ways that you can understand rather than using medical jargon, suggests Dr. Lipkin.

Responsiveness. Your personal physician should be somebody that you feel you can call with a question—somebody you can relate to, says Dr. Lipkin.

Personal interest. Besides being able to treat chronic medical problems, a good personal physician should develop a sensible, preventive health plan for you, says Dr. Lipkin. He will do this by assessing your diet, how much exercise you get, what you do in your leisure time, and other factors. He will then tailor a preventive medicine plan that meets your needs. So, for example, if you are a mailman with a walking route and your doctor recommends that you get more walking exercise, you might have reason to think that your doctor hasn't devised a program specifically for you.

BE PREPARED

It's unfair to put all the onus for a solid doctor-patient relationship on the physician. Dr. Lipkin suggests that men prepare for a visit to the doctor: Know your parents' medical history. Be prepared to disclose what medications you are already taking. Write down questions so that you don't forget to ask them.

A good doctor values a patient who asks questions and wants a say in his treatment, says Dr. Lipkin. These patients benefit physically and emotionally, he says. Doctors also gain. "It's the difference between having to do the heavy work and row and simply having to steer the boat," Dr. Lipkin says.

It's also important for men to let a doctor know what kind of working relationship they want with him, Dr. Lipkin says. "Some people want a doctor who tells them what to do. Other people want to make their own choices. Some people want options explained. You have to find a doctor who is right for you that way; otherwise, you'll both waste time," he says.

All of this can be trickier if you are in a managed-care health insurance plan that limits what doctors you can see. The most restrictive of these allows you to choose only from doctors in a particular health center. Even there, you might find a doctor you like a lot. Finding a personal physician is like finding a wife, Dr. Lipkin jokes: "Most of us only need one most of the time."

Maybe, but as Dr. Lipkin acknowledges, doctors and patients often move in and out of various plans, making continuity in medical care ever more difficult. If you must be in a managed-care plan, he recommends that you choose one that gives you flexibility. Some plans, for example, offer a sizable list of doctors to choose from. Others allow you to go outside their list of doctors, with the proviso that they will pay only 80 percent of the bills. No matter what type of medical plan you have, be aggressive about changing doctors until you get one who is right for you, says Dr. Lipkin.

GET PHYSICAL

Even if a visit to a doctor seems scarier than a brain surgeon with the jitters, you ought to make appointments for certain regular checkups, says Dr. Goldberg. "You need to do things even when you feel fine," he says. Dr. Goldberg recommends the following exams.

Physical exam. Men ages 20 to 39 should get a physical every three years; those 40 to 49 should get one every other year. Starting at age 50, a physical should be an annual event.

Blood pressure. It should be checked every year to determine if you are developing hypertension.

Blood and urine tests. These should be done with the same frequency as a physical exam. Cholesterol and glucose levels and how efficiently your kidneys are functioning are among the things that these tests will show.

Electrocardiogram (EKG). An EKG should be done every three to five years for men over 50, or after 30 if you're at high risk for heart disease. It will reveal your heart's health by tracing the heart's rhythms and other actions.

Tetanus booster. Have one of these every 10 years to protect against bacteria found in soil and dust and spread by animal and human feces that enter the body through a puncture in the skin, such as from a nail or splinter.

Rectal exam. This exam should be performed annually after age 40. The sound of a doctor snapping on a rubber glove while a guy's bent over, pants down, could make even Superman tremble. But it's an important test to check for prostate and rectal cancer.

Prostate-specific antigen (PSA) blood test. Have this test every year after age 50. For men who are at high risk for prostate cancer, have this test annually after age 40. Elevated levels of prostate antigens are a sign that something's wrong with your prostate.

Sigmoidoscopy. This should be done every three to four years after age 50. Men at high risk of colon cancer should get one when they turn 40. A sigmoidoscopy is even less fun than a rectal exam and harder to say. The doctor uses a lighted, thin, flexible instrument to look inside your rectum, colon, and large intestine. More precise than a rectal exam, it is used to diagnose colon cancer and polyps.

If one of these or another exam turns up a problem, your doctor may instruct you to alter your lifestyle or your diet or to take a medication. But too often, patients fail to heed the doctor's advice. We don't mean to mess up; we just get it wrong. Here are a few ways to get it right.

Get it in writing. Ask your doctor to list main points as you discuss them. Take notes during your visit, and ask for pamphlets or other written materials.

Ask questions. Ask why a test is ordered, what it will involve, whether there are any risks, and when you'll learn the results.

Understand your prescription. Make sure that you know how to take a drug correctly, why that drug is best, and what results you can expect from it, including any side effects.

Repeat what you hear. By repeating what your doctor has told you, it allows him to elaborate on any instructions that aren't clear.

Stress teamwork. Solve problems together with your doctor. If some advice he gives you isn't doable, explain why and see if the two of you can come up with an alternative plan.

New Approaches to Healing

There's a lot of baggage attached to the word *alternative*.

Something alternative belongs on the margins. That's fine if you're starting a rock-and-roll band, but getting called alternative in medicine can mean that you won't be taken seriously or trusted.

That's changing, though. Alternative medicine is becoming less "alternative" and more mainstream every day. There has been huge growth in the sale of herbs and other alternative health-care products and a huge amount of attention devoted to alternative medicine in the popular press. Both suggest that the number of people using alternative methods can only have gotten larger.

Meanwhile, the federal government has established an Office of Alternative Medicine to coordinate and fund research into alternative methods. And dozens of the nation's best university medical schools—including Harvard, Yale, and Stanford—have added courses on alternative medicine to their curricula.

All these developments are evidence of three central facts about American health care today.

1. Conventional "mainstream" medicine is increasingly recognizing that it doesn't have all the answers.
2. Patients are demanding kinder, gentler alternatives to surgery and drugs, which for 50 years or so have been the nearly exclusive mainstays of mainstream medicine.
3. There is growing evidence that alternative medicine works. It doesn't work for every ailment, but it works often—which isn't that different from the track record achieved by mainstream medicine.

John La Puma, M.D., an internist and director of CHEF (Cooking, Healthy Eating, and Fitness) Skills at Alexian Brothers Medical Center in Elk Grove Village, Illinois, thinks that there is much in alternative medicine that is good. So he edits a newsletter for medical professionals called *Alternative Medicine Alert* with the latest research in the field. He's convinced that traditional doctors will eventually integrate the best of alternative remedies with Western medicine, if for no other reason than their patients will demand it.

That's why throughout this book you'll find hundreds of so-called alternative solutions in addition to more mainstream remedies. Some of the alternative methods—eating healthy foods and taking vitamins to help ward off illness, for example—aren't big departures from what we're used to. Others are less familiar; some may seem downright strange. To help set the scene, here are brief explanations of the alternative disciplines and remedies that you'll encounter on the pages that follow.

HEALING DISCIPLINES

Aromatherapy. This system of caring for the body with aromatic botanical oils (such as rose, lavender, and peppermint) has been around since the time of the Pharaohs. Whether these powerful oils are added to bath water, massaged into skin, or inhaled directly, aromatherapy has been used to treat pain and reduce tension and fatigue.

Ayurveda. This 5,000-year-old Indian discipline of holistic healing aims to restore physical, mental, and spiritual harmony, enlisting in that pursuit an array of treatments including herbal remedies, yoga, and meditation.

Ayurveda's healing methods are based on the sorts of Eastern religious concepts that many Americans find hard to swallow—the body, for example, is seen as an expression of divine intelligence. Nevertheless, its holistic approach is a good example of how modern medicine is catching up to the ancient healing philosophies. The idea that the mind can influence health is now a widely accepted part of conventional health care.

Chiropractic. Today, more and more patients with mild back pain are being referred to chiropractors by their doctor. The Agency for Health-Care Policy and Research in Rockville, Maryland, concluded that spinal manipulation is an effective short-term treatment for lower-back pain.

Chiropractors manipulate joints and bones to correct misalignments and restore health. Very traditional chiropractors believe that all illness is the result of misalignments and rely on manipulation alone to treat all health problems. Less traditional chiropractors, however, treat mostly muscular and skeletal problems and refer patients with other types of health problems to physicians for treatment. A doctor of chiropractic (D.C.) and a doctor of osteopathy (D.O.) are each trained to perform spinal manipulation.

Flower essence therapy. Why do women love to receive flowers? Perhaps it's because flowers seem to have a therapeutic effect when your spirits are low or when you're fighting illness. Flower essences are created by soaking flowers in water, which is then mixed with alcohol. These are said to convey an "energetic imprint" of the flower, which can be used to address emotional (not physical) problems. Treatment consists of ingesting a bit of the mixture on the tongue or mixing a few drops in a small glass of water. There's no scientific evidence that flower essences work, but practitioners claim that they can gently help to restore emotional well-being.

Herbal medicine. It's likely that herbal medicine is older than man: Zoologists have noticed that apes will chew on certain medicinal herbs if they're feeling poorly. Research has since verified the healing properties of numerous herbal remedies. In fact, some of our most common medicines (aspirin, for one) are based on active ingredients derived from plants.

Be aware that the healing action of herbs is usually far more subtle than drugs: Expect a tap on the shoulder rather than a kick in the pants.

Most herbs are available in tablet or capsule form, but a more economical approach is to make a tea. Simply pour a cup of boiling water over one teaspoon of dry or fresh herb leaves or flowers and steep for about 10 minutes. Tinctures, also known as extracts, are made by soaking fresh herbs for days or weeks in alcohol with varying amounts of water. The mixture is then shaken regularly, strained, and rebottled for use. Herbal ointments and creams are also available for external use and should always be applied according to the label instructions.

Homeopathy. You've probably heard of the hair-of-the-dog cure for a hangover, in which drinking a bit in the morning of what got you sloshed last night is supposed to quiet those jackhammers drilling in your head. Homeopathy is a bit like that. It's based on the principle that what can create a certain set of symptoms in a healthy person can cure that same set of symptoms in someone who is ill.

Here's how it's supposed to work. Homeopaths have tested more than 1,000 substances—taken from plants, mostly, although some are derived from mineral and animal sources—that produce certain specific symptoms when given to healthy people. According to the homeopathic "law of similars," a sick person who displays those same symptoms can kick-start his healing mechanism (including his immune system) by taking a tiny dose of that same substance. By doing this, he'll be on his way to being cured.

Sound weird? It gets weirder. Some of these substances, if taken straight, can be toxic. But homeopaths dilute them in water over and over again, often hundreds of times. In theory, the remedy's medicinal effect grows stronger the more it's watered down.

Remedies come in various concentrations, marked with a number and either a "C," for the centesimal scale, which means potencies are diluted 100 times each time that they are shaken, or an "X," for the decimal scale, which means that potencies are diluted 10 times each time that they are shaken. The higher the number, the more powerful the substance will be, yet the more dilute it is, according to proponents of homeopathy.

Whether homeopathy is hokum or healthy is much debated. It has been around for more than 200 years—ever since a German physician named Samuel Hahnemann wondered why quinine cured malaria. He ingested quinine bark and experienced malaria symptoms, leading him to conclude that a substance that can cause certain symptoms when given to a healthy person can cure those same symptoms in someone who is sick.

Although many in the medical community are skeptical of homeopathy, says Dr. La Puma, various studies in Europe have shown that homeopathic remedies bring positive results for certain illnesses or symptoms such as diarrhea and hay fever. While homeopathy is used by a small but growing number of people in the United States, it is widely practiced in Europe, Latin America, and Asia. Three states require homeopaths to be licensed, while others allow them to practice as a specialty under another medical license, such as that of an M.D. or D.O.

Naturopathy. Naturopaths are the general practitioners of alternative medicine. They pride themselves on being conversant with a broad spectrum of natural treatments, from diet and acupuncture to herbal remedies and homeopathy. Typically, they will concentrate in one or two of these areas, referring patients to other specialists when necessary. But the naturopathic approach is intentionally eclectic. It also emphasizes the ability of the body to heal itself, with gentle, rather than dramatic, remedies.

To be licensed, a naturopathic doctor (N.D.) must complete a four-year degree program at one of the four naturopathic medical schools in North America. Some licensed naturopathic doctors can prescribe certain pharmaceutical drugs, depending upon the state where they practice. For acute or life-threatening illnesses, a naturopathic doctor should refer patients to conventional physicians, says Dr. La Puma. Because naturopathy uses so many different treatments, it's difficult to compare its effectiveness to conventional medicine. Studies that have analyzed some of the individual therapies used have reported favorable results, however. Eleven states and several Canadian provinces currently grant licenses to practice naturopathic medicine, and some states have specific provisions for naturopaths to practice.

Traditional Chinese Medicine. As it is practiced today, Traditional Chinese Medicine dates back to 476 B.C., and there's archeological evidence that its methods were in use many hundreds of years before that.

Traditional Chinese Medicine is a system combining acupuncture and herbal medicine as well as other elements, including the meditative exercise routines of tai chi and chi gung. Philosophically, Chinese medicine is based on the idea that health results from the proper balance of energy, symbolized by the yin/yang sign.

Doctors who practice this ancient discipline may have the designation O.M.D., for doctor of Oriental medicine, after their names. This means that they received their medical training specifically in Oriental medicine. The O.M.D. can be a degree granted by a school or earned through extensive training; however, it does not guarantee training in conventional medicine.

MENTAL TECHNIQUES

Meditation. The public image of meditation got seriously skewed in the 1960s. There were too many grinning gurus in saffron robes and too many rock stars sitting at their feet in the lotus position.

That's a shame, because meditation's fundamental concept—that it's healthy to shut off the ceaseless chatter of our minds for awhile—isn't all that far out.

It has been around for thousands of years in one form or another. Most techniques have come to the West from Eastern religions, but Christian contemplation—such as saying the rosary or repeating the "Hail Mary"—is similar to meditation.

Meditation is believed not only to bring peace of mind but also to aid in physical healing. Cardiologists often recommend it as a means of reducing high blood pressure. Insurance statistics for a group of 2,000 meditation practitioners compared with 600,000 people who didn't meditate showed that the use of medical care in 17 of 18 health categories was 30 to 87 percent less for those who meditate. Another study found that patients who attended a six-week behavioral medicine group that included meditation made substantially fewer visits to doctors during the six months that followed. The savings were estimated at $171 per patient.

Meditation entails making a concentrated effort to focus on a physical experience, sound, or thought. For example, you may focus on breathing or repeating a certain word or mantra. There also are moving meditations, such as the Chinese martial art of tai chi and the Japanese martial art of aikido.

And just in case you're still wondering, sitting in the lotus position isn't required.

Visualization. By using your imagination, you can better control pain or illness. It's called visualization. Skeptical? Let's say that you want to will yourself to have an erection. You might do so by imagining yourself buck-naked in a hot tub with Tyra Banks, smooching Sharon Stone, or whatever image turns you on. That's visualization.

Almost any serious athlete uses visualization on a regular basis, whether he's picturing his tee shot heading straight down the fairway or his forehand skimming perfectly into the backcourt. Corporate competitors also use visualization techniques to help build their confidence before a big presentation. The exact same idea can be applied to health: By visualizing yourself well when you're sick, or free of pain when you're hurt, you can succeed at getting better. Visualization techniques are used most commonly for colds, headaches, cancer, asthma, and allergies.

PHYSICAL TECHNIQUES

Acupressure. This is acupuncture without the needles. Hands and fingers do the healing, pressing at strategic points on the body to alleviate everything from sports injuries to eyestrain and stress. The theory is that there are channels running through the body that direct its vital energy. Acupressure (like acupuncture) is said to clear blockages in those pathways. That's why putting pressure on one point can produce an effect somewhere else.

Research suggests that acupressure may relieve some symptoms of illness by producing neurochemicals, which are transmitters of information between the brain and the rest of the body. It may also improve circulation. Even if you're still skeptical, it can't hurt to try it as long as you've been to your doctor to make sure that your condition is not serious, says Dr. La Puma. Acupressure has virtually no side effects.

Massage. Anyone who has ever had a decent massage doesn't have to be convinced that it's good for you: How could something that relaxing *not* be good for you?

Given that stress can have a major impact on health, that might be enough. But professional massage therapists will tell you that their skills include a long list of other benefits. They include improved blood circulation, reduced swelling and inflammation, improved digestion, and improved joint mobility.

There are all sorts of massage techniques and many different ways to enjoy them. You can have a pro knead you like pizza dough, massage and be massaged by your partner, or rub yourself in a pinch. It's a practice that truly feels good from head to toe.

Yoga. Here's another victim of 1960s excess. You don't have to be a guru or a guru wannabe to practice yoga. Yoga is an effective system that can help you think more clearly while becoming more supple and flexible. Yoga can be a wonderful way to reduce stress, control tension, and bring all your mental faculties into sharp focus, says Dr. La Puma. *Then* you'll be ready to ponder the cosmos.

Universal Remedies

The secret to a healthy life really isn't all that much of a secret. More than 2,000 years ago, the Roman philosopher and statesman Cicero said: "Exercise and temperance can preserve something of our early strength even in old age."

In all the years since, doctors and researchers have spent a lot of time and money proving Cicero right. While you'll find hundreds of useful tips in the pages of this book to cure common health problems, the plain fact is that you probably have more control than you think over whether you are faced with most of these illnesses, ailments, and injuries.

Men, for example, are more inclined than women to engage in risky behavior such as smoking and driving fast and to be more remiss in taking care of themselves.

"There is much more social pressure on women at all ages to be thin, to be attractive, whereas men are rated more on their status and earning power and achievements," says Robert Kolodny, M.D., medical director of the Behavioral Medicine Institute in New Canaan, Connecticut. But it's not like you have to choose between being successful and looking and feeling good. In fact, they go together quite naturally.

Here are the basics of a healthy lifestyle.

EAT LIGHT AND RIGHT

"Eat to live and not live to eat," goes an old proverb. It's still good advice, says Mack Ruffin IV, M.D., associate professor in the department of family medicine at the University of Michigan Medical Center in Ann Arbor. Chow down like a hog at the trough and before you know it, you're jiggling more than a bowl of gelatin. And your personal appearance isn't the worst of it. Obesity—being 20 percent or more over your ideal weight—can also lead to the following:

- Hypertension
- Heart disease
- Adult-onset diabetes
- Certain cancers

• A worsening of arthritis because of the additional stress on joints and bones

When guys do pork out, the pounds usually go directly to our bellies, which makes us especially prone to heart disease, says Richard Honaker, M.D., a family physician in Carrolton, Texas. So to avoid a gradual slide into obesity, maintain a healthy weight by following the U.S. Department of Agriculture's Food Guide Pyramid eating plan:

Grains should be the foundation of your diet. Strive for between 6 and 11 servings per day of bread, cereal, rice, and pasta. That sounds like a lot, but a slice of bread counts as one serving, so a sandwich is the equivalent of two servings. Similarly, a mere one ounce of ready-to-eat cereal counts as one serving, and a dinner portion of spaghetti would amount to two or three servings of pasta. Choose foods in this group that are made with little fat or sugars, such as bread, English muffins, rice, and pasta.

Vegetables should account for three to five servings each day. One cup of raw, leafy vegetables; ½ cup of other vegetables, cooked or chopped raw; or ¾ cup of vegetable juice each count as one serving. Try to eat a variety of vegetables because you will get different nutrients from each. Dark green, leafy vegetables and legumes are especially good sources of vitamins and minerals. Legumes provide protein and can be substituted for meat.

Fruits should add up to two to four servings per day. Juices containing 100 percent fruit count as a serving, but not punches, -ades, and most so-called fruit drinks, which have little juice and lots of sugar.

Dairy products such as milk, yogurt, and cheese should be eaten two or three times a day. Choose skim milk and nonfat yogurt when possible. One cup of milk, 8 ounces of yogurt, and 1½ to 2 ounces of cheese each count as one serving.

Meat, poultry, fish, dry beans, eggs, and nuts should account for two to three servings a day. Two to three ounces of cooked lean meat, poultry, or fish; one egg; and a half-cup of dried beans, such as navy, black, pinto, and kidney, are each equal to one serving. When preparing meats, trim away all the fat you can see. Broil, roast, or boil these foods rather than frying them.

Fats, oils, and sweets should be eaten sparingly. Go easy on fats and sugars added to foods in cooking or once they are served—butter, margarine, gravy, salad dressing, sugar, and jelly. If you aren't already doing so, scale back on candy, desserts, and soda.

And it's not just what you eat but when that's important. Dr. Honaker stresses the importance of eating breakfast. Those people who start their day with a meal tend to live longer, healthier lives, he says. He thinks that the ideal meal in the morning should include a banana. "The banana is probably the best form of food there is in the world," he says. "It's the perfect mixture of vitamins, antioxidants, fiber, and trace minerals."

BREAK A SWEAT

A snapshot of many American men as we near the twenty-first century: Wake up, drive to work, sit at a desk all day, drive home, eat dinner, and watch television. On weekends, watch sports and maybe go to a movie or a concert. Their heaviest exertion all week is popping a cap off a bottle of beer. And their bodies are as soft and pliant as that of the Pillsbury Dough Boy.

The U.S. Surgeon General estimates that more than 6 of 10 American adults are not physically active on a regular basis. One in four aren't active all.

Should we be concerned? Yes. And not just because that dough boy bod is about as sexy to women as dandruff. Exercise seems to be good for practically every aspect of a guy's health—physical and mental. Here are some examples, courtesy of the American Medical Association.

Heart. Like other muscles, your heart becomes stronger and more efficient when it's given a workout.

Arteries and veins. Exercise reduces the amount of bad cholesterol (called low-density lipoprotein, or LDL) and fats in your blood. It also helps reverse hardening of the arteries, which lowers blood pressure, and may prevent blood vessels from becoming clogged with the plaque that cuts off blood flow and that is a major cause of heart attacks and strokes.

Lungs. Regular exercise helps prevent the decline in oxygen uptake that occurs naturally with aging and from inactivity.

Weight control. If you sit on your butt all day, you will take in more calories than you burn. Those excess calories are stored as fat and excess weight. Exercise burns calories and helps you keep your calorie intake in balance.

Cancer. Guys who exercise regularly have lower incidences of cancer, including cancer of the prostate and colon. The reason is that exercise accelerates digested food through the colon so that it can't ferment and cause irritations that may become cancerous.

Mental health. Men who exercise are usually less tired, more productive at work, and even more interested in sex. There may be a chemical reason for this. One theory is that exercise elevates levels of serotonin, a hormone and neurotransmitter associated with feelings of well-being.

The good thing about exercise is that you don't have to do that much of it to reap benefits, and it needn't be boring. The Centers for Disease Control and the American College of Sports Medicine recommend 30 minutes a day, including at least 20 minutes of sustained aerobic exercise that increases your heart rate, at least three times a week. Aerobic activities include cross-country skiing, ice hockey, jogging, jumping rope, running in place, stationary cycling, and uphill hiking.

If you do begin an exercise program, check with a doctor first if you are middle-aged or older, have a heart condition that requires supervision, or have another medical condition, such as insulin-dependent diabetes or high blood pressure, that requires special attention. Other exercise that isn't aerobic but useful to your health includes such routine tasks as mowing the yard and gardening.

SLEEP DEEPLY

Don't yawn; this is a serious problem. More than 200 sleep disorders centers have sprung up across the country, and slumber is the subject of thousands of studies and more than a few books. A poll commissioned by the National Sleep Foundation found that 47 percent of U.S. workers have trouble sleeping, and two-thirds of these groggy souls think that this adversely affects their job performance. The cost of this sleeplessness could be more than $18 billion in lost productivity, the survey concluded.

Sleeplessness and sleep disorders have also been blamed, in part, for some stupendous disasters, including the Exxon *Valdez* oil spill and the Chernobyl and Three Mile Island nuclear mishaps and the 1972–1973 Philadelphia 76ers. Okay, we made up the last one, although the 76ers did appear to be sleepwalking as they posted a 9-73 record to set the NBA standard for futility. Keep in mind too that there are at least 100,000 sleep-related auto accidents in the United States every year.

Those late hours you keep may not result in a calamity, but sleep deprivation can harm your physical and mental health in very real ways. Quite simply, sleep is necessary in order to live. Get too little and you may have some of the following problems, says Peter Hauri, Ph.D., administrative director of the insomnia program at the Mayo Clinic and co-director of the Mayo Clinic Sleep Disorders Clinic, both in Rochester, Minnesota.

- Your immune system may suffer. When that happens, you are more susceptible to colds and other illnesses.
- You are less able to concentrate, and your memory is muddled. You feel like you have the mental sharpness of Gomer Pyle.
- You get stressed more easily.
- You have an energy crisis. You're so sluggish that you give inertia a bad name.

Generally, the deeper your rest, the more energy you have. So how much sleep do you need? It varies from person to person. If you "catch up" on sleep on the weekends, get drowsy during long meetings, or have trouble getting out of bed when you should, you aren't getting enough quality sleep, says Dr. Hauri. To find the right amount of sleep for you, Dr. Hauri recommends getting up at the same time every day—including weekends—but varying your bedtime until you find the amount of sleep that seems to be the most restorative for you.

KEEP COOL WHEN YOU'RE HOT

Dr. Honaker needs no convincing that managing stress is crucial to one's health. In his forties, Dr. Honaker, who is president of Family Medicine Associates near Dallas, is a tournament racquetball player who takes pride in the top-notch condition he keeps himself in. But one April day in 1997 he experienced chest pain and learned he had a 90 percent blockage in the main artery to his heart—despite the fact that he had no family history of heart disease or cholesterol problems.

"The only risk factor I have is that I am an extreme type A person that runs a medical practice of seven doctors with a high stress level," Dr. Honaker says. Now the doctor is trying to limit his stress-inducing events to ensure a long life for himself.

Chronic stress may also contribute to the following:

- Reduced immunity to disease
- Fatigue
- Weight gain or weight loss
- Constipation, diarrhea, or both
- Headaches

Some stress is normal, of course. A death in the family, a divorce, or job-related worries might even put Mr. Rogers in a funk. If it all becomes too much, there are various relaxation techniques that you can try, ranging from meditation to progressive muscle relaxation. Some of them are mentioned in part two, which deals with specific problems. Here are a few other things that can also make a day less gray, says Dr. Honaker.

Get your Zzzs. If you're not getting enough sleep, you are more prone to feeling stressed.

Get soaked. A hot bath or a soak in a whirlpool can melt away tension, provided that you don't have a health condition that makes this dangerous, such as circulatory problems.

Get active. Regular aerobic exercise lowers blood pressure and makes people feel calmer, studies show. Even a short walk during a break or on your lunch hour at work can help.

Get a pet. Several studies have found that owning a pet helps reduce blood pressure or stress levels. One study suggested that people performed stressful tasks better with a dog present than with their spouse.

TAKE A HEALTHY INTEREST IN SEX

At some point, almost every man surely has felt that having sex was a matter of life and death. It turns out that that's not far from the truth. A study of 918 middle-aged men in Caerphilly, South Wales, found that those who had orgasms twice a week or more had half the mortality risk of those who had orgasms fewer than once a month.

Dr. Kolodny is among those who think sex provides health benefits for most men. "The question is, is it really necessary to have an active sex life with a partner?" he says. "Probably the answer is no. From a health point of view, a male who is masturbating as often as his counterpart is having intercourse, may be perfectly fine."

Here are some benefits of sex other than the fact that it feels mighty good—which, of course, is benefit enough for most of us.

- If you have an inflamed prostate, ejaculation combined with antibiotics is the way to cure it. Tough medicine, we know.
- Ejaculating improves sperm quantity and quality for many men, which can be useful if you are trying to start or expand on a family.
- Sex is an effective stress-reducer, says Dr. Kolodny. He adds this caveat: For someone in a rotten relationship, sex can make stress worse, not better.
- Men who regularly have sex may experience an overall sense of well-being, says Dr. Kolodny. That's pretty clear by the goofy grin on your face when it's over.
- Older men need to have sex occasionally in order to continue being able to produce erections. Doing so can postpone the inevitable tapering off of erections, says Dr. Kolodny. In other words, use it or lose it. "Once or twice a week being preferable to once or twice a month, being preferable to once or twice a year," he adds.

So have sex. Whether you make it a team sport or play solo is up to you. But if it's the former and you're not in a monogamous relationship, take these precautions, says Dr. Kolodny.

- Limit your number of sexual partners. From a health point of view, monogamy is clearly safer than the alternative.
- Always use a latex condom and spermicide, regardless of the need for contraception, if you're not in a monogamous relationship or if you and your partner haven't been tested for AIDS or other sexually transmitted diseases.
- Be aware that women who have had multiple partners are at considerably higher risk for sexual infections that they may not even realize they have.
- Avoid sex with anybody being treated for a sexual disease.

STUFF YOUR BUTTS

By now you realize that nicotine is addictive . . . and deadly. "Cigarettes are killers that travel in packs," a wit once said. "Of the things a man can do for himself, clearly the single most important one from an overall health standpoint is not to smoke," Dr. Kolodny says. Yes, smoking can make your lungs look like burnt toast, but there are other reasons to kick the habit. Here are a few.

Other cancers. In addition to lung cancer, smoking can also cause cancer of the throat, larynx, mouth, esophagus, kidney, bladder, and pancreas. And while penile cancer is uncommon, smokers are far more likely to contract it than nonsmokers, says Dr. Honaker.

Other diseases. Smokers are at greater risk for heart disease, emphysema, and chronic bronchitis.

Sperm damage. Nicotine reduces sperm concentration, movement, and shape, making it more difficult to father a healthy child.

Erection-erasers. Smokers are more likely to have erection problems than nonsmokers.

Skin damage. Smoking is a major contributor to wrinkled skin. The chemicals in tobacco constrict blood vessels, reducing blood flow to the skin and causing wrinkles. And smokers' wrinkles are deeper and more numerous, says Dr. Honaker.

Harm to others. Nonsmokers exposed to smokers also are at increased risk of contracting smoking-related diseases. Studies show that nonsmoking spouses of smokers are at a 30 percent higher risk of dying of lung cancer than those who have nonsmoking partners.

Maybe you think that you've been smoking so long that quitting now won't help you. Wrong. Regardless of age, not smoking for 7 to 10 years makes your health risks comparable to those of nonsmokers. Quitting after age 50, for example, cuts your risk of heart disease in half.

SHUN THE SUN

Sure, there's no better feeling than dozing off on a beach, the sun's warm rays penetrating every pore, cooking you gradually like a chicken in a Crock-Pot. And there's no denying that a golden tan looks great. But it can be a look to die for—literally.

When you get a sunburn, ultraviolet light bores deep into the skin, injuring several layers of cells. The skin loses elasticity, making it more vulnerable to premature wrinkling and increasing the risk of skin cancer. Sun exposure accounts for about 90 percent of skin cancer.

It's a cumulative process. Skin cancer can take up to 20 years to develop. Fair-skinned men and those with a family history or repeated exposure to x-rays and industrial chemicals are most susceptible.

Skin cancer isn't the only repercussion from sun exposure—only the most serious. If you catch as many rays as George Hamilton, your skin may wrinkle and age prematurely. One day, that golden glow is gone, and your face is as craggy and creased as an old baseball glove. Even if you're a young man, you can get age spots if you have constant unprotected exposure to the sun. The sun is also considered a major source of cataracts.

There are times, of course, when prolonged periods in the sun are unavoidable. Maybe your job is outdoors. You like to go fishing or skiing. Regardless, here are a few things that experts say you can do to minimize damage to your skin.

Slather up. Use a waterproof sunscreen that has an SPF (sun protection factor) of at least 15 about 30 minutes before you go outside. Reapply it every two to three hours, even more often if you go swimming or sweat like an NBA player.

Cover up. Wear long sleeves and pants. And don't go topless; wear a hat.

Impose a curfew. Try to avoid being in the sun between 11:00 A.M. and 3:00 P.M. in the summer, when the sun's strength is the greatest.

Monitor medications. Be aware that some medications, such as antibiotics, can make your skin more sun sensitive. If you're not sure about your medicines' side effects, ask your doctor.

DRINK UP

Experts recommend drinking eight, eight-ounce glasses of water a day. Nonalcoholic beverages count toward meeting this goal. But alcoholic beverages, coffee, tea, and caffeinated sodas—though sources of fluid—are diuretics that actually cause you to *lose* fluid through the kidneys as urine. Why are fluids important? They aid digestion, elimination, and the building of tissue. And water regulates your body temperature through perspiration and lubricates your joints.

Water also helps prevent a number of ailments or conditions that may plague you. Among them are the following:

Kidney stones. Drinking plenty of fluids dilutes the concentration of calcium and magnesium salts in urine, which can otherwise cause one of the most painful conditions to curse a man.

Obesity. When water mixes with the food you've eaten, you feel full more quickly and for a longer period of time, making you less tempted to snack.

Constipation. Combined with more fiber and regular exercise, drinking more water can relieve constipation.

Jet lag. Airplane cabins are extremely dry, leaving many passengers feeling dehydrated by the end of the flight. Drinking plenty of water before boarding helps combat the feeling.

The Healthy Man's Toolbox

To do a job right, you have to have the right tools. Every man knows this. It's one of the first things we learned in Manhood 101. That's why men always have a toolbox in the house. Even if its main function is to collect dust. The idea is that when something breaks, you don't want to have to run down to the hardware store to pick up what you need to fix it—especially if it's 3:00 in the morning, and especially if what breaks is the plumbing and your basement is quickly filling with water.

The same goes for your body. When something goes wrong, you don't want to have to run down to the drugstore to pick up what you need to fix it—especially if it's 3:00 in the morning, and especially if you're coughing, running a fever, and you generally feel like death warmed over.

So what should a man have in his health toolbox? We're glad you asked. Just like in home repairs, there are numerous ailments and injuries that you can treat yourself if you have the right stuff.

Here are some of the things our experts recommend throughout this book to help you feel better, faster.

MEDICINES

The following are items that come up again and again in this book, so they're worth keeping in your medicine cabinet.

Acetic acid. For athlete's foot and poison ivy. Example: Domeboro.

Alpha hydroxy products. Use a moisturizer with alpha hydroxy acids to relieve dry skin and to prevent acne. Use a cream for ingrown whiskers, to prevent scarring, to make wrinkles less apparent, and to help eliminate a double chin. Example: Alpha Hydrox.

22

Antacid. To relieve heartburn and to soothe canker sore pain. A good choice is Mylanta, which contains a combination of magnesium and aluminum.

Antibacterial soap. To prevent burns and open wounds from becoming infected; to treat chafing, jock itch, and boils; and to prevent body odor. Example: Lever 2000.

Antihistamine. For eczema, poison ivy, and motion sickness. Example: Benadryl.

Baby powder. To relieve rectal itching and to prevent various skin problems such as blisters, boils, and chafing. Generic brands are readily available.

Calamine lotion. For itchy skin caused by poison ivy or sunburn. Generic brands are readily available.

Colloidal oatmeal bath. To relieve itching caused by sunburn, rashes, shingles, and psoriasis. Example: Aveeno Bath Treatment.

Cotton swabs and cotton balls. For applying medicines topically. Generic brands are readily available.

Cough medicine. For a productive cough (one that gets rid of phlegm), use a brand containing guaifenesin, such as Robitussin. For an unproductive cough (a dry cough that keeps you up at night), use one that contains dextromethorphan, such as Robutussin DM.

Decongestant. To relieve a stuffy head caused by allergies, a sinus infection, or a cold. Our experts recommend brands that contains pseudoephedrine, such as Sudafed.

Elastic bandages. For treating knee pain, sprains, tendinitis, and bursitis. Example: Ace bandage.

Fiber supplement. For occasional use, when eating foods high in fiber doesn't relieve constipation. Metamucil, which contains psyllium fiber, is a good choice. Taken with meals, a fiber supplement can also prevent you from overeating.

Hydrocortisone cream. For itching and inflammation caused by rashes, poison ivy, or razor burn. Generic brands are readily available.

Nasal spray. For a stuffy nose, use one containing oxymetazoline, such as Afrin.

Pain medicine. For headaches and minor pain. Because certain pain medications are better for certain conditions, you should keep three different kinds on hand: acetaminophen, aspirin, and ibuprofen. For example, you should take acetaminophen rather than aspirin or ibuprofen if you have an ulcer, an earache, or pain associated with a bruise or open wound. You should also avoid aspirin if you have a fever or suffer from gout. But if you're having chest pains that may be from a heart attack, chewing one aspirin may help save your life.

Pepto-Bismol. For a stomachache, diarrhea, or nausea. The pink stuff's active ingredient, bismuth, is also available in generic brands.

Petroleum jelly. To treat chapped lips and psoriasis and to prevent scarring, chafing, saddle sores, and hangnails. Generic brands are readily available.

Thermometer. To take your temperature to determine whether you are running a fever.

FIRST-AID KIT

You should also keep a well-stocked first-aid kit on hand so that you're prepared for any emergency. Here's a list of items discussed in this book to get your kit started.

Antibiotic ointment. To prevent blisters, burns, cuts, and other open wounds from becoming infected. Example: Polysporin.

Butterfly bandages. To keep the edges of a wound together.

Disposable latex gloves. To wear whenever administering first-aid to another person to protect yourself from picking up diseases such as hepatitis and HIV.

Face mask. To wear when doing cardiopulmonary resuscitation or when giving mouth-to-mouth resuscitation.

Hydrogen peroxide. To clean an open wound or to use as a mouthwash to disinfect irritated gums.

Ipecac syrup and activated charcoal. For treatment after swallowing certain poisons.

Reusable, instant-activating ice bags. For icing injuries.

Rubbing alcohol. To sterilize tweezers before using them or to clean your bike seat after a ride to prevent saddle sores.

Saline solution for contact lenses. To moisten sterile gauze used to bandage a broken bone that breaks through the skin or to wrap up a severed appendage so that you can take it to the hospital and possibly have it reattached.

Sterile gauze. To bandage open wounds, burns, blisters, and corns.

Tweezers. To remove dirt or debris from an open wound, a tick that is attached to your skin, or a splinter.

VITAMINS AND MINERALS

A multivitamin serves as an insurance policy, says Cathy Kapica, R.D., Ph.D., assistant professor of nutrition and dietetics at Finch University of Health Sciences/Chicago Medical School. "It doesn't excuse you, however, from eating a well-balanced diet."

One caution: Make sure that the multivitamin you choose does not contain extra iron, says David Meyers, M.D., professor of internal medicine and preventive medicine at University of Kansas School of Medicine in Kansas City. Most men get too much iron in their diet already, and excess iron has been linked to higher risk of heart disease and cancer in men.

For each nutrient that follows, we list the Daily Value for men established by the Food and Nutrition Board, which is the minimum amount you need of each nutrient every day to keep you healthy at the most basic level. Throughout this book, our experts recommend getting more than the Daily Value for many of these nutrients to help in healing, to combat fatigue, and to prevent illnesses such as heart disease.

The optimal amounts we list below are recommended by two of the leading experts in the field—Shari Lieberman, Ph.D., co-author of *The Real Vitamin and Mineral Book*, and Alexander Schauss, Ph.D., author of *Minerals, Trace Elements, and Human Health*—to help men live life to the fullest. In addition to a multivitamin, you might want to consider eating foods that are good sources of these vitamins and minerals to help you reach the optimal amounts recommended by our experts.

Vitamin C. Strengthens resistance against infection, and helps form collagen, which fortifies blood vessel walls and forms scar tissue. Daily Value for men: 60 milligrams. Optimal amount: 1,000 milligrams a day. Food sources: oranges, cranberry juice, cantaloupe, broccoli, red and green peppers, pink grapefruit, kiwifruit.

Vitamin E. Combats heart disease and certain cancers. Daily Value for men: 30 international units. Optimal amount: 400 international units. Food sources: vegetable and nut oils, sunflower seeds, whole grains, wheat germ, spinach.

Calcium. Builds strong bones and teeth. Daily Value for men: 1,000 milligrams. Optimal amount: same, until age 65 and older. Then it's 1,500 milligrams. Food sources: milk, yogurt, cheese.

Magnesium. Involved in metabolism and nerve functions. Daily Value for men: 400 milligrams. Optimal amount: 500 milligrams a day. Food sources: meats, poultry, dairy products, cereal, and dark green, leafy vegetables.

Zinc. Strengthens immune system, helps in sperm production and the healing of wounds. Essential for brain function. Daily Value for men: 15 milligrams. Optimal amount: same. Food sources: red meats, poultry, eggs, oysters.

HERBS

Among the healing herbs that our experts recommend throughout this book are the following:

Aloe. For burns, including sunburn, and to relieve rectal itching. An aloe poultice can draw a splinter to the surface of the skin. Aloe vera juice can also help relieve constipation.

Arnica. For sprains and muscle soreness, and to speed the healing of bruises—like that black eye that is so embarrassing—as well as other injuries due to trauma.

Calendula. Also known as garden or pot marigold, this herb can help soothe razor burn and is effective in treating blisters, canker sores, and chafing.

Chamomile. To help settle an upset stomach and to relieve gas.

Echinacea. Also known as cone flower, echinacea strengthens the immune system and helps fight off colds, ear infections, the flu, pneumonia, and perhaps even Lyme disease.

Ginger. Contains anti-inflammatory properties that make it useful for people with arthritis, bursitis, or tendinitis. It can also help relieve gas, diarrhea, nausea, motion sickness, allergies, bad breath, and hiccups.

Ginkgo. Improves blood flow to the brain, keeps you mentally sharp, and elevates your mood. May help relieve impotence, depression, back pain, and absentmindedness.

Ginseng. May boost energy and libido. Can help relieve stress, burnout, and impotence.

Goldenseal. To help fight ear infections, pneumonia, and a cough associated with a cold. It can also ease the pain and speed the healing of canker sores and gum ailments.

Kava. To relieve muscle cramps, muscle soreness, and restless legs that keep you up at night.

Saint-John's-wort. For moderate depression, seasonal affective disorder, and fatigue associated with mild depression.

Saw palmetto. For frequent urination or incontinence caused by an enlarged prostate.

FOODS

Keeping the right stuff in your kitchen can keep you healthier. Here are a few foods that our experts suggest keeping in your refrigerator and pantry.

Bananas. To help relieve diarrhea and muscle cramps. Eating potassium-packed bananas as part of your regular diet can also help relieve the pain associated with sciatica and can even help bring down high blood pressure.

Cayenne pepper. To help relieve congestion, a stubborn cough, a sore throat, and bad breath. Cooking with cayenne on a regular basis can help lower cholesterol. Our experts also recommend taking cayenne pepper capsules to relieve migraine headaches and to prevent frostbite.

Chewing gum. To help relieve bad breath, dry mouth, heartburn, and even an in-flight earache.

Chicken soup. To unclog a stuffy nose and to slow your body's phlegm production. Homemade chicken soup would be better, but condensed, canned chicken soup does work.

Fish. The omega-3 fatty acids in fish such as salmon, mackerel, tuna, herring, and sardines may relieve depression, skin rashes, and eczema; can reduce the pain and stiffness of rheumatoid arthritis; and may prevent and even reverse heart disease.

Flaxseed oil. To help relieve constipation, dry skin, eczema, and rashes. Also available in seed and supplement form.

Garlic. Can help fight off colds and flu as well as athlete's foot, relieves a nagging cough and diarrhea, and helps lower cholesterol, making your blood less likely to form dangerous clots. Of course, fresh garlic is best, but if you're worried about repelling your friends and co-workers as well as vampires because of garlic's notorious odor, fear not. Odor-free garlic capsules are readily available.

Hard candy. For a sore throat or hiccups.

Honey. To help relieve constipation, heartburn, a sore throat, bad breath, and even a hangover.

Horseradish. To relieve congestion.

Lemon. To soothe wasp stings or to get rid of body odor. It is also an ingredient in remedies recommended by our experts to relieve a cough, a sore throat, bad breath, and the hiccups.

Milk. To relieve and prevent muscle cramps, to prevent kidney stones from forming, and to soothe sunburn. Just make sure that you're drinking nonfat or low-fat milk so that you're not clogging your arteries or putting on extra pounds.

Olive oil. Use as your regular cooking oil for a healthy heart. It is also the main ingredient in an aftershave used to soothe razor burn.

Orange juice. To help curb your nicotine cravings, prevent kidney stones from forming, and help soften the stools of those with diverticular disease of the colon.

Sports drinks. To prevent muscle cramps, replenish fluids lost during a bout of diarrhea, or prevent symptoms caused by inflammatory bowel disease. Gatorade is one brand to try.

Vinegar. White vinegar as a remedy to soothe wasp stings, as eardrops to help dry up moisture and stop any itching, and as a soak to get rid of foot odor. Apple cider vinegar as a digestive aid to ease heartburn and as a rinse to fight dandruff and dry hair.

Wheat germ. To help restore coenzyme Q_{10} levels in the hearts of people with angina and to relieve restless legs that wake you up in the middle of the night.

Yogurt. For an energy boost to relieve that early-afternoon slump. Eating yogurt is also a good way for those who are lactose-intolerant to get their calcium. They generally can tolerate yogurt because the lactose is digested by the live bacteria found in most yogurt.

OTHER STUFF

The following items don't fall under the other categories but are recommended by experts elsewhere in this book for problems that you're likely to face. So add these to your healthy man's toolbox.

Art supplies. To work through emotional and psychological problems such as bad dreams, a midlife crisis, and envious feelings. All you need to give art therapy a try is an unlined pad of paper and some colored pencils or markers.

Condoms. To delay ejaculation and to protect yourself from sexually transmitted diseases, especially if you have multiple sex partners.

Date book. Keeping better track of your appointments and scheduling weekly chores can help you change bad habits such as sloppiness, chronic lateness, and absentmindedness. It can also help when you're trying to kick an addiction. And if your sexual desire is down, try setting a date for sex. You will find that it's a real libido-lifter—and the one appointment that you're most likely to keep.

Heating pad. To speed the healing of bruises and to relieve back or neck pain, arthritis pain, heartburn, or an earache.

Humidifier. To keep your skin and nasal passages moist, especially during the winter months. It will help relieve dry mouth, dry skin, eczema, bronchitis, laryngitis, and nosebleeds.

Part Two

REMEDIES

Abdominal Fat

▶PROBLEM

As unhealthy as it is unattractive, the pot-belly has long been the bane of men who love to eat but don't get enough exercise. We *know* we should lose it. We *want* to lose it, but it's not easy. In a typical survey, abs were the overwhelming choice of respondents asked to name the area of the body they wanted most to tone.

▶CAUSE

It's a simple equation: Take in more calories than you expend, and you're going to put on weight. And for a guy, one of the first places you're going to see evidence of the added pounds is on your stomach. A big part of this story is genetics. Just as women are predisposed to packing extra weight on their hips and waists, men tend to store it in their gut—prominently, for all the world to see.

▶HOW SERIOUS

In a word, very. Study after study tells us that fat between the shoulders and hips (read: abdominal fat) is bad news for the heart. It helps raise cholesterol levels, which blocks arteries and leads to coronary heart disease. Fat around the midriff has been linked to insulin resistance, which can raise blood pressure. There's also evidence to suggest that it puts you at increased risk for diabetes. Felicia Busch, R.D., spokesperson for the American Dietetic Association and a dietitian in St. Paul, Minnesota, calls it the most critical weight to lose. "You can be only 10 to 15 pounds overweight, but if it's all in the ab-

DO THIS NOW

Any exercise that moves the body through space will help lose that gut, says Peter D. Vash, M.D., executive medical director of Lindora Medical Clinics in Costa Mesa, California. "Isometrics with weights is great for building muscle mass and certainly shouldn't be ignored, but if you want a toned stomach, you have to lose fat mass. And you do that by regular and frequent aerobic exercise—anything from treadmill walking or running to swimming or cycling," Dr. Vash says. Aim for a minimum of 30 minutes, four days a week, he adds.

domen, it's much more serious than if you were 30 to 40 pounds overweight with the pounds spread out," she says.

▶SOLUTIONS

Exercise and eat. It may seem that cutting back on how much you eat is the quickest way to get rid of a pot belly. But it's not. Dieters who severely restrict their caloric intake may lose fat, but they can actually lose *muscle* as well.

In a study done at Tufts University in Boston, 11 men and women age 60 and older were divided into an exercise group and a diet group. The exercise group rode a stationary bike for two 45-minute sessions to burn 360 calories a day, and closely monitored their diets to be sure that they ate exactly the same amount of calories as before the program began. To make the match even, the dieters ate 360 fewer calories a day than before.

After 12 weeks, the dieters had lost an average of about 11 pounds, but more than 6 of those pounds were muscle. The exercisers dropped an average of 16 pounds, all of it fat. The moral of the story: If you're cutting calories, only cut between 200 and 400 calories a day, says William J. Evans, Ph.D., professor of physiology, nutrition, and geriatric medicine at the University of Arkansas for Medical Sciences in Little Rock and director of the nutrition, metabolism, and exercise laboratory at the University of Arkansas for Medical Sciences/Veteran Affairs Medical Center's Donald W. Reynolds Center on Aging in North Little Rock. Any more than that and you risk losing muscle, warns Dr. Evans, who conducted the study with his former colleagues at Tufts.

And for someone trying to lose weight, muscle can be your best ally. That's because even when you're not using your muscles, they burn more calories than fat stores do. So the more muscle you have, the easier it is to lose weight.

Break up your workouts. Two or three short bouts of exercise throughout your day can help melt that belly fat away. "Breaking up your workouts helps you to increase your fitness while expending more calories at the same time," Dr. Evans says. "Because you're not doing the activity for as long, you're able to keep up your intensity throughout your workout without getting as tired."

Try to work two or three 20-minute sessions into your day, five days a week, Dr. Evans recommends. A morning jog and brisk walk at lunch will suffice. Just make sure that you're doing aerobic exercise—the kind that gets your heart pumping and your lungs huffing and puffing. "Aerobic exercise is probably the very best way to target abdominal fat," says Dr. Evans. "It is the only kind of exercise shown to pull fat stores more directly from your abdominal region."

Exercise squatter's rights. The exercise known as "squats" engages lots of muscles—the gluteus maximus (the largest buttocks muscle), quadriceps, hamstrings, inner thighs, outer hips, abdominals, lower back, and shoulder girdle—all the while elevating your heart rate. "There's no such thing as spot reduction; you have to work your entire body to lose the belly," says Annette Lang, a certified personal trainer at Equinox, a fitness club in New York City.

Lang offers the basic free-standing squat as an excellent starter exercise. Stand with your legs at least shoulder-width apart and your feet slightly pointed out to keep your hips, knees, and ankles in alignment.

Cross your arms in front of your chest. As you slowly lower your body, keep your abs and lower back stable. Make sure that your rear end goes back, rather than your knees going forward, making sure that your knees do not extend out over the tips of your toes. It should feel like you're sitting in an imaginary chair. Lower your butt until your thighs are parallel to the floor, then slowly rise back up. Start out doing 8 to 12 repetitions every day, work up to two or three sets, and add dumbbells or a barbell later. Keep in mind that you should always check with your doctor before starting a new exercise program.

Be true to form. Abdominal crunches won't melt belly fat; only sufficient aerobic exercise and proper nutrition will. But they are a great exercise for strengthening the muscles below the belly fat. And that can certainly aid your appearance and help keep your back healthy. But you have to do crunches properly. "Don't get locked in to the 'more is better' way of thinking," says Ann Marie Miller, a certified personal trainer and fitness training manager at New York Sports Clubs in New York City. "Doing 500 crunches quickly and in haphazard fashion won't do you as much good as 20 done with perfect form. There are no ab muscles in your neck or legs, but I still see guys jerking their heads and swinging their torsos. Your goal is to stimulate as many muscle fibers as possible, and you do this by executing your crunches slowly."

Here's how to get the most out your crunches, Miller says: Lie flat on your back, arms folded across your chest or hands behind your head, elbows out. Bend your knees at a 45-degree angle, feet flat on the floor. Slowly curl your torso upward. Lift your shoulders off the floor while your lower back remains flat on the floor. Your pelvis and rib cage will come toward each other.

Eat less fat. It's a no-brainer, but so important. And it's easier for men to make the small dietary changes that add up over the long haul than it is for women, Busch says. "Ironically, the fact that men, in general, have worse eating habits gives them lots of room to improve. Switching to low-fat milk and salad dressings, eating pretzels instead of potato chips, and skipping the cheese on your sandwich all are very small changes that can make a big difference over time," she says.

Tense up. Your stomach muscles, that is. Lang likens it to the way that you'd instinctively tighten up if someone tried to punch you in the stomach.

A tip that Busch gives her patients is to get in the habit of consciously holding in your stomach as you walk. "Or when you're driving, suck in your gut at every stoplight. These are just a couple small things you can do to engage your abdominals as much as possible in order to tone the underlying muscle," Busch says.

▶ALTERNATIVE APPROACHES

Get your kicks. You don't have to be a black belt or even join a karate class to benefit from the martial arts. Try this "tae kwon do kick with a tai chi approach" advocated by Tim Hoover, owner and operator of the Hoover Karate Academy in Allentown, Pennsylvania, and 27-year veteran of the martial arts. It's a great exercise for your obliques, the stomach muscles that make up your waist. To gain the most benefit, the exercise should be performed slowly and deliberately, utilizing balance and a fluid motion. As with any exercise program, take a few minutes to warm up before beginning. Jumping jacks are a great way to get the blood flowing and to warm up the muscles before a workout.

Here's how Hoover says to get your kicks: When you first try this movement, stand next to a wall or a stable object and hold on with your left hand for balance if you need to. In slow motion, bring your right knee straight up in front of you as high as you can, with your thigh parallel to the ground. Pull the toes up to flex the foot. Now, keep your knee high and look right. Extend your right leg out to the right while you pivot the foot you are balancing on so that your toes face the wall. Your eyes, right shoulder, and right heel should form a straight line. Your fully extended right leg should now be pointed away from the wall or object that you are using for balance. In this position, count to five slowly, then reverse the move. Retract your leg back to the bent-knee position, then slowly lower it to the floor. Breathing is another important facet of this exercise. As you bring your knee up, inhale; as you push your leg out, exhale. When you retract your leg, inhale; as you lower it, exhale.

Hoover recommends three to five repetitions with the right leg, then shake out the muscles for a few seconds. Repeat with three to five repetitions using the left leg. Do this every other day and work up to 10 repetitions on each side, he adds.

▶PREVENTIVE MEASURES

Limit the libations. Not only is alcohol very calorically dense but also it targets the abdomen, hence the term *beer belly*. If you're going to keep your waistline under control, you must cut back on the booze. Busch recommends that when you're out on the town, make your first two drinks club sodas or something else nonalcoholic. "Not only does this help fill you up before you've touched any alcohol but also it prevents you from lowering your inhibition, which always makes it easier to overdo it on the food and drink," she says.

Absentmindedness

▶PROBLEM

Forget an appointment? Can't find where you put your book? Relax. Being absentminded usually just means that you're knee-deep in the muck of life. Middle-aged men are notoriously overworked, overstressed, and, on the whole, a little off balance mentally. And one way it manifests itself is absentmindedness. Yes, some drop in memory ability does occur naturally in the twenties or thirties. Exacerbated by the stress of everyday life, this drop can be worrisome or annoying.

▶CAUSE

Even before you blame your lifestyle, look at your learning habits. Frankly, the main cause of forgetfulness is not learning information well the first time around. If something's fuzzy coming in, it's going to be fuzzy coming out. That said, a lot of things can make you absentminded: the daily grind, lack of physical and mental activity, poor nutrition, insufficient sleep, and booze. People also may have bouts of forgetfulness when they experience trauma, such as when mourning the loss of a loved one. One culprit of absentmindedness specific to men is the unconscious mind: Men seem to forget things that they have an intolerance for, like instructions from their wives. Strangely enough, we can forget things on purpose without being conscious that we're doing it.

▶HOW SERIOUS

Everyone has occasional episodes of forgetfulness. On the other hand, a man who notices a gap in memory or has repetitive absentmindedness for three to five days or more should see a doctor, says Kenneth Manges, Ph.D., a psy-

> ### DO THIS NOW
> Take a jog around the block. Do a dozen jumping jacks. Get down and give me 20 pushups. Any kind of exercise—in moderation if it has been awhile—will help snap you out of your daze and snap on your thinking cap. Mental function all around, including memory, gets a big boost out of exercise, says Barry Gordon, M.D., Ph.D., author of *Memory: Remembering and Forgetting in Everyday Life*.

chological in private practice in Cincinnati—especially if the memory loss cannot be connected to a traumatic event such as the death of a loved one, job loss, or divorce.

▶SOLUTIONS

Worship the pencil. "Someone once said that a bad pencil is better than the best memory—but I can't remember who," says Barry Gordon, M.D., Ph.D., author of *Memory: Remembering and Forgetting in Everyday Life.* The message: Carry a daily planner. Stuff an index card into your shirt pocket. Buy sticky notes wholesale. Just write it down. This

> ## MEN'S HEALTH INDEX
>
> **We were going to list the top 10 things people commonly forget, but we could only remember 5 of them. As summarized by Barry Gordon, M.D., Ph.D., author of *Memory: Remembering and Forgetting in Everyday Life*, they are:**
>
> 1. **Names**
> 2. **Where we put things (like keys)**
> 3. **Telephone numbers we just checked**
> 4. **Words**
> 5. **Forgetting that we already told something to someone; forgetting what other people have told us (tie)**

memory aid is a guaranteed reminder, a personal secretary of sorts, as long as you can recall where you posted that note. If you're plagued by terrible handwriting, or if you habitually lose pencils, consider carrying a tape recorder instead.

Get out and move. Improving aerobic capacity through a regular exercise program has helped sedentary people sharpen their minds, Dr. Gordon says. In fact, exercise can improve some mental abilities by 20 to 30 percent. "It's vital for people to be as physically fit as they can, and a regular regimen of exercise will increase mental alertness and thereby memory," says Dr. Manges.

Tune in to your learning channel. People remember in different ways. Some people remember best when they hear something; others, when they see it. Some people absolutely have to write it down in order to remember. But all people remember best in the way they learn best, explains Dr. Manges. In general, there are three learning "channels": auditory (learn by hearing), visual (learn by seeing), and experiential (learn by doing or writing). To determine your best learning channel, ask yourself how you learn a new skill best—what steps you take to learn the skill most efficiently, Dr. Manges says. For optimal memory, always try to learn new information through the channel that is most productive for you. Learn well and remember well.

▶ALTERNATIVE APPROACHES

Respect the coffee/chocolate fix. The caffeine in coffee and cola and the caffeinelike compounds in chocolate are tried-and-true brain fuels, the memory boosters that we've all relied on at one time or another. In small amounts, caffeine stimulates our nervous systems, improving attention and making us feel more alert, Dr. Gordon says. That bag of M&Ms, slugged down with a can of Coke, may not be the healthiest of snacks, but an occasional quick fix will improve your ability to learn and remember in the short term.

Think ginkgo. Ginkgo has been found to be useful for improving the memory of older people who suffer from insufficient blood flow to the brain. But, according to Andrew Weil, M.D., director of the Program in Integrative Medicine at the University of Arizona College of Medicine in Tucson and author of several books, including *Eight Weeks to Optimum Health*, it is possible that ginkgo may help younger people as well. You can find ginkgo extract capsules in most health food stores, but the brands vary greatly in how much of the active ingredients they contain.

"An effective dose of ginkgo is 40 milligrams of extract standardized to 24 percent ginkgosides, three times a day with meals," says Dr. Weil. To find out if it helps your memory improve, you will have to try it for about eight weeks before you see any change. If you see an improvement, continue for six months before tapering off. That way, you'll be able to tell if ginkgo really helped solve the problem. If you are taking monoamine oxidase (MAO) inhibitors, check with your doctor before taking gingko.

▶PREVENTIVE MEASURES

Know when to say "when." A couple of drinks may do wonders for your pool game, but it throws a blanket over your memory. Alcohol is a fairly well known deterrent to memory, Dr. Gordon says. If you're a heavy social drinker, you may be able to improve your memory by cutting back. While it is still debated whether a few drinks a day can impair your recall, Dr. Gordon says that drinking to the point of tipsiness every day is a high-risk situation for absentmindedness and memory loss.

Start a routine. Always putting things in the same spot is an easy way to minimize absentmindedness, says Dr. Gordon. So empty your pockets in the same place every day. Make a little hook for your keys next to the front door, and hang them there as soon as you're inside. Create permanent places to store things like business cards, can openers, photo albums, and nail clippers.

Treat your pain. Take care of what ails you. Physical wellness is essential to good memory. If you suffer from any kind of ailment—sinus problems, gastrointestinal difficulties, or migraine headaches—you may become distracted by your pain, limiting your ability to learn, Dr. Manges says. If you have trouble taking in new information, it only follows that your ability to retain or repeat that information is going to be jeopardized. Stress and inadequate rest can have the same effect on memory, says Dr. Manges.

Acne

▶PROBLEM

The basic cause of acne is still a mystery. We do know that many factors contribute to it, and most of these are hormonal and genetic, says Yohini Appa, Ph.D., director of research and development for the Neutrogena Corporation in Los Angeles. Acne's hallmarks rear their ugly heads (black, white, or red) when the pores of your skin become plugged and you "break out."

Acne blemishes are most likely to appear on sebum-rich areas loaded with fat and skin cell debris, especially your nose (blackheads, mostly), the rest of your face (usually pimples and whiteheads), and on your chest and back (blackheads, whiteheads, cysts, or pimples).

▶CAUSE

Blame it on the androgens. Acne is more severe and a little more common in men than women because men produce more androgens—the hormone that fires up sebaceous gland activity. These glands ooze a greasy lubricating substance that can plug up the hair follicles and contribute to an acne attack.

It's in the genes. Experts don't understand how a tendency toward acne may be inherited, but if one or both of your parents were troubled by moderate or severe acne, you're likely to be plagued by it, too.

When you're a teenager, the root of your problem is more likely to be hormones—specifically, testosterone—that trigger sebum production. As a man ages, sebum levels, like testosterone levels, drop but don't stop.

DO THIS NOW

If you have a white pus-filled zit on your face, first clean the area well. Then sterilize a needle by striking a match and holding the tip of the needle in the flame for about three seconds and gently, without squeezing, nick the surface of the pimple. "Use a cotton swab to drain it out, then leave it alone," says Gary White, M.D., chief of the department of dermatology at Kaiser Permanente Hospital in San Diego. "If it's messy, you can use hydrogen peroxide to wash it up, but anything else, especially squeezing, will only make it worse."

Did You Know?

Can a birth control pill help guys fight acne? The question isn't as strange as it seems. A form of the birth control pill Ortho Tri-Cyclen helps combat acne in women. The pill lowers the levels of some of the hormones that contribute both to ovulation and skin eruptions in women. So, can a guy take it?

"No," says Patricia Farris, M.D., a dermatologist in private practice in New Orleans. "It's mostly testosterone that causes acne in guys, but the pill doesn't suppress testosterone. It acts on estrogen and progesterone."

Some medications that effect male hormones are being tested for their anti-acne properties, but nothing is available yet, says Dr. Farris.

▶HOW SERIOUS

"By the time most men are 20 or 25, acne vulgaris (the kind you see on kids) is gone," says Gary White, M.D., chief of the department of dermatology at Kaiser Permanente Hospital in San Diego. "It's much more common for an adult man to have rosacea, which requires very different care than pimples do." (For more information on rosacea, see Red Nose on page 440.)

Getting an occasional zit isn't serious, but if your skin has suddenly started acting up, you might consider seeing a dermatologist to be sure that the problem is really acne and not something that needs to be treated differently, says Eugene Zampieron, a doctor of naturopathy in Middlebury, Connecticut, and a professional member of the American Herbalists Guild.

▶SOLUTIONS

Medicate it. "Apply acne medication at the first signs of a breakout," says Dr. Appa. "The key to gaining control over acne is to apply the medication preventively to acne-prone areas on a regular basis," Dr. Appa says. "Most people think that they're trying to dry up the skin, but acne medications keep pores from clogging up and attack acne-causing bacteria."

You can choose from many over-the-counter acne preparations that contain either benzoyl peroxide or salicylic acid. Benzoyl peroxide products range from 2.5 percent (Neutrogena) to 10 percent (Oxy-10, Clearasil). Salicylic acid (Clean and Clear Moisturizer, Sensitive) can be irritating to sensitive skin, so experiment with the creams to see which one fights your pimples without drying up the surrounding area. Use twice a day.

Leave it alone. If you have one of those red, inflamed bumps sitting under your skin and you're just dying to squeeze it, pop it, poke it, or stab it—don't. "There's nothing you can do, and you can only make it worse by messing with it," says Dr. White. "Putting 5 percent benzoyl peroxide on it might help get rid of some of the bacteria, but other than that, just try to keep your hands off it."

Look for a pattern. Are you breaking out near your ears and mouth? It's probably from a dirty telephone receiver that you use a lot. Do you have lots of pimples on your chest and back? You probably sweat a lot when you work out and wait too long to shower. "Sometimes the solution is to pay closer attention to what's going on in your environment," Dr. Zampieron says.

Phones can be cleaned with a little glass cleaner, for example. Make sure that you wipe off the cleaner well, though, to keep it from irritating your skin. If it's sweat from your workout that's causing the problem, be sure to rinse off after a run or an hour at the gym. If you don't have access to a shower, bring moistened towelettes or at least change your shirt before your sweaty T-shirt dries.

▶ALTERNATIVE APPROACHES

Become the egg man. If John Lennon had followed this advice, maybe he wouldn't have had that forehead zit in his *White Album* photo. To help clear up a pimple, crack an egg, put some of the egg white on a cotton swab, and apply it to the blemish, suggests James Fulton, M.D., a dermatologist in private practice in Newport Beach, California. The egg white tightens the skin and probably has some anti-inflammatory proteins, he says.

Disinfect your razor. Just rinse it in some alcohol to prevent any bacteria that have developed on it from being transferred to your face, says Dr. Zampieron. Remember, too, that ingrown hairs can cause clogged pores, which will lead to pimples. Shaving properly, with plenty of warm water and a good shaving cream, will help solve this problem. (For more tips, see Ingrown Whiskers on page 317.)

▶PREVENTIVE MEASURES

Wash right. In other words, don't scrub. "The pore is a hole, and scrubbing only irritates the surface. You can't dig into it," explains Dr. White. "Using a cleanser with salicylic acid is a better idea." He suggests Neutrogena's Oil-Free Acne Wash or Sal-Ac, both of which are found in drugstores.

You can put 5 percent benzoyl peroxide on afterward, says Dr. White, especially on those areas that might be prone to breakouts.

Fight wrinkles. Alpha hydroxy acids, which are used to combat wrinkles, also have been proven effective in fighting acne. "If you're using a product that will increase the cell turnover rate, then you'll have a good chance at clearing up any problem skin," says Patricia Farris, M.D., a dermatologist in private practice in New Orleans. Some over-the-counter moisturizers contain alpha hydroxy acids up to 8 percent. (For more tips, see Wrinkles on page 569.)

Afternoon Slump

▶PROBLEM

It's like clockwork. Every day after lunch, your eyelids feel heavy. *Productivity* becomes a word that you can barely spell between 2:00 and 4:00 P.M., according to James Maas, Ph.D., professor of psychology at Cornell University in Ithaca, New York.

▶CAUSE

Our bodies are programmed for naps, and the urge to lay our heads on our desks after lunch is a normal function of our circadian rhythms, the built-in biological clocks that regulate our sleep-wake cycle. No matter what you do, there's going to be a dip in the middle of the afternoon. But the fewer winks you get at night, the harder you'll be hit by afternoon slump, says Michael Bonnet, Ph.D., professor of neurology at Wright State University School of Medicine and director of the sleep laboratory at the Dayton Veterans Affairs Medical Center, both in Dayton, Ohio.

▶HOW SERIOUS

Besides putting a crimp on your productivity, those midafternoon slumps don't usually signal a medical problem. But if handling heavy equipment or driving is part of your job description, afternoon slump can be dangerous and even deadly. Nodding off at your desk is also risky business if you're trying to climb the corporate ladder. If you can't manage your slump with any of the following remedies, or if your urge to nap becomes an all-day event or you're snoring loudly, see your doctor, says Dr. Bonnet, to determine what other factors may be causing your fatigue.

▶**SOLUTIONS**

Minimize the caffeine. You'd think that having a pot of coffee every day might give you some en-

ergy to get you over the hump, but your body gets used to the caffeine jolt over time, making it less effective. If you really want to jolt yourself in the afternoon, switch to decaf in the morning and give yourself a cup of high-octane java in the afternoon, where the more judicious use of the caffeine in coffee can really offer a boost, says Elizabeth Ward, R.D., nutrition counselor with Harvard Vanguard Medical Associates.

Have a snack. Any snack between 2:00 and 4:00 P.M. is going to help, but your best bet is something high in carbohydrates with a little protein, says Ward. Yogurt or graham crackers with a smidgen of peanut butter are good alternatives to your usual chocolate chip cookies, and both will satisfy your taste buds, too. A yogurt-based dip and fresh veggies for dipping is a super choice. It's especially convenient if you make it ahead of time and have access to a refrigerator at work, says Ward.

Go to the john. Drop your pants, get comfy, and close your eyes. Try to tune out the sound of toilets flushing as you nap surreptitiously in the comfort of your favorite stall. It sounds silly, but in some jobs, the men's room is the only place you can catch 10 to 15 minutes worth of Zzzs without being canned, so to speak. The john's as good a place as any for a catnap if your boss frowns on snoozing in the office or if you don't have the privacy to get some genuine shuteye, says Dr. Maas. No matter where you nap, though, make sure that you keep it short—20 minutes at the most, or you may have trouble falling asleep at night.

Customize your day. If you're sitting in front of a computer or doing some similarly draining task, use your slump time to do something more active, such as making phone calls, talking to your co-workers, or straightening up your office or work area, suggests Dr. Bonnet. If you switch off and on between the usual stuff and more active work, you'll stoke up your level of arousal and avoid slumping altogether.

▶**ALTERNATIVE APPROACHES**

Meditate. Besides allowing you to escape that pile of paperwork, your imaginative powers can really revitalize you during an otherwise dreadfully dull day. If you missed a few winks last night and can't take a nap, then try a technique called meditative relaxation once or twice a day, suggests Dr. Maas. Here's how you do it: Sit quietly in a comfortable position, then close your eyes and relax your muscles. Breathe easily through your nose. As you exhale, silently say one word, such as "one." Continue this procedure for 10 to 20 minutes. Done once or twice a day, meditative relaxation can relieve restlessness, tension, and fatigue. In fact, many people who practice meditative relaxation regularly probably need less sleep at night since they enter into what is technically a very light sleep, says Dr. Maas.

Lighten up. To stave off the afternoon slump, increase your exposure to sunlight throughout the day, suggests Dr. Bonnet. If you work inside, scoring a nice big window office may be a bit of a pipe dream. But you can install an extra bright light to help keep you awake. Having more lights on in your office space can increase alertness all day long, says Dr. Bonnet. Noon-time strolls in the sun can also energize you—heck, even on cloudy days, you can still soak up a lot of those revitalizing rays. Just be sure to apply a sunscreen with an SPF (sun protection factor) of at least 15 on your face and other exposed areas before you step out.

▶PREVENTIVE MEASURES

Sleep tight. Tonight and every night this week, go to bed a half-hour earlier than usual, suggests Dr. Bonnet. That midday coffee break or even an afternoon bout of exercise has its perks, but getting a normal night's sleep is what'll really keep you perked up. Dr. Bonnet simply recommends going to bed when you feel sleepy at night and letting yourself wake up naturally in the morning. Of course, the alarm clock's always a good backup; but with enough sleep, you'll be up before that alarm even starts buzzing.

Lunch right. And that means lunch light. A heavy meal in the middle of the day can be a real energy-drainer, says Ward. That low-fat turkey sandwich may seem smart compared to McDonald's, but the company cafeteria usually offers sandwiches two to three times the size of the kind you slap together yourself. Your best bet is to eat a light lunch (600 calories or less and mostly carbohydrates and protein) and then snack on something later, says Ward. If you pack a lunch, you can spread it out over the day, beginning at 11:00 A.M. or whenever you start getting the growls. And, oh yeah, don't even think about having a beer with that sandwich. The sedative powers of alcohol are sure to make you slump.

Alcoholism

▶PROBLEM

Someone who's addicted to alcohol is preoccupied with drinking, finds himself drinking more or for longer periods of time than planned, and continues to drink even when it wreaks havoc on his personal life, causing trouble at home or work and even leading to legal, financial, or health problems. Alcoholism isn't just the guy who drinks until he's in the gutter every night. People develop tolerance to alcohol, requiring more and more to have the same effect. The booze affects the person's judgment, inhibitions, and impulse control. If you drink alcohol to give yourself permission to do things you ordinarily would not do, you have the problem of alcoholism. Just understand that self-diagnosis is tricky: A person with alcoholism may not recognize his dependence on alcohol and deny that he is dependent on it.

▶CAUSE

Why some of us can take a drink without a problem and others get hooked is still a mystery. Evidence points to a genetic link that may be passed on from generation to generation, leaving you more inclined to become addicted than others, says Max A. Schneider, M.D., director of education at the Positive Action Center at Chapman Medical Center in Orange, California; past president of the American Society of Addiction Medicine; and chairman of the board of the

DO THIS NOW

People with alcoholism tend to shirk their responsibilities, forcing others to pick up the slack, says Max A. Schneider, M.D., director of education at the Positive Action Center at Chapman Medical Center in Orange, California, and chairman of the board of the National Council on Alcoholism and Drug Dependence. Have you stopped taking out the trash? Does your housemate now do what used to be your chores? Do coworkers admonish you because they are always covering up for you? If drinking leads you to neglect your responsibilities and the people you love, then you probably have alcoholism and need some help, says Dr. Schneider.

National Council on Alcoholism and Drug Dependence. The genetic disposition may skip generations. It is important, therefore, for the person who has a family history of alcohol dependence to be more alert to the early warning signs for themselves and their children. Other possible causes include environmental factors such as your home life, social life, and the prevalence of alcohol in your life.

▶How Serious

Alcohol abuse ravages the body in many different ways. Estimates show that 9 to 22 years of life are lost for a person with alcoholism who dies of liver disease. Compare that with 2 years lost for cancer and 4 years for heart disease. The liver isn't the only organ to suffer. Every body tissue is negatively affected by alcohol—the pancreas becomes inflamed, as does the heart muscle. But alcoholism also destroys marriages, family relationships, friendships, and professional opportunities. If a person with alcoholism wants to prevent or reverse these problems, he needs to get help—the sooner the better. As your first step, call a local Alcoholics Anonymous (AA) chapter or an addiction-recovery program at a hospital, Dr. Schneider says. Their numbers should be listed in the white pages of the phone book.

▶Solutions

If you think that you might have a problem but aren't sure, take this simple test, developed by John Ewing, M.D., professor emeritus in the department of psychiatry at the University of North Carolina at Chapel Hill Center for Alcohol Studies, to screen for alcoholism.

- Have you ever felt the need to cut down on your drinking?
- Has your drinking ever gotten out of control?
- Have people ever annoyed you by criticizing your drinking?
- Do you get angry when people talk about your drinking?
- Have you ever felt guilty about your drinking?
- Has your drinking ever given you grief?
- Have you ever needed an eye-opener: a drink first thing in the morning, or lots of coffee to get you going?
- Have you ever taken an early-morning drink to recover from a hangover or to steady your nerves?

If you answered yes to two or more of these questions, you may have an alcohol problem and should seek professional help.

Go cold turkey. People who truly have alcoholism can't just cut back, Dr. Schneider says. The alcohol will just suck them back in. And they shouldn't rely on substitutes such as nonalcoholic beer; people with alcoholism should stay away from the atmosphere of drinking altogether, says Ken Leonard, Ph.D., senior research scientist and clinical psychologist at the Research Institute on Addictions in Buffalo.

History Lesson

Perhaps the ultimate attempt at eradicating alcoholism came on January 16, 1920, when the U.S. government adopted the "out-of-sight, out-of-mind" policy of Prohibition. Pushed by rural Protestant moralists who viewed alcohol as the root of sin and evil in American society, Prohibition banned the production, transportation, and sale of liquor in the United States.

But just like a teenager who's told by his parents that he isn't allowed to do something, people rushed out and actually drank more hard liquor. (It was easier to smuggle.) High-class speakeasies replaced corner bars. Less affluent Americans turned to their own kitchens, brewing up sometimes-poisonous moonshine made with wood alcohol. After only six years, the "noble experiment" created a $3.6 billion underground bootleg industry.

Despite its failure, Prohibition wasn't repealed until the Great Depression, when our country's leaders realized that liquor could help boost the country's wounded economy.

The only way to recover is to stop drinking, Dr. Schneider says. If you have medical complications from alcohol withdrawal, many hospitals or clinics have programs to help you stop drinking. Then many people need a program such as AA to not start again.

Overhaul your social life. Take a good look at your social circle. Do all your favorite hangouts have bar stools in them? Does a friendly get-together always revolve around the liquor cabinet? "It's often the case that the social life of a person with alcoholism revolves around drinking and that most of his friends are drinkers," Dr. Leonard says.

Say goodbye to your drinking buddies and find a new group of people to have fun with. Joining a support group such as AA will give you an instantaneous sober social circle. Change your hangouts where you can meet new and sober people and find healthier ways to spend your time, Dr. Schneider says. People, places, and things in your drinking life must be changed. *Change* is the key word.

Reward yourself. You probably want to beat alcoholism to make your life happier and more enjoyable. Yet the actual act of recovery may seem like a merciless rite of penance. "At some point your personality is going to rebel against recovery and set off the whole thing. That's why it's important to build in rewards so that your recovery process is enjoyable," says Aviel Goodman, M.D., director of the Minnesota Institute of Psychiatry in St. Paul. Treat yourself to something special for every milestone, whether it be each week you stay sober or when you resist a strong urge. The types of rewards suggested by Dr.

Goodman include going out to dinner, taking a warm bath, or buying a CD. "Part of the process of recovery is discovering what else you enjoy besides alcohol," he says. Just make sure that you don't exchange one addiction for another (eating, shopping, and the like).

Chew on a pen. If you need to develop a habit or a diversionary tactic to curtail your drinking, go right ahead, says Dr. Leonard. "Anything you do that doesn't involve drinking is the best thing. Do whatever works for you," he says. Chew on pens, suck on a toothpick—whatever does the trick. If you really want to turn over a healthier leaf, take a walk or exercise whenever you get a drinking urge, he suggests.

▶ALTERNATIVE APPROACHES

Buy an organizer. Some people drink to cope with a hectic, out-of-control lifestyle, says Jay L. Glaser, M.D., medical director of the Maharishi Ayur-Veda Medical Center in Lancaster, Massachusetts. But scheduling your day will let you fit everything in without killing yourself, he adds. Go to bed and wake up at the same time every day, which will ensure that you're well-rested, he says. Block time out of each day for nutritious meals. Plan for work, exercise, leisure activities, even watching TV. Getting your day organized will help keep your life under control, leaving you less likely to turn to the drink, Dr. Glaser says.

Listen to your body. According to the Vedic approach to health that has been around since ancient India, your body sends you messages, telling you what it needs to stay healthy, says Dr. Glaser. But many people with alcoholism interpret all messages—whether they be "I'm stressed out" or "I need sleep"— to mean, "I need a drink." The next time you want to drink, lie down on your back and close your eyes for five minutes. Quietly think about the sensations you're feeling. "One might actually feel hungry or tired, overstimulated or depressed," he says. Once you've heard your body's desires, fulfill them without taking a drink, Dr. Glaser says. If you are under stress, take a walk. If you are tired, go to bed.

▶PREVENTIVE MEASURES

Reorganize your time. If alcohol is the be-all and end-all for you, find a purpose in life other than drinking. Volunteer work builds up your self-esteem and gives you less time to think about the booze, Dr. Schneider says. Consider joining organizations such as service, nondrinking social, or community support clubs so that you can build up your nondrinking social circle and help others at the same time. Whatever volunteer activities you choose, make sure that you enjoy them soberly, Dr. Schneider recommends.

Work on your comeback line. You'll be faced at some point with someone offering you a drink. Rehearse how you will react so that you'll be prepared. Popular decline lines include: "Thank you, but I choose not to drink"; "I'm allergic to it"; and Dr. Schneider's personal favorite, "I'm too young to drink."

Allergies

▶PROBLEM

We inhale up to 2½ tablespoons of solid crud every day. Car exhaust, pet dander, smoke, pollens, and smog are just some of the culprits. For certain people, that leads to trouble when their respiratory system goes haywire. You sneeze, snort, drip, hack, and cough; your eyes are red and watery; and you generally feel crummy. You have an inhalant allergy, your body's response to something you breathed in. Hay fever also falls into this category.

▶CAUSE

Consider your immune system the Jedi warriors of the biological world. When Darth Vader and the Stormtroopers come near, the minions of evil get a blasting. But in some people, the sensory gear gets fouled up and they can't recognize good guys from bad guys. When this happens, harmless things such as pollen, dust, and cat hair cause an immune system response that mimics a respiratory infection.

▶HOW SERIOUS

Much of the time, the most serious effect of inhalant allergies is the dent in your wallet from buying tissues. But these allergies have been known to trigger asthma attacks, especially if the person already has asthma that is poorly controlled, says Patricia McNally, M.D., an allergist with the Kaiser Permanente Allergy Clinic in Springfield, Virginia. And asthma attacks can be fatal. If you can't get a handle on your allergies with home remedies, seek out a board-certified allergist. Simple skin tests can identify exactly what you're allergic to, and doctors can formulate a plan of treatment.

▶SOLUTIONS

Get steamed. "I frequently tell people to buy a steam inhaler or to boil water in a pot," says Ralph T. Golan, M.D., a general practitioner in Seattle and author of *Optimal Wellness*. A steam inhaler is a small, personal vaporizing device available at some drugstores. Drape your head in a bath towel over the pot, or use the inhaler and breathe deeply. Breathe until you feel your sinuses loosening, says Dr. Golan, which may take up to 15 minutes. You can repeat this as needed.

Caution: Take the pot off the stove before you do this, and stay far enough back from the steam. You don't want to add facial or nasal burns to a runny nose.

Adding a drop or two of eucalyptus oil to the water will help, too, if you don't mind the scent. Eucalyptus oil is widely available at health food stores and stores that carry natural skin and hair-care products.

Snort salt water. A good follow-up to the steam treatment, adds Dr. Golan, is a saline solution you can put up your nose. Take a cup of warm water, add a half-teaspoon of salt and a pinch of baking soda and dissolve. Put the mixture in a medicine dropper or squeeze/spray bottle and drop or squirt it into one nostril. Close off the opposite nostril, and sniff deeply. Repeat with the other nostril. Do this three or four times a day during allergy attacks. Not only does it lubricate a war-torn nasal passage; it can help you avoid sinusitis, an infection of your sinuses.

Wash that mustache. It gets the soup out, too, but regular mustache washing can lessen your allergies. Dr. McNally and her fellow physicians did a small, uncontrolled study in which they asked each man sporting handlebars who had hay fever to wash his mustache twice a day—in the morning and before bed. "Pollen grains impact your mustache, and it's like a reservoir," explains Dr. McNally. In each case, the men reported having to use less decongestants and antihistamines for their allergies and increased comfort in breathing, especially while sleeping. She suggests washing your mustache twice a day, using a liquid soap or shampoo to get out the pollen grains.

Show your mite. If cleaning the whole house is more than you can handle on a regular basis, concentrate on the bedroom. For one thing, it might help the odds of having a woman actually want to join you there. Even if it doesn't, clean sleeping quarters will help you breathe easier. "We spend so much time in the bedroom that that's really the important room," says Dr. McNally. On top of that, little critters called dust mites thrive in your bed because they eat the skin you shed when you're rolling around. It's not the mites themselves but their little feces that cause allergy attacks. You can buy dust mite covers to isolate the mattress, their favorite nesting spot.

History Lesson

Buddy Ebsen of *The Beverly Hillbillies* and *Barnaby Jones* fame was originally slated to be the Tin Man in the 1939 movie *The Wizard of Oz* until an allergic reaction to his makeup nearly killed him.

MGM had no idea how to dress the Tin Man, so the studio experimented with several choices. It was finally decided that Ebsen's face would be painted with clown white and aluminum dust applied over the top. A month later, Ebsen was in an oxygen tent in a California hospital after his lungs failed. An allergic reaction to the aluminum dust left him bedridden for six weeks.

Typically sympathetic, Hollywood replaced Ebsen during his sickness with Jack Haley. The aluminum dust was changed to a paste that was painted on.

You can still hear Ebsen's voice in the movie, though, when the foursome of Dorothy, the Scarecrow, the Tin Man, and the Cowardly Lion sings "We're Off to See the Wizard."

Wash your sheets. Dust mites die if you wash your sheets in hot water of 130°F (55°C) or warmer. If you can't get your water that hot, Australian researchers have found another equally effective method. Mix eucalyptus oil with liquid dishwashing detergent (one without bleach) at the ratio of one part detergent to three to five parts oil. Fill your washer with warm water first then add the oil-detergent mixture, followed by your sheets. Let them soak for 30 minutes, then finish the wash cycle. This kills just as many of the bugs. Not all dishwashing detergents are equal, though. You'll have to experiment a bit. You need a soap that holds the oil in the solution. Stir a teaspoon of the oil and soap combination into a glass of water. If the oil floats to the top within 10 minutes, it won't work. Eucalyptus oil is widely available at health food stores.

Bare your floor. Carpet is another favorite harbor of dust mites, dust, and pet dander, Dr. McNally says. Get rid of wall-to-wall carpet permanently, at least in the bedroom, and put down area rugs that can be washed.

Book 'em, Dan-o. Remove any bookshelves from the bedroom; the books gather dust. And use roll-up shades, suggests Dr. McNally. They're much easier to dust than blinds. Keep your bedroom dust-free, and try to keep the clutter to a minimum.

▶ALTERNATIVE APPROACHES

Pinch yourself before breakfast. Before you eat in the morning, grate a pinch of fresh ginger, mix it with a pinch of salt, and put it in your mouth where it can stimulate digestive enzymes, suggests Helen Thomas, D.C., owner of an Ayurvedic center in Santa Rosa, California, and co-author of *Ayurveda*. She has also trained with Deepak Chopra, M.D., one of the forerunners in bringing Ayurveda to North America. Drink some warm water and swish the ginger around for 10 seconds. "It's just like putting a few logs in the fire," she says, and will get your immune system primed. This can be done every morning, especially during the allergy seasons.

Fight fire with fire. Dr. Thomas also suggests adding hot and spicy foods to your diet on a regular basis. Ground red pepper, chili peppers, and other hot-pepper sauces are good examples. Not only will they keep the mucus flowing freely but also they'll bolster your immune system, Dr. Thomas says. "It's like putting your foot on the accelerator."

▶PREVENTIVE MEASURES

Pack it in. As if there weren't enough good reasons to kick cigarettes. "Smoking just makes things so much worse," says Dr. McNally. See your family doctor if you need help; there are more ways than ever now to assist you in getting off the lung darts.

Choose health. There comes a time when you have to consider which is more important: your health and that of family members with allergies, or owning a pet. Dr. McNally says that she regularly sees patients who refuse to get rid of Bowser or Mittens, even though they, and sometimes their children, are suffering greatly. "Find a nice, safe home for the pet where you can go visit sometimes," she suggests.

Anger

▶ PROBLEM

For years, medical experts have argued over whether it's better to express or suppress anger. We now know that anger is bad for your health, period. Rage, fury, ire, wrath, resentment—whatever you want to call it—anger is a strong feeling of displeasure experienced on the gut level that sometimes leads to aggressive, violent behavior.

▶ CAUSE

Anger has two essential prerequisites, says Matthew McKay, Ph.D., clinical director of Haight Ashbury Psychological Services in San Francisco and co-author of *When Anger Hurts*. First, you need to experience stress or pain of some kind. Second, you must have a "trigger thought"—a flash in your brain that says that someone or something has caused you pain, embarrassment, stress, or loss.

▶ HOW SERIOUS

Whether you clench your teeth, scream and yell, or walk away in a huff, angry feelings have been associated with many health problems, particularly cardiovascular diseases such as stroke, hypertension, and coronary heart disease. At the Western Electric Company in Chicago, a study of almost 2,000 men revealed that men who scored high on a hostility scale were 1½ times more likely to have a heart attack than men who scored lower. A 25-year follow-up study of male physicians found six times more cases of coronary heart disease among angry men than among their less-angry counterparts. Moreover, anger takes a serious toll on relationships. If you're chronically angry or hostile, you may damage supportive relationships, which also can harm your health, says

> **DO THIS NOW**
>
> When you find yourself getting angry, take a deep breath through your nose, tighten up every muscle in your body, and then slowly let everything relax as you exhale, suggests Cary Rothstein, Ph.D., psychologist and co-director of the Crossroads Center for Psychiatry and Psychology in Doylestown, Pennsylvania. Breathing techniques like this one reduce the physical arousal caused by angry feelings.

Christopher Peterson, Ph.D., professor of psychology at the University of Michigan in Ann Arbor.

▶SOLUTIONS

Take your finger off the trigger. Trigger thoughts are the matches that ignite angry feelings. Pay attention to your inner voice that says that *they* did something to you, or that labels someone as crazy, stupid, or a selfish jerk. Catch yourself using words that magnify the situation (*terrible*, *awful*, *disgusting*) or words that overgeneralize (*always*, *all*, *every*, *never*). Be conscious of any sentence that begins with "You should not have" or "You should have." Without these blaming thoughts, global labels, and "should" statements, your pain wouldn't express itself in anger, Dr. McKay says. To undermine anger, replace your negative interpretation of the situation with a more positive outlook. For example, instead of assuming that your waitress is surly and rude, consider that she has been on her feet all day and that her last customer probably stiffed her on the tip.

Listen to your body. The signs of anger vary from man to man, but some may include balling up your fists, raising your voice, feeling hot, tightening in your abdomen, clenching your teeth, and feeling your heart pumping faster. Recognizing these physical warning signs of anger will help raise the red flag to begin quick relaxation techniques to prevent an outburst, Dr. McKay says.

Relax. There are all kinds of instant relaxation techniques, most involving deep breathing. Here is Dr. McKay's six-step strategy for quick, temporary relief from an onslaught of anger.

1. Spend 10 seconds rubbing a tense part of your body.
2. Take 10 slow, deep breaths.
3. Change your posture and stretch.
4. Talk more slowly.
5. Go get a cold drink (nonalcoholic).
6. Sit down and lean back.

Talk to yourself. As with any relaxation technique, it helps to think a "coping thought" as you concentrate on your breathing. Coping thoughts need not be elaborate, as long as they are calming and reassuring, says Cary Rothstein, Ph.D., psychologist and co-director of the Crossroads Center for Psychiatry and Psychology in Doylestown, Pennsylvania. For example, "It'll be okay," "Not a problem," or "I can handle it." Coping thoughts also can replace the negative thoughts that trigger anger, Dr. McKay says.

▶ALTERNATIVE APPROACHES

Take a time-out. To stop anger on the spot, try calling time-out. And do it just like the big guys in the NBA. Make the T sign with your hands and take a breather. Of course, this requires that the other person not only understands the sign but also has the same right to call time-out. The idea, Dr. McKay says, is

History Lesson

Golf can teach us much about life. Here's one small lesson on anger.

Following a particularly poor shot one day, a 40-year-old duffer got really teed off and broke his graphite driver across his leg. The shaft left an ugly gash on his thigh, which seemed to heal normally. But things are not always as they seem. Two months later, the wound was painful, red, and swollen. An exam showed that graphite particles from the golf club had become embedded in the skin and caused inflammation.

So next time your club fails you—which, no doubt, will be the next time you play golf—take a deep breath and walk it off.

that when two people with a history of conflict sense that things are escalating, one can call for an end to all talking. Then separate for a predetermined period of time (perhaps an hour). No parting shots allowed.

Dr. McKay suggests doing something physical or relaxing during this time to work out some of your stress before you meet again and to absolutely stay away from drugs or alcohol. When you get back, check in with each other. "Indicate whether you feel ready to return to a discussion of the conflict, and do so," says Dr. McKay. "If you're not ready, set a specific time when you both feel willing to resume an exploration of the issue. This helps to maintain trust and establishes your willingness to communicate."

▶PREVENTIVE MEASURES

Be realistic. It's difficult never to be angry, but it is possible to be angry less—as soon as you start expecting less, says Dr. Peterson. Kicking a soda machine when it eats your dollar isn't unreasonable, but when you constantly blow up at your wife, it's time to figure out what unfulfilled expectation is getting you so worked up. It's possible that you may be expecting too much. Even if you believe that your expectations *are* realistic, you should still temper yourself. Approach her with one issue at a time, identifying the specific behavior you want her to change, Dr. McKay says. Reciting a long list of grievances will only make *her* angry.

Live the good life. To prevent our short fuses from sparking angrily, we need to lower the stress levels in all areas of our lives, Dr. Rothstein says. When we're stressed, we have little tolerance. To de-stress, we need to live well. We need good nutrition, the right amount of exercise, just enough fun, and plenty of love. One of the most important life improvements you can make to minimize angry feelings is to have a strong connection to others. "Warm, supportive relationships go a long way in giving us more ability to withstand the pains and frustrations in the outside world," says Dr. Rothstein.

Angina

▶PROBLEM

Angina is a recurring pressure in the chest that occurs when the heart fails to get enough oxygen-rich blood. Often, the pressure is temporary and will go away once oxygen needs return to normal. It's not a heart attack, which occurs when the flow of blood to the heart is completely blocked. But it is a warning sign that cannot be ignored.

▶CAUSE

Various factors can make your heart demand more oxygen than your arteries can provide. The most common is narrowed arteries. If blood can't easily make its way to the heart, you'll feel it every time your heart rate speeds up. Mental stress and exercise often can trigger angina attacks because they increase the heart's oxygen needs. However, with angina, once you stop exerting yourself, the pressure in your chest will subside.

▶HOW SERIOUS

There are four classes of angina and the lower classes are relatively harmless, with the chest pressure only lasting two to three minutes. But by the time you get to Class 4 angina, you need to worry. At this stage, people are often at rest and even asleep when the attacks occur. Class 4 angina often requires intense medical treatment.

If you suspect that you have angina, you should see your doctor about it as soon as possible, says Peter M. Abel, M.D., director of cardiovascular disease

DO THIS NOW

Aspirin can thin the blood and prevent death from heart attack when used in conjunction with the clot-busting drugs you'll get at the hospital, says Mark J. Eisenberg, M.D., assistant professor of medicine at Jewish General Hospital in Montreal. Chewing gets the aspirin in your system faster than swallowing, but the important thing is the intake of 325 milligrams.

Taking an aspirin every day—even when you are not feeling pain—is an even better strategy, but only if you suffer from chronic coronary disease and you've talked to your doctor about it.

Did You Know?

The human heart is amazingly resilient. All the way back in the 1800s, sur-geons realized that some foreign objects—the old-style round bullets, fish bones, wood splinters, even hat pins—were better left alone once they had pierced the heart. It could take a licking and keep on ticking for years, even with those objects lodged inside. The heart's Achilles' heel, however, is its oxygen supply. When you deprive your hardest working muscle of oxygen, its cells die. That's why angina hurts so much.

and prevention at the cardiovascular Institute of the South in Morgan City, Louisiana. It may turn out to be something minor, but a heart disorder is not something that you want to self-diagnose. Making a mistake can be disastrous, he cautions. If you have chest pain, as opposed to chest pressure, that lasts for 15 minutes or is accompanied by shortness of breath and a sick-to-your-stomach feeling, go to the emergency room immediately. You may be having a heart attack instead of an angina attack. The longer your heart goes without oxygen, the more likely you'll end up with heart damage, Dr. Abel warns. Heart disease and angina are caused by the same problem—pinched, clogged arteries. (For more home remedies, turn to Heart Disease on page 281.)

▶SOLUTIONS

Sit down. Some angina attacks are brought on by exercise, when the heart needs too much oxygen too quickly. So sitting down and resting for a few min-utes can ease the pain, Dr. Abel says.

Calm down. Mental stress can cause chest pain for the same reasons as physical stress: It increases the oxygen demands of the heart. So if you feel chest pain when you argue with your wife, worry about your taxes, or chastise your kid for his bad report card, call a mental time-out and lie on the couch, Dr. Abel says.

Get a daily massage. Having your partner's hands against your skin can heal your heart, says Stephen T. Sinatra, M.D., director of the New England Heart Center in Manchester, Connecticut, and author of *Optimum Health* and *Heartbreak and Heart Disease*. Her touch will help you let go of artery-clogging negative emotions such as anger, sadness, stress, and fear. It also will reduce your heart rate, creating less oxygen demands on your pinched arteries.

Quit smoking. Smoking constricts your blood vessels, creating even less room for blood to flow to your heart, Dr. Abel says. It also robs your heart muscle of oxygen. If you want to eliminate angina, ban the butts—now.

▶ALTERNATIVE APPROACHES

Try coenzyme Q$_{10}$. When functioning normally, your heart has the highest concentration of the vitamin-like coenzyme Q$_{10}$ in the body, Dr. Sinatra says. The heart needs the enzyme to heal injured cells and transfer energy. The problem is that when frequent angina deprives your heart of oxygen, coenzyme Q$_{10}$ levels fall. You can get some coenzyme Q$_{10}$ from food, such as fatty fish, liver and organ meats, and wheat germ. But to get the levels that Dr. Sinatra recommends, you'll need to take supplements, found at health food stores. Take 120 to 180 milligrams a day to supplement conventional methods to treat angina. To help prevent angina and other heart problems, take 60 to 100 milligrams a day, says Dr. Sinatra.

Forgo the fat. Though the American Heart Association recommends keeping your fat intake to less than 30 percent of your daily calories, there's some evidence that you should slash much more dietary fat to reverse heart disease and the chest pain that accompanies it. "We found a reduction in the frequency of angina or chest pain within weeks of making severe changes in diet and lifestyle," says Dean Ornish, M.D., president and director of the nonprofit Preventive Medicine Research Institute in Sausalito, California, and author of *Dr. Dean Ornish's Program for Reversing Heart Disease.*

Dr. Ornish recommends holding dietary fat to 10 percent of your calories and eliminating animal products. The move will do more than soothe your chest pain. Progressively over time, it will open up your clogged arteries, preventing heart attack. Studies by Dr. Ornish have shown that a super-low-fat diet (less than 10 percent), when combined with exercise, giving up cigarettes, and reducing stress, not only lowers cholesterol but also may actually reverse existing blockages in the arteries.

▶ PREVENTIVE MEASURES

Watch *Old Yeller*. You know the saying, "Men don't cry." Dr. Sinatra strongly believes that dry eyes are one of the reasons that men get heart attacks. "We have found that men who don't cry, who don't reach out, who don't hug other men, who deny their feelings, have higher amounts of breakdown products, like the stress hormone cortisol, in their urine," Dr. Sinatra says. "The body tells the truth. All those men had heart disease." He believes that crying gets rid of heart-damaging chemicals as well as pent-up emotion. The women studied who reached out and nurtured one another had no signs of heart disease and no cortisol by-products in their urine. Surprisingly, the women who were in traditionally male-dominated roles, those who had to "act like a man" and shut off their women's intuition, were not only predisposed to heart disease but also showed an increased level of cortisol in their urine, says Dr. Sinatra.

So, you still don't want do cry, do you? That's okay. One easy way to get those tears out of your system and still preserve your masculinity is to watch a really sad movie by yourself. Sob. Be done with it.

Anxiety Attack

▶PROBLEM

When you have an anxiety attack, your body reacts to being in a crowded mall the same way it would react to a tiger lunging at you. Your heart may speed up, blood pressure may rise, your breathing may get labored, you may feel dizzy and faint. It's an overreaction of the nervous system that leaves you worrying that you're going crazy or are about to suffer a heart attack.

▶CAUSE

Anxiety attacks tend to first appear after a period of unusual stress, such as an illness, a death, or a divorce, says Cary Rothstein, Ph.D., psychologist and co-director of the Crossroads Center for Psychiatry and Psychology in Doylestown, Pennsylvania. As your resistance is overwhelmed, all that anxiety comes to the fore. The hypothalamus in your brain releases hormones that cause the adrenal glands (two glands near the kidneys) to release more hormones. These hormones may slow digestion and speed up your heart rate, blood pressure, and breathing, leaving you with a sense that something terrible is going to happen to you. It's your body's fight-or-flight response kicking into action, but there's nothing physical for you to fight off or flee from.

▶HOW SERIOUS

When someone has an anxiety attack for the first time, he may end up in the emergency room, only to find out that there's nothing medically wrong with him. If the attacks continue, he may avoid places or situations where he could get stuck, such as bridges, bank lines, supermarkets, turnpikes, parties, crowds,

DO THIS NOW

If you're having an anxiety attack right now, breathe slowly, in and out, then rapidly read a few sentences in this book aloud. Repeat these steps for five to eight minutes to distract yourself from the symptoms of the anxiety attack, recommends Benjamin Fialkoff, Ph.D., a psychologist in private practice in New York City and Ridgewood, New Jersey.

58

Did You Know?

Anxiety disorders are the most common mental health illnesses in America.

open spaces—any place he can't escape in a hurry. When the avoidance is repeated over time, it becomes a phobia—a persistent, irrational, intense fear of a specific object, activity, or situation. When phobias take over, life becomes more and more restricted. (For more information, see Phobias on page 413.) If you find yourself repeatedly avoiding places and situations because you fear having an attack, then it's time for you to seek treatment, says Dr. Rothstein, either through a self-help program or through a mental health professional or physician.

▶SOLUTIONS

Accept your symptoms. Your heart is pounding, and you feel like you're going crazy. "Tell yourself that it's just anxiety," says Dr. Rothstein. "Tell yourself that you're not in any danger, despite the fact that you feel like hell."

One of the first steps to overcoming anxiety attacks is accepting your symptoms and understanding that they aren't dangerous. "Give your body permission to do what it has to do, allowing it to relax to decrease the symptoms," says Kenneth Reinhard, Ph.D., director of the Hudson Valley Veterans Affairs Hospital Anxiety Disorders Clinic in Montrose, New York.

Stay put. "Don't bolt," says Elke Zuercher-White, Ph.D., a psychologist in San Francisco and author of *An End to Panic.* "Just try to ride through the panic as if you were surfing on the ocean. The wave will pass you by, and so will a panic."

Most people who have anxiety attacks develop phobias because the attacks happen in certain places. Instead of sticking it out when the panic comes on, they abandon the situation, according to Dr. Reinhard. The real trick to overcoming anxiety attacks (and the phobias that go along with them) is to tell yourself that they are not the danger you fear. This may help you stay in the situation a little bit longer, and the panic may thus decrease. Even if you decide to leave, staying just one extra minute is a positive step toward ending anxiety attacks.

Talk kindly to yourself. "When you're having an anxiety attack, you have to tell yourself something other than, 'This is terrible,' 'I look like a fool,' or 'I'm going to die,'" says Benjamin Fialkoff, Ph.D., a psychologist in private practice in New York City and Ridgewood, New Jersey. Say something realistic to yourself to help you cope with the symptoms, like "I can handle it," "It will go away," or "I've dealt with this in the past."

▶ALTERNATIVE APPROACHES

Sing it out. One way to distract yourself from thinking negatively during an attack is by singing, either aloud or to yourself, depending on who's around, says Dr. Fialkoff.

Occupy your mind. Any distraction will help calm you down, says Dr. Rothstein: counting shoes, trying to remember sports statistics, looking for Chevrolets—whatever works.

Practice relaxing. While sitting down, visualize a pleasant scene or even your favorite color and let yourself drift for about 10 minutes. Do this at least twice a day. Each time you practice visualization or any other relaxation technique, you call out the relaxation response in your body, says Dr. Fialkoff. By regularly calling out the relaxation response, you can immunize yourself against anxiety attacks. You can call on this visualization technique to calm yourself during an attack as well. First breathe deeply, then read out loud, then visualize. Repeat this procedure for five to eight minutes.

▶PREVENTIVE MEASURES

Expose yourself. Nearly everyone with anxiety attacks avoids places where attacks repeatedly occur, says S. Lloyd Williams, Ph.D., professor of psychology at Lehigh University in Bethlehem, Pennsylvania. The key to overcoming anxiety attacks forever is to expose yourself to the situation you fear. The concept is simple: Go to the mall. *Drive* across the bridge. Psychologists call this exposure therapy. For maximum benefit, exposures must be frequent—at least three times as week, says Dr. Zuercher-White. While you may start with short exposures, eventually try to stay in them for 1½ to 2 hours. Some people can do exposures on their own; others need a "buddy" for support.

Take a walk. Exercise and good nutrition are both important in warding off anxiety attacks. According to Dr. Fialkoff, exercise metabolizes one of the stress hormones that triggers anxiety attacks. One of the best exercises for men who are prone to anxiety attacks is fast walking. Shoot for 30 to 45 minutes a day. Check with your doctor before you start any new exercise program.

Mitigate the mood-enhancers. Dr. Fialkoff suggests cutting down your caffeine intake to zero because, even in small doses, caffeine triggers anxiety. The same is true for drugs and alcohol. While they can calm you for a moment, drugs and alcohol increase anxiety in the long term and may cause addiction and abuse, according to Dr. Zuercher-White.

Arthritis

▶PROBLEM

Arthritis is a generic name for any disease that causes pain and swelling of the joints and connective tissue in the body. There are more than 100 types of arthritis, afflicting some 42.7 million Americans, more than one-third of them men. Men most commonly get osteoarthritis, (4.1 million), gout (800,000), and rheumatoid arthritis (600,000). (For more information on gout, see Gout on page 258.)

▶CAUSE

Osteoarthritis is associated with a breakdown of cartilage, the shock absorber between bones. It usually occurs in old age, but sport injuries, repetitive stress, and especially obesity can bring it on sooner.

Rheumatoid arthritis is a malfunction of the immune system that causes the body to attack the joints. It usually strikes after age 40.

▶HOW SERIOUS

The main symptoms of arthritis are pain, stiffness, swelling in and around joints, and limited movement that lasts more than two weeks. If you have these symptoms, see your doctor. Don't delay because you think that all you have are minor aches and pains, says Howard R. Smith, M.D., chief of rheumatology at Meridia Huron Hospital and adjunct professor of medicine at Case Western Reserve University School

DO THIS NOW

When arthritis flares up, you can use either cold or heat to help relieve the pain, says Howard R. Smith, M.D., chief of rheumatology at Meridia Huron Hospital and adjunct professor of medicine at Case Western Reserve University School of Medicine, both in Cleveland. It depends on the problem. If your joints and muscles are stiff when you wake up or after a long period of inactivity, take a long, hot shower; dip your hands in a paraffin bath; or apply a heating pad to the stiff area. If your joints are inflamed and swollen, apply ice or an ice pack wrapped in a thin towel. As a general rule, apply the heat or cold for 20 minutes, and repeat as needed, up to several times a day.

of Medicine, both in Cleveland. Often, the sooner you see your doctor, the more options you have and the better the outcome, he says. As an arthritic condition worsens, the joint may become more painful and deformed; and, in some cases, you may need a joint replacement to regain movement and function. While some forms of arthritis can be cured, there are no cures for osteoarthritis and rheumatoid arthritis. But they can often be effectively controlled, says Dr. Smith, and there are things you can do to help manage them.

▶SOLUTIONS

Bone up. After you have been diagnosed with arthritis, learn as much about the disease as you can, suggests Michele Boutaugh, vice president for Patient and Community Services and a spokesperson for the Arthritis Foundation in Atlanta. The more you learn, the more you'll know about nondrug options to help you control the symptoms and manage your arthritis. It also gives you a sense of control, she says, and you can work with your physician to make the choices that are right for you. For more information on arthritis, self-help programs, and exercise programs, contact your local chapter of the Arthritis Foundation; or write to them at P. O. Box 7669, Atlanta, GA 30357-0669.

Lose some weight. There is a strong relationship between being overweight and having osteoarthritis in weight-bearing joints, such as your knees, explains Sarah Morgan, R.D., M.D., associate professor of medicine and nutrition science at the University of Alabama at Birmingham. Losing weight can reduce pain in joints affected by osteoarthritis. If you are overweight, lose the extra pounds; if you are at your healthy weight, maintain it, Dr. Morgan suggests.

Work it out. Exercise, especially exercise that doesn't put a lot of strain on the affected joints, can make arthritis more manageable by building strong muscles and ligaments around weak and diseased joints, says Dr. Smith. Exercise also helps by elevating mood, increasing endurance, improving the range of motion of joints, and easing chronic pain through the release of endorphins (the body's own painkillers), says Dr. Smith.

Walking, cycling, strength training using very light weights, stretching, and, in particular, exercise done in the water—swimming and water aerobics—are beneficial, says Dr. Smith. "The buoyancy of the water supports the body and takes weight and pressure off aching joints," he says.

Eat well. Many folks with arthritis just don't eat very well. Their diets are top-heavy with fat, prepared foods and sodium, says Dr. Morgan. "A good diet improves overall health, boosts your immune system, and provides minerals and vitamins that the body needs," she says. Because many arthritis drugs affect the way you absorb vitamins and minerals, you might get vitamin deficiencies if you don't eat a balanced diet, she explains. Eat lots of fruits, vegetables, and whole-grain cereals, suggests Dr. Morgan.

Munch a mackerel. Try to eat fish, preferably cold-water fish such as salmon and mackerel, two or three times a week, Dr. Morgan advises. Studies

History Lesson

In the early 1800s, physicians recognized rheumatoid arthritis as a separate form of the disease. They believed that it was caused by infections or ailments such as syphilis and tuberculosis. To stop the arthritis from spreading, doctors sometimes pulled the patient's teeth, cut out his tonsils, or even removed the appendix and gallbladder. Considering the crude state of nineteenth-century surgery and operating room hygiene, it was often a case of the cure being worse than the disease.

have shown that omega-3 fatty acids, found in cold-water fish, can help reduce pain and stiffness in some people with rheumatoid arthritis.

▶ALTERNATIVE APPROACHES

Try to relax. When you are feeling stressed, your muscles tense up, which can cause more pain. You can get caught in a destructive cycle where stress, pain, depression, and limited movement all work together to make you feel miserable. Learning how to relax is an important way to handle stress, advises Dr. Smith. It's more than just sitting down and being quiet. It is an active process that takes practice. There's more than one way to relax, Dr. Smith says. Try deep breathing, progressive relaxation, or guided imagery and find out what works for you. Whichever one you try, pick a quiet place where you'll have at least 15 minutes to yourself. Get comfortable. Loosen tight clothing and sit or lie down, without crossing your legs, ankles, or arms. Try to do this daily, or at least four times a week.

Breathe deeply. To begin, sit comfortably with your feet on the floor, your arms at your sides, and your eyes closed, says Dr. Smith. Breathing in, say to yourself, "I am. . . ." As you breathe out, say, ". . . relaxed." Continue breathing in and out silently saying positive things to yourself like "My hands . . . are warm" or "I feel calm . . . and relaxed." Coordinate your breathing with your words.

Be progressive. Progressive relaxation, in which you tense your muscles and then let them relax, is another helpful technique, says Dr. Smith. Close your eyes. Take a deep breath and hold it a few seconds. Breathe out, letting all your stress escape with the breath. Imagine that your muscles feel heavy and let them sink into the chair or floor. Starting with your feet and legs, tense your muscles for a few seconds and then let them relax. Work your way up your body, first tensing and then relaxing various groups of muscles. When you are done, remain sitting or lying quietly with your eyes closed for a few minutes and enjoy the feeling.

Use your imagination. Guided imagery and visualization refocus your attention off stress and pain and on to more pleasant things, such as a day at the beach. Or, better yet, a day at the beach with the entire female cast of *Baywatch*. Start by closing your eyes and taking a deep breath. Hold it a few seconds and exhale, letting go of your stress. Continue taking deep breaths and releasing your stress as you exhale, says Dr. Smith. Now think about a pleasant scene from your past or make one up. Imagine it in detail: the warm water lapping at your pain-free knees, the warm sun easing the aches in your hands and shoulders, the *Baywatch* babes taking turns handing you a tall, cool . . . well, you get the picture. Savor the image and enjoy feeling relaxed for a few minutes before you open your eyes.

You can also visualize painful body parts symbolically. Imagine your inflamed knees as bright red. Then try to change the picture. Make the red color disappear as you imagine all stress and pain fading away.

▶PREVENTIVE MEASURES

See about C. Are you getting enough orange juice? You might want to. Research suggests that vitamin C may slow the development of osteoarthritis. In a Boston University study of 640 people, results showed that those who had higher vitamin C intake had three times less progression of osteoarthritis in their knees than people with the lowest intake. It's thought that the antioxidant properties of vitamin C may help prevent tissue damage when the joints are inflamed. Research is still sketchy in this area, but the news ought to be enough of a nudge to get you to eat and drink enough vitamin C. In the study, men who got more than 119 milligrams a day (twice the Daily Value)—the amount in two oranges—had less disease progression.

Proceed with caution. Since arthritis already makes joints weak, don't give it any help by doing things that will compound the problem. When you exercise, don't do deep knee bends or take a pounding run. Keep the stooping and crouching—and anything that puts undue pressure on your joints—to a minimum, says Dr. Smith.

Don't overload. Don't overload your joints with too much weight. The primary way to prevent osteoarthritis in your weight-bearing joints, such as your knees, is to lose weight, says Dr. Smith. Use your largest joints and strongest muscles for lifting and carrying. Haul your gear in a backpack instead of a briefcase to protect the joints in your arms and hands.

Shape up. You need strong, flexible muscles and tendons to support your joints. A good, balanced workout that combines aerobic and strength training with stretching exercises can help give your joints the support they need and may help prevent osteoarthritis, says Dr. Smith.

Asking for Directions

▶ PROBLEM

You would rather drive miles and miles out of your way than admit you have no clue where you are.

▶ CAUSE

The male ego is the cause. "When you go into a gas station saying that you are lost, psychologically, it's like having your tail between your legs," says Robert Butterworth, Ph.D., a clinical psychologist in private practice in Los Angeles. "Men will do anything to avoid having to ask for help."

Some men argue that they love to get lost. Finding their way out of a maze of roads gives them a sense of accomplishment, they say. Dr. Butterworth—who, by the way, hates to ask for directions—doesn't buy it. "When you are lost, you get angrier and angrier that you can't find your way," he says. "The more you search, the more you have to face the sad truth that you are lost, stupid, and should have listened to your wife when she told you to pull over hours ago."

▶ HOW SERIOUS

In most cases, such drivers only risk embarrassment. In some situations, however, not asking for directions can harm your health, says Mike Morrissey, public relations manager at the American Automobile Association (AAA) in Orlando, Florida. Lost drivers cause car accidents when they stare at maps while driving, back up on in-

DO THIS NOW

Get off the road. Yes, pull over. Right away. Think back to when you last knew where you were, suggests Terradan Landchild, Youth/Scouting Coordinator of the Columbia River Orienteering Club in Vancouver, Washington. (In orienteering, people race through unfamiliar terrain with a detailed map.) Now, pinpoint the spot on your map where you last knew where you were. Then, mentally retrace your steps to where you are now. You have two choices: Either retrace your route back to where you initially got lost or use your map to find another road that will take you where you need to go.

History Lesson

One July weekend in 1997, an elderly New Jersey couple got seriously lost. The husband, of course, was behind the wheel. He drove aimlessly for more than 24 hours, traveling an estimated 800 miles through New York, New Jersey, and Pennsylvania. During the all-night adventure, he stopped twice for gas. But he refused to eat or ask for directions or help.

The couple, both in their mid-eighties, left their home on a Friday. When they failed to show up for a doctor's appointment at noon the next day, family members started to worry. A fender bender at 2:00 in the afternoon finally brought the long, meandering trip to an end—when a police officer at the scene called their family to come pick them up and take them home. There were no injuries, unless you count the bruised male ego.

terstate highways to get to passed exit ramps, or cut across six lanes of traffic to read road signs.

▶SOLUTIONS

Say, "I'm not stupid." Say it again. And again. Just because you're lost doesn't mean that you have no sense of direction or that you're a poor driver. And it doesn't mean that you're stupid, Dr. Butterworth says. As smart as he was, Albert Einstein frequently got lost. Now, start looking for someone to ask for help.

Find full service. You don't want to ask more than once. So pull into a place where you'll find an intelligent human being who knows the area. Gas stations rank as the most convenient places to find such people, though today's versions aren't as good as yesteryear's. "Today you're more likely to find a few pumps with a teenage clerk," Morrissey says. "Those gas stations are still good. But they are not as good as the ones where you get to talk to an adult who lives and works in the area."

If you stop at a station that provides gainful employment for local high school kids, make sure that at least two of them hear your request. Directions from two teens are better than directions from one—unless, of course, the two happen to resemble Beavis and Butt-head.

Other good bets include fire and police stations, though finding either one on an interstate highway could pose as much of a problem as finding where you are going. Rest stops also count as another good choice. Besides lots of people, you'll usually find a little building with maps posted (and a big "you are here") to help you find your way.

Wherever you stop, make sure that the area is well-lit and populated, for your safety.

Know when you've gone too far. When someone gives you directions, make sure he tells you something like: "If you see a building with the American flag painted on the side, you've gone too far." If he doesn't, ask. "That keeps you from getting even more lost," Morrissey says.

Make a note of it. You said, "Yes," "Uh-huh," "Got it," as the pimply faced teen told you: "Turn right out of the parking lot, go down the road to the stop sign, make a left, go over the bridge and fork right, and then go around the circle and look for I-87." Now you're at the bridge and you can't remember if you're supposed to fork right or left. Next time, write down your directions, Morrissey says.

▶ALTERNATIVE APPROACHES

Assign points. So, you think you can find your way without any help. The problem is that your wife doesn't believe you. To keep her from pestering you to pull over, play this game. Every time you are actually lost beyond comprehension and must pull over to ask for directions hours after she suggested, give her a point. Every time she thinks you're lost but you manage to get the car back on course within a reasonable amount of time (let's say before the car runs out of gas), give yourself a point. Now, if you have more points than she does, kindly remind her of your track record. On the other hand, if she's ahead, pull over. This way, you never have to admit that you're lost, Dr. Butterworth says. You're only playing fair.

Follow the sun. A simple method to keep track of travel without a compass is to use the sun. For example, if it is near midday, the sun will be near due south and if you intend to drive to the east, you keep the sun on your right. If you must leave the interstate intending to find a secondary road on which to travel west and it is late afternoon, you should end up driving toward the sun, advises Terradan Landchild, Youth/Scouting Coordinator of the Columbia River Orienteering Club in Vancouver, Washington.

▶PREVENTIVE MEASURES

Be a man with a plan. Figure out your route well before ever thinking about climbing behind the steering wheel. Either whip out your road atlas and write down the various road names or get an individualized map from the AAA that tells you the best roads to take, Morrissey says. These maps are called Triptiks and are available for free to AAA members. To get one, contact your local AAA office at least two weeks prior to your trip.

Put your thumb on it. To make sure that you never get lost, use a trick from orienteering. Have the person in the front passenger seat hold your map as you drive. When you pull out of the driveway, have them put their thumb just below the "you are here" spot so that you can follow along from your present location. Now, as you drive, have your passenger move his or her thumb along your route on the map. If you're driving alone, follow the above advice from Morrissey: Write down the road names you'll need to watch for and glance at them from time to time to keep yourself on track.

Asthma

▶PROBLEM

About five million American men have asthma, a chronic condition that affects the tubes that carry air in and out of the lungs (the bronchi) and their smaller branches (the bronchioles). During an asthma attack, you become short of breath or you can't breathe at all. Your chest feels tight. You wheeze. You might even cough and hack up mucus.

▶CAUSE

Any number of things can spark an asthma attack, but allergies top the list. Half of all people over age 30 who have asthma also have allergies. Asthma attacks are caused by the usual suspects, including molds, pollen, dust mites, pet hair, and some drugs, especially aspirin. Nonallergic triggers include cigarette smoke (yours or other people's); smoke from fireplaces or wood stoves; exercise; certain foods, including eggs and shellfish; emotional stress; and infections such as colds and flu. Whatever the trigger, the process is the same: The inflamed tissues inside the lungs narrow your airways, which become plugged with excess mucus. As these airways swell, the muscles around the airways constrict, which further blocks breathing.

▶HOW SERIOUS

Some people with asthma have mild, infrequent attacks. You might wheeze only when

DO THIS NOW

The next time your chest feels tight, try this imagery exercise recommended by Gerald Epstein, M.D., director of the American Institute for Mental Imagery in New York City and an expert on the use of imagery to treat asthma: Close your eyes. Breathe out slowly three times. Sense a weight on and in your chest. See what it looks like and feel the constriction it causes. Breathe out one time slowly and see yourself removing this weight. Then, see and sense your lungs expanding and filling with white light as you find your breathing becoming easy and flowing, as your chest and rib cage relax. Repeat this breath twice more and then open your eyes.

you hang out in a smoky bar, get a cold, or cut the grass. But for others, who have severe, frequent attacks, asthma can be life-threatening. "In the most severe cases, you can have symptoms virtually every minute of every day and can have life-threatening asthma attacks that land you in the hospital," says Daniel Hamilos, M.D., director of the Asthma Center at Washington University School of Medicine in St. Louis.

Any person who experiences asthma symptoms more than twice a week should be treated with specific medications designed to control the inflammation in his lungs, Dr. Hamilos says. Asthma symptoms typically include shortness of breath, wheezing, chest tightness, chest congestion, and coughing. In addition, asthma symptoms get worse at night, he explains. While most physicians can handle mild asthma, Dr. Hamilos says that an asthma specialist may help greatly to find what's causing it and will be able to recommend the best forms of treatment. Without proper treatment, asthma may get worse over time, he warns.

▶SOLUTIONS

Spray before you play. If you have asthma while exercising, try using a bronchodilator inhaler five minutes before you begin to exercise, advises Dr. Hamilos. "It should protect you for anywhere from four to six hours," he says.

Warm up before you work out. Warm up continuously for 15 minutes before you work out; it may reduce the chemicals that cause the tiny airways in the lungs to constrict, preventing exercise-induced asthma. In a study conducted at the University of British Columbia in Vancouver, six minutes of running induced an asthma attack in 12 people with asthma who didn't warm up. But when they exercised moderately for 15 minutes beforehand, half of them breathed freely afterward.

Watch what you eat. While foods are not considered a common trigger for asthma, certain foods may act as triggers in some people, Dr. Hamilos says. Some people with more serious cases of asthma react to metabisulfites, preservatives added to prepared foods, including instant mashed potatoes, trail mix, pizza dough, and dry-mix salad dressings. Metabisulfites also occur naturally in fish, shellfish, beer, and wine. If you have experienced asthma symptoms with any of these products, you may want to read labels on foods and try to avoid sulfites in any form, Dr. Hamilos says.

Peruse your painkillers. About 5 percent of people with asthma are allergic to aspirin or nonsteroidal anti-inflammatory drugs such as ibuprofen, and many don't know it. "Every month or two, I see someone who has been sensitive to aspirin for months or years without realizing it," says Henry Milgrom, M.D., director of the ambulatory pediatric allergy program at the National Jewish Medical and Research Center in Denver. The allergy can begin after years of taking these drugs. So if you start wheezing after taking a painkiller, tell your doctor, who will probably recommend acetaminophen, Dr. Milgrom says.

Reach your peak. A peak flow meter, the gadget used to measure your ability to push air out of your lungs, is an important part of an asthma-management plan. So use it. "Measuring your peak flow rate can alert you to a potential attack even before you have symptoms," says Dr. Milgrom. He advises that you use the device twice a day—once in the morning, again at midday. These meters are available at most drugstores and medical supply stores, but you should check with your doctor about the type and size that is best for you.

MEN'S HEALTH INDEX

All kinds of weird stuff have been known to trigger asthma attacks. Here are some of the odder ones.

Thunderstorms
Cockroach excrement
Athlete's foot (caused by the *Trichophyton* fungus)
Those smelly perfume-sample strips bound into magazines
Garlic

Grab an emergency cup of coffee. If you're far from home without your inhaler and you feel an attack coming on, have a cup or two of coffee, Dr. Milgrom says. Caffeine and theophylline, which for years was the major drug used to treat asthma, are chemically related. "Theophylline is a fairly good bronchodilator," Dr. Milgrom says. But this is a remedy of last resort, to be used only in an emergency since inhalers are much more effective, he says.

▶ALTERNATIVE APPROACHES

Breathe easier with herbs. Go to a health food store and ask for *tylophora* and *coleus forskohlii*, suggests Richard Firshein, D.O., a physician in private practice in New York City. Both of these herbs, which are available as supplements, have been found in studies to reduce inflammation in the lungs caused by asthma, says Dr. Firshein, who has asthma himself. "I recommend taking 50 milligrams of *tylophora* and 50 milligrams of *coleus forskohlii* two or three times every day," he says. Take the herbs in addition to your regular medication, he says.

Get your kneads met. A 15-minute upper-body massage once a week may help relieve asthma symptoms by helping you identify stress in your life. Just becoming aware of your stress with massage and learning how to relax can reduce the number and severity of asthma attacks, says Mary Malinski, R.N., an asthma researcher and massage therapist at Allergy, Asthma, and Dermatology Associates in Portland, Oregon. In a small study of people with chronic asthma, Malinski found that massage helped reduce these folks' wheezing, chest tightness, and breathing discomfort.

Put the pressure on. Acupressure can help relieve and even prevent asthma attacks, according to Michael Reed Gach, Ph.D., director of the Acupressure Institute in Berkeley, California, and author of *Acupressure's Potent Points*. Put both thumbs on the upper outer portion of your chest (just under your collarbone), pressing on the muscles below your collarbone. You'll find a sensitive, knotted spot on each side of your chest. Let your head hang forward, then breathe slowly and deeply as you press these points with your thumbs for two minutes.

Do this three or four times a day for both prevention and relief of asthma symptoms, Dr. Gach recommends. This exercise is best for people who tend to get asthma or who have had asthma in the past, he says.

▶PREVENTIVE MEASURES

Accept your triggers. Most guys with asthma know what sets them wheezing, but a surprising amount deny their triggers, Dr. Milgrom says. "Many people, for example, deny that their pets trigger attacks," he says. "And you'd be surprised how many people with asthma smoke." So don't just know your triggers, says Dr. Milgrom. Accept them and avoid them.

Track new triggers. Ask your partner to tell you if she switches to a new perfume or scrubs the bathroom with a new cleanser. And be careful if you switch colognes or cleansers; the chemicals they contain could exacerbate your asthma, Dr. Milgrom says.

Muffle an attack. Breathing in cold, dry air can trigger an asthma attack. So before venturing outside in cold weather, wrap a scarf around your mouth so that you breathe in warm, moist air, suggests Dr. Hamilos.

Athlete's Foot

▶PROBLEM

Imagine that your foot is a tree in a dark, wet rain forest, also known as your shoes. Your toes are the roots of that tree. What usually grows near the roots of wet trees? Mushrooms, also known as fungi. And that's what's happening to you. Fungus is growing on your foot (mostly between your toes), and your foot is reacting to these growths with itching, redness, and, possibly, cracked skin and an odor. But there's not a tasty portobello in sight.

▶CAUSE

Athlete's foot is a contagious fungus that thrives in locker rooms and on shower floors (because it's one of the few places we share with others that is wet and filled with germs that touch our feet). However, "the fungus is everywhere," says John Scanlon, D.P.M., chief of podiatric services at Chestnut Hill Hospital in Philadelphia.

Despite its name and love of locker rooms, you can, in fact, get athlete's foot even if the most exercise you ever do is click your remote control. All it takes is exposure to the fungus and having wet feet. If you have it once, you're also predisposed to developing it again.

▶HOW SERIOUS

Even the mightiest athlete can be brought low by athlete's foot. It won't kill you, but it will annoy the heck out of you. More than that, however, is its potential to become something serious.

DO THIS NOW

Saturate a cotton ball with tea tree oil, tape it onto the infected area of your foot with surgical or first-aid tape, and then put a sock on it overnight, advises Christopher Trahan, a doctor of Oriental medicine and licensed acupuncturist in private practice in New York City. "Tea tree is a natural antifungal and antimicrobial essential oil," Dr. Trahan says. "You can find it in health food stores and most drugstores." If you have sensitive skin, you should check with your doctor before using tea tree oil.

Did You Know?

The antifungal clotrimazole, which is the active agent that makes Lotrimin AF effective in fighting athlete's foot, also is the key ingredient in Gyne-Lotrimin. That's right, it does double duty battling vaginal yeast infections.

While yeast is a form of fungus, the two infections are not exactly the same chemically. Needless to say, the products are *not* interchangeable.

"Athlete's foot can lead to a bacterial infection," says Dr. Scanlon. "If an over-the-counter antifungal cream or other remedy doesn't work within five to seven days, you should see a doctor." You should also see a doctor if the skin on your feet is so cracked that it's painful or is beginning to look more like cuts and not cracks.

If the fungus moves to the skin underneath your toenails, then you'll have a very difficult time getting rid of the fungus (which is now a nail fungus) without a prescription for an oral medication, says Richard Braver, D.P.M., a sports podiatrist and head of the Active Foot and Ankle Care Centers in Englewood and Fair Lawn, New Jersey. Nail fungus occurs most often in athletes and people over the age of 65.

▶SOLUTIONS

Think "wet" or "dry." "Sometimes athlete's foot is dry and itchy, and sometimes it's moist and itchy," says Marjorie Menacker, D.P.M., a podiatrist with Chesterfield Podiatry Associates in Midlothian, Virginia. "If it's dry, you want to wet it; and if it's wet, you want to dry it."

So if your feet are dry, use an antifungal cream or ointment, which will add moisture. But if they're wet, use an antifungal powder, which won't add moisture, Dr. Menacker says.

Look for clotrimazole. Want a fast-acting over-the-counter remedy? "I like clotrimazole, which is available over-the-counter in Lotrimin AF and some other athlete's foot medications," says Dr. Scanlon.

Apply Lotrimin AF to the infected area three times a day. If you can, let it air dry for 15 minutes before putting on your socks and shoes, Dr. Scanlon says. And don't stop using a cream or powder until two to three weeks after you notice the infection is gone. The fungus could still be inside your foot.

Soak to dry. If you suffer from the moist variety of athlete's foot, soaking your feet in Domeboro solution (available in drugstores) and water will help pull the moisture out. Domeboro is an astringent, which means that it dries up the skin, Dr. Scanlon says.

"Soak your feet for about 15 minutes a day, following the directions on the package of Domeboro," Dr. Scanlon says. "You can do this every day until the infection seems to be gone."

▶ALTERNATIVE APPROACHES

Cut out the candy. Sugar feeds any sort of yeasty fungus, and that's what athlete's foot is. So if you cut out the sugar, you'll cut out one bit of sustenance to the gunk growing between your toes.

"The remedies you put on the outside of your body will only help long-term if you're also feeding the inside of your body properly," says Nancy Dunne-Boggs, a doctor of naturopathy at Bitterroot Natural Medicine in Missoula, Montana. "You need to cut at least simple sugars out of your diet."

That means no candy, sugar, soda, maple syrup, ice cream, or other sweets, says Dr. Dunne-Boggs. "Do this until you can't see the fungus anymore and then for three weeks after that," she says. If you begin to eat sugar again and the fungus comes back, cut out the sweets again, then experiment with how much sugar you can eat without sending your feet back into fungus land.

Go for garlic. Raw garlic has natural antifungal properties. Put several crushed garlic cloves in a basin with warm water and a little rubbing alcohol. "This is my first-choice treatment," writes James A. Duke, Ph.D., the world's foremost authority on healing herbs, in his book, *The Green Pharmacy*. "A garlic footbath might be malodorous, but it usually relieves itching and burning between the toes."

▶PREVENTIVE MEASURES

Wear shower shoes. "Public showers are the number one source of athlete's foot infection," says Dr. Scanlon. "Fungus gets into the cracks of the shower floor and then thrives. If you have dry skin or cracks in the skin of your foot, then it won't be able to protect you against the bacteria."

If your skin can't protect you, you'll need to find something else that will. And the thing that will help you most are shower shoes made of plastic. Be sure to keep them clean and dry, just like your feet.

Sock it to synthetics. Socks made of Coolmax or Thermax and other materials that wick moisture away from your skin will help keep your feet dry and bacteria-free, says Dr. Menacker. This will help cut off the moisture on which fungus thrives. Look for sport socks or sock liners made of these materials at sporting goods stores and camping outfitters.

Wash and dry. Make sure that you wash your feet, using a washcloth and soap, says Dr. Scanlon. It's the scrubbing action, more than the soap you use, that helps. Then, make sure that you dry your whole foot, especially the spaces between the toes, he adds. "Drying your feet thoroughly is the most important thing you can do," Dr. Scanlon says. Pat dry your feet last so that you do not spread the fungus to other parts of your body. You also want to be sure not to reuse the washcloth or towel until they have been laundered, he adds.

Back Pain

▶PROBLEM

Whether you're a warehouse worker hefting boxes onto a truck or a telemarketer rooted to a chair, headset, and computer, you'll probably have a case of serious back pain sometime in your life. About 80 percent of people do.

▶CAUSE

The back isn't a single anatomic entity like an arm or foot but a rather complex column of bones, disks, and muscles designed to hold your torso erect. Consequently, the causes of back pain are numerous: pinched nerves, weak abdominal muscles, loss of flexibility, tight leg muscles, a big gut, trauma, sitting too long, poor overall fitness, and herniated disks.

▶HOW SERIOUS

Your first bout of back pain will likely clear up within a month or so, no matter what you do, says Philip Greenman, D.O., professor of osteopathic manipulation and physical medicine at the College of Osteopathic Medicine at Michigan State University in East Lansing. But if you've had back pain once, you have a 50 percent chance of having it again.

"Back pain is notoriously recurrent, and the second and third incidences tend to be more severe than the first," says Dr. Greenman. "It's hard to treat, and that's why you really want to focus on prevention." See your doctor immediately if you have severe, debilitating pain, numbness, or pain radiating down a leg; loss of function in your leg, such as not being able to raise up on your toes; or loss of bladder and bowel control, says Dr. Greenman.

DO THIS NOW

Need a break from the pain and discomfort? Simply lie on the floor on your back, bend your knees to a 90-degree angle, and put your legs up on a chair, suggests Philip Greenman, D.O., professor of osteopathic manipulation and physical medicine at the College of Osteopathic Medicine at Michigan State University in East Lansing. "This position takes all pressure off your back, disks, and nerves." he says. "It usually gives you the relief you're looking for." Do this for 20 minutes every couple of hours.

▶**SOLUTIONS**

Loosen the legs. You might think that the problem is in your back, where the pain is, but it could be in your legs. After sitting or bending all day, your leg muscles may be extremely tight or unbalanced (meaning that some muscles may be loose and relaxed but others are contracted or in spasm). Tight leg muscles pull oddly on the torso and put pressure on the back and abdominal muscles, says Jerome F. McAndrews, D.C., spokesman for the American Chiropractic Association. To rebalance your calf muscles, stand flat-footed on a stair step in flat, comfortable shoes with the balls of your feet on the very edge and your heels in the air, advises Dr. McAndrews. Holding on to a railing for support, slowly lower your heels until you feel a tightness up the back of the legs. Hold for a few seconds, repeat 5 to 10 times, and do as needed during the day, says Dr. McAndrews.

Extend those hamstrings. The same is true of those muscles running down the back of your thighs. Sitting for long periods—the bane of office workers—shortens the hamstring muscles in the back of your legs, which then yank on the pelvis and make other muscles compensate. Work your hamstrings by standing up and placing one heel on a steady chair or end table. (Hold on to a nearby table or chair for balance). Keep this leg straight and lean forward until you feel a pulling sensation in the back of your thigh. Hold for about 30 seconds, and then switch to the other leg, suggests Dr. McAndrews. Do this a few times a day, especially after you've been sitting for a long time. Don't try to "lock" the extended leg when first attempting this stretch. As the muscles stretch out, "locking" the leg will come naturally, advises Dr. McAndrews.

Take a hot bath. A heating pad, hot compress, or a warm bath or shower relaxes muscles and brings fresh, healing blood to the injury, says Dr. Greenman. Take a 10-minute warm shower, or apply heat with a heating pad or hot compress for 15 to 30 minutes or until the area has a pink blush, and then remove. Don't do it any longer than that or you'll make matters worse, Dr. Greenman warns. "People will lie on a heating pad for hours and then won't be able to move. That's because the area is just congested with blood," he says. "You should apply heat just a few times a day for short periods."

Get up, lazybones. The old prescription for backache was several days of bed rest, recalls Dr. Greenman. But since most back pain is from muscle strain, tightness, and spasms, being immobile just makes you weaker and more prone to further injury. And bed rest helps convince you that you really are sick and unable to help yourself, says Dr. Greenman. "The sooner you get moving, the sooner you'll feel better," he says. So get up and do some walking and a little stretching. Don't overdo it, though.

▶**ALTERNATIVE APPROACHES**

Pump in the blood flow. Getting fresh blood to an injury brings in nutrients needed for healing and also carries away waste products manufactured by injured cells, says Alison Lee, M.D., a pain-management specialist and acupuncturist with Barefoot Doctors, an acupuncture and natural-medicine resource center in Ann Arbor, Michigan. The herb ginkgo biloba has been shown to dilate blood vessels and may theoretically increase blood flow to your aching back, says Dr. Lee. You can buy the herb in capsule form in health food stores and over the counter in many drugstores. Dr. Lee recommends a product with standardized extract. Follow the package directions for dosage information.

Try a combination. In some cases, a combination approach may be useful. Where ginkgo biloba increases blood flow, curcumin can add an anti-inflammatory effect, suggests Dr. Lee. Curcumin, a highly concentrated form of turmeric sold in health food stores, is a potent anti-inflammatory medicine that is very effective for a soft-tissue injury, like a sore back, says Dr. Lee. Look for a product (capsule form) with standardized extract of 95 percent, and follow the recommended dosage on bottle.

MEN'S HEALTH INDEX

You are not alone in your back pain. The following are basic back facts from the Vermont Back Research Center at the University of Vermont in Burlington.

- **Ten percent of U.S. adults currently have back pain.**
- **Back pain is the number two reason that people visit a medical clinic. (Fatigue is number one.)**
- **Only half of back-injured workers, who have been out for six months or more, ever return to work.**
- **About 2.5 million Americans are permanently disabled by back disorders.**

▶PREVENTIVE MEASURES

Walk it off. There's nothing better for your back than walking, says Dr. McAndrews. Walking gets you moving while you're recovering from back pain. It forces you to assume an anatomically correct back posture, that is, standing straight with a slight curve in the lumbar region of your spine. Walking also builds strength in the large muscle groups that hold the back in the proper position. And it warms up muscles and loosens joints so that you have more range of motion and less stiffness, says Dr. McAndrews.

For your walks, choose level ground rather than hills. Swing your arms with your head up. Walk briskly if you can, but don't overdo it, warns Dr. McAndrews. In time, hills will be fine; but you need to get the circulation into the muscles to normalize them before "pumping" them up on hills, adds Dr. McAndrews.

Lift carefully. To avoid injuring your back or pulling a muscle, be smart about lifting heavy objects: Get close to the object, plant your feet shoulder-width apart, tighten your abdominal muscles, and lift—with your legs. As you stand, make every effort to keep your back and neck straight. If you can't, it's too heavy. Put it down and get a pal or a forklift to help you, advises Dr. McAndrews.

Stretch it out. To help keep your back limber and lessen the chance of future back pain, Dr. McAndrews recommends the following back stretches. While standing, lean forward, hands on your thighs, and arch your back until you feel a gentle pull on the muscles down your back. Hold this for two minutes and then stand straight. Next, reach straight up with your right arm and lean to the left until you feel the muscles stretch along your right hip and waist. Then do the other side. You can do these several times each day depending on how tight the muscles are upon your first attempt. As the muscle tightness decreases, you can reduce the number of times you do these stretches to three or four per day.

Bad Breath

▶PROBLEM

Your mouth emits the bouquet of a rotting carcass on the Serengeti. Great for attracting vultures; otherwise, a major turnoff.

▶CAUSE

Stand in front of a mirror and stick your tongue out. See how its surface gets progressively rougher the farther back it goes? That's where bad breath usually begins. Specifically, in the vast majority of cases—up to 85 percent—the source of bad breath is bacteria in the mouth and the sulfurous gases they produce. "Where the folds of your tongue are deepest, that's where the bacteria collect the most," says Robert Rioseco, D.M.D., a dentist in White Plains, New York. Other causes of bad breath, chronically known as halitosis, include gum disease, sinus problems, and poorly cleaned braces or dentures.

▶HOW SERIOUS

People like to joke about bad breath, but in real life, it's no laughing matter. Having halitosis, or worrying that you have it, can interfere with your love life, your social life, and your career. If you have bad breath that's unshakable, mention it to your doctor, says Dr. Rioseco. Halitosis can be a side effect of serious disease, including cancer, cirrhosis, and diabetes.

▶SOLUTIONS

Get in a scrape. Go after bad breath bacteria where they live by cleaning your tongue twice a day, suggests Jon L. Richter, D.M.D., Ph.D., director of the Richter Center, which specializes in the treatment of breath problems, in Philadelphia. Drugstores sell plastic tongue-scrapers, which are specially de-

Did You Know?

Scientists who study bad breath, chronically known as halitosis, consistently report that people have wildly mistaken ideas about how pleasant or unpleasant their own breath is. One study found that women tend to worry about bad breath when they shouldn't, while men are more likely to think they smell sweet as a rose when they don't. Researchers are also familiar with a condition called halitophobia, a morbid fear of having bad breath. "In extreme cases," as reported in the *Journal of the American Dental Association,* "people with halitophobia are driven to social isolation, may have their teeth extracted, and occasionally even commit suicide.

signed for the job. You can also try a plastic or metal spoon, inverted so that the bowl side is up.

Place your scraper of choice on the back border of the tongue and drag it forward four or five times. To be thorough, give the sides of the tongue a couple of scrapes, too, using the same back to front motion. "Rinse with water afterward and you'll have a dramatic reduction in breath odor that will last a couple hours or more, depending on the person," Dr. Richter says.

Keep it clean. Visit your dentist regularly for a teeth cleaning and examination, the American Dental Association recommends. Many dentists suggest that you see them at least every six months. If needed, your dentist can also prescribe sterner measures to fight bad breath, such as a prescription mouthwash that can curb the guilty bacteria for as long as 24 hours, when combined with tongue scraping.

Eat something. The bacteria that cause bad breath flourish in dry mouths, which is why your breath is rankest in the morning. That's also why there's some truth to the stereotype about old people having bad breath: Our salivary glands naturally lose some of their effectiveness as we age. Chewing stimulates the flow of saliva and helps wash dragon breath away. "Eating will cause a physical removal of the stagnant material on the back of the tongue, and the increase in saliva will wash away the gases already in your mouth.," Dr. Richter says. Chewing gum is another way to get the salivary glands flowing.

Beware mints and mouthwashes. Americans spend more than $500 million a year on mouthwashes and other breath potions, and most of it is wasted money. "Study after study shows that most of these products only mask the odor for 20 minutes to a half-hour at most," Dr. Rioseco says. He adds that mouthwashes containing alcohol can actually damage the delicate lining of the mouth.

Check your medicine cabinet. Some prescription drugs can cause bad breath, Dr. Rioseco says, among them are antidepressants, stimulants, and high blood pressure medications. A review of your pill regimen and a phone call to your doctor may be in order.

▶ALTERNATIVE APPROACHES

Grease the works. Use toothpastes containing tea tree oil, recommends Andrew Weil, M.D., director of the Program in Integrative Medicine at the University of Arizona College of Medicine in Tucson and author of several books, including *Eight Weeks to Optimum Health*. "It's a powerful disinfectant that smells a bit like eucalyptus," he says. Look for it in health food stores or herb stores.

Flush the problem. Keeping your nasal passages clean can help get rid of bad breath, says Brenda Gordee, a dental hygienist and certified naturopathic doctor in Madison, Wisconsin. She recommends starting your day by swallowing a sinus-clearing mixture of fresh-squeezed lemon (a half-teaspoon), honey (two teaspoons), a slice of fresh ginger, and hot water (six ounces). The kicker? An eighth- to a quarter-teaspoon of ground red pepper. "If your head is full of mucus," she says, "this will instantly dissolve it." It'll also wake you up faster than a cup of espresso, we'd wager.

▶PREVENTIVE MEASURES

Don't ask for trouble. Certain substances generate bad breath on their own, without the help of bacteria. High on the list are cigarettes, alcohol, onions, garlic, and pastrami. Avoid them when you're expecting intimate contact with other humans.

Find a confidante. The only sure way to know if you have bad breath is to ask someone you trust to tell you. "It's not an easy task, but it's necessary," Dr. Richter says. "You simply can't identify your own bad breath."

Baldness

▶PROBLEM

Man's battle with baldness began way before rugs, plugs, Rogaine, and Sy Sperling. Through the ages, we've rubbed our scalps with a variety of gross stuff—including chicken droppings—in a desperate attempt to keep our hairlines from heading south. But there's still no magic pill or potion. Two out of three American men develop some form of balding, and half of us are markedly bald by the time we're 50.

▶CAUSE

Androgenetic alopecia, the medical term for male-pattern baldness, is the condition responsible for 95 percent of hair loss in men. It can begin as early as puberty, starting with a loss of hair from the top of the head or a receding hairline. Eventually, all that may be left is a monklike fringe around the sides and back of the head. Male-pattern baldness is thought to be caused by a combination of two factors: heredity plus a sensitivity to something called dihydrotestosterone (DHT), which is derived from androgen, a male hormone. It's thought that DHT shuts down the hair follicles on the scalp in men who are genetically destined to go bald, says Richard S. Greene, M.D., a dermatologist in private practice in Hallindale, Florida, who has performed more than 9,000 hair transplants. Less-common causes of hair loss include a high fever, some medications, chronic illness, and major surgery.

▶HOW SERIOUS

It depends on your attitude. Some guys have an easy-come-easy-go attitude about hair, while others equate a balding pate with the passing of their youth

> ### DO THIS NOW
>
> Go get a haircut. "Men who are losing their hair tend to wear their hair the way they did when they were younger—to cling to a style that's just not working anymore," says Vaughn Acord, a senior hairstylist at Bumble and Bumble Hair Salon in New York City. "You have to face the problem and work with what you have." His recommendation is to go short, especially if you have a receding hairline.

History Lesson

October 24, 1973: Striking a blow for the hair impaired the world over, Telly Savalas debuts as Lieutenant Theo Kojak, the gritty prince of the New York City's Manhattan South precinct, in *Kojak*. Who loves ya, baby?

and vigor. The seriousness of losing your hair also depends on how far you're willing to go to get it back since some treatments involve considerable expense and risk.

▶SOLUTIONS

Switch shampoos. If your hair is thinning, try using a "body-building" or "hair-repairing" shampoo, suggests Dr. Greene. "These products often contain protein, which coats the hair and makes it appear thicker," explains Dr. Greene.

Try minoxidil. Studies have shown that 2 percent minoxidil grew moderate amounts of hair for 25 percent of the men who used it. The newer "extra-strength" kind, which contains 5 percent minoxidil (marketed as Rogaine Extra Strength for Men), can grow 45 percent more hair for men than the 2 percent minoxidil version, according to studies conducted by the company that makes Rogaine. You can get either formulation in most drugstores. You should know that Rogaine doesn't work for everyone, that hair growth will be light to moderate rather than luxuriant, and that it takes at least four months of twice-a-day use to see results. One more thing: You have to keep using it, says Dr. Greene, because if you don't, any hair you've managed to grow will fall out.

Consider a hairpiece. A well-made hairpiece or hair weave "is the best and safest hair-replacement system there is right now," in the view of Vaughn Acord, a senior hairstylist at Bumble and Bumble Hair Salon in New York City. A hairpiece consists of human or synthetic hair implanted into a fine nylon mesh and is attached to the scalp with glue, tape, or metal clips. By contrast, a hair weave involves sewing a wig into existing hair. While a good hairpiece can cost thousands of dollars, they don't carry the risks of surgery, and they're virtually undetectable. "You'd be surprised at who's wearing hairpieces," says Acord.

▶ALTERNATIVE APPROACHES

Take some sage advice. Sage has had a long-standing reputation as a hair preserver. In the old days, people often used sage extracts in hair rinses and shampoos. The herb allegedly had the ability to prevent hair loss and maintain color. Since this use of sage is unlikely to cause any harm, add a few teaspoons of sage tincture to your shampoo, suggests James A. Duke, Ph.D., the world's foremost authority on healing herbs and author of *The Green Pharmacy*.

Oil up. If you're up for it, you can make a hair oil that stimulates hair growth from the Ayurvedic herbs amla and ashwaganda, according to Partap Chauhan, an Ayurvedic physician in Haryana, India. Here's how. Crush 1 ounce each amla and ashwaganda herb (available through mail order) into a rough powder (not a fine powder). Combine the powder with seven cups of water and soak overnight. The next day, boil the mixture until it's reduced by 75 percent. Strain it and add a small amount of sesame oil—approximately one-quarter the amount of the herb-water mixture. Boil again, until everything evaporates and only the oil remains. Cool, strain, and bottle. Some fragrance oils can be added at this time. Massage the oil into your hair and scalp twice a week.

▶PREVENTIVE MEASURES

Go with it. Okay, so if you're genetically predestined to lose your hair, there's not a lot you can do to prevent it. But you can prevent baldness from making you look or feel bad. Don't shy away from baldness. Embrace it. Work with it. Perhaps grow facial hair; it'll offset the dome effect. And if you've lost everything on top, consider shaving off the rest, suggests Acord. "I know a guy who shaved 15 years off his age when he shaved his head," he says. "He looks like a whole different guy."

Being Henpecked

▶PROBLEM

In the Philippines, a henpecked man is said to be "under the skirt." Over here, we call him whipped. But whatever you call him, a guy who lives with a domineering woman has a tough gig. But before we go any further, let's get our terms straight: Being henpecked isn't the same as being nagged. "Nagging is a subset of henpecking," says William F. Fitzgerald, Ph.D., a psychotherapist who specializes in marital and sexual psychotherapy at the Silicon Valley Relationship and Sexuality Center in Santa Clara, California. "A man can be nagged without being dominated. But a henpecked man is both nagged and dominated." (Since we know you want ways to stop the nagging, we've included advice about that, too.) The classic sign of henpecked behavior is being unable (or unwilling) to make even the smallest decision without checking with the wife first.

▶CAUSE

It may be tough to swallow, but a man who tolerates henpecking in silence is as much to blame for his predicament as his wife, says Dr. Fitzgerald. "Somebody has to break the cycle of nagging: silence, resentment, inaction or begrudged action, nagging." Your job is find out the reason for her shrewish behavior so that you can work to change it—together.

DO THIS NOW

Deny her the payoff. "When a man gives in to his wife's nagging, he's telling her that nagging works," says William F. Fitzgerald, Ph.D., a psychotherapist who specializes in marital and sexual psychotherapy at the Silicon Valley Relationship and Sexuality Center in Santa Clara, California.

So the next time your partner carps, tell her loud and proud that you're not going to take it anymore. But make sure that you tell her what you propose as an alternative. Dr. Fitzgerald suggests something along the lines of: "I won't reward your nagging by doing what you want. When you're ready to make a respectful, reasonable request, then we can talk."

History Lesson

November 4, 1842: Abraham Lincoln marries Mary Todd in Springfield, Illinois. The ceremony kicks off 23 years of domestic terror.

Lincoln was more than henpecked by his wife. He was battered, according to Michael Burlingame, author of *The Inner World of Abraham Lincoln*. One day, for example, Abe didn't put wood on the fire as soon as Mary would have liked. She hit him with a piece of firewood. The next day, the Great Emancipator showed up for work with a bandaged nose. Mary "was seen frequently to drive [Abe] from the house with a broomstick," according to a neighbor of the Lincolns. On other occasions, Mary let him have it with books, hot coffee, and potatoes. She also blackmailed him, once making him late for a Cabinet meeting by refusing to let him have his pants until he conceded to her demands.

In 1864, a year before his assassination, Lincoln pardoned a soldier who had deserted the Union army to marry his sweetheart. As he signed the pardon, Lincoln made an aside to a witness: "I want to punish the young man. Probably in less than a year, he will wish I had withheld the pardon."

▶HOW SERIOUS

For some men, mild henpecking may not be a problem at all. But an extremely dominating partner can do damage, says Dan Jones, Ph.D., director of the counseling and psychological center at Appalachian State University in Boone, North Carolina. "Most men don't like to think of themselves as being abused," Dr. Jones says. "But henpecking is abuse when it starts to erode self-esteem." When she berates your worthiness as a husband, father, or breadwinner, you may not feel that you can sit down with your partner and discuss the situation calmly. If that's the case, consult a minister or marital therapist, recommends Dr. Jones. "A third party can keep the situation from escalating and getting out of hand," he says.

▶SOLUTIONS

Tell her how you feel. Men who feel nagged half to death are likely to fight back with anger, "which isn't very productive," says Dr. Jones. If you really think about it, you'll most likely find that you're probably more hurt than angry. If you find that this is the case, "the best thing to do is to say, 'You're hurting my feelings,'" says Dr. Jones. "Most men aren't comfortable saying things like this. But if you can do it, most women will be receptive because they don't want to hurt the people they love."

Teach her to ask, not order. You know the difference between a request and a demand, but your wife may not. "When she starts to nag, tell her, 'Please don't make demands—make requests,'" says Willard Harley Jr., Ph.D., a clinical psychologist and expert on marital therapy in Whitebear Lake, Minnesota, and author of several books on marriage, including *Give and Take*. "If she can learn to do that, a lot of the problem will be solved."

Call a time-out. Once you have your partner's tone squared away, it's time to work on her timing. If she usually begins yapping the second you walk in the door, for example, "tell her that you'll be more receptive once you've had time to unwind," suggests Dr. Harley. "So you might say, 'I know you want these things done, but the time to talk to me about them isn't now, when I've just come home. I need a chance to relax. So let's talk about them after dinner.'"

Make the best of it. If nothing you say or do silences your partner's incessant harping, take inspiration from the great Greek philosopher Socrates. His wife, Xanthippe, is one of the best-known fishwives of Western civilization—so famed that she rates a mention in Shakespeare's play *The Taming of the Shrew*. But Socrates never let Xanthippe's carping get to him. "I have gotten used to it," he reportedly said. "You do not mind the cackle of geese."

▶ALTERNATIVE APPROACHES

Tense up to relax. Being henpecked can put even a patient, mild-mannered guy on edge. But a technique called progressive relaxation, in which you systematically tense and relax the body's major muscle groups, can help relieve tension, says Sundar Ramaswami, Ph.D., a clinical psychologist at the F. S. DuBois Community Mental Health Center in Stamford, Connecticut. The whole exercise should take about 10 minutes and should be done twice a day—once in the afternoon around lunchtime and once in the evening.

Here's how to do it, says Dr. Ramaswami: Go to a quiet spot and sit in a comfortable chair. Clench your right fist as tightly as you can. Keep it clenched for about 10 seconds, then release. Feel the looseness in your right hand and notice how much more relaxed it is than when it's clenched, as though you had just flicked a "tension switch" from "on" to "off." Now, repeat the process with your left hand, then with both hands at the same time. Continue to alternately tense and relax the muscles in your arms, shoulders, and neck. Then, squeeze your eyes shut and clench your jaw. Finally, tense and relax the muscles in your stomach, lower back, butt, thighs, calves, and feet.

▶PREVENTIVE MEASURES

Anticipate her cluck. If your partner is always after you to mow the lawn, it's possible that her squawking is the only way she has found to get you off the couch and onto the riding mower. "If she's nagging about something that you know you should be doing, accept responsibility for it and get it done before she can comment on it," Dr. Fitzgerald says.

Belching

▶ PROBLEM

Belching is the sudden, involuntary, and sometimes loud eruption of air from the stomach through the mouth. Although those inopportune burps can be somewhat embarrassing, belching is simply your body's way of relieving itself of uncomfortable excess gas in the digestive system. Some men, however, experience what is known as repetitive belching, which can be little more annoying than an occasional burp. Fortunately, repetitive belching is a habit that can be broken.

▶ CAUSE

The number one cause of belching is swallowed air. Each time we swallow, small amounts of air enter in the stomach, where it either accumulates to be belched out or travels through the intestinal tract to be absorbed or passed out the rectum. With repetitive belching, swallowed air doesn't even reach the stomach. It simply collects in the esophagus and is belched almost immediately back out. There are many causes of air swallowing: eating too quickly, chewing gum, drinking carbonated beverages, and even wearing poorly fitting dentures.

▶ HOW SERIOUS

Burping occasionally, especially during or after a good meal, is a normal and sometimes very satisfying event. In some men, of course, excessive belching may be linked to a medical problem such as hiatal hernia (signaled by a burning pain in the chest), gastroesophageal reflux disease, or peptic ulcer disease. On

History Lesson

The 1990s: As the Internet evolved into the World Wide Web, the world moved one giant step closer to becoming the global village that futurists were always chattering on about. And as people began to use this vast network of computers to exchange ideas and information around the globe, more than a few cybernauts saw the Internet as the ideal venue for some rip-roaring, window-rattling, belching action. It turns out that there are scores of Web sites on the Internet that contain sound bytes of some of the most profound belches around the world. You can immortalize your emissions, too. Some burp sites ask for real audio "submissions" of your more musical eructations. To find these and other sites, simply turn on your browser software, click on the search button, and type in the word *belch*.

the other hand, swallowing air without realizing it—perhaps as a nervous habit—is more than likely the reason behind all that excess gas. If the problem worries you, however, consult your doctor to rule out the possibility of problems in the gastrointestinal tract, advises Harris Clearfield, M.D., professor of medicine and section chief of the division of gastroenterology at Allegheny University of the Health Sciences MCP–Hahnemann School of Medicine in Philadelphia.

▶SOLUTIONS

Fight heartburn right. Men who suffer from heartburn often unconsciously swallow air as a defense against acid reflux, the backward flow of stomach acid up the esophagus that causes the burn, says Roger Gebhard, M.D., professor of medicine at the University of Minnesota Medical School in Minneapolis and staff physician at the Minneapolis Veterans Administration Medical Center. When we feel heartburn coming on, we often swallow a little saliva along with some air, creating a contraction wave down the esophagus that pushes acids back down to the stomach. The side effect may be some belching. Instead of gulping down air, treat heartburn with an antacid or other acid-reducing substance; the less acid reflux, the less tendency there is to swallow air. (For more tips, see Heartburn on page 277.)

Visit your dentist. If you wear dentures, that is. It sounds odd, but poorly fitting dentures may cause inadequate chewing and result in excess air being swallowed, according to Dr. Clearfield. If you wear them, a few adjustments might help temper the amount of air you swallow—and the number of times you need to burp.

Nip postnasal drip. People also tend to swallow air when they have postnasal drip because of an allergy or a cold. Treat the postnasal drip, and you may notice a dip in your need to belch, says Dr. Clearfield. The remedy for postnasal drip usually consists of an over-the-counter nasal decongestant (such as Sudafed), which shrinks the nasal membrane.

Ease with simethicone. Antacid preparations containing simethicone (such as Mylanta) may be useful in relieving belching in some men, although their effectiveness has not been established. Remember, though, if acid reflux is behind your belching, antacids—with or without simethicone—will help, says Dr. Clearfield.

▶ALTERNATIVE APPROACHES

Pick papaya and pineapple. To beat the indigestion that can lead to excessive belching, eat more fruits like papaya and ripe pineapple, says James A. Duke, Ph.D., the world's foremost authority on healing herbs, in his book *The Green Pharmacy.* The juices from these "neutral-based" fruits can soothe your stomach and keep you from being more bubbly. Other fruits to try are peaches, pears, honeydew, cantaloupe, and mangoes. Stay away from citrus fruits, unripe pineapple, strawberries, and grapes. The acid in these fruits could cause more belching.

Be air-aware. People often swallow when they're nervous, often gulping down quite a bit of air as a result. Simply being conscious of the fact that you do have this anxiety reflex can help you minimize air-swallowing and belching, says Dr. Gebhard. Regular exercise and plenty of rest also go a long way in reducing the anxiety behind that urge to swallow.

▶PREVENTIVE MEASURES

Let coffee cool down. Avoiding extremely hot or cold drinks will help stave off swallowed air, too, says Dr. Gebhard. The sucking action of gingerly sipping an ice-cold glass of lemonade or a piping-hot mug of java makes us swallow the air that cools (or warms) the liquid before it goes down the hatch.

Forgo the fizz. By downing a few carbonated beverages, you're setting yourself up for some uncontrollable rumblings. To reduce your daily burp count, do away with the fizz. With every can, you're downing bubble after bubble of carbon dioxide. Some of this gas doesn't even reach the stomach; it gets lodged momentarily in the esophagus before it causes belching, says Dr. Clearfield. If the air bubbles do accumulate in your stomach, you'll either belch it out, or it'll pass through the rest of the gastrointestinal tract, where it'll undoubtedly take form in another kind of gas.

Black Eye

▶PROBLEM

Damaged tissue and blood vessels cause blood to pool around your eye, making you look like Petey the dog from *The Little Rascals.* Oh yeah, and it hurts, too.

▶CAUSE

The cause of a black eye is trauma, usually from something (like a ball) or someone (with a good right hand). Basically, you've been clocked, which breaks the skin or the small veins under the skin near your eye. Blood leaks into the skin around the eye. All that collected blood causes swelling and makes you look like Rocky Balboa faster than you can say, "Yo, Adrian!" However, sometimes people can get black eyes from sinus infections or allergic reactions.

▶HOW SERIOUS

Black eyes look pretty nasty, but like any other bruise, they respond to ice and rest, and usually fade away in two to three weeks. However, if you're experiencing vision problems, have trouble moving your eye, or your eyes are very sensitive to light, get to your doctor immediately. Sometimes a blow to the eye area can break the bones around the eye and cause an orbital blowout fracture, which is serious and requires immediate medical attention.

DO THIS NOW

Get something cold on that eye. Besides reducing swelling, the cold will narrow blood vessels, limiting the amount of blood that will get pooled under the skin and cause a shiner, says Kevin Ferentz, M.D., associate professor of family medicine at the University of Maryland School of Medicine in Baltimore.

Wrap the ice in a towel and apply for 15 minutes every 2 to 3 hours. You can also try a bag of frozen corn or peas wrapped in a thin towel since it'll mold to your eye area well. Don't leave the ice on for longer than 20 minutes, or your body will send blood over there to warm things up, which actually increases swelling.

Did You Know?

Boxers use Inswell for their black eyes. To stay in the ring after a well-landed punch, the cornerman applies pressure with the flat side of this metal band, which is kept on ice ringside. The cold and pressure keep the eye from swelling shut (which would end the fight) and give the boxer a fighting chance.

▶SOLUTIONS

Warm it up. After three or four days of ice, put heat on your eye, says Kevin Ferentz, M.D., associate professor of family medicine at the University of Maryland School of Medicine in Baltimore. The pooled blood from the original shot you took needs to be reabsorbed back into the body so that your black eye will go away, and Dr. Ferentz says that heat will help. Soak a washcloth in comfortably warm water, wring it out, and then apply it for 15 minutes 2 or 3 times a day, suggests Dr. Ferentz.

Pass on aspirin. The basic thing you need to do to heal a black eye is to stop the bleeding above or below the skin's surface and get that blood out of the area. Clots are what the body uses to stop bleeding, and the platelets in your blood stick together to form them, says Flip Homansky, M.D., a ringside physician in Las Vegas who has worked more than 250 championship boxing matches. But if you take aspirin for the pain, your broken blood vessels will take longer to clot and heal. Instead of aspirin, take 500 to 650 milligrams of acetaminophen every four to six hours for as long as you have pain.

This kills the pain without interfering with the blood clotting, says Richard Roberts, M.D., associate chair and professor of family medicine at the University of Wisconsin Medical School in Madison. People with liver disease must be careful about taking acetaminophen, so check with your doctor if you have liver problems, he cautions.

Take your medicine. If you haven't walked into any doors or fists lately, and you have allergy symptoms like itchy eyes and sneezing, then your allergies are more than likely the source for your shiner, says Dr. Roberts. If your skull is pounding and your sinuses hurt along with the black eye, then it's probably a sinus headache that's causing it. In both cases, see your doctor and have him or her treat these conditions with the proper medications, which should also clear up the black eye.

▶ALTERNATIVE APPROACHES

Pop some pellets. Arnica is a homeopathic remedy that would make you sick if you took it in massive doses. But in a diluted, pellet form, it actually stimulates your body to heal itself. It's "an all-purpose trauma remedy known to reduce hemorrhaging or bleeding from any particular area," says Kristin Stiles, a doctor of naturopathy in private practice in Great Bend, Pennsylvania. You can get arnica at most health food stores. Dr. Stiles recommends taking one to three pellets of 30C potency arnica three or four times a day for two or three days. Dr. Stiles says that contact with your skin can reduce the homeopathic arnica's effectiveness, so for best results, shake out the pellets onto the lid of the bottle and tip them into your mouth without touching them.

Be a poultice guy. For black eyes, Dr. Stiles recommends an herb poultice made from comfrey leaves, which she says soothes the eye, lessens pain, stops bleeding, and promotes wound healing. You can buy dried comfrey leaves at most health food stores. Boil four ounces of water, add a tablespoon of leaves, and stir. Shut off the heat, and put the mix in the refrigerator for 10 to 15 minutes so that it cools and steeps. Then soak a piece of cheesecloth or washcloth in the mix, wring it out, and apply to your eye for 20 minutes four times a day.

▶PREVENTIVE MEASURES

Protect your peepers. Since sports-related trauma can cause the black eye, Dr. Ferentz says that it's very important to protect those delicate orbs when playing sports like racquetball or basketball. He suggests using a pair of sports goggles. If you wear glasses, these goggles are even available with prescription lenses. Look for goggles with polycarbonate lenses; they're far more impact-resistant than their plastic counterparts.

Stop and think. If you have a black eye from a fight, and it was in a bar or alley instead of a ring, Dr. Roberts says that you may want to sort through what got you in that situation. Sometimes it can be a problem dealing with anger, alcohol, or a domestic violence issue. He suggests facing the problem realistically to prevent future black eyes and seeking help if you need it because the next go-around in a bar might lead to something a lot more damaging than a black eye.

Bladder Shyness

▶ PROBLEM

It's halftime at the football game or intermission at the theater, and you join the herd heading to the head to relieve your bursting bladder. But once you find a urinal, you realize that you can do nothing more than stand there. Then you slink sheepishly back to your seat, having to urinate worse than ever.

▶ CAUSE

About 4 to 5 percent of men have problems using the rest room away from home. Many find that they just cannot make their bladder relax so that they can urinate when they are near others doing the same thing in a public rest room, says Joseph Himle, Ph.D., assistant clinical professor of psychiatry at the University of Michigan Medical School in Ann Arbor.

It's uncertain why this happens, but Dr. Himle says that a combination of low self-esteem and general social anxiety—coupled, perhaps, with physical factors—may be the best explanation.

▶ HOW SERIOUS

Mostly, it's pretty embarrassing if you think it's obvious to those urinating blithely on either side of you that you've come up empty. Don't despair, says Raul Parra, M.D., professor and chairman of urology at St. Louis University School of Medicine. "It's a normal condition. There is nothing wrong with you," he reassures.

In older men, having difficulty urinating can be a symptom of prostate problems such as benign prostatic hyperplasia or an enlarged prostate, adds Dr. Parra. If your bladder shyness is associated with other symptoms, you should see a doctor, he says.

DO THIS NOW

If your bladder gets stage fright in a public rest room, use one of the doored stalls instead, says Raul Parra, M.D., professor and chairman of urology at St. Louis University School of Medicine. Just that little bit of privacy may be all that you need to let loose.

▶SOLUTIONS

Scope out the facilities. Before you need to use a men's room at an arena or concert hall, do a little reconnaissance, suggests A. Scott Klein, M.D., a urologist at the Gundersen Clinic in La Crosse, Wisconsin. One bathroom may have those long troughs where men stand side by side like cows waiting for milking, while another could have individual urinals with a privacy partition between them. "If you know what the status is, you may choose to use one bathroom as opposed to another," Dr. Klein says.

Beat the rush. You know that bathrooms are going to be packed during intermission, halftime, or the seventh inning stretch. So relieve yourself during less-hectic times at the event you are attending, Dr. Parra says.

Empty the tank before it's full. Maybe you think that if you wait until you're about to pee your pants, you'll be able to go more easily in a public rest room. Just the opposite is true, Dr. Klein says. "Sometimes it's harder to go when you have an extremely full bladder than when you have a medium-full bladder," he says.

MEN'S HEALTH INDEX

Believe it or not, there are guys concerned about public rest room etiquette. Here are 10 things they say you should never do at a urinal.

10. **When waiting for a urinal, don't ask if the guy using it is almost finished.**
9. **Don't peer at the guy standing at the next urinal. If you must look, don't glance *down there*.**
8. **Don't sing.**
7. **Don't read.**
6. **Don't show off by using the look-ma-no-hands technique.**
5. **Don't show off by using *two* hands when your urinate.**
4. **Don't fart while you urinate.**
3. **If you do pass gas, don't pretend somebody else is guilty.**
2. **Don't touch anybody but yourself.**
1. **Don't try and retrieve coins. Remember, it's a urinal, not Rome's Trevi fountain.**

▶ALTERNATIVE APPROACHES

Practice. Using bathroom stalls and restricting your visits to the men's room to nonpeak hours only avoid the problem rather than overcome it, Dr. Himle says. He favors a strategy whereby a guy with a bashful bladder drinks lots of fluids, then visits public rest rooms and repeatedly practices doing what should come naturally.

Start with an isolated bathroom, urinating 10 to 15 times for a few seconds each time during the course of an hour. Once you've mastered that, you graduate to a slightly more crowded rest room before eventually going on to conquer, say, a lavatory at halftime during the next Super Bowl. "Start out with easy situations and work up to more challenging ones," advises Dr. Himle. "It works quite well."

▶PREVENTIVE MEASURES

Have one for the road. Just before you head off to an event where you might have to use a public rest room, pee one last time. It may tide you over throughout the event, allowing you to skip a trip to a crowded men's room, Dr. Parra says.

Stay dry. If you're not trying Dr. Himle's tactic, then quaffing several brews or soft drinks at a ballgame doesn't make much sense. "Unfortunately, a lot of people go to games and start drinking beer and sodas and they get a full bladder and have to go to the bathroom," Dr. Parra says. So it's your choice: Work on becoming comfortable enough to urinate in a public rest room, or learn to enjoy not drinking during events. Just think of all the money you'll save.

Blisters

▶PROBLEM

These bubbles of skin and liquid can make walking or working with your hands a painful experience.

▶CAUSE

Blisters pop up when something, whether it be a shoe or a wooden rake handle, rubs against the skin again and again. The constant friction separates the outside layer of skin from the other layers. Eventually, the skin layer starts to bubble from the constant irritation, and fluid that usually lies unnoticed between skin cells collects inside.

▶HOW SERIOUS

Almost everyone during their lifetime will experience the woes of a blister. Though painful and inconvenient, rarely do they cause any real harm. But if they turn red, get infected, or don't heal, you should go see a doctor, says Pamela Colman, D.P.M., a medical officer for the American Podiatric Medical Association in Bethesda, Maryland. People with diabetes and other chronic illnesses should be especially vigilant that the blister does not become infected. Also, if your skin develops blisters—especially a rash of them—for no obvious reason, you should see a doctor, Dr. Colman adds.

▶SOLUTIONS

Keep the roof on. If you've popped the blister, keep the "roof" intact—don't rip it off. This layer of skin is meant to protect the irritated area from get-

History Lesson

A blister is usually considered a fairly minor medical issue for most people. But for the tallest man in history, a blister proved to be David to this Goliath. Robert Pershing Wadlow measured a towering 8 feet 11 inches, making him the tallest man ever, according to the *Guinness Book of World Records*. The 22-year-old was born a normal 8½ pounds but soon grew by leaps and bounds. At age 10, he stood 6 feet 5 inches tall. Wadlow enjoyed good health but always had problems with his feet—a size 37AA (18½ inches). While wearing a poorly fitted ankle brace, Wadlow developed a blister, which then became infected. The infection spread quickly, and after 11 days in the hospital, Wadlow died on July 15, 1940.

ting infected, says David C. Novicki, D.P.M., president of New Haven Foot Surgeons in New Haven, Connecticut, and past president of the American College of Foot and Ankle Surgeons in Chicago.

Use an antibiotic. For an open blister, clean the area and apply a layer of antibiotic cream such as Neosporin. Then cover it up with a bandage, says Dr. Colman. Reapply the cream every time you take off the bandage or put on a new one.

Give it air and water. You want to keep the blistered area protected with a bandage when you wear shoes all day. But when you can, take off your shoes, socks, and bandages and give the blister some breathing room. "The best thing you can do for a blister is give it some air because the air will help it heal faster," Dr. Colman says. A good 20-minute soak in lukewarm water will also speed up the healing process, she adds.

▶ALTERNATIVE APPROACHES

Aid it with aloe. This plant, usually used for burns, can also treat blisters, says Eric A. Weiss, M.D., assistant professor of emergency medicine at Stanford University Medical Center and author of *Wilderness 911*. Aloe vera will help heal and protect a blister because it contains both anti-inflammatory and antibiotic properties, he says. But be certain that you use pure aloe vera gel, because some prepared products contain additives such as alcohol, which may sting, says Dr. Weiss. Smear some on before you bandage the area. For added benefit, put a thin coat of aloe on the blister and a thin coat of honey (it's a natural antibiotic) on a piece of gauze and tape it down with first-aid tape, says Dr. Weiss

Be blister-free with comfrey. The herb comfrey contains allantoin, a compound that helps heal wounds, says Kathleen Maier, director of the Dreamtime Center for Herbal Studies in Flint Hill, Virginia, and a professional member of the American Herbalists Guild. You can buy an already-made comfrey cream at an herbal or health food store, or you can make a poultice by using the following recipe: Take a small handful of comfrey leaves and cut them up. Cover them with boiling water and let steep for 10 minutes. Let cool. Remove the leaves from the water and gently squeeze out excess water. Place a piece of gauze over the blister, put the moistened herb on top of the gauze and cover with another piece of gauze. Keep the gauze in place with an elastic bandage for a minimum of 20 minutes. Do this two times daily, Maier says.

Let E help. A mixture of the herb calendula and vitamin E will speed up the healing of your blisters, says Andrea D. Sullivan, Ph.D., a doctor of naturopathy; president of Sullivan and Associates Center for Natural Healing in Washington, D.C.; and author of *A Path to Healing*. Both calendula and vitamin E can reduce inflammation of the blister. They also contain compounds that promote wound healing, Dr. Sullivan adds. How much of the mixture you need depends on the size of the blister. Mix equal parts of calendula and vitamin E oil (which can you can get by poking a vitamin E capsule with a pin if you don't have the actual oil on hand) and spread it on the blister. Reapply as needed for about a week. If you have a burn as well as a blister, add some honey.

Make a blister-busting cocktail. Obviously, vodka can relieve the pain of a blister—if you drink enough so that you can't feel your feet anymore. But there's another way that vodka can help soothe a blister, according to James A. Duke, Ph.D., the world's foremost authority on healing herbs and author of *The Green Pharmacy*. Mix a handful of each of the following herbs: fresh thyme, rosemary, a mint that contains menthol such as peppermint or spearmint, and either cherry birch or wintergreen. Crush the herbs and put them in a glass jar and cover with vodka. After a few days, strain out the herbs and keep the liquid in your medicine chest or first-aid kit. Apply the liquid on your next blister. The mixture will help fight infection.

▶PREVENTIVE MEASURES

Wear padded socks and gloves. Some sock companies now make socks with extra material around the areas where you normally get blisters, Dr. Novicki says. The extra-padded socks such as the Thor-lo brand are also made of a special material that wicks away perspiration, which can also lead to blisters. "These help to combat blisters just enormously," Dr. Novicki says. To protect your hands from blisters, wear thick gloves.

Powder your feet. Giving your feet a baby-powder rubdown before putting on shoes will absorb sweat and lessen the friction, Dr. Novicki says.

Get shoes that really fit. You're bound to get a blister if your shoes don't fit properly, Dr. Colman says. To buy the right-size shoes, get your feet measured for length and width every time you buy, always try on shoes before you buy them, shop for shoes in the afternoon because your feet swell later in the day, and wear the socks you will actually wear with the shoe.

Body Odor

▶PROBLEM

You don't have to work up a sweat to work up a stink. Sure, you may notice a foul smell after a hard workout, but that's to be expected. And you can usually leave it in the locker room, provided you shower.

When you're nervous about giving a speech or asking a woman out on a date for the first time, however, the last thing you need is flop sweat under your armpits and a malodorous scent.

▶CAUSE

There are about two million sweat glands in the body, and they are divided into two types: apocrine, which release steroids that interact with bacteria to produce body odor, and eccrine, which release moisture to cool down our body temperature.

Eccrine glands are located all over your body, while apocrine glands are concentrated around your underarms, navel, anus, and pubic area.

Scientists theorize that apocrine odors, which we usually emit when we're sexually excited or nervous, play a role in mutual attraction and physical defense. For example, a small study conducted in Switzerland found that women are attracted to men whose body odor differs from their own, seemingly because this helps a woman choose a mate whose immune system is complementary to her own.

The eccrine glands produce sweat that cools the skin as it evaporates. That helps keep you from overheating during a workout.

History Lesson

Louis XIV reeked. That's not a commentary on his long reign as king of France. It's a historic fact. The "Sun King" considered baths unhealthy and loved women who smelled as foul as he did. Like other aristocrats of his time, Louis the Great fancied himself as a man of the land and wanted sex to smell the way it does with animals.

▶How Serious

If good hygiene and healthy eating don't help you smell appealing, you should see a doctor. Some diseases actually have particular scents that accompany them as a symptom, or you could have hyperhidrosis (excessive sweating) or another problem that requires a prescription-strength deodorant or antiperspirant.

If you just experience occasional problems with wetness and body odor, the following tips should help. "No solution works 100 percent by itself, but if you combine all of these habits, you'll have an almost foolproof shot at getting rid of body odor," says Debra Wattenberg, M.D., a dermatologist in private practice in New York City.

▶Solutions

Pick proper protection. Deodorants fight odor, and antiperspirants fight wetness. If you're a guy whose shirts are damp at the end of the day, but you don't smell bad, pick an inexpensive antiperspirant. If you are a bit ripe but not wet, then go with the deodorant. And if you're both, choose a combination deodorant/antiperspirant. "There is no reason to get something expensive or excessively scented," says Patricia Farris, M.D., a dermatologist in private practice in New Orleans. "Almost all of these products contain the same active ingredients—aluminum chloride or triclosan." These ingredients are also found in deodorant soaps.

Remember though, when wetness meets bacteria, the result is odor. You might need to fight wetness, too, even if it's only the odor that bothers you. And if you wear cologne, it's a good idea to use either an unscented deodorant or one that matches your fragrance so that the two scents don't clash.

Use antibacterial/deodorant soap. Lever 2000 is Dr. Wattenberg's first choice in antibacterial soaps. "It's both deodorizing and moisturizing," she says. "Most other deodorant soaps dry the skin too much."

If your skin is oily, you can even use it on your face, although the fragrance and deodorizing properties may be harsh for sensitive skin.

Act fast. Eventually, you won't smell your own odor, but everyone else will.

"Our noses smell something for a few moments and then we get desensitized to it," says Vail Reese, M.D., a dermatologist with the Dermatology Medical Group in San Francisco. "So, at the first whiff, it's a good idea to take care of the problem."

▶ALTERNATIVE APPROACHES

Put in the scrubs. When you shower, use a loofah or clean washcloth to scrub the underarm and remove excess dead skin, says Eugene Zampieron, a doctor of naturopathy in Middlebury, Connecticut, and a professional member of the American Herbalists Guild. That will give the bacteria and moisture a chance to "breathe" a bit more.

Change your diet. Don't underestimate the power of food. "People who eat a lot of excess meat may experience body odor," Dr. Zampieron says. "You can alter your diet to see if that helps." Spicy foods, particularly those made with garlic, also can increase body odor.

Squeeze out odor. You can find relief in the fresh fruit section of your grocery store. "Rub cut lemons in your armpits every day to change the pH level of your skin," Dr. Zampieron advises. There's no need to rinse; just pat dry. "The more acidic the body moisture, the less likely it is to be a problem."

▶PREVENTIVE MEASURES

Wash every day. "You'd be amazed how many people shower every other day and then wonder why they smell on the second day," says Dr. Reese. "It seems like an easy solution, but a lot of guys just don't do it."

Dress smart. Wearing workout clothes that wick moisture away from the skin will prevent water from settling near the bacteria in your pores. Some newer garb even have triclosan, the antibacterial agent found in deodorants, mixed into their threads. Check out sporting good stores and camping equipment retailers for high-tech underwear, T-shirts, and tights (for running). Mountain Hardwear's ZeO$_2$, Marmot Mountain's DriClime, and the North Face's Alpine all passed a three-day stink-control test by backpackers. It's undie innovation worth investigating.

Boils

▶PROBLEM

Boils can be simply described as red, hot, painful infections. They originate deep in the layers of your skin but make their presence known as they rise to the surface.

▶CAUSE

Any number of irritants can cause strains of the bacteria *Staphylococcus aureus* to get inside a hair follicle or pore and cause an infection. The body responds by deploying white blood cells to kill the infection. In some people—especially those with diabetes, compromised immune systems, and certain skin problems—the body's attack on the bacterial invaders causes pus, which gathers into an abscess right below the skin.

▶HOW SERIOUS

Many boils can be safely brought to a head right at home. But if you develop a fever, chills, or an increasing red area surrounding the boil, you should see a doctor immediately because the infection may have spread, says Karl Kramer, M.D., clinical professor of dermatology at the University of Miami School of Medicine.

Also, if the boil is extremely painful, you may want to see your doctor. "I've seen men really put this off. But relief can be in seconds when treated," says Vail Reese, M.D., a dermatologist with the Dermatology Medical Group of San Francisco.

DO THIS NOW

Box in that boil by applying an antibiotic ointment that contains an ingredient called bacitracin zinc to the boil itself and especially the area around the infection.

The ointment may destroy some of the infectious agents and keep the boil from spreading, says Don W. Printz, M.D., president of the American Society of Dermatology and a dermatologist in Atlanta. Apply the ointment two times daily with one application immediately after taking a shower or bath.

Did You Know?

As the popularity of men having hair-free chests increases, so do boils. Dermatologists in the San Francisco area are seeing more patients who develop boils because they shave or wax their chest and abdominal muscles, says Vail Reese, M.D., a dermatologist with the Dermatology Medical Group of San Francisco.

▶SOLUTIONS

Apply warm compresses. Soak a washcloth or a compress in warm water and place it on the boil for 15 minutes three times a day, Dr. Reese says. The warm compress brings the boil to a head, causing it to drain naturally.

Take a bath. If you have the time to spare, take a warm bath for 20 minutes a few times a day, says Michael Carlston, M.D., assistant clinical professor in the department of family and community medicine at the University of California, San Francisco, School of Medicine. The warm water will bring the boil to a head and soothe your pain.

Keep it clean. The infection that causes a boil can easily spread to other areas of your body. Clean the boil area regularly with antibacterial soap, Dr. Reese says.

Leave it alone. Pinching, squeezing, or popping a boil yourself will only lead to a bigger chance of infection, says Don W. Printz, M.D., president of the American Society of Dermatology and a dermatologist in Atlanta. The squeezing motion will actually push the pus down deeper into the skin, possibly spreading the infection.

Popping a boil can also lead to scarring, Dr. Reese adds.

▶ALTERNATIVE APPROACHES

Force it to the surface. Silica, a homeopathic remedy, helps bring stubborn boils to the surface. Use silica when the boil is red and swollen but pus isn't present. Take one dose of a 12C potency silica product once or twice a day until the boil comes to a head, Dr. Carlston says. Silica is available at health food stores.

Make room for rumex. The herb *Rumex crispus* can help calm an erupting boil, says Steven Bailey, a naturopathic doctor at the Northwest Naturopathic Clinic in Portland, Oregon, and a member of the American Association of Naturopathic Physicians. You can find the herb in capsule form in drugstores or health food stores. Take two 100-milligram capsules three times a day for three to four weeks during and for three to four days past the boil's inflammatory stage, Dr. Bailey suggests. The inflammatory stage is over when the pain, redness, and swelling are gone. If your inflammation does not show improvement within two weeks, it's time to see your doctor, says Dr. Bailey. *Rumex crispus* may have a mild laxative effect.

▶PREVENTIVE MEASURES

Wash your own clothes. The infection that causes boils may be able to travel from clothing, Dr. Printz says. Quarantine your clothes when you have a boil so that they don't come into contact with other clothes, especially those of other family members. Wash clothes that have come into contact with the boil separately.

Bathe away bacteria. Besides keeping the boil clean, washing with antibacterial soap on a daily basis may kill the bacteria that causes boils, Dr. Reese says. But you have to use the soap regularly.

Protect with powder. Parts of your body often can rub uncomfortably against things—other body parts and certain types of clothing and equipment—causing friction that can facilitate a boil, Dr. Carlston says. Working out or activities like bike riding can even make the friction worse, he adds. Dr. Carlston suggests applying powder to areas where you often experience rubbing, especially before working out.

Boredom

▶PROBLEM

You have time on your hands, and you can't think of any particular way you'd like to enjoy it.

▶CAUSE

Boredom is a result of too much free time. Before 1750, no one ever said that they were bored. The word hadn't even been invented. That's because people were working 70-hour weeks; they didn't have time to twiddle their thumbs. "Now, go anyplace and you will find people claiming that they are bored," says boredom expert Mounir G. Ragheb, Ph.D., professor of recreation and leisure services administration at Florida State University in Tallahassee.

Numerous technological advances and changes in labor laws during the late 1800s and 1900s increased productivity, reducing the average workweek to 35 to 40 hours. Though few of us would complain, the shorter work hours can leave us with time to kill, if we are not prepared for it.

▶HOW SERIOUS

In its most benign form, boredom means that you need to get a life. In some people, however, boredom can be a symptom of an underlying psychological problem, says Paul Wink, Ph.D., associate professor of psychology at Wellesley College in Wellesley, Massachusetts. For instance, narcissistic guys—the self-absorbed

> **DO THIS NOW**
>
> Try different hobbies, activities, sports, and other leisure pursuits. Possible choices run the gamut from reading to attending theater performances to playing tennis to skydiving. Each time you try a new activity, write in a notebook what you thought about it. Did you feel like a klutz? Did you have a good time? Did you feel challenged? Try as many activities as you can. Then look at your notes and pick the one you ranked highest. Then do that activity on a regular basis, says Andrew Yiannakis, Ph.D., professor and director of the laboratory of leisure, tourism, and sport at the University of Connecticut in Storrs.

types who feel more important than others—tend to bore easily. For such men, boredom may result in poor work performance or stormy social relationships. Also, some people resort to alcohol and drug abuse when bored. If you are chronically bored and see your work and home life deteriorating, you may want to seek the help of a physician, suggests Dr. Wink. Also, Dr. Wink cautions that if you have had a history of only occasional boredom, and you suddenly develop chronic boredom, it may be a sign of depression. If this is the case, you should seek a doctor's counsel.

▶**SOLUTIONS**

Mind your hands. Bore-proof hobbies, careers, and sports force you to think and move your hands at the same time, Dr. Ragheb says. The more body parts you involve, the better. That's why golfers can get lost in a game for hours. They must concentrate mentally as well as move various body parts. The same holds true with chess masters, artists, and video game players (especially the kind that involve complex button mashing).

Compensate for your job. If you have a boring job and don't want to change careers, make up for it with superexciting hobbies and sports, Dr. Ragheb says. The more boring your career, the more consciously you must choose exciting activities for your free time, he says.

Move on. If you participate in plenty of hobbies and sports and still feel bored, it's time to try something new. "The initial excitement of a new activity can wear off," says Andrew Yiannakis, Ph.D., professor and director of the laboratory of leisure, tourism, and sport at the University of Connecticut in Storrs. "Once that happens, you need to move on to something else."

Challenge yourself. Activities that pack the longest boredom prevention for your buck involve increasing levels of skill, Dr. Yiannakis says. Such activi-

MEN'S HEALTH INDEX

Two researchers at North Dakota State University in Fargo wanted to know how people with absolutely nothing to do would entertain themselves. So they took a group of 44 college students and, one at a time, asked them to sit in a room and do nothing for 12 minutes. Behind a one-way mirror stood a video camera, recording a student's every movement. According to the study, here are the top five activities we resort to when we have about 12 minutes too many on our hands.

1. **We pick up and handle anything we can find, from pencils to staplers to paper clips.**
2. **We repeatedly do the same thing over and over: foot tapping, leg shaking, finger drumming.**
3. **We do stuff to our faces such as pulling on the lower lip and rubbing the nose.**
4. **We move our hair around.**
5. **We stick stuff in our mouths such as fingernails and pens.**

ties are nearly impossible to master. Yet you always feel somewhat competent at your personal level. Examples include martial arts, billiards, and golf.

Talk to yourself. Simply asking yourself, "Why do I feel bored?" can help you come up with an entertaining solution to your problem, Dr. Wink says.

▶ALTERNATIVE APPROACHES

Tempt fate. Guys with a higher need for excitement and stimulation will quickly feel bored when they don't get it. Such guys need to plan thrill seeking—skydiving, rock climbing, drag racing—into their lives on a regular basis. "You know how much you need," Dr. Yiannakis says. For instance, if you choose skydiving, do it once and wait to see how long it takes before the urge strikes again. If you only get through a week, then plan a weekly jump. If you get through two, plan them biweekly, he says.

▶PREVENTIVE MEASURES

Tune out. People who watch three or more hours of television a day more often complain of boredom than people who don't, Dr. Ragheb says. So try to hold your television time to less than two hours a day , he recommends. "If you overdo anything, especially something mechanized, you'll find it boring," Dr. Ragheb says. "Yes, television can be very entertaining. But it also can hurt. The analogy is like eating. We cannot survive without food. But if we eat too much, overeating can hurt us."

Plan wisely. Boredom prevention takes planning. Don't assume that fun activities will knock on your door and ask you to play. You must consciously seek them out and plan them into your life, says Dr. Yiannakis.

Bronchitis

▶PROBLEM

The thin membrane lining your bronchi—the tubes that connect your windpipe with your lungs—is swollen and irritated. This inflammation narrows or shuts off the smaller airways in the lungs, the bronchioles, making it hard to breathe. You also cough up lots of phlegm. There are two types of bronchitis: acute and chronic, says Michael Niederman, M.D., a pulmonologist and professor of medicine at the State University of New York at Stony Brook, and chief of the division of pulmonary and critical care at Winthrop-University Hospital in Mineola, New York.

▶CAUSE

Acute bronchitis is usually caused by a virus—less often, by bacteria—and strikes mostly in the winter. It comes on like a cold but progresses to chest pain and a dry, irritating cough that later produces mucus. With chronic bronchitis, the culprit is most often smoking, and the rattling cough and shortness of breath can occur year-round (although they're usually worse in the winter). Men are three times more likely to have chronic bronchitis than women because more men smoke, says Barbara Phillips, M.D., professor of pulmonary and critical care medicine at the University of Kentucky College of Medicine in Lexington.

▶HOW SERIOUS

If you are a healthy person with no underlying lung disorders and you develop bronchitis, chances are that it is a viral infection, and no antibiotics are needed, says Dr. Niederman. This is acute bronchitis, and it should clear up within a week. If you experience increased shortness of breath, increased volume of sputum coughed up, and a change in the color of the sputum (from

History Lesson

The first advertisement for Andrew and William Smith's homemade cough drops ran in a Poughkeepsie, New York, newspaper in 1852: "All afflicted with hoarseness, coughs, or colds should test [the drops'] virtues, which can be done without the least risk." In 1866, the Smith brothers, realizing their product needed a "hook," put their own stern faces on the glass jars from which the drops were dispensed. The boxes came later; they debuted in 1872 and were the first factory-filled candy package to be made in America. Today, the Smith brothers' stern and hirsute faces are reputed to be the most reproduced bearded mugs in America—except for Abraham Lincoln's.

clear to yellow/green/black) or any combination of the above, see a doctor. You probably have a bacterial infection, which would require antibiotic treatment, says Dr. Niederman.

Most of the solutions below are for acute bronchitis; chronic bronchitis requires continuing treatment by a doctor coupled with smoking cessation, says Dr. Phillips. Chronic bronchitis can be very serious. If left untreated, it can be associated with emphysema and, ultimately, heart failure. See a doctor if you cannot sleep because of coughing, if you have shortness of breath or chest pain, if you cough up blood, or if the illness lasts longer than seven days without improvement, she cautions.

▶SOLUTIONS

Crawl into bed. Call in sick and sleep. "There's increasing evidence that our immune systems function better when we get adequate sleep," Dr. Phillips says. "It's during sleep that the body best fights infections."

Give your bladder a workout. It's tough enough to drink eight glasses (eight ounces each) of water a day when you don't have acute bronchitis. It's even tougher when you do. But try. When you're battling fever, you need to keep hydrated, says Dr. Phillips.

Take C. Taking extra vitamin C in supplement form may help your body fight off acute bronchitis, says Dr. Phillips. "There's good evidence that high-dose vitamin C reduces the frequency and severity of viral infections," she says. "I think the reason that we haven't proven this with bacterial infections is that no one has really studied it." She recommends 2,000 milligrams of vitamin C a day. "It's a safe dose since you'll excrete what you don't use in your urine," she says. Don't take this much C if you're prone to kidney stones or gout; there's some evidence that higher levels of vitamin C can contribute to stone formation or flare-ups of gout. Excess vitamin C may also cause diarrhea in some people.

Suppress it. If coughing keeps you up at night, try an over-the-counter cough suppressant that contains dextromethorphan, such as Robitussin DM. "Dextromethorphan is a fairly effective cough suppressant," says Dr. Phillips.

Don't use cough suppressants if you have chronic bronchitis, however, advises Dr. Niederman. "If you have a lot of mucus that you need to expectorate, using a cough suppressant will just keep it in your chest," he says.

▶ALTERNATIVE APPROACHES

Treat your feet. "It sounds so simple, but soaking your feet is one of the best ways to treat for respiratory tract symptoms," says Amy Rothenberg, a doctor of naturopathy in Amherst, Massachusetts, and editor of the *New England Journal of Homeopathy*. Sit on the edge of the tub and fill it with hot water so that it's just past your ankles. "Make the water as hot as you can stand," Dr. Rothenberg says, but be careful not to burn yourself. Soak your feet for 10 minutes, then run them under cold water. The hot soak helps draw congestion from the head, neck, and lungs, says Dr. Rothenberg. Don't try this if you have diabetes or any other condition that affects your circulation.

Sock it to your bug. After your hot footbath, dry your feet very well. Dip the foot part of a thin pair of cotton socks in very cold water (ice water, if possible). Wring out the socks and put them on. Then don a pair of wool socks. We know what you're thinking. "But it really works," says Dr. Rothenberg. What's happening is that your body gets the message that there's something cold and wet on your feet, which it doesn't like. "In an attempt to dry them out, it sends heat—that's blood—to the area," explains Dr. Rothenberg. "And in the process of drawing blood to heat the feet, you're drawing the congestion away from your lungs." Yes, you have to wear the socks all night. "But they'll dry in a few hours," says Dr. Rothenberg.

Take your thyme. The herb can ease bronchial spasms—contractions of the muscles surrounding the bronchi, according to Varro E. Tyler, Ph.D., distinguished professor emeritus of pharmacognosy and dean emeritus of Purdue University School of Pharmacy and Pharmacal Sciences in West Lafayette, Indiana. To make thyme tea, steep one teaspoon of the dried herb in a cup of hot water for 5 to 10 minutes. Strain the tea, then drink. Dr. Tyler suggests drinking a cup of the tea three times a day, adding a bit of honey for sweetness.

▶PREVENTIVE MEASURES

Don't smoke. Just don't do it, especially if you have chronic bronchitis. Even if you don't, smoking increases your risk of developing acute bronchitis, Dr. Niederman says.

Eat right. A balanced diet can help your immune system prevent bronchial infections, says Dr. Niederman. Try to eat at least five servings of fruits and vegetables, six servings of grains, two servings of dairy products, and a couple of servings of fish, poultry, or lean meat each day, he suggests.

Bruises

▶PROBLEM

Various shades of blues, browns, blacks, purples, and a bit of red may be all right for an impressionist painting, but not for your skin tone. Not only can a bruise hurt but also it can be mighty unflattering.

▶CAUSE

A bruise is a symptom of an injury. Because of a fall or a fist to the eye, the blood vessels underneath the skin rupture, leaking blood out into the surrounding tissues. The blood then discolors the skin on top of the injury.

▶HOW SERIOUS

Everyone this side of Superman gets bruises from time to time. Even if it takes weeks for a bruise to clear up, it's not a sign of trouble and you still can take care of it from home, says Vail Reese, M.D., a dermatologist with the Dermatology Medical Group of San Francisco. Some people bruise more easily than others, so you shouldn't be worried if you've always tended to get black-and-blue.

But you should be concerned if you *suddenly* start to bruise easily and frequently. Easy bruising could be a sign of a blood disorder. In such a case, you should consult a doctor, says Karl Kramer, M.D., clinical professor of dermatology at the University of Miami School of Medicine.

▶SOLUTIONS

Give it a little squeeze. By pushing down with a small amount of pressure on the injured area, you can cut off some of the flow from the busted blood ves-

> ## DO THIS NOW
>
> Ice your bruise. Ice will constrict the broken blood vessels under the skin, slowing blood flow and lessening bruising, says Vail Reese, M.D., a dermatologist with the Dermatology Medical Group of San Francisco. Place the ice pack wrapped in a towel on the area for 15 minutes. Apply it again every hour for the first four hours, and then as needed for the rest of the first day.

Did You Know?

Bruising is the number one injury reported among professional jugglers, according to a survey published in *Juggler's World*.

sels. Apply the pressure as soon as possible after the injury. The less blood that spills internally, the less bruising will develop, Dr. Reese says.

Avoid aspirin. Aspirin thins the blood, making it easier for more blood to gather underneath the injured skin. Other nonaspirin pain medications, such as ibuprofen or naproxen, can also thin the blood. If you need pain relief, take acetaminophen, Dr. Reese says.

Raise your hand. Or foot, elbow, or whatever body part you bumped. Elevating the bruised area above your heart will curtail the blood flow to the area, reducing the bruise, Dr. Reese says.

Heat it up. After using ice for the first 24 hours, switch to heat, says J. Greg Brady, D.O., a dermatologist and partner at Advanced Dermatology in Allentown, Pennsylvania. The heat increases the circulation to the bruised area, helping the scavenger cells to reabsorb the blood that has leaked from the broken vessels into the skin. Apply a heating pad or a warm compress for 20 minutes a few times a day.

▶ALTERNATIVE APPROACHES

Alleviate with arnica. "The thing in homeopathy that you always think of when it comes to a bruise is arnica," says Michael Carlston, M.D., assistant clinical professor in the department of family and community medicine at the University of California, San Francisco, School of Medicine. You'll find this herbal remedy in a health food store or homeopathic drugstore. Look for an arnica product that has a potency of 30C. Take one dose every four hours the day you get your bruise. Lower the number of dosages you take each day as the soreness goes away. You should stop using it in a few days, Dr. Carlston says.

Caution: Do not use arnica when you have open, bleeding wounds.

Banish bruises with bilberry. The bilberry herb helps heal the broken capillaries that caused the bruise, Dr. Carlston says. You can find bilberry capsules in health food stores or even your local drugstore, Dr. Carlston says. Take a 60-milligram bilberry capsule three or four times on the day you get your bruise.

▶PREVENTIVE MEASURES

Pump up your capillaries. Grape seed extract contains bioflavonoids, which strengthen capillaries, making them less likely to break under pressure, says Kenneth Singleton, M.D., a physician in private practice in Bethesda, Maryland. Take 20 to 50 milligrams of grape seed extract, Dr. Singleton suggests.

Pad yourself up. If your sport or activity calls for padding or protective gear, use it. A little bit of padding can go a long way to prevent a bruise after a fall or impact, says Dr. Brady.

Be careful out there. One of the only surefire ways to prevent bruising is to use caution and common sense. Bumping into cabinets, walking into furniture, dropping a can on your foot are all things that cause bruising—and things you avoid if you pay attention, says Dr. Brady.

Burnout

▶PROBLEM

New York City psychologist Herbert J. Freudenberger, Ph.D., coined the term *burnout* in the 1970s when he noticed a common psychological syndrome in many of his patients. Those fatigued, frustrated patients had lost the sense of meaning in their lives. They were unable to get along with family members, friends, and co-workers. And they felt disillusioned. The discovery prompted Dr. Freudenberger to write *Burn-Out: The High Cost of High Achievement*. And the name stuck. "At the time, I certainly didn't know the extent the term would be dealt with in society," says Dr. Freudenberger. "It has become a word everyone uses."

Burnout often starts with fatigue. You feel drained, even when you get a good night's sleep or a long weekend of rest. Eventually, small demands such as getting new wiper blades seem overly taxing. Then you become irritable or depressed. Other problems can include loss of concentration, forgetfulness, and decline in motivation.

DO THIS NOW

At the moment, exercise probably sounds as enticing as cracking open your old college calculus book and solving a few integrals. "Usually, when people get badly burned out, the only thing that'll make them feel good is working out," says Ahnna Lake, M.D., a physician in private practice who specializes in and counsels on burnout and work stress issues in Stowe, Vermont. Combining a good heart-pumping aerobic workout with resistance training will bring you the best results, she says.

▶CAUSE

Lots of stress and a poor ability to cope with it in a healthy way. "People who are highly idealistic and who get a great sense of who they are from their jobs are most likely to burn out," says John-Henry Pfifferling, Ph.D., director of the Center for Professional Well-Being in Durham, North Carolina. That's because people who suffer from burnout tend to hold themselves to extremely high standards—so high that they set themselves up for failure. Regardless of your personality type or your coping skills, a sustained stressful lifestyle will eventually affect the levels of brain chemicals, says Ahnna Lake, M.D., a physician in private practice who specializes in and counsels on burnout and work stress issues in Stowe, Vermont. This produces a tired, irritable, scatterbrained feeling. So the guy with burnout may start dreading and avoiding important appointments, have no patience with his wife, or cut corners at work. He falls increasingly behind and starts feeling down on himself, which creates more pressure and a vicious spiral downward.

▶ HOW SERIOUS

Some people deplete their brain chemicals so badly that they need prescription medication to boost those levels back to normal, says Dr. Lake. If you have already tried some of the solutions listed below and you still feel tired and irritable, consider seeing a doctor for drug therapy, she says.

MEN'S HEALTH INDEX

Ever wonder who's at fault—you or your job? Now you can put your job to the test. Here, according to John-Henry Pfifferling, Ph.D., director of the Center for Professional Well-Being in Durham, North Carolina, are 10 items that tend to create a "burnout" environment.

1. Repetition
2. No say in decision making
3. Long, stress-packed hours with few breaks
4. Not enough resources to do your job well
5. Little encouragement
6. Low pay
7. Isolation
8. Too few or poorly run office meetings
9. No performance appraisals
10. A dead end—little ability to move up or sideways

▶ SOLUTIONS

Take time off. If you are burned out, you probably already know that a weekend off isn't enough to revitalize you. You need a vacation. And we're not talking about one of those jam-packed, see-the-world vacations where you need to rest when you return. No, we're talking about the kind of vacation that Henry David Thoreau would crawl out of his grave for. You need pure rest. Do as close to nothing as you can. The time off will help your battered neurotransmitters to recover, boosting your spirits and your energy levels, says Dr. Lake.

Cut back. Maybe you can't afford to take time off. Then your major strategy is to cut back on what you do. And even if you could take a week or two off work, you aren't cured yet. You may feel refreshed and revived, but you have few reserves. So if you jump full force into your usual hectic schedule, you'll quickly use up whatever energy you managed to recuperate. Strike everything off your schedule that you don't absolutely have to do, suggests Dr. Lake. The more you strike off, the better.

"You need to reduce your demands to a minimum for several weeks longer than it takes to feel better," Dr. Lake says. "Simplify your routine as much as possible." That means no big projects at work, no shuttling here and there with your kids, fewer nighttime meetings—just relax.

Sleep often. You may need more than the regular eight hours a night, says Dr. Lake. Take a nap if you need one. Don't feel guilty. Let yourself recuperate.

Redefine yourself. If you define yourself by your job, you'll feel like a total and utter failure when something goes wrong at work, Dr. Pfifferling says. That's why developing interests outside your line of work can keep work-related stresses and strains from plummeting you right back into rock-bottom burnout. Join a softball league. Or serve on a church committee. But whatever you do, really engage in something passion-producing, he says. That way, when one area of your life takes a nosedive, you can find self-esteem from another.

▶ALTERNATIVE APPROACHES

Take a time out. To get your energy back, you need to eliminate as much stress as you can. One area to de-stress, in particular, is how you handle questions. When you give people immediate answers, you feel anxious and usually agree to more responsibility than you need. So learn the artful habit of saying, "Let me think about it." "Unless you are a brain surgeon faced with a leaking artery, you usually can pause to think something through," says Leonard Tuzman, doctor of social work and director of social work services at Hillside Hospital of Long Island Jewish Medical Center in Glen Oaks, New York. "Take time out. Collect yourself. Think through your pros and cons."

Usually, you can buy time just by asking for it. Other times, however, you'll need a more calculated approach, like when your boss demands immediate answers. You can always buy a few seconds by taking a really deep breath. But if you need 5 or 10 minutes to think things through, politely excuse yourself and head to the men's room. (No one can argue with nature's call.) Lock yourself in a stall until you figure out your response.

Surround yourself with upbeat people. Burnout is contagious. So if you know or work with someone who's a perpetual downer, stay away from the guy. Be positive yourself, taking the initiative to complement co-workers, and stick with people who energize you, Dr. Pfifferling says.

Tune up with a tonic. Try taking ginseng to turn up your energy level, suggests Varro E. Tyler, Ph.D., distinguished professor emeritus of pharmacognosy and dean emeritus of Purdue University School of Pharmacy and Pharmacal Sciences in West Lafayette, Indiana. Look for capsules of American or Asian ginseng in your health food store. Make sure that you buy a product with the active ingredient ginsenosides, standardized to between 4 percent and 7 percent. If you are using a product with 4 percent ginsenosides, the daily dose is two 100-milligram capsules daily. Otherwise, follow label instructions. Take it daily to combat stress and fatigue, or, suggests Dr. Tyler, if you need an extra energy boost, take it when your life gets too hectic. If you have high blood pressure, check with your doctor before taking Asian ginseng.

▶PREVENTIVE MEASURES

Avoid stimulants. Don't depend on caffeine, sweets, or stimulants to keep you going, says Dr. Lake. Eventually, they will just make you feel more fatigued.

Seek the light. If you notice that you usually only feel burned out in the winter, you could be suffering from seasonal affective disorder (SAD). Light therapy may be what you need to get your energy back, says Dr. Lake. (For more information, see Seasonal Affective Disorder on page 456.)

Plan a sustainable lifestyle. Sustainability is the key. If your lifestyle is causing burnout, something needs to change, says Dr. Lake. Decide what you are going to do differently about your work and life so that burnout does not happen again. This is a highly personal process, she says. You may need to make only minor changes, such as fewer clients and more delegation of work. Sometimes major changes such as career change are needed.

Pursue true success. While corporate ladder climbing may earn you money and prestige, it probably won't earn you peace of mind. Usually, more money comes with a big price tag—more hours at the office. "The more successful you are, the more difficult your job, and the higher your failure or disappointment potential," Dr. Pfifferling says.

Besides, is it really success if you are too burned out to enjoy it? Is it really success if you have destroyed your relationships in the meantime? asks Dr. Lake. "You have to ask yourself what success is," she says. Instead of always looking up, consider lateral moves, she says. "You want to do work you love. You want to do work that's energizing, not exhausting. If it's more exhausting than energizing, in spite of your efforts to improve things, you are not in the right line of work."

Set limits. Keep a stress diary. Whenever you feel disorganized, resentful, or confused, write down the events that led to those feelings. Eventually, you'll be able to take a look at the diary and pinpoint exactly what saps your energy. "You need to know your stress quotient so that you can control the responsibilities, choices, purchases, and relationships you enter into," says Dr. Tuzman.

Bursitis/Tendinitis

▶PROBLEM

Tendinitis is an inflammation of the tendon and the tendon-muscle attachment, while bursitis is an inflammation of a bursa, a fluid-filled sac positioned over the bony projection of a joint, says Alison Lee, M.D., a pain-management specialist and acupuncturist with Barefoot Doctors, an acupuncture and natural-medicine resource center in Ann Arbor, Michigan.

▶CAUSE

Tendons connect muscles to bone. When you contract a muscle, it pulls on the tendon, which, in turn, moves the bone. You may get tendinitis when you undertake an activity that your tendons and muscles aren't accustomed to, like throwing a Frisbee after a winter's layoff or playing your son in a knock-down game of one-on-one basketball. Or, it can come from repetitive motion, such as painting your house or sliding around a computer mouse, says Dr. Lee.

The bursa, which acts as a cushion between the bone and tendon, may become inflamed at the same time. You can also get recurrent bursitis from bone spurs—tiny but rough outgrowths that chafe and irritate the bursae, says Dr. Lee.

▶HOW SERIOUS

These injuries take time, but they do heal on their own. In the meantime, you shouldn't repeat the offending activity. If you do, you'll get inflammation not only of the tendon but also of the sheath that houses the tendon. In its worst case, you could develop a long-lasting pain syndrome, says Dr. Lee.

DO THIS NOW

Give it an ice massage. Tendinitis and bursitis pain generally is localized, so there's no need slap a big bag of ice over a large area. Instead, fill a paper cup with water, freeze it, peel off the upper edge to expose the ice, and then massage the ice up and down the tender area, says Jon Kluge, physical therapist, certified athletic trainer, and director of the Sports Injury Center in Waterloo, Iowa. Massage for 8 to 10 minutes until the skin is just reddened and numb to the touch.

Did You Know?

When you run, you might think that you're using your leg muscles. But new research by scientists shows that your tendons are doing most of the work. After studying turkeys running on a treadmill on level ground, they found that tendons act like powerful springs. When your foot lands on the ground, the muscles maintain enough tension on the tendon to allow it to store the energy of the impact. Then the muscles release the tendon so that the stored energy propels you forward. The muscle isn't doing much heavy work at all.

So the next time someone says that you run like a turkey, you really do.

▶SOLUTIONS

Flame out the pain. You'll get some pain relief and bring down the inflammation by taking an over-the-counter anti-inflammatory like ibuprofen (Advil, Nuprin), says Jon Kluge, physical therapist, certified athletic trainer, and director of the Sports Injury Center in Waterloo, Iowa. Follow the package directions for dosage, he says.

Wrap it up. It's a good idea to give your sore tendon some support by wrapping it in an elastic bandage, says Dr. Lee. "The pressure of the bandage will hold down the swelling and probably make it feel better, says Dr. Lee. "And it's a reminder that you're hurt, so you'll be more careful."

Stretch out the pain. Tendinitis is usually the result of tension in the muscles attached to a particular tendon, so you have to eliminate the tension in the muscle in order to relieve the pain in the tendon, says James Waslaski, sports massage therapist at the Center for Pain Management and Clinical Sports Massage in Tampa, Florida, and author of *International Advancements in Event and Clinical Sports Massage*. For example, he says, try stretching your calf muscles if you have tendinitis in your Achilles tendon. Icing the inflamed and tight tendon will help the symptoms, but you need to stretch regularly to address the underlying cause, he says.

▶ALTERNATIVE APPROACHES

Make for the manganese. When bursitis strikes, you can have chronic inflammation that forms waste products (oxidants) in the body. Dr. Lee recommends taking a manganese supplement of 50 to 100 milligrams per day in divided doses to help build up the body's antioxidant-fighting properties. Take this amount for one to two weeks, then cut back to 15 to 30 milligrams of manganese per day for up to a month if your pain persists. But after that, it's time to go back to an everyday-size dose of 2.5 to 5 milligrams of manganese per day, Dr. Lee says.

Treat your joints gingerly. A gentle way to combat inflammation from chronic tendinitis and bursitis is to drink a tea made of ginger and sarsaparilla root, says David Winston, professional and founding member of the American Herbalists Guild and a clinical herbalist in Washington, New Jersey.

"Ginger and sarsaparilla are both good systemic anti-inflammatory herbs," says Winston. "They're a good combination for chronic inflammation." For each eight-once glass of tea, you'll need about one teaspoon of the dried ground-up herbs, says Winston. Mix two parts sarsaparilla to one part ginger, and steep for about 45 minutes. Drink three cups a day for several weeks, says Winston. Don't use dried ginger without medical supervision if you have gallstones.

▶PREVENTIVE MEASURES

Stop when it hurts. If you're doing any activity that has recurrent motion, you're prone to tendinitis, especially if you are not conditioned for the movement or you haven't warmed up adequately. As soon as you feel pain in a specific area—an elbow, wrist, or knee—stop what you're doing because you're already doing damage, says Dr. Lee.

"Pain is the body's signal to take it easy. It knows when enough is enough, and so should you," she says. "The price you pay for trying to paint your entire garage in single day is that you're too sore to go near it for a week."

Caffeine Addiction

▶PROBLEM

Four out of five Americans use caffeine at some point in the day, and it's the most widely used stimulant in the world. There's nothing wrong with a morning cup of coffee or an afternoon jolt to keep you going every so often. But when you come to rely on caffeine day in and day out, and you can't function without it, then you probably need to cut down. "If you miss your usual soda, coffee, or tea, and you get headaches, feel lethargic, and start to feel tired—like you have the flu—you have a caffeine addiction," says Jo-Ellyn Ryall, M.D., a psychiatrist in private practice in St. Louis. Other common withdrawal symptoms include drowsiness, fatigue, nausea, and vomiting.

▶CAUSE

When caffeine enters the brain, it knocks out a brain chemical called adenosine while providing its own jolt of energy. Adenosine is a neurotransmitter—a chemical that sends messages from your brain to your body—that produces sedation, making you tired. Caffeine blocks adenosine, thus fighting off sedation. Your brain, however, can grow dependent on that java fix. When you deprive the brain of its caffeine jump start, it fights back by making you tired and sleepy, producing headaches and occasional nausea.

DO THIS NOW

The best way to cut back on caffeine is to do it gradually. If you quit cold turkey, you'll most likely suffer from flulike withdrawal symptoms for days as your body tries to survive without its daily fix, says John Hughes, M.D., professor of psychiatry at the University of Vermont in Burlington. Dr. Hughes recommends cutting back about 25 percent of your caffeine intake every two to three days. For instance, if you drink four cups of coffee a day, drop it down to three cups for two or three days. After you feel comfortable, cut back to a two cups a day, or whatever level you can handle without problems, for awhile.

History Lesson

Coffee wholesaler Ludwig Roselius feared that his profits would sink when he received a shipment of coffee beans in 1902 that had been drenched by salt water. In a desperate attempt to save his beans, he used a process that inadvertently removed the caffeine from the coffee.

He still wanted to make some money off the caffeine-free bean, so he tried some early twentieth century marketing techniques. He came up with a catchy name for his "sans caffeine" coffee. (Sanka—get it?) About 20 years later, it was launched all across the United States, and thus the term *decaf* became part of the American vocabulary.

▶HOW SERIOUS

Caffeine hasn't been shown to be physically harmful, even if you are addicted, says John Hughes, M.D., professor of psychiatry at the University of Vermont in Burlington. The drug causes more behavioral problems than physical ailments. People addicted to caffeine often experience insomnia, the jitters, and an overall feeling of increased anxiety, Dr. Hughes says.

There is some evidence, however, that consuming more than four cups of coffee a day—or the equivalent amount of other caffeinated beverages—may be linked to higher risk of heart disease and high blood pressure.

▶SOLUTIONS

Read the fine print. You've cut down on your coffee and your head is pounding, so you reach for an Excedrin. Well, just two tablets of that painkiller contain 130 milligrams of caffeine—only 5 milligrams less than an eight-ounce cup of coffee, Dr. Ryall says. Since many over-the-counter medications include caffeine, you need to read the labels. Otherwise, you'll unwittingly feed your addiction. "Look for all the hidden sources," Dr. Ryall says. Pay special attention to painkillers, diet pills, and any medication name with the letters "ACP." (The "C" stands for caffeine.)

Mix it up. If you really enjoy your coffee, cheer up. You don't have to cut back. In fact, you can continue to drink the same number of cups that you do now. Just start slipping in some decaf, Dr. Hughes says. On the first day, make one of your four cups decaf. Then, a couple of days later, make it two cups decaf and two regular, Dr. Hughes suggests.

Don't be a soda jerk. Coffee consumption is going down, but caffeine intake isn't, Dr. Hughes says. Why? It seems that as we turn away from the joe, we end up in the arms of cola and other caffeine-laden soft drinks, he says.

"About 80 percent of sodas are caffeinated," Dr. Hughes says. Don't thwart your attempt to break free of caffeine by drinking lots of soda, he says. A 12-ounce can of Mountain Dew, for instance, packs 55 milligrams of caffeine, while the average cola has 35 milligrams.

Sample the substitutes. There are a lot more decaffeinated choices out on the market these days, so be adventurous if you're trying to kick the java jones. Most soft drinks come in a decaf version. And herbal teas provide a tasty punch without any caffeine, Dr. Hughes says. Try out different decaf products and find what you enjoy.

▶ALTERNATIVE APPROACHES

Take a snooze. Through the ages, caffeine has been used to keep people awake and alert. But instead of feeding your body a drug when you feel tired, maybe you should listen to what your body is telling you—that it needs rest, says Jay L. Glaser, M.D., medical director of the Maharishi Ayur-Veda Medical Center in Lancaster, Massachusetts. The next time you feel the need to down a pot of java, lie down for a few minutes and think about why you are tired, he says. You probably aren't getting enough sleep, he says. Your body will feel more refreshed and relaxed after it gets the proper rest than it will from a quick shot of caffeine.

Wake up with sesame oil. Try an ancient Indian Ayurveda technique to wake you up and keep you refreshed without caffeine. Massage yourself with cold pressed sesame oil each morning before your shower, giving special attention to your head, ears, and feet, Dr. Glaser says. The oil will bring balance to your day. And after your shower, a fresh, soft layer of oil will stay with you and keep you soothed and refreshed all day long, he says. Sesame oil is available at health food stores and through mail order.

▶PREVENTIVE MEASURES

Stick to a schedule. Perhaps you tend to stay up late and wake up early. There's no time for breakfast, so you grab your cup of coffee and doughnut and run. Skip lunch, grab a quick dinner. All the while you inhale cups of coffee or cans of soda to keep your engines running. Instead of relying on caffeine to keep you on time, set a strict schedule, Dr. Glaser says. Go to bed and wake up the same time each day so that you develop a consistent sleeping pattern that will give you more energy. Set aside time for nutritious meals, which will keep you fueled. By planning a schedule, you're more likely to get everything done without exhausting yourself and counting on caffeine to do the job for you, Dr. Glaser says.

Calluses

▶PROBLEM

One part of the uppermost layer of your skin, the epidermis, has begun to multiply and build up on your heels and palms. Now you're stuck with rough patches of dry, thick, scratchy, and layered skin, most likely on your fingers and the fleshy parts of your palm, or on your heels and the soles of your feet, says Andrew Pollack, M.D., chief of dermatology at Chestnut Hill Hospital in Philadelphia.

▶CAUSE

"Calluses are the result of friction," says John Venson, D.P.M., chairman of the department of medicine and surgery at the Dr. William M. Scholl College of Podiatric Medicine in Chicago. "It's letting you know that there's abnormal pressure on a specific area of your body."

Your skin reacts to the increased friction or pressure by building up a protective layer, says Dr. Venson.

If you have a callus on your hand, you've probably been doing lots of yard work, gardening, or manual labor. Either all of this hard work is new to your sensitive hands, says Dr. Pollack, or you've been doing it so long that your hands are in a constant state of defensiveness.

If the callus is on your heel or the ball of your foot, you may be wearing shoes that don't fit correctly. Loose shoes rub back and forth across your skin, while tight shoes exert consistent pressure on the skin, Dr. Venson says.

DO THIS NOW

Cover the callus with a wart-remover patch or a wart-remover medicated strip, says Andrew Pollack, M.D., chief of dermatology at Chestnut Hill Hospital in Philadelphia. "They contain salicylic acid, which will loosen and dissolve the extra layers of skin," Dr. Pollack says.

Apply the wart-remover patch or medicated strip after you shower. Keep it on for a day, take it off before you shower again, and reapply a new one after the shower. You'll probably need to do this for a week or so, Dr. Pollack says. They are sold at most drugstores.

Did You Know?

Hard work can make a man horny, but not the way you think. A layer of skin cells that's made today takes 28 days to work its way up to the top of your body and then shed away. While the outermost layer of your skin is called the epidermis, it actually contains layers within itself; and one of these, the "horny" layer, builds up to develop a callus.

"The horny layer of your skin is mostly dead cells that, microscopically, look like little granules," says Andrew Pollack, M.D., chief of dermatology at Chestnut Hill Hospital in Philadelphia. "When friction hits that layer, it begins to thicken. So now there are, for example, 30 horny layers rather than 10; and it no longer takes 28 days, but three months, to shed."

▶HOW SERIOUS

For many men, callous hands are a point of pride, tangible proof that they're not afraid of hard work. And because they protect the skin, calluses are actually a good thing in many cases. A callus only becomes a problem when it grows big enough to become its own source of pressure and discomfort. Avoiding calluses on your hands or feet may be as simple as buying a good pair of work gloves or better-fitting shoes, says Dr. Pollack.

Most men can take care of calluses themselves. However, if you suffer from bad eyesight, have a doctor handle the problem, rather than doing it yourself, advises Andrea Cracchiolo III, M.D., an orthopedic surgeon and director of the University of California, Los Angeles, Adult Foot and Ankle Clinic. Men with bad eyesight can't see the problem on their foot well enough to be sure that it's a callus or to treat it properly, or they may not be able to easily reach their foot, explains Dr. Cracchiolo. Men with diabetes should also see a physician because their foot problems may stem from their diabetes, he adds.

▶SOLUTIONS

Rock it. If you have calluses, follow Bob Dylan's advice: "Everybody must get stoned." Just be sure to use a pumice stone, says Dr. Pollack.

Pumice, which is actually volcanic glass, looks like a gray rock with air holes. It's very rough and grainy to the touch, so it can rub off the dead skin of the callus, leaving smoother skin exposed. It works on your hands or feet, Dr. Pollack says. You can find pumice stones at drugstores, beauty supply stores, and some health food stores.

Bring the pumice stone into the shower with you, and use it, wet, on your wet foot or hand. Just rub it back and forth, not too aggressively, across the callus, Dr. Pollack says. "Nothing will make a callus go away quickly," Dr. Pollack adds. "It will take as long to go away as it did to develop." Therefore, you have to be gentle and patient with removing the callus.

Use the right lotion. Lotions made with urea, such as Carmol, will help get rid of dead tissue before it develops into a hard callus, says Marjorie Menacker, D.P.M., a podiatrist with Chesterfield Podiatry Associates in Midlothian, Virginia. Look for lotions containing urea at drugstores and large supermarkets. If you can't find any, ask your pharmacist if he can order one for you. Just be aware that in some people, urea-based lotions can cause stinging or burning of the skin.

The other major ingredient you'll find in moisturizers is lanolin, which isn't as effective as urea-based lotions, Dr. Venson says.

Think thick. If your hands are developing calluses, cover them up with something thick and cushiony—namely, gloves—when you're working. The thicker the better. The same goes for your feet. "It's all a matter of personal comfort, but if you're prone to getting calluses, you might want to wear thicker socks that have extra cushioning built in," says Dr. Venson.

▶ALTERNATIVE APPROACHES

Walk barefoot in the sand. Sand is a natural skin-smoother. It exfoliates, or rubs off, the dead skin. If, during the summer, your feet have calluses on them from walking barefoot, take a hike on the beach. It will soften up your skin, says Kathy Driscoll, a licensed aesthetician and owner of the Spa at the Houstonian in Houston.

▶PREVENTIVE MEASURES

Soak once a week. Water softens the skin cells, which allows pumice stones and lotions to do their work more effectively. "Take a good long, hot soak in a bathtub once a week," says Driscoll. "The soaking is accomplished in 10 to 15 minutes, but the relaxation continues," she adds.

Water is so good for your skin, in fact, says Driscoll, that you should look for it in the ingredient list of your moisturizer. "Get products that have a high concentration of water rather than oils," Driscoll advises. "One ingredient to look for is dimethicone, which aids in the lotion's spreading ability." It's the main ingredient in Eucerin lotion.

A moisturizer is effective when it doesn't leave a film behind on your skin. Why? A filmy residue indicates that the lotion's moisture content has not been absorbed, Driscoll says.

Canker Sores

▶PROBLEM

Canker sores afflict 20 percent of Americans. They nestle between the folds of your inner cheeks and lips, on the base of your tongue, the floor of your mouth, or on your soft palate. Eat anything acidic, and they'll burn like fire. These painful critters, also called recurrent aphthous ulcers, are yellowish-gray or white with bright red borders. They're tiny, round, and pop up individually or in clusters. Fortunately, they're not contagious and usually heal within 7 to 14 days. But when they do crop up, they can make talking, eating, and even brushing your teeth a hair-raising experience.

▶CAUSES

Stress, heredity, and certain foods such as chocolate, nuts, tomatoes, green peppers, strawberries, oranges, and other citrus fruits are top canker sore triggers. Sharp-edged corn chips and pretzels are just as guilty. They can irritate and injure your mouth's lining and produce an ulcer, says Terry D. Rees, D.D.S., chairman of the department of periodontics and director of the Stomatology Center at Baylor College of Dentistry in Dallas. Studies show that vitamin and mineral deficiencies in B_6, B_{12}, folate, iron, and zinc are linked to the nasty sores. In rare cases inflammatory bowel disorders such as colitis, celiac, and Crohn's disease are the culprits.

▶HOW SERIOUS

In general, canker sores aren't serious, except for the discomfort. But if they recur more than once a month, show up in bunches, appear very large, or last longer than 14 days, see your doctor, says Sol Silverman, D.D.S., professor of

DO THIS NOW

Place one teaspoon of table salt in four ounces of warm water. Swish the solution in your mouth for 20 to 30 seconds and then spit it out. Salt water will keep your mouth clean and helps soothe the pain, says Terry D. Rees, D.D.S., chairman of the department of periodontics and director of the Stomatology Center at Baylor College of Dentistry in Dallas.

oral medicine at the University of California, San Francisco. He can determine whether you really have canker sores or something more serious. "If your sore isn't painful, looks like a white or red and white patch or a lump, and it doesn't seem to heal, it may be the first sign of mouth cancer," says Dr. Silverman.

▶SOLUTIONS

Gargle with antacids. Grab some Mylanta, Maalox, or milk of magnesia from your medicine cabinet. Chew the tablet or, if you have the liquid form, shake the bottle, take a swig, and swish it around in your mouth. Just don't swallow it. "The thick, milky solution coats the canker sore and helps protect it from irritation and abrasion," says Ara DerMarderosian, Ph.D., professor of pharmacognosy and medicinal chemistry at Philadelphia College of Pharmacy and Science.

Numb the pain. If your canker sore is full-blown, dab on a topical anesthetic gel or cream designed for oral use containing benzocaine. Zilactin-B and Orajel are good choices to buy at a drugstore. Use the anesthetic before meals and more often, if necessary, for comfort. But you probably should not apply it more than three or four times a day. "They won't make your canker sore go away any faster, but they'll quell the pain instantly," Dr. Rees says.

Go for vitamin E. Instead of swallowing the gelcap, crack it open and rub the oil on the ulcer, says Craig Zunka, D.D.S., past president of the Holistic Dental Association in Front Royal, Virginia. You can use plain vitamin E liquid for convenience. Four times a day, just saturate a cotton ball and dab it on the sore. "This will cut healing time by 40 percent," says Dr. Zunka.

▶ALTERNATIVE APPROACHES

Wash it away. Wash out your mouth with goldenseal. Prepare a tea to be used as a mouthwash by using two teaspoons of the herb (available at health food stores) and one cup of water. Rinse with the tea three or four times a day. The mouthwash will ease the pain and speed healing, says Varro E. Tyler, Ph.D., distinguished professor emeritus of pharmacognosy and dean emeritus of Purdue University School of Pharmacy and Pharmacal Sciences in West Lafayette, Indiana.

MEN'S HEALTH INDEX

The following is a list of the top eight foods that trigger canker sores (listed in no particular order), according to Terry D. Rees, D.D.S., chairman of the department of periodontics and director of the Stomatology Center at Baylor College of Dentistry in Dallas.

1. Tomatoes
3. Strawberries
4. Pineapple
5. Lemons
6. Chocolate
7. Peanuts
8. Sharp, hard foods like potato chips

Soothe it with calendula. Calendula as a tincture—a solution of the herb steeped in drinkable alcohol or a similar substance—is sold at some health food stores. Buy the water-based or glycerin-based variety; the alcohol-based tincture will sting, says Dr. Zunka. The water-based tincture is available through Washington Homeopathic Pharmacy, 124 Fairfax Street, Berkeley Springs, WV 25411. Smear the liquid right on the canker sore or dilute it with water to use as a mouth rinse. To dilute, use 25 drops of calendula and four ounces of water. "Within 30 seconds, your pain will subside and healing will begin," says Dr. Zunka.

▶PREVENTIVE MEASURES

Say so long to SLS. Studies suggest that the foaming agent sodium lauryl sulfate (SLS), found in toothpastes, may cause canker sores. Study participants who brushed with an SLS-free paste for three months reduced canker sore outbreaks by 70 percent. So find a paste without SLS, recommends Dr. Rees. You can start with Biotene, available at drugstores.

Try triclosan. Switch to a toothpaste containing triclosan, an analgesic and anti-inflammatory agent that may reduce canker sore recurrences, says Dr. Rees. Colgate Total is one product to try.

Police your food. Keep a food diary to determine which foods trigger the sores. That way you'll know what to avoid. If you get canker sores often, cut down on citrus fruits, sweets, and sharp-edged salty snacks to see how you do, suggests Dr. Rees.

Load up on vitamin C. Take 500 to 1,000 milligrams of vitamin C with bioflavonoids twice a day in pill form for five to seven days, says Dr. Zunka. "You'll notice that your canker sore recurrences will drop dramatically," Dr. Zunka says. "If this doesn't work, up the dosage. But don't exceed 3,000 milligrams in a day. Megadoses of vitamin C can cause diarrhea in some people," Dr. Zunka adds. In fact, taking more than 1,200 milligrams of vitamin C daily may be enough to cause diarrhea in some people.

Pop some lysine. Lysine is an amino acid supplement that works wonders for some guys. Take a 500-milligram tablet one to three times a day to prevent the canker sores, says Dr. Zunka. "Some people just need to take the lysine when they begin to get a canker sore," he says. If you're one of those guys, taking lysine for five to seven days should help it clear up fast. If you get canker sores often, taking one or two tablets daily can stop them from starting, adds Dr. Zunka.

Carpal Tunnel Syndrome

▶PROBLEM

The median nerve—the communication cable for the muscles of the hand—and the nine tendons for flexing your fingers pass through the carpal tunnel, a narrow passage of bone and ligaments in your wrist. It's like a six-lane highway narrowing down to two lanes where the tunnel goes through a mountain. If the tunnel closes or narrows, then you have a problem.

▶CAUSE

The median nerve becomes compressed within the carpal canal in the wrist. Inflammation of the tissues or tendons in the carpal canal or increased fluid within the carpal tunnel can intensify the pressure placed on the median nerve. The results are pain, tingling, numbness, sometimes a loss of grip and pinch strength, and impaired coordination.

If you work a lot with your hands—pounding nails, typing at a keyboard, or working with small parts for long periods—you're susceptible to carpal tunnel syndrome, says Robert Harrison, M.D., associate professor of occupational medicine at the University of California in San Francisco.

DO THIS NOW

Ease off on the work a little bit. If you can't stop what you're doing entirely, then cut back when you can and take frequent, short breaks, says Mark Bracker, M.D., clinical professor of sports medicine in the division of family medicine at the University of California, San Diego, School of Medicine in La Jolla.

And when you go home, don't launch into another hand-intensive activity like painting your garage.

"Repetitious work is often to blame. When the tendons swell, they compress the median nerve. And if that swelling is not relieved, you'll eventually have loss of function," Dr. Harrison adds.

▶HOW SERIOUS

At first it may be just a temporary tingling and soreness after an afternoon of leaf raking or long day of typing. But carpal tunnel often arises on the job where you have to repeat the activity day after day. Without prevention or treatment, the problem nearly always gets worse, says Houshang Seradge, M.D., assistant professor of orthopedic surgery at the University of Oklahoma Science Center and director of the Orthopedic and Reconstructive Center, both in Oklahoma City.

You should see your doctor if you have any or all of these symptoms, says Dr. Seradge: numbness in your hands that wakes you at night; clumsiness and a tendency to drop things; tingling and numbness in the thumbs, index fingers, or long fingers during work or at night. Ignore the problem too long and you may have trouble telling warm from hot with your hand, have difficulty buttoning your shirts, or when reaching in your pocket feeling for change, be unable to distinguish between a dime or a quarter, says Dr. Seradge.

"The hand essentially becomes dull, blind, and weak," Dr. Seradge adds.

Surgery may relieve the pressure. In advanced cases, however, the nerve damage can be permanent.

▶SOLUTIONS

Work at right angles. We've become a nation of desk jockeys and computer geeks, which puts us more at risk for carpal tunnel because of the intensive hand work. But often, all it takes is a simple change of posture or better ergonomics at our "workstations" to relieve the symptoms, says Dr. Seradge. You should sit in a 90-90-90 position, meaning your elbows, back, and knees should be at 90 degrees. That position evenly distributes body weight and makes you sit up straight, he adds. And it keeps your wrists straight.

See eye-to-eye. Keep your monitor at eye level, says Dr. Seradge. It'll help ensure that you maintain a good working posture.

Mickey with your mouse. Put your mouse in a position where you don't have to reach. Or trade in that mouse for an alternative, like a touch pad or track ball, suggests Dr. Seradge.

Go ergo. "There are a lot of good ergonomic products and advice out there. I would experiment and see what helps you," says Dr. Seradge. A simple example of one is using a wrist pad on your keyboard to alleviate pressure on the carpal tunnel. A rolled towel or a strip of hard sponge under your wrist can work well. There is no need for expensive commercial equipment.

Sleep with a splint. Carpal tunnel frequently wakes you up at night with pain and tingling sensations. That's because in sleep, you often fold your wrist and put pressure on the already in-flamed nerves and tendons, says Dr. Harrison. Try sleeping with a wrist brace or wear one during the day to limit your hand movement and hold your wrist in a "neutral" position, suggests Dr. Harrison. You can find the braces at most drugstores.

Bring down the swelling. To help ease the pressure in your inflamed wrist, you can take over-the-counter nonsteroidal anti-inflammatory drugs (NSAIDs) like aspirin or ibuprofen. Dr. Seradge suggests taking two 200-milligram doses three times a day with meals. See your doctor if this doesn't seem to be providing enough relief.

Lose weight. Being overweight can aggravate repetitive strain injuries, says Margaret Cullen, a registered occupational therapist, certified hand therapist, and director of hand therapy at the University of California, San Diego, Hand and Upper Extremities Center, in La Jolla. When you are overweight and sedentary, there's a greater chance that less oxygenated blood and nutrients will be delivered to your tissues. If your muscles don't receive the food and oxygen they need to function correctly, they tire quickly. Extra pounds also add to the weight that the muscles must support to move your hand and arm.

▶ALTERNATIVE APPROACHES

Go natural. Many foods contain natural anti-inflammatory chemicals, called proteolytic enzymes, that may help relieve the pain and swelling of carpal tunnel syndrome. In his book *The Green Pharmacy*, James A. Duke, Ph.D., the world's foremost authority on healing herbs, recommends eating his Proteolytic CTS Fruit Salad made of pineapple, papaya, and grated ginger. Liberally spice your other food with sage and cumin, and you will have added even more natural anti-inflammatory and pain-relieving chemicals to your diet.

Rub it in. You can make your own pain-relieving lotion by adding several teaspoons of ground red pepper to a quarter-cup of skin lotion, suggests Dr. Duke. Ground red pepper contains several compounds that ease pain and inflammation. He also suggests adding several drops of lavender oil—another natural anti-inflammatory that has a relaxing scent—to the lotion. He cautions that some people may be sensitive to the chemicals in ground red pepper, so test the lotion first on a small area and stop using it if it irritates your skin.

Get your blood moving. Aerobic exercise increases the flow of oxygenated blood to your hands while removing the waste products from inflammation, says Cullen. Exercise also releases endorphins, your body's natural mood-enhancers. Aim for 30 to 40 minutes of aerobic exercise at least three times a week.

Don't smoke. Smoking can make repetitive strain injuries such as carpal tunnel syndrome worse. Nicotine constricts your blood vessels and replaces oxygen with carbon monoxide, explains Cullen. So the blood flow to your tissues is reduced.

▶PREVENTIVE MEASURES

Take a break. Workers who use their hands intensively on the job should do this three-minute stretching routine every hour, or at least once after the lunch break, says Dr. Seradge, developer of the routine: Start with your right hand, hold each position for a count of 10, and let your motions flow from one position to the next. Remember to keep breathing normally as you do these. Stop if you feel pain. Stand with your arms relaxed at your side, feet shoulder-width apart. Bring your right arm up straight in front of you to shoulder level with your palm facing up. Spread your fingers and bend your wrist down until your fingers point toward the floor. Then, bring your hand up and make a fist. Keeping your arm straight, flex your wrist toward yourself. Bend your arm at the elbow and pull your fist toward your shoulder. Keeping that position, rotate your arm out to the side from the shoulder and turn your head to look at your fist. With your arm still out to the side, straighten your arm, and—with your palm facing up—extend your fingers and bend your wrist down until your fingers point to the floor. Turn your head slowly to look over the opposite shoulder. Repeat the sequence with your left hand.

"That gets those muscles, nerves and tendons ready," Dr. Seradge adds. "If you're having symptoms of carpal tunnel, you should see a physician and do this routine every hour or so."

For a free copy of Dr. Seradge's complete exercise program, send a stamped (single first-class stamp), self-addressed envelope to Houshang Seradge, M.D., Director, The Hand Institute, The Orthopedic and Reconstructive Research Foundation, 1044 Southwest 44th Street, Oklahoma City, OK 73109. The Foundation also has a videotape with exercises and ergonomic tips for about $50. For more information, write to Dr. Seradge.

Chafing

▶PROBLEM

Somewhere in elementary school you must have done the pencil experiment—the one where you rub two number twos together until the wood heats up and the yellow paint peels off. The same thing happens with your thighs (regardless of whether they still resemble pencils) as you run, only you lose skin instead of yellow paint.

As your right thigh travels forward and your left thigh back, scra-a-a-ape—some skin cells flake off. As they rub past one another over and over, more and more skin drops away. The same thing can happen under your arms or when your nipples rub against your shirt during exercise.

Scrape enough skin cells off and your body responds with the usual immune system arsenal of killer blood cells and swelling, leaving the rubbed area red and raw.

▶CAUSE

Elementary physics. Remember the definition of friction? It's the force that resists two objects from moving in different directions. In this case, either already-dry, scaly skin or sweaty, wet skin creates friction as one part of your body rubs against another, ripping those poor little skin cells from their homes. This itches.

So we scratch, ripping off more skin cells and further inflaming the area. As we make our way down to raw, bloody skin, the bacteria, yeast, and fungi that naturally live on our skin's surface make their way under our skin, causing infection.

▶How Serious

Usually, you can cure chafing and its related infections with simple home care and over-the-counter medication. If you follow the tips in this chapter and don't see relief within a couple of weeks—or if the chafed area gets worse—consult a physician for prescription medication, advises Richard A. Miller, D.O., a dermatologist in private practice in Port Richey, Florida.

▶Solutions

Soften after your shower. If your skin is raw but not bloody, rub in a moisturizer after bathing. The moisturizer will trap the water on your skin, preventing the evaporation of moisture and further drying of your skin, says Daniel Groisser, M.D., a dermatologist at Clara Mass Medical Center in Belleville, New Jersey. Also, moisturizer will help reduce the itchy feeling that results from chafing, keeping you from scratching and worsening the chafed area. Dr. Groisser recommends using Curel moisturizer for your body, Eucerin Light on your face, and Cetaphil as a wash instead of soap. Use as needed and as directed on the package.

Cream yourself. If you've rubbed yourself bloody, apply an over-the-counter antibiotic ointment such as Polysporin once you've washed and dried your raw skin, Dr. Miller says.

Cover it up. If you are bleeding somewhat heavily, place a nonstick bandage (such as Telfa pads) over the wound, says Dr. Miller. You can secure the bandage with netting (such as Gauztape or Ace Wraps), available at most drugstores or medical supply stores. If you use a regular adhesive bandage or tape, you may further irritate the wound when you remove the covering. Change your bandage once a day.

Don't be rash. Your shower and antibiotic ointment should take care of bacteria. But if you notice a bumpy rash forming on or near the chafed area, you may have developed a yeast or fungal infection. This usually happens on the inner thigh and groin, says Dr. Miller. You can combat such infections by using an over-the-counter anti-yeast or antifungal medication, such as Lotrimin

---

MEN'S HEALTH INDEX

So you go to the store to get antibacterial ointment. You stare at ointment after ointment. Which one to buy? Is one better than another? Not to worry. The American Pharmaceutical Association foresaw your quandary. They asked 100 pharmacists to name the products they personally use. Here are some of the ones they recommended, with the percentage that use it.

Neosporin (original): 57 percent
Neosoprin Plus (maximum-strength): 24 percent
Polysporin (first-aid antibiotic): 8 percent
Betadine (solution): 2 percent
Bactine (first-aid antiseptic): 1 percent
Campho-phenique (pain-relieving antiseptic): 1 percent

AF cream or powder or Micatin cream, twice a day for two to three weeks. If you sweat a lot, stick to powders instead of creams. If the rash persists or gets worse, see a doctor for a prescription ointment or pill.

▶ALTERNATIVE APPROACHES

Oil your skin. The Australian tea tree makes an oil that can speed healing and protect your chafed skin from infection. You don't have to travel to Australia and chop down a tree. Just go to your local health food store and buy a bottle of tea tree oil. Soak a cotton ball in water, apply just a few drops of the oil to the cotton ball, and then press the cotton ball into the chafed area several times a day until your skin heals, says Eve Campanelli, Ph.D., a holistic family practitioner in private practice in Beverly Hills, California. Some people with very sensitive skin may experience an irritation or allergic reaction to tea tree oil. If you have sensitive skin, be sure to do a patch test before using the oil: Place a drop of the oil on a patch of clean skin on your arm, wait 24 hours, and if you don't experience any irritation, then the oil is safe to use.

Concoct your own skin-saver. You can make a soothing ointment by mixing an ounce of vitamin E cream or olive oil, which is naturally high in vitamin E, with 5 drops each of lavender and geranium essential oils, 15 drops each of bee propolis and poplar bud tinctures, and a quarter-teaspoon of a low-alcohol calendula tincture. Apply the mixture to the chafed area three times daily. The ointment is safe, even on sensitive skin, says Pamela Taylor, a doctor of naturopathy in private practice in Moline, Illinois. Ingredients such as vitamin E help soothe skin and promote healing, while others such as bee propolis—a natural antibiotic substance made by bees to protect their hives—fight infection. Most of these ingredients can be found at your local health food store. Poplar bud tincture is often sold as Balm of Gilead. If you can't find it, substitute 15 drops of tincture of comfrey (its use should be limited to 4 to 6 weeks' daily application) or double the amount of calendula tincture to a half-teaspoon, Dr. Taylor recommends.

▶PREVENTIVE MEASURES

Try some lube. Smear petroleum jelly or some other gooey lubricant between your thighs, under your arms, on your nipples, and along any other area that tends to chafe, says Dr. Miller. The lubricant will allow your thighs and other body parts to glide past one another.

Powder your puff. If you're carrying around a few extra pounds, your skin rolls may rub together. Of course, losing those extra pounds will help. But that takes time. In the interim, sprinkle cornstarch or baby powder between the folds of your skin every morning, says Dr. Miller.

Chapped Lips

▶ PROBLEM

Your lips are dry, red, and burning. They may even be cracked or blistered, depending on the degree of chapping. A smile quickly turns into a pained grimace.

▶ CAUSE

You could be forgiven if you think of lips as a flaw in the flow of evolution. Despite the wear and tear your lips receive, they are remarkably unprotected. Lips lack the natural oils that the rest of our skin employs to stay supple. They also lack melanin, the pigment that protects us from the sun and turns us tanned. It's no wonder that the environment often smacks us right in the kisser—strong winds, indoor heating, the blazing sun, and cold, dry winter days all conspire to take the wet out of our whistle.

▶ HOW SERIOUS

There's no question that chapped lips can put a damper on your love life. Who wants a passionate peck when it seems the Mojave Desert has relocated just below your nose? Aside from the comfort factor, there are certain times when you should treat chapped lips with due seriousness. If you have persistent dryness, redness, or scaling, it could be a sign of premalignant activity, says Alexander H. Murray, M.D., head of the division of dermatology at Dalhousie University Faculty of Medicine in Halifax, Nova Scotia. It looks like a bad case of chapping, but if it resists healing and hangs around more than a couple of weeks, get yourself checked by a doctor. Plus, if your lips

> ## DO THIS NOW
>
> "If you don't have anything else in the house, use Crisco. That will moisturize your lips," says Judy Johnson, R.N., a nurse in a dermatology office in Anchorage, Alaska. Dunk your finger into that familiar blue can or box and slide a thin coating on your parched puss. You don't have to be brand-conscious either, she says. Any vegetable shortening you have will do just as well. Not only will you get some instant relief but also you'll be able to grease up the cookie sheet in a whole new way.

crack and get infected when they're chapped, a doctor can prescribe antibiotics to get you back in shape.

▶SOLUTIONS

Tap into hydro power. Hydrocortisone in a 1 percent balm comes in a little tube available over the counter at any drugstore and most supermarkets. It promotes healing and can stave off infections in cracked lips, says Abraham R. Freilich, M.D., a dermatologist and assistant clinical professor of dermatology at Downstate Medical Center in Brooklyn, New York. Apply to your lips a couple of times a day when you have chapped lips.

Turn to old faithful. Who can imagine the uses that the old standby, Vaseline, has seen? It has never been put to better use than as a treatment for chapped lips, says Dr. Murray. Apply as needed to your parched lips, and give dryness the kiss-off.

Change toothpaste. Certain

MEN'S HEALTH INDEX

Here are some balms that got the thumbs-up during an informal survey of *Men's Health* staffers. These may be worth paying lip service to when you have chapped lips.

- **Sun Stick SPF15 by Polo Sport:** Contains mineral oil so that it glides on easily. Ideal for sore lips in winter. Water- and sweat-resistant.
- **Bull Frog Sunblock Stick:** Originally developed for surfers, it's waterproof for up to six hours. Has an SPF (sun protection factor) of 18.
- **Dermalogica Solar Shield SPF15:** Contains beeswax to guard against winter drying and soothes with menthol and grapefruit oil. Only available at select salons.
- **Un-Petroleum Citrus Sunscreen Lip Balm:** All-natural ingredients and fruity taste, with an SPF of 18.
- **Neutrogena Lip Moisturizer:** Taste- and fragrance-free, with an SPF of 15.

toothpastes can promote chapping in some sensitive people, Dr. Freilich says. The flavoring agents seem to be the main culprit. He suggests brushing with just water or with baking soda when your lips are chapped.

Try Aquaphor. Aquaphor is available at most drugstores. "It's like a heavy-duty Vaseline," says Judy Johnson, R.N., a nurse in a dermatology office in Anchorage, Alaska. It stays on longer than Vaseline, she adds, but is extra greasy. Use it when you need relief. Just be sure to warn your woman before you plant one on her.

▶ALTERNATIVE APPROACHES

Thumb your nose at it. If you're stuck at the top of the ski hill and feel your lips withering, use your head. Or nose. Run your finger over the side of your nose or forehead and borrow some skin oil. Transplant it to your lips. "If you have oily skin, that will work in the short term," Johnson says.

Get in touch with your feminine side. Women get chapped lips far less frequently than men. Why? Lipstick, says Dr. Murray. They also get skin cancer on their lips much less for the same reason. You don't have to look like an escapee from *The Rocky Horror Picture Show* to reap the same benefits. There's a more manly alternative—zinc oxide balm. It's the really cool stuff you see sailors, lifeguards, and skiers wearing on their noses and lips. "It's impregnated with various colors—neon greens, yellows, and pinks," says Dr. Murray. Not only do you look ultra chic but also it stops sun damage and holds in moisture.

▶PREVENTIVE MEASURES

Be like Tricky Dick. Always cover up. Why do you have chapped lips anyway? Because you went out into the elements without protection. Always put on a lip balm with at least an SPF (sun protection factor) of 15 before heading outside for any length of time, Dr. Murray recommends. "It's like wearing a seat belt," he adds. So buckle up your lips and make it a habit of slathering on some protection.

Lick your problem, not your lips. A dry and dusty cowboy hitches his horse to a saloon. He walks around back of the critter, raises its tail, and plants a kiss straight on its nether region. "What'd ya do that fer?" asks the saloonkeeper. "Got chapped lips," says the cowpoke. "Does that help?" the saloonkeeper asks. "No, but it sure keeps me from licking 'em."

That's a good point. "You cause a lot more irritation by licking your lips when they're chapped," warns Dr. Freilich. Resist the urge and keep your tongue in your mouth.

Chicken Legs

▶PROBLEM

Chicken legs, skinny legs, thin legs. All mean the same thing—a pair of pins that just won't pump up. While your gym buddy develops a pair of powerful pistons after a minimum of work, yours are still toothpick-thin.

▶CAUSE

"There's a clear genetic component involved," says Frederick C. Hatfield, Ph.D., president of the International Sports Sciences Association in Clearwater, Florida, an organization that certifies personal fitness trainers worldwide. "Some guys with little or no training will have reasonably muscular legs, while others won't." It all comes down to the body type you inherited and the type of muscle fibers you have in your legs. A majority of slow-twitch fibers lend themselves to endurance, while fast-twitch fibers are better-suited to bulk and brute strength. If you have more of the fast-twitch kind, the technical term for your body type is *mesomorphic*. If your legs have more slow-twitch fibers, you are probably more ectomorphic," he explains.

▶HOW SERIOUS

Chicken legs isn't one bit serious, except that it makes it harder to fill out a pair of pants. "In fact, the ectomorphs are the ones who tend to be better aerobic athletes," says Dr. Hatfield. This body type also tends to live longer, he adds. "On the

---

DO THIS NOW

"Running backward, just like a football linebacker would do, is very good," says Frank Zane, three-time Mr. Olympia; owner of Zane Experience, a training facility in Palm Springs, California; and author of *Mind, Body, Spirit* and *Fabulously Fit Forever*. "It's a good way to strengthen the lower back, firm up the buttocks, and even work the hamstrings and calf muscles." You can also do this walking and reap some of the same benefits. "When I walk my dog, I always walk backward for the last portion," Zane says. How far you go is up to you. You'll feel the burn when your leg muscles are getting a good workout.

Did You Know?

Looks (and legs) can be deceiving. When you look at a chicken standing on what appears to be spindly legs, you are actually looking at a part of its feet. A chicken (like most birds) has a thighbone that is imbedded in muscle close to the body. That's the part you rip off for a drumstick. The leg really begins to move freely at the knee, which is also hidden in feathers. The part you see sticking down is a bone called the tarsus, which connects the toes and the heel.

other hand, mesomorphs tend to be better athletes at all other sports not requiring great endurance."

▶SOLUTIONS

Squat for success. Squatting exercises are among the best ways to beef up your thighs, says Dr. Hatfield. He should know. At age 45, he squatted 1,014 pounds—more weight than anyone in history had ever lifted in competition.

Here's an easier one to get you started: Hang on to your bedpost, doorknob (make sure that the door is locked), or anything else steady and about hip height. This will allow you to keep your balance and to maintain proper posture while exercising. Keeping your feet flat on the floor and shoulder-width apart with your torso erect and straight, bend your knees slightly and squat down. Do not allow your knees to extend past your toes. Continue the movement until your thighs are parallel to the floor. You should begin with three or four sets of 10 repetitions, but over the first month, work up to three or four sets of 40 to 50 repetitions every day, Dr. Hatfield says. You can then start doing squats while holding a dumbbell in each hand at your side. Start with 10 pounds per hand and work up from there. Eventually, Dr. Hatfield says, you'll reach the point where you can hold a barbell with weights on your shoulders as you do the squats.

Make like Rocky. There's a good reason why the Italian Stallion did his little victory dance after running up the stairs at the Philadelphia Museum of Art in the original *Rocky* film. Stairclimbing is a perfect way to put some extra beef on your leg bones, Zane says. Shun the elevator at work and spend some extra time beside the banister at home. Walk or jog the stairs until you feel the muscles in your legs getting pumped. But please, whatever you do, *don't* start yelling, "Yo, Adrian!"

Raise a calf. The stairs can help you build bigger calf muscles even while you stand. Place the balls of your feet on the edge of a stair with your heels hanging off the end of the stair, and do some calf raises, says Zane. Lower yourself down as far as you can, and then lift yourself until it looks like you're standing on tiptoe. Pause there for just a second or two before you start your descent. Start with two sets of 15 repetitions and move up to three sets of 15 reps from there. Make sure that you don't bounce. Concentrate on slow, fluid lifts.

Play the swashbuckler. "One of my favorite exercises is lunge walking," Dr. Hatfield says. To do this, envision yourself as one of the Three Musketeers. (Not the guys on the candy bar wrapper—the real thing.) Thrust your lead leg forward, bending at the knee so that your crotch gets nice and low to the ground. Your trailing leg should not bend, and the knee should not touch the ground. The knee to your front leg should not extend past your toes; otherwise, you'll hurt your knees. Now repeat with the other leg, turning this into a lunge walk.

"You don't need to do much," Dr. Hatfield says. "Just the equivalent of once or twice around the pool each day. Start with three or four sets of 15 to 20 lunge steps, or about five to six minutes of exercise, and you'll be amazed at the musculature your legs will begin to develop." Besides, he adds, it's fun. "You'll feel good. It'll make you feel young again." The muscles of your groin, thighs, lower legs, and hips all become stronger and more flexible, enabling you to enjoy an active lifestyle without becoming stiff or injured, Dr. Hatfield explains.

▶ALTERNATIVE APPROACHES

Engage in a cover-up. One way of dealing with thin legs is simply to hide them. "You want pants that are cut on the full side," says Alan Flusser, owner of a custom shop in Saks Fifth Avenue in New York City and author of *Style and the Man*. He also suggests pants that rest more on the natural waist rather than lower on the hip. This will cause the fabric to hang better. "I'd also wear chunky fabrics," adds Flusser. "That will give you a sense of bulk." Look for thicker corduroy fabrics and flannels.

▶PREVENTIVE MEASURES

Get out of your jeans. If you're self-conscious about your thin legs, jeans are the worst thing to wear, Flusser says. They're too fitted and accentuate skinniness, he says.

Go slow. Bulking up is going to mean some hard work, says Zane. You want to take it slow so you don't injure yourself. At the same time, you want to maximize your efforts. "Just make sure that you're doing something that is a fair bit harder than you're used to doing," he says. Listen to your muscles, he adds. If you're working too hard, they'll tell you. Back off for a few days.

Chronic Lateness

▶PROBLEM

Whether it's going to a meeting or an appointment, a movie or a golf date, you seem to always make a not-so-grand entrance by arriving late.

▶CAUSE

Some guys are simply irresponsible, while others need a crash course on time management, says Mack Ruffin IV, M.D., associate professor in the department of family medicine at the University of Michigan Medical Center in Ann Arbor.

Then there are men who are habitually late because of fatigue that leaves them sluggish, dull, and struggling to keep on schedule, says Claire Etaugh, Ph.D., professor of psychology and dean of the College of Liberal Arts and Sciences at Bradley University in Peoria, Illinois.

▶HOW SERIOUS

Being repeatedly late can be simply annoying to others, or it can seriously disrupt their plans or schedules. When it occurs regularly in the workplace, it can signal that a man is bordering on burnout or is already there, says Dr. Ruffin. He recommends that a man seek help from his family physician if lateness is a significant problem that is disruptive to his professional or family life.

▶SOLUTIONS

Cut waste. Sure, you look forward to playing solitaire on your computer after lunch, or shooting the bull with a buddy down the hall. But if you're always running late, these are the sorts of the things that you should curtail. Elim-

DO THIS NOW

Allow yourself extra time to get where you're going, advises Claire Etaugh, Ph.D., professor of psychology and dean of the College of Liberal Arts and Sciences at Bradley University in Peoria, Illinois. For example, if you have to drive across town for an appointment, leave a few minutes earlier than you think is necessary in case heavy traffic or a detour makes the trip longer than you expect. You'll also spare yourself considerable stress by doing so.

Did You Know?

If you've ever heard or used the expression "Johnny-come-lately," you might think that guys have a history of chronic lateness. But in fact, the expression refers to somebody who is a newcomer to a situation or status. So if the kid clerking down at the 7-Eleven store wins the lottery, you might say that he is a Johnny-come-lately to the ranks of the rich. Since being a Johnny-come-lately has nothing to do with tardiness, it would not preclude you from being a Johnny-on-the-spot—a person who is present at a crucial time.

The term *Johnny-come-lately* originated in the early nineteenth century British navy as *Johnny Newcomer*, meaning a seaman new to a ship. In America it was changed to *Johnny-come-lately*. It first appeared in print in an 1839 novel by Charles F. Briggs, titled *The Adventures of Harry Franco*.

Maybe you already knew all of this. If not, better late than never.

---

inate one unimportant, time-wasting activity from your life each week, suggests Nepha Franks, R.N., a retired health educator who developed time-management guidelines for the Fronske Health Center at Northern Arizona University in Flagstaff in order to help the students manage their time more effectively.

Make use of down time. When you're standing in line at the bank or sitting in a doctor's waiting room when you have an appointment, use that time productively, advises Franks. Review notes, read a report, draft a memo.

Delegate. "One of the major problems with men who tend to be workaholics is that they believe that no one else can do the job as well as they can," Dr. Ruffin says. If that describes you, start trusting colleagues more. Set priorities as to what only you can do and delegate other tasks if you are in a position to do so, Dr. Ruffin suggests. By lightening your workload, you are more apt to make it on time to meetings and appointments.

Get enough Zzzs. If you are habitually late because of fatigue, go to bed earlier, Dr. Etaugh says. If you routinely fall asleep within seconds of hitting the lights, you probably should be turning in sooner.

Dr. Etaugh gives the following advice for a good night's sleep: Go to sleep and wake up at the same time every day, even on weekends. Establish a relaxing bedtime routine that might include meditating or taking a hot bath. Do not read or watch TV in bed. Get out of bed if you don't fall asleep within a half-hour. If you have trouble falling asleep at night, avoid daytime naps. Engage in moderate physical activity two to four hours before bedtime.

Cut it loose. Don't waste time trying to make every project absolutely perfect, Franks advises. Procrastination is often the result of fearing that your effort won't be perfect.

Use a planner. Use a planning guide or day log to plan your time, at least daily and weekly, Franks recommends. Schedule key events, projects, and deadlines. Make tasks manageable by dividing larger ones into smaller parts. Complete one part at a time. Update your list daily, crossing off finished tasks and adding new ones.

Control interruptions. Drop-in visitors, telephone calls, or television can control your time. Control them, tactfully, but assertively, says Jon Rudy, senior health educator at Fronske Health Center at Northern Arizona University in Flagstaff. He suggests that you greet unexpected guests at your home or office warmly, but let them know from the outset that you're busy. Ask them to reschedule if the visit can't be concluded in a few minutes.

You may want to screen your telephone calls with an answering machine, Rudy says. Try standing up while talking on the telephone: It will be a constant cue to bring the conversation to an end.

As for television, don't turn it on as soon as you walk in the door at home. Tune in only when you want to watch a specific program, and then turn it off immediately afterward, Rudy suggests.

▶ALTERNATIVE APPROACHES

Keep a time log. Carry a notebook for a week, suggests Franks. Jot down what you're doing every 30 minutes. Then review the log to determine whether deadlines were met without a crisis and to identify habits that keep you from achieving goals in a timely manner.

▶PREVENTIVE MEASURES

Prioritize. If you've committed yourself to taking on extra projects at work, coaching a Little League team, taking a college course in the evenings, and volunteering at the local public radio station, your plate may be too full. Learn to say no, advises Franks. Set priorities and do a few things efficiently and on time rather than spreading yourself thin.

Colds and Flu

▶PROBLEM

You know that you feel lousy, but you're not sure whether you have a cold or the flu. Here's how to tell the difference.

- Cold: nasal congestion, scratchy throat, sneezing, coughing, blocked sinuses, slight fever, if any
- Flu: All of the above, plus fever of 102° to 104°F; headache; muscle aches and pains; exhaustion; dry, hacking cough; and stomach problems like diarrhea, nausea, or vomiting

The biggest difference between a cold and a flu is that a cold isolates in your head and chest, while you feel the flu all over your body. "People can usually function with a cold, but it's hard to function properly when you have the flu," says David Rooney, M.D., a family physician with Southern Chester County Family Practice Associates in Oxford, Pennsylvania.

▶CAUSE

Although they share some common symptoms, the flu is not simply a more severe version of a cold. You "catch" a cold when you inhale virus-containing droplets expelled by someone else or rub your eyes or nose with contaminated fingers. The virus—rhinoviruses cause about half of all common colds; coronaviruses take credit for most of the rest—latches onto a mucous membrane in your nose, eyes, or throat. To fight this invasion, your body unleashes the cold symptoms (runny nose, sneezing, cough, and the like) to get rid of the virus. Colds generally last for three to seven days.

The flu, on the other hand, comes in three different strains: A (which has many subgroups), B, or C. Most of us catch the A strain, as Duke Ellington (almost) said. The flu incubates in the body for one to three days, but lasts for three to seven days.

▶HOW SERIOUS

Colds and the flu aren't serious, but if you don't take care of your symptoms, they can both lead to more serious problems like pneumonia. Certain people are more likely to develop pneumonia from a cold or the flu, including the elderly; those with chronic conditions like asthma, emphysema, diabetes, or heart disease; and people whose immune systems have been weakened by such things as chemotherapy or by taking drugs like prednisone, says Dr. Rooney. Pneumonia develops when someone is lying down a lot (like you do when you're sick) and there's a lot of mucus in your body, which can't clear easily.

"You should see a doctor if any of your symptoms last more than five days," Dr. Rooney says. "Other than that, there's really nothing a doctor can do because colds and the flu cannot be helped by antibiotics."

If, however, your cold or flu is accompanied by an extremely high fever (105°F or above) or out-of-the ordinary symptoms (chest pain, blood in the mucus from your nose, or if your phlegm or mucus is green, brown, or bloody) don't wait: See a doctor pronto, Dr. Rooney advises. Of course, seeing a doctor each year between mid-October and mid-November to get a flu shot can help you avoid a trip to the doctor's office during flu season. And every person over 65 as well as those mentioned earlier who are more likely to develop pneumonia should get the shot, says Dr. Rooney. "There are three things to know about the flu shot," he says. "You need to get it once every year, it will only protect you against three types of flu, and it doesn't work until two weeks after you get it. So you can still get the flu during those two weeks, and you can also get a flu that isn't included in the shot." The shot is good for six months.

▶SOLUTIONS

Be selective. You're a guy who wants to cover all your bases, so you look for those cold and flu remedies that promise to erase every symptom, even ones you aren't sure you have. Think again.

"I tell my patients to simply ease each symptom with one medication," Dr. Rooney says. "And there's no reason to buy a brand name instead of generic."

Dr. Rooney recommends the following: To relieve the pain of headaches or muscle aches, use ibuprofen (Advil, Motrin). Do not take ibuprofen if you are allergic to aspirin or if you've had a recent ulcer, Dr. Rooney warns. To fight phlegm, look for guaifenesin (found in cough syrups such as Robitussin). If you're congested but don't have a cough, use pseudoephedrine (Sudafed). And to suppress a cough that keeps you up at night, use dextromethorphan (Vicks 44D or Robitussin DM). Once again, you should feel free to use the generic equivalents.

Follow the package directions on all medications. The perfect accompaniment to these medications is water, which will help thin the mucus that's plugging you up, Dr. Rooney says.

Did You Know?

Here are the makings of a great science project: 20 men in a windowless room, a poker game, vitamin C, and . . . a cold virus.

A few years ago Elliott Dick, Ph.D., now a retired professor of preventive medicine and former chief of the respiratory virus research laboratory at the University of Wisconsin Medical School in Madison, wanted to study vitamin C's effect on the common cold. He and his colleagues got 20 guys together to play a game of poker. They infected 8 of the men with a cold virus and watched it spread to the other 12 guys through sneezing, coughing, and passing cards among each other.

Now that they knew how colds spread, the good doctor and his colleagues conducted three more studies to find out if vitamin C could protect the men from the virus. In the three following studies, half of the guys took 2,000 milligrams of vitamin C, while the rest took placebos, for 3 ½ weeks. The men then resumed their poker playing. Vitamin C really did make a difference. Although everyone came down with colds, the vitamin C guys had less-severe cold symptoms, and those symptoms stuck around for less time. In fact, only one guy in the vitamin C group came down with an honest-to-goodness cold, while the placebo guys got what Dr. Dick calls real humdingers. Just be aware that some people experience diarrhea when taking more than 1,200 milligrams of vitamin C.

Supplement with vitamin C. Vitamin C can shorten the length of time your cold stays with you, but only if it's used right. "Take 500 milligrams of vitamin C every two hours at the first sign of a cold," says Devra Krassner, a doctor of naturopathic medicine and homeopathy in private practice in Portland, Maine. "You can decrease the frequency to three times a day as you improve. If you're not feeling better after four to five days, you should consult a doctor," advises Dr. Krassner.

Some people may experience diarrhea when taking more than 1,200 milligrams of vitamin C. "If you experience any stomach discomfort or diarrhea, decrease the dosage to a level at which you are no longer experiencing these symptoms," adds Dr. Krassner.

Think zinc. Suck on some zinc gluconate lozenges, which have been shown to decrease the length of time a cold lasts, Dr. Krassner says. Look for lozenges made without added sugars because that renders the zinc useless. Just remember that these lozenges are meant to be taken only for a short period of time, so don't exceed the manufacturer's directions.

And in case you're wondering, the zinc in your multivitamin and mineral tablets will not provide the same cold- and flu-fighting punch as the lozenges.

You need to let the zinc gluconate lozenges dissolve in your mouth, flooding your throat with zinc ions that help prevent the rhinoviruses from going on a rampage in your body.

▶ALTERNATIVE APPROACHES

Try an herbal remedy. When you feel the first symptoms of a cold or the flu coming on, take echinacea. This immune system–boosting herb fights colds and flu and could shorten the virus's stay, says Adriane Fugh-Berman, M.D., former head of field investigations for the Office of Alternative Medicine at the National Institutes of Health in Bethesda, Maryland.

Take two 100-milligram capsules of echinacea three or four times a day, or take 20 to 40 drops (40 drops equals about one dropperful) of tincture—a solution of the herb steeped in drinkable alcohol or a similar substance—three or four times a day, recommends David Edelberg, M.D., assistant professor of medicine at Rush Medical College; section chief of holistic medicine at Illinois Masonic Medical Center and Grant Hospital, all in Chicago; and founder of the American Whole Health Centers in Chicago, Denver, and Bethesda, Maryland. Just drop it in about a quarter-cup of water and drink, he says. You can find echinacea capsules and tincture at drugstores and health food stores.

"It's very important to take echinacea every few hours instead of just once a day because it doesn't stay in your system for very long," adds Dr. Fugh-Berman. Continue to take echinacea until you feel better, but no longer. You should not use echinacea for more than eight weeks in a row.

Add garlic. Garlic has shown itself to be a great aid to the immune system. "If you feel yourself starting to get sick, make a big pot of vegetable soup and add some fresh garlic, ginger, and onion, " says Elson Haas, M.D., director of the Preventive Medical Center of Marin in San Rafael, California, and author of *Staying Healthy with Nutrition* and *The Detox Diet*. "To have a more active effect, press two or three cloves and drop them straight into your bowl of soup."

If fresh garlic is a little too much for your stomach or breath, simply take two or three odorless garlic capsules three times a day. Look for 300- to 500-milligram capsules at a health food store, says Dr. Haas.

Obtain Oscillococcinum. No, you will never, ever be able to spell it. There's a good chance that you'll never even be able to pronounce it, but this homeopathic remedy does work to reduce the severity of flu symptoms. And really, isn't that all that matters?

"It's fabulous for the flu, especially when you are experiencing muscle aches, alternating feelings of hot and cold, and fever," says Dr. Krassner. "It works best when taken in the first 24 hours after onset of the symptoms."

It comes in packages of three or six vials and is available in many health food stores. Dr. Krassner recommends getting a three-vial pack and taking one vial every six hours. "If this is the correct remedy for your flu, you should feel better after three doses," she says.

Cook chicken soup. You don't have to actually pluck the feathers from the bird, but making yourself a nice pot of chicken soup as long as you're home alone feeling crummy will probably make you feel better.

"It's not a cure, but the steam coming up from the bowl will definitely make you more comfortable," Dr. Rooney says. Actually, there may be more to chicken soup's nose-clearing affect than just the steam. In a study done a few years ago by researchers at the University of Nebraska Medical Center in Omaha, chicken soup did seem to open airways and decrease phlegm production, at least for a little while. The researchers explained it this way: When a cold hits, blood cells called neutrophils rush to the troubled area to fight the invading virus or bacteria. It's the extra traffic in that spot that leads to your stuffed-up head and nose. In this study, the researchers discovered that chicken soup actually slowed the neutrophil attack, but which ingredient gives the soup its nose-clearing ability remains a mystery.

▶PREVENTIVE MEASURES

Pick your friends. A study conducted at Carnegie Mellon University in Pittsburgh has suggested that people with abundant social ties don't come down with colds as readily as people who have smaller social circles.

The key is to have lots of friends and activities in different aspects of your life. For example, studies have shown that people who are married but also take part in activities with friends, extended family, fellow workers, and social and religious groups live longer than their less-social counterparts. The theory is that having lots of friends and being involved with a variety of activities in life may help us deal more effectively with the stresses that lower immunity.

Don't pick your nose. "You pick up the virus from another hand, a doorknob, or some other object; then you unconsciously touch your nose and—wham!—you just put a cold virus in touch with your mucous cells," Dr. Rooney says. The same goes for your eyes or mouth. It's hard for your body to fight off an invitation like that. So keep your hands off your face.

Ease off the sweets. An excessive intake of sugar can lower the bacteria-killing effect of your white blood cells, says Dr. Haas. That means that it may be more difficult to fight off possible infections that come your way. Also, if you're eating a lot of sugar, you're probably not eating nutritious foods that contain the vitamins and minerals that will help your body stay healthy. "Sugar used consistently will undermine your health," Dr. Haas warns.

Wash your hands. By wash, we mean soap and water around every part of your hands, including under your fingernails. "Viruses live on hands," says Dr. Rooney. "If you wash your hands frequently, then you'll be less likely to catch a bug."

And if you're a father who doesn't want to catch whatever virus is going around your kids' school, make sure that your children get in the habit of scrubbing up at an early age.

Commuter Strain

▶PROBLEM

While traveling to and from work you become bored, irritated, frustrated. You might feel some stiffness in your back, rear-end, and legs from sitting too long.

▶CAUSE

Sometimes it seems as if your life consists of driving, driving, and more driving. The average American commute is just slightly more than 22 minutes one way, but we can think of lots of people who spend a couple of hours a day in their cars.

"There are two types of commuter strain," explains Robert Butterworth, Ph.D., a clinical psychologist in private practice in Los Angeles. "The first is someone who struggles with boredom because it takes him a long time to get from point A to point B. The second is someone who doesn't have far to go but is consistently stuck in traffic. He has to deal with a lot of frustration."

Meanwhile, both commuters have to cope with being physically confined to the interior of an automobile.

Or, perhaps you're one of the 5 percent of American commuters who take public transportation. Of course, that number is an average, reflecting the 25 percent of New Yorkers who ride trains and buses and the 0.3 percent of South Dakotans who do.

DO THIS NOW

Start humming. This will help counteract the effects of stress or a monotonous commute.

"It's like two to three minutes of sonic caffeine," says Don Campbell, a music researcher, director of the Mozart Effect Resource Center in St. Louis, and author of *The Mozart Effect.* "You're massaging your brain from the inside out."

Campbell says that you should stay on one pitch with a relaxed jaw when you begin to hum and don't think about using words. Then try to make an "a-a-ah" or "e-e-ee" sound. "This deepens your breath and releases tension, which recharges your body and brain," Campbell says.

Did You Know?

It's every guy's dream: Wake up, smell the coffee drip, read the sports page, then go to work—downstairs, in your bathrobe and slippers.

Oh, and earn a couple hundred thousand a year.

Well, anywhere from 9 million to 14 million people lived at least part of that dream in 1997. They telecommuted or worked at home during all or some of their workweek. And no, most of them didn't earn $200,000, although most telecommuters do earn more than the average $36,000 salary.

"Anyone who is a 'knowledge worker' is a good candidate for telecommuting," says Eddie Caine, president of TAC, the International Telework Association based in Washington, D.C.

So, who is a knowledge worker? He's someone whose job focuses on the processing of information. He may do a lot of phone work, scheduling, and thinking but requires minimal supervision to get his job done. That would include writing, telemarketing, auditing, data analysis, data processing, and other similar careers.

"Basically, if you're someone who drives to work, sits in front of a computer, and then drives right back home, you could telecommute," Caine says. "Remember, work is not just a place you go. It's a thing you do."

▶How Serious

It can ruin your day. And that can ruin your week. And before you know it, your commute has taken over your life. "If you're commuting 2 hours a day or 10 hours a week, then it can interfere with your family life," Dr. Butterworth says. "You can become a slave to your drive."

▶Solutions

Share the stress. More than 84 million Americans drive to work alone, while 15 million carpool, according to the U.S. Census Bureau. That's a shame, because carpooling can solve so many problems at once: energy consumption, boredom, and loneliness, just to name a few. One idea is to carpool a couple of times a week, rather than every day, in order to give yourself some "free" days to run errands after work or come in earlier or stay later, Dr. Butterworth says. Also, the variety of driving with someone else every couple of days will help combat some of the boredom associated with commuting.

Feed your head. Learn French, memorize inspirational speeches made by Vince Lombardi and Paul "Bear" Bryant, listen to Clive Cussler's new novel. When you're bored it's a sign that you need to stimulate your mind, so listening to books on tape is an almost-perfect solution to the problem.

"As long as a book on tape doesn't take away from your concentration, then it's a great way to eliminate boredom," Dr. Butterworth says. "I studied my graduate program work that way for almost a year."

Tune in to a variety show. If you find yourself getting upset or agitated during a drive, it's your body's way of saying, "You've been doing this too long," and even a 10-minute drive can become routine. "You can get complacent about short commutes and not even remember driving from one place to the other," Dr. Butterworth says.

Try to find a way to vary your routine: Find an alternate route; leave a half-hour earlier and see if the traffic is different; take a walk for 20 minutes before you ride home to see if you feel better during your drive. "Change something about your commute," Dr. Butterworth says. "Even a slightly longer route might make a positive difference in your life."

▶ALTERNATIVE APPROACHES

Be a wheel man. Next time you're stuck in rush-hour hell, simply squeeze the steering wheel as hard as you can for a count of five, then relax. "Really focus on the release part," says Charles Kuntzleman, Ed.D., professor of kinesiology at the University of Michigan in Ann Arbor. "That stimulates a relaxation response in the body, which will help you be more loose and limber when you get to work or head to the gym." This one simple exercise not only helps relieve rush-hour stress but also is a good grip-strengthener.

Don't be a stiff. We know that you're in a small space, but move as much as possible. One way is by doing simple isometric exercises that alternately tense and relax muscle groups like your arms and legs. These exercises allow the driver to get some relief from muscle tension without endangering driving, says Dr. Butterworth. And if sitting still is causing you to feel edgy during your drive, then park at a nearby mall and walk around a store for a few minutes, he adds.

▶PREVENTIVE MEASURES

Do the math. "Commuters should take a look at how much their time on the road is taking away from their quality of life," Dr. Butterworth advises. "Is it worth the extra $5,000 you're earning? You might not even be making up that difference when you consider wear and tear on your car, not to mention on your nerves."

In other words, don't assume that an aggravating commute is simply a part of living in today's world. "Try to come up with a mathematical formula, figuring in what you're spending on babysitters and other extra things, as well as how much it costs you to be away from your family and friends for long periods of time, to determine if your commute is worth the hassle," Dr. Butterworth says.

Congestion

▶PROBLEM

You can't breathe, but you're not underwater. Your nose feels as if it's partially stuffed with cotton and you're coughing a bit. Sneezing? You only wish you owned stock in Kleenex.

What's happening? The technical explanation is that the mucous membranes in your mouth and throat are discharging increased amounts of mucus, says Miles Greenberg, a naturopathic and homeopathic physician with the Natural Health and Pain Relief Clinic in Kauai, Hawaii. Mucus—the thin, clear substance that lines the airway—is made of fat, protein, enzymes, and infection-fighting white blood cells. Its purpose is to keep inhaled dust, fumes, pollen, bacteria, and viruses from entering your lungs. Your body, which always produces various forms of mucus in numerous sites throughout your body, is now overproducing it to defend against an allergy, virus, or bacterium that has begun to invade your head, nose, throat, or chest. If the congestion is in your head, then you also have swelling of those membranes.

▶CAUSE

Congestion is a symptom of another problem, most likely a cold, flu, sinusitis, or allergy.

"If you wake up congested in the morning without other accompanying symptoms, then you may have an allergy to something in your bedroom," says Devra Krassner, a doctor of naturopathic medicine and homeopathy in private practice in Portland, Maine. "You should consider your pets, dust, pollen, the down feathers in your comforter, or even the detergent you use." You could also be sensitive to certain foods that you are eating

On the other hand, if you also have a yellow or green discharge from your nose and pain in your face or a headache, then you probably have sinusitis.

"Sometimes physical obstructions cause congestion," says David Rooney, M.D., a family physician with Southern Chester County Family Practice Associates in Oxford, Pennsylvania. "It's pretty common for a guy who has been hit in the nose to be congested, especially in one nostril."

▶HOW SERIOUS

Congestion itself is annoying but not serious. More important to assess is the underlying cause. A cold or flu just requires soothing remedies, not a cure. But sinusitis, for example, needs to be treated; and allergies need to be dealt with.

Also, there is the possibility that enlarged adenoids or polyps are causing the problem, especially if you're having difficulty breathing. If you are congested for more than five days, see your doctor.

▶SOLUTIONS

Get the right un-stuff. The main ingredient in Sudafed and other decongestants, pseudoephedrine, will unstuff your stuffiness. "Take 60 milligrams every six hours, and feel free to use the generic brands rather than the more expensive brand names," Dr. Rooney says. He also advises his patients to take this medication at the first sign of congestion if they are predisposed to developing sinus infections, and to continue using it for four or five days or until congestion is gone or nearly gone. It could ward off more serious problems.

Sip a steaming cup of chicken soup. It may help uncork your clogged nasal passages and turn off your phlegm-making machinery. In an experiment at the University of Nebraska Medical Center in Omaha, chicken soup (homemade, using a real grandma's recipe) was found to slow the action of infection-fighting white blood cells, called neutrophils, in test tubes. Slowing this onslaught of neutrophils may help reduce inflammation, a trigger for phlegm production, speculates Stephen Rennard, M.D., professor of pulmonary and critical medicine at the University of Nebraska Medical Center. Add a dash of ground red pepper or fresh ginger, too. Hot spices will speed up the soup's phlegm-cutting power.

Steam it out. Take a hot, steamy shower. "Warm, moist air helps loosen secretions, both in the chest and in the head," says Ronald Greeno, M.D., co-director of respiratory therapy pulmonary function at Good Samaritan Hospital in Los Angeles. "It opens your airways and helps stimulate coughing, which helps loosen phlegm so that you can cough it up."

Stay hydrated. If you have very thick mucus, drink at least eight, eight-ounce glasses of water a day, recommends Dr. Greeno. Water will help thin the phlegm so that it's easier to cough out, he says.

History Lesson

Shiki Masaoka, a Japanese poet, died of tuberculosis at age 35 on September 19, 1902, after being bedridden for seven years. During this time, one of Shiki's most bothersome symptoms was coughing up phlegm, which, according to legend, was treated with the fluid from a plant called the sponge gourd. Liquid collected during a full moon was supposed to be especially powerful.

Apparently, the sponge-gourd juice didn't work, at least not for Shiki. (Or maybe his relatives collected the last batch on a moonless night.) The day before he died, coughing and weak, Shiki wrote a final haiku:

gallons of phlegm
even the gourd water
couldn't clear it up

Spray salt in your nose. Saline nasal sprays are a great temporary source of relief, especially if you're congested because of dry conditions at night. "I tell my patients to keep it near their bed and use it before they go to sleep," Dr. Rooney says. "It helps them breathe, and there's no downside."

Hand over the handkerchief, chief. A neatly folded handkerchief in the breast pocket of a blue blazer makes a striking fashion statement. Just make sure that you leave it there. When you have to blow your nose, grab a tissue instead. "I can't even imagine why a guy would use a handkerchief," Dr. Rooney says. "It's gross, and it's even grosser for the person washing it."

They're more than just gross, though, Dr. Rooney warns. Handkerchiefs also are unsanitary and the perfect way to spread your germs to another human being, or to even possibly reinfect yourself if what you're sneezing out is infected mucus.

▶ALTERNATIVE APPROACHES

Start your day with cayenne. Put a quarter-teaspoon to a half-teaspoon of ground red pepper in a four-ounce glass of water and drink that every morning for about a week, or until the congestion goes away, says Christopher Trahan, a doctor of Oriental medicine and licensed acupuncturist in private practice in New York City. This may cause a burning sensation in your throat, so use your personal taste and tolerance.

Find some fenugreek. Make a tea by simmering about a tablespoon of fenugreek seeds in a couple of cups of water for 10 to 15 minutes, says Dr. Trahan. "Drink parts of that during the day; it doesn't have to be hot. If you don't like the taste, feel free to add some cinnamon," he says. You can also buy it ground up as powder, then add it, to taste, to grains or soup. Fenugreek is a component of curry powder and can be used daily. It is available in grocery stores or specialty gourmet shops.

Mull the benefits of mullein. Take 7 to 10 drops of mullein tincture (available in health food stores) in a quarter-cup of water every two to three hours, suggests Amy Rothenberg, a doctor of naturopathy in Amherst, Massachusetts, and editor of the *New England Journal of Homeopathy*. In herbal lingo, mullein is a demulcent, which means that it soothes irritated mucous membranes and helps mucus slide out a little bit easier.

▶PREVENTIVE MEASURES

Eliminate dairy products. This is a very common food sensitivity, and often an allergy to dairy will reveal itself as stuffiness. "If you take dairy products (milk, cheese, yogurt, ice cream, and butter) out of your diet for 7 to 10 days and notice an improvement, then you've probably just discovered the cause of your congestion," Dr. Krassner says.

Even if you think that you might be allergic to dairy, it's unlikely that you'll have to give it up forever. "We all have a different threshold for how much of any certain food or allergen we can tolerate," Dr. Krassner explains. "During the winter, for instance, a dairy sensitivity may combine with the stresses of exposure to viruses, a closed home, and heating systems to push you over the allergy threshold to the point at which you become symptomatic."

To see if you can tolerate dairy in your diet again, Dr. Krassner suggests adding a few servings for a day and then wait a couple of days to see if you have any symptoms.

Avoid over-the-counter medicated nasal sprays. We're talking serious addiction here, with serious side effects. These sprays aren't the same as saline sprays, which say "saline" right on the package. Instead, these are medicated sprays available over-the-counter.

"We actually have to wean people off those sprays," says Dr. Rooney. "If you rely on a nonprescription nasal spray to relieve your congestion, you develop a medically induced chronic runny nose." In other words, your nose is going to wait for the spray in order to decongest. They are not a solution to the problem and, in fact, will make you even more congested in the long run.

Constipation

▶PROBLEM

Constipation could mean that you have bowel movements so infrequently that you become uncomfortable. Or it could mean you have regular bowel movements—but with stools that are difficult, even painful, to pass. Either way, the National Center for Health Statistics reported in 1997 that more than a million men in the United States complained of constipation in a recent two-year period, and 71.6 percent of these cases involved at least one visit to the doctor.

▶CAUSE

Usually, it's a shortage of fiber and fluid in your diet. Both are essential if your stool is to have the right consistency for a timely, comfortable trip through the bowel. But a few other culprits can tighten you up, too. Certain medications can cause irregular bowel function, leaving you with either constipation or diarrhea. Constipation is also common in men who lead hectic, stressful, unhealthy lives. And constipation can beget constipation; continual straining on the toilet stretches and damages the nerves in the muscles that you use to go.

▶HOW SERIOUS

If you find yourself on the throne reading *Sports Illustrated* cover to cover just once in awhile, don't sweat it. An uptake in fiber and fluids likely will get things moving again, says James Scala, Ph.D., a nutritionist in Lafayette, California, and author of *Eating Right for a Bad Gut*. But if constipation keeps recurring, it might mean that you have irritable bowel syndrome, colitis (inflam-

---

DO THIS NOW

Stir two teaspoons of honey into a 10-ounce glass of warm water. Drink this lubricating liquid on an empty stomach and you'll be relieved within a half-hour, says Maoshing Ni, Ph.D., a doctor of Oriental medicine, licensed acupuncturist, and director of Tao of Wellness, a professional acupuncture corporation in Santa Monica, California. Dr. Ni recommends repeating this treatment as needed up to three times a day.

mation of the colon), or diverticulitis (swelling in the walls of the large intestine). When constipation causes stop-what-you-are-doing pain or is accompanied by severe cramping or abdominal swelling, it's time to see a doctor, Dr. Scala says.

▶SOLUTIONS

Hit the bottle. Get a water bottle and constantly sip from it; in time, the water should help soften things up. The average man needs to drink about a gallon of water daily. But that amount can vary by person and by circumstance; if you are in the sun all day, you could need twice as much, says Dr. Scala.

Hug a mug. Hot beverages such as coffee also are favorites for relieving constipation, as warm liquids help relax the bowel walls, says Maoshing Ni, Ph.D., a doctor of Oriental medicine, licensed acupuncturist, and director of Tao of Wellness, a professional acupuncture corporation in Santa Monica, California. He recommends drinking only one cup of coffee or some other warm liquid a day and suggests using it as a last resort—only if other constipation treatments don't work.

Probe your prescriptions. If you're taking any medications, check with your doctor about the possibility of them causing your problem. Many commonly used drugs, including some heart disease medications, cause constipation as a side effect. If the drug is essential, you may need to pay extra attention to your eating and lifestyle habits to stay regular, says Sidney Phillips, M.D., professor of medicine in the Gastroenterology Research Unit at the Mayo Clinic in Rochester, Minnesota.

Look into laxatives. If your stool becomes small, hard, and difficult to pass, a simple saline laxative like milk of magnesia is harmless in the short term, says Dr. Phillips. But if constipation is a recurring problem, look to your diet and lifestyle and use laxatives regularly (two times a week) only as a last resort. If you feel the need to use them more frequently, you should consult with your doctor. Overuse may weaken your bowels, making you dependent on the laxative.

Suppositories also can be habit-forming. They're useful when you have normal movement of material all the way through the colon and down to the rectum but can't complete that final step of pushing out the stool. Over-the-counter medicines like glycerin suppositories can give you relief, and they should only be used to help you get back into good habits, says Dr. Phillips. "When used for several weeks on a daily or every-other-day basis, stimulation of bowel movements may lead to a better-trained bowel, which will continue without the use of stimulating agents," he says.

▶ALTERNATIVE APPROACHES

Swallow some seeds. The lubricating effect of pine nuts, flaxseed, and sesame seeds can all help ease a mild case of constipation, says Dr. Ni. Eating a handful of any of these, now available in many grocery stores, should do the trick. Dr. Ni recommends eating a handful once a day, chewing them well, and drinking a glass of water afterward.

Become a juice man. Apple juice is a tried-and-true elixir for mild constipation, but it'll work even better when you mix four ounces of apple juice with four ounces of aloe vera juice (which can be found in most health food stores), says Dr. Ni. Drink it up on an empty stomach first thing in the morning for the quickest relief. Make this juice mixture part of your daily regimen to keep your bowel healthy. You can drink one glass a day without any side effects, Dr. Ni says.

Find the pressure point. In the ancient disciplines of acupressure and acupuncture, the miracle point for relieving constipation is the "hegu," located in the web between the index finger and the thumb. About a thumb's width down from the web on either hand, squeeze the hegu with the thumb and index finger of your other hand. Breathe deeply and continue periodically throughout the day until you feel the urge to visit the men's room, says Robert Rakowski, D.C., a chiropractic physician, acupuncturist, and clinic director of the Natural Medicine Center in Houston.

MEN'S HEALTH INDEX

Sitting on a toilet with your favorite magazine can be a relaxing way to wait for poop to come, but if the men's room just isn't doing it for you, here are five movies that will remind you to do your duty.

1. *Monty Python and the Holy Grail* **(Great Britain, 1975)— Frenchmen empty several chamber pots (and catapult a few cows and other farm animals) from the top of a castle onto the heads of King Arthur and the knights of the Round Table.**
2. *Dances with Wolves* **(1990)— Union soldiers wipe themselves with pages of Kevin Costner's journal.**
3. *The Holy Mountain* **(Germany, 1974)—An alchemist transforms feces into gold. Incentive enough for you?**
4. *Back to the Future* **(1985)—In a traffic accident, a truckload of manure is dumped into a convertible.**
5. *The Discreet Charm of the Bourgeoisie* **(France, 1972)—Guests sit around the "dinner" table on toilets, talking, defecating, and passing around toilet paper on silver trays. Occasionally, the guests excuse themselves and go into a little room to eat something.**

Rub it out. Massage the area around the belly button in a clockwise fashion to stimulate bowel movement, suggests Dr. Ni. Concentrate on the abdomen, and repeat this circular motion 100 times, or even more, until you feel the urge to go.

Another useful massage technique that Dr. Rakowski recommends is actually a direct stimulation of the colon itself. The colon begins on your right side just above the hip bone and travels up the right side to about the rib cage, across the bottom of the rib cage to your left side, and, finally, down the left side to the hip bone. If you massage along this path, which follows the motion of flow inside your colon, you can stimulate bowel movement. Do this massage in one-minute intervals and repeat as needed until you feel relief.

▶PREVENTIVE MEASURES

Feast on fiber. Two types of dietary fiber, soluble and insoluble, work together to keep your bowel movements regular. Insoluble fiber, found in vegetables and wheat bran, absorbs water and increases in bulk as it passes through your bowel. This makes for a speedy journey through your colon. To ensure that your diet is rich in this bulk-forming fiber, get on it first thing in the morning, says Dr. Scala. A breakfast of whole-grain cereal such as All Bran or Fiber One will provide 10 to 13 grams of fiber before you even walk out the door. (The American Dietetic Association recommends eating 20 to 35 grams total of dietary fiber daily.)

Soluble fiber—found in fruits, some beans, and grains such as oats, rye, and barley—dissolves in water to form a gel within the digestive system that helps soften stools and keeps them from moving too quickly through your bowel. This gel also helps increase the rate at which nutrients from food are absorbed into the bloodstream. Ripe bananas, apples, prunes, figs, and raisins are all handy snacks of soluble fiber.

Try supplements. Fiber supplements such as psyllium, which can be bought in health food stores and drugstores, are also good bowel regulators. Psyllium supplements come in powder and capsule form. Dr. Scala doesn't recommend taking capsules because you have to take so many to get the fiber you need. Mixing one tablespoon of a powdered psyllium supplement in a glass of water two or three times a day is a more convenient way to get extra fiber, Dr. Scala says. Dr. Scala also recommends commercial supplements such as Metamucil and Perdiem, which contain psyllium and other gums that ease bowel movement. Take these as you would other powdered psyllium supplements.

People with chronic constipation should take these supplements every day, Dr. Scala says.

Move to keep moving. Although it hasn't been easy to prove that exercise helps move material through the colon more rapidly, there is evidence that not moving enough can cause constipation, says Philip Miner, M.D., a gastroenterologist with the Oklahoma Center for Digestive Medicine and president and medical director of the Oklahoma Foundation for Digestive Research, both in Oklahoma City. It's also fairly well known in running circles that running may give you "runner's trots." In other words, exercise—especially running—appears to speed up bowel movement.

Corns and Bunions

▶ PROBLEM

Repeated pressure from ill-fitting shoes aggravates the toe or the irritated area and speeds up the production of hardened, callused skin, forming a corn. A bunion is a big bump on the side of the foot just below the big toe or the smallest (baby) toe—the result of an out-of-line toe joint.

▶ CAUSE

Corns are caused by shoes that don't fit. As men reach their forties and fifties, ligaments in the foot may start to stretch and expand, which may cause a jump up in size and width. But because their shoe size hasn't changed since high school, many men keep shoving those feet into shoes that don't fit, and that can cause corns. If you develop bunions, though, your family history probably has more to do with it than your footwear. You inherit the shape of your foot from your ancestors. If they had certain foot deformities that made them more susceptible to bunions, you may be destined to develop them as well.

▶ HOW SERIOUS

Both corns and bunions can be unbelievably painful. Most corns can be managed from home, although those that cause major pain should be seen by a doctor. Anyone who has diabetes or any other vascular problem should never try to self-treat corns and bunions. They may ulcerate, get infected, and eventually lead to amputation, says Pamela Colman, D.P.M., a medical officer for the American Podiatric Medical Association in Bethesda, Maryland. People can live with the discomfort of a bunion. But severe bunion pain can put a damper on your lifestyle, making it impossible for you to enjoy physical activity as

> **DO THIS NOW**
>
> Put a bandage, a piece of gauze, or a nonmedicated corn pad around the corn. Bunion pads, which can be made of cotton or bought in a drugstore, cushion the bunion, protecting it from further irritation while wearing shoes, says Pamela Colman, D.P.M., a medical officer for the American Podiatric Medical Association in Bethesda, Maryland.

Did You Know?

Corns were one of the most reported injuries of 265 surveyed runners in the 1994 New York City Marathon.

simple as walking. You should consider bunion surgery when the pain is unrelieved by properly fitted shoes, when the toe deformity gets progressively worse, and when you can no longer fit into any reasonable shoes, says Dr. Colman.

▶SOLUTIONS

Change your shoes. For shoes to fit well, you should be able to wiggle your toes. Although a change of footwear won't rid you of bunions, it may make them less painful. If you can get away with it, wear athletic shoes as often as you can, says David C. Novicki, D.P.M., president of New Haven Foot Surgeons in New Haven, Connecticut, and past president of the American College of Foot and Ankle Surgeons in Chicago. They provide excellent comfort and support for people with bunions.

Give them a good soak. Soak both your corns and bunions after a long day on your feet. The warm water softens the corns, making them easier to remove, Dr. Colman says. A relaxing foot bath for 20 minutes in lukewarm water may also help soothe painful bunions.

Keep a file. After a shower or a foot soak, use a pumice stone to file down your corns. A pumice stone is a piece of hardened lava rock that gently files down and smoothes out hardened skin. Don't file down the entire corn in one sitting because it will irritate the area, Dr. Colman warns. Work at it a little bit each night, she advises.

Avoid corn treatments. Over-the-counter corn treatments contain acid and could cause more damage to your foot, says Dr. Novicki. "Corn plasters are very dangerous. A concentrated amount can eat its way through the skin. It can create an ulcer with a secondary infection," he warns.

▶ALTERNATIVE APPROACHES

Cover your feet in castor oil. Massage your feet with castor oil every night, says Andrea D. Sullivan, Ph.D., a doctor of naturopathy; president of Sullivan and Associates Center for Natural Healing in Washington, D.C.; and author of *A Path to Healing*. Castor oil softens the corns, making them less painful and easier to file down. The oil and massage will reduce the tension and pain in the bunion as well.

Pick pineapple. Take a little of the peel from a fresh pineapple and wipe it directly on your bunion, recommends James A. Duke, Ph.D., the world's foremost authority on healing herbs and author of *The Green Pharmacy*. Pineapples contain a compound called bromelain, which is often used as an anti-inflammatory agent. Bromelain reduces swelling and pain in irritated bunions, Dr. Duke says. Taking 250 to 500 milligrams of pure bromelain in capsule form three times a day can provide the same relief, he says. The capsules are available at health food stores and in some drugstores.

▶PREVENTIVE MEASURES

Give your toes room. Both corns and bunions are aggravated by not having enough room in the toe area. Buy shoes with a wide toe box, Dr. Colman says. A wider, roomier toe box keeps the toes from rubbing against the shoe, which will prevent corns. A wider toe box will also be more comfortable and help quell the inflammation and pain of a bunion. To get the right-size shoe, have your feet measured for length and width every time you buy a shoe. As you get older, your feet may expand, meaning that you may have to go up in size, Dr. Colman says. Also, buy shoes in the afternoon or evening because your feet swell later in the day, she adds.

Listen to your feet. Corns don't just show up one day. When you start to feel pain or start developing a callus on your feet or toes, act immediately. "You'll start feeling discomfort initially, and that's an indication that the foot is being irritated," Dr. Colman says. Change your shoes, pad the irritated area, and soak and soften the foot.

Treat your feet to special shoes. People predisposed to developing bunions can buy special orthopedic shoes. These are designed to give support or keep bunion pain from becoming unbearable. The shoes are deeper and wider than regular footwear, Dr. Colman says. Check out an orthopedic footwear store or see your podiatrist to get this therapeutic shoewear.

Coughing

▶PROBLEM

Coughing is, most often, a natural reflex that clears the throat and helps keep irritants out of the lungs. A productive cough brings phlegm up so that you can spit it out. And that's just what you want to do.

However, a dry, hacking cough is one that doesn't bring up phlegm. It only irritates your throat, making you cough more, and that's when the cough isn't "natural," says Douglas Lakin, M.D., a physician with the Town Center Medical Group in Scottsdale, Arizona.

"If you keep coughing unproductively, you're further irritating those passages, which makes it harder to stop coughing," Dr. Lakin says.

▶CAUSE

"A nonproductive cough is usually associated with irritation from above the throat, such as postnasal drip," says Miles Greenberg, a naturopathic and homeopathic physician with the Natural Health and Pain Relief Clinic in Kauai, Hawaii. "The discharge irritates your throat and causes coughing."

"A productive cough indicates an infection or the production of increased secretion," says Leif Christiansen, D.O., a physician with the Perkiomen Internal Medicine Group in Mount Penn, Pennsylvania. "An unproductive cough can also be infectious, but not usually. It most often represents an irritant, such as smoking or asthma."

▶How Serious

Coughing is, most often, a symptom of a cold, flu, or allergy. But it can also be the first sign of a serious illness, such as asthma (if you're coughing at night and wheezing), lung cancer, pneumonia, tuberculosis, or heart disease. Barring those scenarios, however, a cough is like all those athletes who refer to themselves in the third person—just plain annoying.

How do you determine if your cough is a sign of something more serious? Look at the phlegm you're producing. "Clear, watery, foamy phlegm usually signifies a viral infection and you don't need to see a doctor about that," says David Rooney, M.D., a family physician with Southern Chester County Family Practice Associates in Oxford, Pennsylvania. "But if your phlegm is yellow or brown, or if you've been coughing for a long time and have a high fever, you need to see a doctor."

It's also time to see a doctor if your cough sticks around for more than five days, Dr. Rooney says. This is especially true if you smoke.

▶Solutions

Know your syrups. If you have a productive cough, reach for an over-the-counter syrup with guaifenesin, which is found in Robitussin and many generic brands. "It's an expectorant that will help get the junk out of your chest," Dr. Rooney says. Follow label directions.

If, however, you need to quiet your cough in order to sleep or are experiencing a dry, hacking cough, try one of the syrups that lists dextromethorphan as an ingredient (Robitussin DM, for example). "It's very mild and won't squash your phlegm production too much," Dr. Rooney says. Again, follow label directions.

Just because a syrup has lots of other ingredients doesn't make it a better buy, Dr. Rooney says. Most combination remedies either have side effects or target symptoms that you don't even have, he says. "I prefer single solutions to problems," says Dr. Rooney. "There's no reason to pull out a whole arsenal of medications just for a cough."

Rub it in. Vicks VapoRub, which uses the scents of oil, camphor, and eucalyptus, among others to help clear congestion, probably won't cure anything, Dr. Rooney says. But it will probably provide some relief to irritated respiratory passages, which is reason enough to give this blast-from-the-past remedy a try. Follow label directions.

Breathe steam. Fill your bathroom sink with hot water, put your head over it, and breathe the steam for about 10 minutes, Dr. Lakin advises. For greater effectiveness, use a towel over your head to keep the moisture contained. The steam will ease the irritation, and that will help reduce the urge to cough. This technique is particularly helpful if your cough wakes you up at night. An unproductive cough is not worth a lost night of sleep.

Did You Know?

They're the words no man likes to hear: "Turn your head and cough." Given where your doctor's fingers are when he asks that question, exactly what, you'd like to know, does this have to do with coughing?

"Actually, we're checking for a hernia," says David Rooney, M.D., a family physician with Southern Chester County Family Practice Associates in Oxford, Pennsylvania. "There is increased pressure in that area when you cough, so we're feeling for a weakness because that usually means you have a hernia."

So why do you have to turn your head? "So that you don't cough in the doctor's face," Dr. Rooney explains.

▶ALTERNATIVE APPROACHES

Lick it with licorice. Suck on a licorice lozenge. "Make sure that you're getting a lozenge that has real licorice in it, not just anise oil. It will say that it contains either licorice or licorice root" says Miles Greenberg, a naturopathic and homeopathic physician with the Natural Health and Pain Relief Clinic in Kauai, Hawaii. Sorry, guys, but that means that Twizzlers don't count. Licorice root breaks down the phlegm and also soothes the irritated passageways throughout your respiratory tract.

You can also find licorice teas in health food stores, but once again, be sure that it's the real thing. (It should list licorice root as an ingredient.) You'll want to use the lozenges and teas rather than licorice in a capsule because that way, it will touch the irritated areas of your throat.

Lozenges can be used every two to four hours, and you can drink four to six cups of licorice tea a day. These herbal remedies are best used during an acute period of coughing and not daily. If you want to make a tea of leaves and ground roots, steep it for 5 minutes. If you are using whole roots and stems, boil it for about 15 minutes.

Be aware that prolonged use or high doses are not recommended except under the supervision of a qualified health practitioner. Don't take it at all if you have diabetes, high blood pressure, liver disorders, severe kidney insufficiency, or abnormally low potassium levels in your blood. It can cause potassium depletion and sodium retention, resulting in such symptoms as high blood pressure, edema, headache, and vertigo.

Drink your meals. If your nagging cough kills your appetite for solid foods, just drink clear broths or miso soup because your body still needs nutrients to fight what's ailing you, Dr. Greenberg says. Also, cook a base of carrots (about 60 to 70 percent) in some water and add beets, zucchini, celery, or parsley. Blend it or juice it and drink as much as you're thirsty for during the day until the congestion is gone. This is usually two or three days.

Try home sweet homeopathy. There is a homeopathic remedy for different kinds of coughs, Dr. Greenberg says. Here are three that Dr. Greenberg says you'll be likely to find at your local health food store.

- Antimonium crudum. Use if a cough is slow to resolve, you have a red throat, and you feel irritable; also if your cough gets worse in a warm room and your voice sounds different, especially if its hoarse.
- Arsenicum album. Use if you feel chilly and thirsty, exhausted, but restless; also if your cough is worse when you're lying down and you have a burning sensation in your chest with very little expectoration.
- Carbovegitalis. Use if your cough is accompanied by low vitality, a pale complexion, and wheezing and you crave open air or fanning.

You should take one dose at the 12C or 30C concentration of these medicines every three to four hours until symptoms improve, then take less often until the congestion clears, says Dr. Greenberg. If the symptoms change or existing symptoms become aggravated, the homeopathic remedy should be discontinued. If you don't experience relief within a day or two, then the medicine you've chosen may not be the right one. You can feel free to try another remedy without any risk. Just follow label directions.

▶PREVENTIVE MEASURES

Open the window. If you don't have other symptoms such as fever or runny nose, coughs are often a sign that something in the air is irritating your lungs or the lining of your throat. Simply getting out in the fresh air or using a humidifier in a dry room will help keep your lungs soothed, says Dr. Greenberg.

Play the daily double. Echinacea and goldenseal are two herbs that are becoming more familiar in family medicine chests to help fight colds, flus, coughs, and sore throats, says Elson Haas, M.D., director of the Preventive Medical Center of Marin in San Rafael, California, and author of *Staying Healthy with Nutrition*. You can use both during the winter or when you feel that you might be coming down with something. They are equally good on their own or in a combination that's ready-made. (Zand makes a good product called Insure Herbal, which is a tincture that features both herbs, Dr. Haas says. You can find this remedy in health food stores and many drugstores.) Use a dropperful in water or straight on your tongue three or four times a day, says Dr. Haas.

Note that echinacea should not be taken for more than eight weeks straight. Also, do not take it if you have tuberculosis, leukoses, collagenosis, multiple sclerosis, AIDS, HIV infections, or other autoimmune diseases.

Dandruff

▶PROBLEM

Dandruff is a catchall word used to describe any flaking or scaling of the scalp, says Steven S. Greenbaum, M.D., director of the Skin and Laser Surgery Center of Pennsylvania in Philadelphia. The use of the word *any* here is key. Some guys might have only a few errant flecks of white on their shoulders, while others look like they've been sprinkled with grated cheese.

▶CAUSE

The cause is dead skin cells. Normally, you shed old cells from your scalp as new ones push their way to the surface, a process that should take 28 days. For some reason, some folks who have dandruff (and that's about 20 percent of us) may shed the cells on their scalps twice as fast as people who don't. Guys also tend to have problem dandruff more often than women. That's because male hormones, such as testosterone, can lead to an over-oily scalp, resulting in increased flakiness.

▶HOW SERIOUS

A few flakes now and again are nothing much to worry about, but severe dandruff can affect a guy's social or professional standing. Dandruff can also signal other skin problems. If your scalp is red, inflamed, or extremely scaly, experts recommend that you consult a dermatologist. You may have a condition such as seborrheic dermatitis or psoriasis and need a prescription-only medication to clear it up.

There's also some evidence that certain types of dandruff are caused by elevated levels of a common yeast, *Pityrosporum orbiculare*, that feeds on body

DO THIS NOW

Get a silicone-based styling spray, spritz it through your hair, and brush, says Richard Michael, owner of the Richard Michael Salon in Fountain Valley, California. These sprays (often called glossers or luminators) won't make your hair oily, says Michael. What they will do is make your hair just slick enough for the flakes to slide out of your hair.

Did You Know?

Even bald men can have dandruff.

oils. So if the following tips don't stem your blizzard of flakes, ask a doctor about using a prescription antidandruff shampoo, such as Nizoral. This product contains ketoconazole, an antifungal medication that kills this yeast.

▶SOLUTIONS

Work yourself into a lather. Wash your hair every day, says Robert Schosser, M.D., chief of the division of dermatology at the University of Kentucky A. B. Chandler Medical Center in Lexington. A daily shampoo will help dislodge the scalp flakes that ultimately end up on your shoulders.

Try stronger medicine. If a daily shampooing with your regular brand doesn't help, switch to an over-the-counter medicated antidandruff shampoo, says Dr. Schosser. These nonprescription products contain a variety of active ingredients that either slow cell growth or loosen and remove cell overgrowth. Finding a dandruff shampoo that works for you is a matter of trial and error, so if one doesn't show results in about two weeks, try another.

Shampoo right. To bring out the full power of a medicated dandruff shampoo, let it sit on your head for a full 10 minutes, says Dr. Schosser. To save time, shampoo while you shave: Wet your hair with warm water and lather up at the sink. Let your scalp marinate while you shave. Then, step into the shower, rinsing away the shampoo just before you get out.

Switch shampoos. If your medicated dandruff shampoo isn't working as well as it used to, switch to another brand with a different active ingredient, suggests Dr. Greenbaum. Products that contain selenium sulfide (Selsun Blue) remove the buildup of cells on your scalp, slow cell growth, and have an antifungal effect. Those formulated with pyrithione zinc (Head and Shoulders) or coal tar (Tegrin, Denorex) slow cell growth. Shampoos that contain salicylic acid (Scalpicin) remove excess cells and retard cell growth.

Give the gel a rest. If you slick back your hair with gel, or control it with a dollop of mousse, stop using these products for a few days and see if your dandruff improves. Gels and mousse tend to flake as they dry, and it's easy to mistake these flakes for dandruff, says Dr. Schosser.

▶ALTERNATIVE APPROACHES

Rub in *brahmi*. Massage your scalp with *brahmi* oil, suggests Scott Gerson, M.D., an expert in Ayurvedic medicine in private practice in Brewster, New York, and New York City. The oil's main ingredients—sesame oil and the juice and leaves from an aquatic plant called *brahmi*—help cool and moisten the scalp, prevent dryness, and dislodge flakes, says Dr. Gerson. Before you go to bed, rub a small amount of the oil into your scalp. Put a towel over your pillow so that the oil doesn't leave a stain. Wash out the oil in the morning during your regular shampooing. You'll find *brahmi* oil through mail-order companies that specialize in Ayurvedic herbs.

Rinse with vinegar. After you shampoo, rinse your hair with a mixture of one tablespoon apple cider vinegar and one quart of water, suggests Dr. Gerson. The rinse helps fight dandruff by normalizing the scalp's natural pH balance, he says.

▶PREVENTIVE MEASURES

Try a low blow. Use the lowest heat setting on your blow-dryer, suggests Dr. Greenbaum. Blow-drying on "high" may dry your hair faster, but it can also parch the skin on your scalp and make dandruff worse.

Cover up. If your dandruff tends to get worse in the winter, wear a hat when you're outdoors, suggests Dr. Greenbaum. Exposure to cold, dry air can leach the moisture from your scalp, causing flakiness.

Delayed Ejaculation

▶PROBLEM

During intercourse, it takes you a lot longer to ejaculate than either you or your partner would like.

▶CAUSE

In older men, "it may just be one of the consequences of aging," says Robert Birch, Ph.D., a sex therapist in Columbus, Ohio, and author of *Male Sexual Endurance*. Certain medications, such as antidepressants, may delay ejaculation. So can injuries to the nervous system. Some men find that they require a long time to ejaculate when wearing a condom because of reduced sensitivity. Others are uncomfortable with intimacy. But the most common cause in younger men is simply excessive masturbation, says Dr. Birch.

DO THIS NOW

Some guys have trouble ejaculating because their partner is too dry, and sandpaper sex just doesn't do it for them. Try using a water-based lubricant such as Astroglide, advises Robert Birch, Ph.D., a sex therapist in Columbus, Ohio, and author of *Male Sexual Endurance*. Slather it all over your equipment and hers.

▶HOW SERIOUS

Delayed ejaculation, also called inhibited or retarded ejaculation, can be particularly nettlesome if a couple is trying to make a baby and perhaps having intercourse more than usual. It can play on a guy's mind, perhaps to the point where he frets so much about ejaculating that he now starts having problems getting erections, says Dr. Birch. And the partner of a man who is slow to ejaculate may blame herself in the belief that she doesn't excite him. If a man becomes concerned about his inability to ejaculate easily, he should consult a doctor, Dr. Birch adds.

▶SOLUTIONS

Take a hands-off approach. For younger guys, the best advice may simply be to masturbate less, says Dr. Birch. "If they're masturbating excessively,

Did You Know?

The flap over foreskins continues. The foreskin keeps the glans, or head, of the penis more sensitive than that of a circumcised penis. Proponents of an uncut member say that a fully intact penis affords more sexual pleasure because the foreskin has a knobby mucous membrane that is stimulated during sex as the foreskin glides back and forth over the glans and the penis shaft. Some circumcised men feel so strongly about their loss that they undergo a painstaking process aimed at creating a faux foreskin.

Circumcision advocates say that there is no difference in sexual responsiveness. And they point out that penile cancer, while rare, occurs more often in the United States among uncircumcised men. Urinary tract infections also are far more common among intact men. Guys with foreskins also can develop an unappealing buildup of secretions with the equally unappealing name of smegma. By regularly pulling back the foreskin and washing it, however, this can be avoided.

---

they've gone to the well too often," he says. "They've pumped the well dry, so they have to work a little harder to reach an ejaculation." Excessive, vigorous masturbation may also numb nerve endings in the penis and render men less sensitive to the gentler stimulation of a vagina. And by masturbating a lot, some men inadvertently condition themselves to reach a sexual climax with their hand rather than a vagina, says Dr. Birch. "There isn't a vagina in the world that's going to grip your penis the way you grip it when you're masturbating."

Ration your sex life. If you and your partner have intercourse a lot, you might slack off just a bit, says Dr. Birch. Just as with excessive masturbation, frequent intercourse can result in difficulty ejaculating because a man is not recognizing the fact that he has a refractory period—the length of time it takes to recover from an ejaculation.

Be creative. Try experimenting with different sexual positions, says Dr. Birch. Many men find that the rear-entry position gives them a feeling of greater tightness because the woman's pubic bone rubs the underside of their penis during thrusting, he says.

Drink in moderation. Alcohol is a depressant and can impede an ejaculation, says Dr. Birch. On a night that you're likely to have sex, try to keep your drinking to a minimum.

Towel off. While many men suffer from delayed ejaculation because of dryness concerns, there is a flip side: Some guys don't get enough friction because their partners lubricate so much. Pause to wipe your penis dry now and again, then carry on, advises Neil Baum, M.D., associate clinical professor of urology at Tulane University Medical School and Louisiana State University School of Medicine, and director of the Impotence Foundation, all in New Orleans.

Junk the junk food. A diet heavy in saturated fats can, over time, harden your arteries, impeding blood flow to the penis, perhaps making it more difficult to ejaculate, says Willard Dean, M.D., medical director of the Center for Self-Healing in Santa Fe, New Mexico. Try to get less than 30 percent of your calories from fat, and make more room in your everyday eating for foods like pasta and vegetables.

▶ALTERNATIVE SOLUTIONS

Play longer. Extend the time you devote to foreplay, advises Dr. Baum. This is especially worthwhile for older guys who simply need more physical stimulation to become erect and to ejaculate than they did when they were younger, he says.

▶PREVENTIVE MEASURES

Ban the porn. Looking at a pornographic video or magazine probably won't help you ejaculate faster and could do more harm than good, says Dr. Birch. "If it's truly inhibited ejaculation, the guy already is excited," he says. "He just can't get over the brink. If the woman is already feeling inadequate because she's not getting him off, that can actually make it worse. She may be saying, 'He can do it with a video, but he can't do it with me.' If it doesn't work, it's very disappointing. If it does work, it's very disappointing."

Look in the medicine cabinet. Some medications, believe it or not, can make it more difficult for a man to ejaculate. These include some antihistamines, certain blood pressure medications (Diuril, Lozol, and Enduron), and some antidepressants (Prozac, Paxil, and Zoloft). If you're taking a medication and are having a noted difficulty in ejaculating, the two may be linked, says Dr. Baum. Ask your doctor about switching prescriptions, he says.

Depression

▶PROBLEM

As many as one in eight men may need treatment for depression during their lifetimes. The telltale signs include loss of interest in activities that used to be pleasurable, excessive irritability, becoming socially withdrawn, sleep disturbances, loss of appetite or increased appetite, flagging sexual desire, lethargy, and feelings of worthlessness or excessive guilt. Suicidal thoughts are present in at least 40 percent of individuals with clinical depression, says Jonathan Alpert, M.D., assistant professor of psychiatry at Harvard Medical School and associate director of the Depression Clinical Research Program at Massachusetts General Hospital in Boston.

▶CAUSE

Nerves in your brain use chemical substances called neurotransmitters to communicate with one another. Your brain holds 80 or so different kinds of neurotransmitters, all with hard-to-spell names such as norepinephrine, dopamine, endorphins, histamine, acetylcholine, and serotonin. These brain chemicals work together in a delicate balance to help you concentrate, remember, and perform other mental tasks. When levels of some are too high and levels of others too low, you can feel confused, tired, edgy, or depressed.

Neurotransmitter levels run amok for various reasons. You may have inherited a delicate brain chemistry from your parents or grandparents. Or var-

DO THIS NOW

When we're depressed, we see the world through negative lenses, says Leonard Tuzman, doctor of social work and director of social work services at Hillside Hospital of Long Island Jewish Medical Center in Glen Oaks, New York. To change your outlook, tap into the running commentary in your head. Listen for negative thoughts—stuff like "She hates me," "I'm a crappy father," or "I can't get anything right." When you catch yourself thinking such thoughts, do a reality check. Just because your kid failed chemistry doesn't mean that you're a bad dad. Now, remind yourself of the things you do right.

ious feelings, especially unrelieved anger, unrealistic guilt, and loneliness, could have altered these brain chemicals. The cause might even be something you ate. One theory is that a delayed-onset food allergy—one where symptoms surface anywhere from 2 to 72 hours after eating—can trigger depression, says James Braly, M.D., medical director of Immuno Laboratories in Fort Lauderdale, Florida; editor of *The Food Allergy Advisor*; and author of *Dr. Braly's Food Allergy and Nutrition Revolution*.

▶HOW SERIOUS

Everyone feels a little down now and again, but untreated major depression can result in social and occupational disability and can even lead people to suicide. If depression keeps you from performing your job or if you sometimes think about killing yourself, seek professional help. If you suspect a food allergy, see a nutritionally oriented physician and request a blood test or guidelines for an elimination diet.

▶SOLUTIONS

Supplement with folate. A deficiency in this B vitamin can bring you down, says Dr. Alpert. You can eat more folate by boosting your intake of leafy green vegetables, orange juice, liver, avocados, and beans. Unfortunately, many depressed men have a habit of indulging in fast food or junk food rather than preparing healthy meals. So don't rule out supplements, says Dr. Alpert. Aim for at least 200 micrograms of folate (folic acid) a day between your diet and supplements. Certain conditions that often accompany depression increase folate requirements such as alcoholism and possibly even stress, adds Dr. Alpert. So ask your doctor about your folate needs.

Go to bed on time. Going to sleep and getting up at the same time every night and day may help keep levels of important brain chemicals consistent, says Dr. Alpert.

Pump yourself up. Numerous studies have revealed the antidepressant effects of weight lifting and aerobic exercise. Exercising three or more times a week in short 20- to 30-minute sessions may help improve sagging energy or depression, says Dr. Alpert.

Talk it out. It's important to focus on your negative thoughts and emotions, says Leonard Tuzman, doctor of social work and director of social work services at Hillside Hospital of Long Island Jewish Medical Center in Glen Oaks, New York. So letting a good friend or support group hear you out could be the release you really need. The National Depressive and Manic Depressive Association (NDMDA) can help you locate self-help groups in your area. Contact them by writing to the NDMDA at 730 North Franklin Street, #501, Chicago, IL 60610-3526.

Be a family man. Just because you may sometimes feel like you're on a sinking ship doesn't mean that you have to take your family down with you.

"Men have a tendency to keep problems to themselves. But if you are open about your condition, your wife and kids will know that Dad's irregular moods are not their fault," says Dr. Tuzman. "They may also be a great encouragement." Remind your family (and yourself) that your condition is treatable and that there are steadier waters ahead.

Count your lucky stars. Remind yourself that there are galaxies of people who have conquered depression, many of whom are famous, says Dr. Tuzman. According to the National Association for Mental Illness, some stars who shine, despite bouts with various forms of depression, include journalist Mike Wallace, writer and humorist Art Buchwald, media personality Dick Cavett, actor Jim Carrey, comedians Robin Williams and Rodney Dangerfield, musicians James Taylor and Lou Reed, baseball players Dwight Gooden and Pete Harnish, football player Lionel Aldridge, basketball player Kendal Gill, and astronaut Buzz Aldrin.

▶ALTERNATIVE APPROACHES

Bow to Saint John. The herb Saint-John's-wort (also called hypericum) may boost spirits by stopping brain enzymes from destroying various feel-good chemicals such as serotonin, epinephrine, and dopamine, says Varro E. Tyler, Ph.D., distinguished professor emeritus of pharmacognosy and dean emeritus of Purdue University School of Pharmacy and Pharmacal Sciences in West Lafayette, Indiana. Look for a standardized herb extract at a health food store. To ensure that you buy a supplement with the right active ingredients, look on the label for the word *hypericin*. Follow package directions.

Separate the wheat from the chaff. It's not clinically proven but worth considering that a delayed food allergy can cause depression. And gluten—a protein found in wheat, rye, oats, and barley—ranks as one of the most common allergy-triggering foods, says Dr. Braly. To positively determine whether gluten is responsible for your problem, you'll need either a special blood test from your doctor or some patience. You can pinpoint the problem at home by completely avoiding foods with wheat, rye, oats, and barley in them and monitor your mood. If you feel better after a week or so, chances are that you can blame gluten.

Permanently living a gluten-free existence can pose quite a challenge. Fortunately, an amino acid supplement called glutamine may alleviate symptoms of gluten sensitivity, says Dr. Braly. Try 10 to 20 grams a day of the powder. That's about one rounded teaspoon two to four times a day. The theory is that a person can continue to eat grains while taking glutamine and that, if taken while eating gluten, the allergic reactions may actually be reversed, he explains.

Mix up some NADH. Just in case you're ever playing the chemistry category on Jeopardy, we'll let you know that NADH stands for nicotinamide adenine dinucleotide. A coenzyme naturally found in the body, NADH can boost production of some mood-enhancing brain chemicals. Some people naturally

Did You Know?

Men are so good at masking their clinical depression that it often goes unde-
tected for a very long time. "Doctors make poor mind readers," says
Jonathan Alpert, M.D., assistant professor of psychiatry at Harvard Medical
School and associate director of the Depression Clinical Research Program
at Massachusetts General Hospital in Boston.

"Just because you've seen your doctor for a variety of aches and pains,
don't expect him or her to diagnose your depression without your help. If
you experience symptoms of depression that persist for more than a few
weeks, you should communicate that as directly as possible to your doctor
without delay. The earlier you recognize it, the easier it is to treat, and the
sooner you will be on the track toward getting better," says Dr. Alpert.

---

have more of the coenzyme than others. And the more you have, the happier
you feel. You can up your natural stores by taking the coenzyme in supplement
form, says Dr. Braly. Try 5 to 10 milligrams a day. You should feel its benefit in
one to two months, Dr. Braly says. If you don't mind NADH's relatively high
price, you can continue taking it for life to maintain the good-mood enzymes
as well as reap the benefit of NADH's anti-aging properties. Otherwise, discontinue taking it once your moods improve, he says.

Try tyrosine. This amino acid seems to boost levels of the feel-good brain
chemical dopamine. It is ideal for people who are not severely or clinically depressed but feel blue sometimes. "In my experience, 3 to 6 grams a day can reverse depression in people who don't respond to prescription medication," says
Dr. Braly. For tyrosine to work effectively, you'll also need optimal levels of vitamin B_6. Look for a B-complex vitamin that contains between 25 and 50 milligrams of B_6, says Dr. Braly. Tyrosine is safe to take indefinitely. But this amino
acid is not recommended for people with schizophrenia (who are thought to already have high dopamine levels) or melanomas (which thrive on tyrosine), he
cautions.

Go for ginkgo. Like Saint-John's-wort, the herb ginkgo biloba seems to
work by keeping those bad brain enzymes from destroying your happy-go-lucky
brain chemicals, says Dr. Braly. When you go to the health food store, however,
don't plop down money for just any ginkgo supplement. Look at the label. You
want a product with a guaranteed potency. So make sure that the words *flavo-
glycosides* and *terpenes* are listed. "Some products contain the right herb, but
they don't contain the active ingredients," warns Dr. Braly. For depression to
lift, you'll need to take somewhere between 120 and 240 milligrams a day. Start
with 120 and slowly increase the dosage until you feel better, says Dr. Braly.

Ginkgo works slowly, so allow three to six months for maximal benefits. Check with your health-care practitioner before taking ginkgo if you are taking any monoamine oxidase–inhibiting drugs (depression or anxiety medication) because of possible interactions. Otherwise, Dr. Braly says that ginkgo can be taken safely and indefinitely.

▶PREVENTIVE MEASURES

Boost moods with seafood. If you are cutting back on total dietary fat and cholesterol to protect your heart, an unfortunate side effect can be depression. It seems that our brains need a type of fat called omega-3 fatty acids to keep levels of neurotransmitters at optimal levels. Cholesterol-lowering drugs such as cholestyramine resin (Questran) and simvastatin (Zocor) may also cause depression for similar reasons.

But preliminary evidence shows that you can protect your heart and uplift your spirits by boosting your intake of fish, a food source naturally high in omega-3's. More research is needed to determine the optimal fish intake to prevent depression, says Joseph R. Hibbeln, M.D., chief of the outpatient clinic at the National Institute on Alcohol Abuse and Alcoholism in Rockville, Maryland, and co-author of a study that explored the link between depression and fatty acids. For now, stick with the amount that will protect your heart—two servings a week, he says. "Two servings will virtually eliminate the risk of dying from arrhythmia after a heart attack. The data suggest that this also may be beneficial to reduce depression—at least hostility," Dr. Hibbeln says.

Jump on the wagon. You probably already know from your days of junior high drug education that alcohol is a depressant. So it makes good sense to hang up your shot glass for good, says Dr. Alpert. "In fact, alcoholism is far more common than food allergies or nutritional deficiencies as a cause of depression. As few as two or three drinks a day can markedly contribute to depression. I can't stress enough how important it is to avoid," says Dr. Alpert.

Cut back on coffee. Overconsumption of coffee can suppress feel-good brain chemicals, causing depression, says Dr. Braly. Keep your cups of brew to two or less a day, he says. A healthier alternative to the java fix is green tea, which has powerful antioxidant and perhaps anti-cancer benefits (not to mention less caffeine), Dr. Braly adds.

Diabetes

▶PROBLEM

There are two main types of diabetes: type I, or insulin-dependent diabetes mellitus; and type II, or non–insulin-dependent diabetes mellitus. Type I accounts for 5 to 10 percent of diagnosed diabetes in the United States. If you have increased thirst and urination, constant hunger, weight loss, blurred vision, or extreme fatigue, you may have type I diabetes. It develops most often in children and young adults but can appear at any age. A person with type I diabetes needs daily injections of insulin in order to live.

Type II diabetes accounts for 90 percent or more of diabetes cases. The symptoms for type II are similar to those of type I, but they develop gradually and are less noticeable than in type I diabetes. It usually strikes people over age 40 and is most common after age 55. By then, other conditions are often thought to be responsible for the symptoms. If you are over age 60 and have frequent urination, you'd probably blame it on your prostate. Think again; it could be diabetes. Both types of diabetes can be managed, but currently there is no cure for type I diabetes. If you inherit the potential for type II diabetes, you may be able to delay its onset and maintain normal blood glucose control by keeping active, maintaining a reasonable weight, and eating balanced meals throughout the day.

▶CAUSE

Diabetes occurs because the pancreas, a large gland behind the stomach, produces no insulin (type I) or the body cells don't produce enough insulin or don't respond to the insulin that is produced (type II). Insulin is a hormone that moves glucose from our blood into our cells. Glucose is a simple sugar created by digestive juices and is the main source of fuel for the body. In a person with diabetes, the glucose or blood sugar can build up in the bloodstream, spills into the urine, and passes out of the body, depriving the body of this vital fuel source. Type I diabetes is more common in Whites than non-Whites, but African-Americans, Hispanics, and Native Americans and some Asian-Americans and Pacific Islanders are at greater risk for type II.

▶HOW SERIOUS

If you notice increased thirst or urination; have unintended weight loss; feel fatigued; or have cuts that heal slowly, you should see your doctor, says Frank Vinicor, M.D., director of diabetes at the Centers for Disease Control and Prevention in Atlanta. Diabetes is a serious illness. It's estimated that diabetes costs the United States $98 billion annually in direct medical costs and in indirect costs, such as loss of wages and productivity and premature death. Heart disease and stroke are two to four times more common in people with diabetes. It is the leading cause of new cases of blindness among people between ages 20 and 74. It can cause kidney and nerve disease, causing the need for kidney dialysis or transplantation and the amputation of lower limbs. Because they tend to be on their feet more and take care of their feet less, men tend to have more foot problems and amputations. People with diabetes have more periodontal disease and with more severity.

If all that doesn't scare you, maybe this will: Diabetes can rob you of your erections, or cause some loss of sensation, so you need to be stimulated longer to get an erection. Sometimes these changes are not reversible. For men with diabetes over age 50, the rates of impotence can be as high as 50 to 60 percent. Still there are things you can do at home to minimize the effects of diabetes.

▶SOLUTIONS

Get off your duff. Exercise or less structured physical activity such as walking and gardening has a positive impact on blood sugar levels, says Dr. Vinicor. Being physically active helps people with type II diabetes lose weight—an important benefit because most people with type II diabetes are overweight. But it's also beneficial to those with type I, who typically are of average weight or are thin, says Dr. Vinicor.

"The more fit a person is, the less insulin they need to produce from their pancreas or by injection," says Pat Schaaf, a research dietitian and diabetes educator at Stanford University's General Clinical Research Center.

Be balanced. People with diabetes are encouraged to eat balanced meals throughout the day for overall good nutrition, weight management, and control of blood sugar and fat levels, says Schaaf. What's not balanced? Skipping breakfast and lunch and overeating at dinner and selecting foods from only one food group would be considered not balanced.

You should select a variety of foods from all food groups at every meal and throughout the day, Schaaf says. About 50 percent of each meal should be carbohydrates such as breads, cereals, rice, pasta, fruits, and vegetables. The rest should come from lean sources of protein—such as meat, poultry, fish, dry beans, eggs, and nuts—and from fat. Monounsaturated fats, such as olive oil, canola oil, olives, avocado, and nuts, are good sources of fat. For example, a balanced lunch could be a turkey sandwich on whole-grain bread with a couple slices of avocado and some lettuce and tomato with a glass of low-fat (less than 2%) or nonfat milk.

These are general guidelines. The exact percentages of carbohydrates, fats, and proteins need to be worked out on an individual basis with your dietitian. If you need to lose weight to improve your blood glucose level, don't eliminate meals or certain kinds of foods. Just eat smaller portions, says Schaaf—especially at night, when most people overeat.

Lower your cholesterol. Studies show that people with diabetes get an even bigger boost to their health from lowering their cholesterol than folks who don't have the condition, says Dr. Vinicor. Usually, only about 30 percent of your calories should be from fat, adds Dr. Vinicor.

Of that, notes Schaaf, only 10 percent should come from saturated fats. Keep your intake of cholesterol under 300 milligrams per day.

▶ALTERNATIVE APPROACHES

Become a mellow fellow. Yoga, meditation, exercise, and other methods of stress reduction can help control diabetes. That's because stress can cause blood sugar levels to rise, says Dr. Vinicor. Also, the hormones released when we're stressed tend to oppose the effects of insulin, making it harder to manage diabetes, he says.

Try some chromium. The chemical element chromium may help regulate blood sugar levels, particularly if you are chromium-deficient, says Dr. Vinicor. Deficiency is rare in the United States, but you could try a supplement of 200 micrograms a day. But before you take any vitamin or mineral, check with your doctor, since they may affect your medication.

MEN'S HEALTH INDEX

Here are 10 famous men who have had diabetes.

1. Arthur Ashe
2. Menachem Begin
3. James Cagney
4. Paul Cézanne
5. Thomas Edison
6. Jerry Garcia
7. Dizzy Gillespie
8. Ernest Hemingway
9. George Lucas
10. Jackie Robinson

▶Preventive Measures

Be a team player. Work with your health-care team and develop a game plan to identify trouble early, suggests Dr. Vinicor. There is strong evidence that serious complications of diabetes, including eye, kidney, and nerve damage, can be prevented if you control your blood sugar and blood lipid levels.

Take care of your feet. One of the first signs that you've had diabetes for a long time is nerve damage, which often starts in the feet. That loss of feeling can cause a barefoot person to be oblivious to a cut on his foot. And because of diabetes, the cut can be more troublesome to heal, leading to infection and, in some extreme cases, amputation. If you control your blood sugar and follow simple foot-care rules such as wearing comfortable shoes, not going barefoot, and examining your feet every day for cuts and sores, your risk of amputation could be cut in half, says Dr. Vinicor.

Diarrhea

▶PROBLEM

You have the all-too-frequent passing of loose, sometimes watery stools.

▶CAUSE

It's a long list. Diarrhea may be either acute, which comes on suddenly, or chronic, which lasts for weeks. Usually, acute diarrhea results from an infection of some kind, most often a virus (such as the stomach flu), bacteria (food poisoning), or parasites (in travelers). It can also be a symptom of food allergies or a response to certain types of medications. Chronic or intermittent diarrhea (the runs) is also a hallmark of many intestinal problems, including irritable bowel syndrome (in which stress can be a contributing factor) and inflammatory bowel disease (ulcerative colitis or Crohn's disease). Blood or fever associated with diarrhea is due to some type of inflammation—either infection or inflammatory bowel disease—and requires communication with a doctor, says Stephen B. Hanauer, M.D., professor of medicine and clinical pharmacology at University of Chicago Pritzker School of Medicine. Antibiotics are sometimes needed to treat infectious diarrhea, and people with ulcerative colitis or Crohn's disease require long-term medications to stop the inflammation.

> ### DO THIS NOW
>
> **Have a cup of black tea. The astringent property of tea will help slow down diarrhea, says Maoshing Ni, Ph.D., a doctor of Oriental medicine, licensed acupuncturist, and director of Tao of Wellness, a professional acupuncture corporation in Santa Monica, California. Tea contains tannin, which tones and tightens the intestinal lining, helping to prevent toxins that caused the diarrhea from being absorbed back into the bloodstream, he says. Be sure to drink plenty of other fluids to stay fully hydrated.**

▶HOW SERIOUS

Diarrhea generally isn't dangerous or long-lasting, but it can make you awfully uncomfortable. Most cases are what doctors call self-limited—if you wait two or three days, it'll go away on its own. In prolonged cases, diarrhea can be serious, even life threatening, since it drains your body so quickly of essential fluids

and nutrients. If the diarrhea lasts more than three days, you have rectal bleeding, or you alternate between constipation and diarrhea, contact your doctor to rule out more serious intestinal ailments.

▶SOLUTIONS

Stop it up. Diarrhea is your body's way of getting rid of something it identifies as toxic to you, so when possible, you want to let it run its course. But sometimes, you just need to put up the flood gates, says Dr. Hanauer. Over-the-counter antidiarrheals like Pepto-Bismol, Kaopectate, or Imodium AD come in handy in such situations. Dr. Hanauer warns, however, that these remedies should not be used if you have a fever or bloody diarrhea.

Keep drinking. A case of the runs can really sap your body of fluids, so it's important to drink up—at least one eight-ounce glass of water or other liquid per hour. Sports drinks like Gatorade or All Sport are good choices because they contain glucose and minerals, which are lost during a bout of diarrhea, and salt to help you retain fluid, adds Dr. Hanauer. Avoid milk products or large amounts of fruit juice, warns Dr. Hanauer. The sugar in fruit juice and lactose in milk will aggravate diarrhea, as they can be difficult to digest.

Follow the BRAT diet. Eating bland, easily digestible foods is one of the oldest and simplest home remedies for diarrhea. The BRAT diet is perfect: banana, rice, applesauce and toast. Rice, applesauce, and (dry) toast are kind to your bowel because they're low-fiber and easily digested, giving your whole digestive system a chance to rest and heal itself, according to Dr. Hanauer. The bananas work to bind the stool together, slowing down bowel movement just enough without causing gastrointestinal distress. Stick with this diet until your diarrhea symptoms stop and your bowel movements firm up.

Steer clear of coffee. Fill that morning mug with a brew a little less loaded with caffeine, suggests James Scala, Ph.D., a nutritionist in Lafayette, California, and author of *Eating Right for a Bad Gut*. Any kind of stimulant is a bad idea when you have the runs since it only makes diarrhea worse. Instead of that morning cup of brew, try tea or juice instead, says Dr. Scala.

Double-check your Rx. Some kinds of chronic diarrhea can be linked to a medication you're taking, says Dr. Hanauer. Anti-inflammatory drugs and aspirin-related drugs often cause diarrhea or inflammation of the bowel. Talk to your doctor if you think that a drug may be causing your chronic case of the runs.

▶ALTERNATIVE APPROACHES

Try a garlic tea. Bake two unpeeled garlic cloves in foil at 350°F for 10 minutes until they're brown and make a tea with them, recommends Maoshing Ni, Ph.D., a doctor of Oriental medicine, licensed acupuncturist, and director of Tao of Wellness, a professional acupuncture corporation in Santa Monica, California. To make the tea, boil the baked cloves in 10 ounces of water for 7 to 8 minutes, strain, cool, and drink. Do this every three hours until the diarrhea stops, says Dr. Ni. Garlic is an antimicrobial, which means that it kills microorganisms such as bacteria and viruses—or at least keeps them from multiplying. And believe it or not, garlic tea is a homemade remedy you can actually stomach. When browned, garlic has a pleasant odor, says Dr. Ni.

Eat gingerly. Fresh ginger, a staple of the Chinese diet, can also soothe the gastrointestinal tract when you have a case of diarrhea, says Dr. Ni. You can buy commercial ginger capsules in a 500-milligram dosage in health food stores. Follow label instructions. Or make a ginger tea using two teaspoons of ground or grated ginger per cup of boiling water, steeped for 10 minutes. Drink this tea once every three hours until the diarrhea stops.

Forage for porridge. A bowl of this soupy mush (white rice or Cream of Rice cooked with water until it is soft and soupy) with a teaspoon of ginger and a half-teaspoon of black pepper is just right for a case of diarrhea. The porridge will rehydrate you, while the warming powers of the black pepper will help to stimulate contraction in the intestinal walls to slow down bowel movement, says Dr. Ni. Eat one 10-ounce bowl of this mixture once every four hours.

▶PREVENTIVE MEASURES

Watch out for water. When you're traveling outside the United States, and especially in developing countries, assume that all water is contaminated (including ice cubes), says Dr. Hanauer. Always boil before you drink. If you opt for soft drinks, choose canned over bottled, as the bottled beverages may not have been filled under sanitary conditions.

Forget raw fruits and vegetables. Dr. Hanauer suggests another tip for avoiding traveler's diarrhea: Watch the vegetables; they may be infested with microorganisms or handled by people who are. The only way that they're safe is if you carefully peel away the skin or boil the heck out of them.

Stay away from sorbitol. Sorbitol, the sweet stuff you savor in sugar-free gum and candy, is a common instigator of diarrhea. What it saves you in calories it costs you in intestinal distress, says Dr. Hanauer. Our bodies just aren't equipped to digest large amounts of this chemical. For some people, just three little sticks of sugarless gum could mean trouble, he says. Since our small intestines can't absorb sorbitol very well, the bacteria in our colons ferment it, causing gas, swelling of the colon, and cramping. The worst are the by-products of the fermentation, which cause water to flow into the gastrointestinal tract. The result is diarrhea.

Diverticulosis

▶PROBLEM

Little pouches sometimes develop in weak spots of digestive organs such as the esophagus, duodenum, small intestine, or colon. These pouches are called diverticula, and the presence of them is called diverticulosis. Diverticula in the small intestine can cause complications just by their presence, but these cases are relatively rare. The most common type of diverticulosis (the kind that strikes the colon) is much less serious, that is, as long as the pouches don't get infected, causing a disease known as diverticul*itis*.

▶CAUSE

Weaknesses in the wall of the colon can cause diverticula to form there. Constipation is a risk factor for the formation of these out-pouchings in the colon. A likely suspect for constipation and the formation of diverticula is—you guessed it—your diet. Eating processed, refined, and other low-fiber foods make for small, hard, dry stools that are difficult to pass. Under these conditions, the colon has to squeeze much harder to eliminate waste than it does to pass the softer, bulkier stool left over from fiber-rich foods. The hard stools put so much pressure on the walls of the colon as it squeezes that little pouches protrude through the wall's weak spots.

▶HOW SERIOUS

The mere presence of diverticula is not a medical problem unless there is bleeding or leakage from a small perforation, which may cause fever, cramping,

DO THIS NOW

Drink water or orange juice with pulp at mealtimes—especially if you have a high-fiber meal— to keep your stools from drying up and hardening, says James Scala, Ph.D., a nutritionist in Lafayette, California, and author of *Eating Right for a Bad Gut.* **This will ensure that your waste has a smooth and pleasant trip through the colon and will prevent any new potholes (diverticula, that is) from being formed along the way.**

abdominal pain, and possible blockage of the colon. Then there's diverticulitis, a whole other story. If you experience muscle spasms and cramping in the lower left por-

tion of your abdomen, you may have diverticulitis, which is an infection around a diverticula. That's when it's time to see a doctor, says Philip Miner, M.D., a gastroenterologist with the Oklahoma Center for Digestive Medicine and president and medical director of the Oklahoma Foundation for Digestive Research, both in Oklahoma City. Serious infections may require surgery, but you can take care of some mild cases with antibiotics and rest. Bleeding from a blood vessel near the perforation can also be severe enough to require surgery, says Dr. Miner.

▶SOLUTIONS

Sip, slurp, and guzzle. No man should skimp on water, but it's an absolute must if you have diverticulosis. James Scala, Ph.D., a nutritionist in Lafayette, California, and author of *Eating Right for a Bad Gut*, recommends drinking at least two quarts of fluid daily to soften stools and help prevent constipation, a symptom associated with diverticulosis. Diverticulosis never goes away, so you will need extra fluids for the rest of your life. In fact, as you age, you might need more fluid because your body passes it more easily.

Outrun it. Or head for the gym. In a study of more than 47,000 men, guys who exercised the most reduced their risk of diverticulosis by one-third, compared to guys who exercised the least. Of all exercisers, runners and joggers decreased their risk the most, causing some experts to reason that the motion of running may decrease pressure in the colon by loosening up the materials inside of it.

Find your sensitivity. After a while, people with diverticulosis may suspect that a particular food causes new flare-ups—with good reason. Food sensitivities often develop when we have chronic inflammation of the intestinal tract, says Steven Bailey, a naturopathic doctor at the Northwest Naturopathic Clinic in Portland, Oregon, and a member of the American Association of Naturopathic Physicians. If flare-ups seem to follow certain foods, take a break from those foods. Reintroduce your staple foods one at a time. As you get nausea, cramping, or other symptoms of diverticulosis, you'll know that this flare-up is due to undigested bits of that particular food, says Dr. Bailey.

While food allergies cannot be reversed, sensitivities can, Dr. Bailey believes. Give your digestive tract a chance to repair itself by forgoing your trigger food for a couple months, suggests Dr. Bailey. *Then* rechallenge. "You have to get the digestive system working normally before you have hope of breaking down these foods adequately," says Dr. Bailey.

▶ALTERNATIVE APPROACHES

Go seedless. Seeds often sneak through your gastrointestinal tract unnoticed, showing up later on—completely undigested—in your stool, says Dr. Bailey. If you have diverticulosis, however, seeds can get stuck in those little pouches in your colon, potentially causing an infection. Sunflower and sesame seeds are big-time troublemakers, but some people with diverticulosis need also to avoid the seeds found in fruits and vegetables, such as cucumbers and tomatoes, says Dr. Bailey. Regardless of your medical condition, be certain to chew seeds well.

Rejuvenate with juice. Vegetable juices are a nutritious replacement for the fiber-rich raw vegetables that are tough for your stomach to churn. Drinking any amount of vegetable juice instead of crunching on vegetable sticks will rest your gastrointestinal tract, but an actual juice fast will help clear the road to recovery even quicker, Dr. Bailey says. He suggests a five-day juice fast of five to six quarts of fluid daily (half juice, half water). Talk to a doctor before trying this one.

▶PREVENTIVE MEASURES

Foil it with fiber. The formation of diverticula can be prevented with one key remedy: a high-fiber diet. According to Dr. Miner, one of the major causes of diverticulosis is the American diet, which consists of refined food products that have lost their fiber content during processing. If you have diverticulosis, prevent further damage by reintroducing fresh fruits and vegetables, beans, and whole grain breads and cereals into your diet. And do it gradually to minimize the gas symptoms that can go along with upping you fiber intake, says Dr. Miner.

Note: If you've been diagnosed with diverticulitis, your doctor may recommend a *low*-fiber diet to rest your colon until the infection is handled with antibiotics or, in more serious cases, surgery.

Double Chin

▶PROBLEM

That bulging deposit of fat under your chin was cute when you were two months old and bouncing on your mama's knee, but as an adult, it's another matter altogether. Along with wrinkles and sagging skin, a double chin completes the facial aging trifecta.

▶CAUSE

It's basically one of two things: Either you're one of those unlucky guys who's genetically predisposed to a double chin, or else it's one of the consequences of being overweight.

▶HOW SERIOUS

In and of itself, a double chin is nothing to worry about. For lots of guys, it's just part of aging; as you put on extra pounds, your neck is one of the places some of it will settle. If your double chin is a result of being seriously overweight, however, then much more than your vanity is at stake. You need to lose those extra pounds or risk all of the attendant health problems, including heart disease, high blood pressure, and diabetes, says John Altobelli, M.D., senior attending plastic surgeon at Lehigh Valley Hospital Center in Allentown, Pennsylvania.

▶SOLUTIONS

Get real. Forget about quick fixes and fads. "Those chin strap devices they try to sell you

---

DO THIS NOW

Good skin care is one of the keys to defeating a double chin, says Jim Gilmore, M.D., a facial plastic and cosmetic surgeon in Dallas. "Your skin's elasticity breaks down naturally as you age, and this looser skin compounds a double chin," Dr. Gilmore says. "But there are factors that speed up this process. For example, smoking causes loss of collagen, and too much sun also works to break down the elasticity." Dr. Gilmore recommends vitamin C creams and alpha hydroxy acids to help retain your skin's youthfulness. Apply to clean skin, both morning and evening. Follow the directions on the label, Dr. Gilmore recommends. You should see results within two weeks.

Did You Know?

It's well-known that the camera adds a few pounds to all of us. But you can hide that double chin from posterity by simply putting your tongue on the roof of your mouth just before the picture is snapped, says Margaret Voelker-Ferrier, associate professor of fashion design at the University of Cincinnati.

don't work. Facial exercises don't work; there's no such thing as spot reduction, for a double chin or any other part of your body," says Dr. Altobelli.

Hit the right tone. Although spot reduction won't work, you can tone the underlying muscle, says Kevin Maselka, certified conditioning specialist and president of both Elite Physique and Planet Fitness in Rockville, Maryland. Here's a simple exercise he recommends: Lie on your back on the floor with your head up and repeatedly touch your chin to your chest. Two or three sets of 8 to 15 repetitions is sufficient, two or three times a week.

A simple variation of this exercise will work the sides of the chin, says Maselka. Just lie on your side and touch your chin to your shoulder. Do two or three sets of 8 to 15 repetitions, and then switch sides and repeat. When your muscles are toned and conditioned, your skin simply hangs better, he explains.

Once you've lost the weight, toning can help lessen what Dr. Altobelli calls the turkey neck effect—the loose skin that hangs under your chin after the fat has been lost.

Aim for overall weight loss. It's the most foolproof solution, but not what many guys want to hear. "We don't want to hear the obvious things. We all want to believe in magic solutions, but these serve only to encourage denial and delay instituting legitimate remedies," says Peter D. Vash, M.D., executive medical director of Lindora Medical Clinics in Costa Mesa, California. In other words, the best way to banish a double chin is to do it the old-fashioned way: Lose weight. In the simplest terms, that means reducing your caloric intake (especially fats) and getting regular exercise, Dr. Vash says.

▶ALTERNATIVE APPROACHES

Camouflage with clothes. Shedding pounds takes time. So what's a well-intentioned guy to do in the meantime? Margaret Voelker-Ferrier, associate professor of fashion design at the University of Cincinnati, has a few ideas. "A high collar hides a double chin very nicely, but many men find these to be uncomfortable. A better option might be a dark blue or black cotton-knit turtleneck," she says. "It creates a long, lean line from your chin to your belt. Don't fold it down; go longer with the turtleneck and tuck it under at the top just an inch or so."

Don't be concerned that this look won't cut it for more formal wear. "A black turtleneck with a dark gray jacket is both fashionable and classic, or you can go with a silk turtleneck for evening wear," says Voelker-Ferrier. And one more thing: *Never* wear a shirt that's too tight in the neck.

Get the right haircut. The longer you wear your hair, the more attention will be drawn to a double chin, says hairstylist Susan Mengle of Port Carbon, Pennsylvania. "The best strategy is to wear it short and closely cropped, and combed back at the sides," she advises.

▶PREVENTIVE MEASURES

Develop an action plan. To prevent a double chin recurrence, your first priority must be weight control. Annette Lang, a certified personal trainer at Equinox, a fitness club in New York City, advocates a "thought process of movement" for her clients. "With our increasingly sedentary lifestyles, working out for an hour three times a week just isn't enough," she says. "We have to get used to moving our bodies more—period." Lang suggests such simple changes as taking the stairs instead of elevators, standing instead of sitting at your desk (when feasible), and walking whenever possible.

Dry Hair

▶PROBLEM

If you only know sheen as that guy in *Apocalypse Now*, you probably have dry hair. Dry hair looks dull, feels rough, is frizzy, and breaks easily. Instead of stroking your hair, your woman buffs her fingernails on it.

▶CAUSE

Some people—particularly those with coarse, thick hair—may be predisposed to dry hair because they may have fewer or less active oil-producing glands on their head, says David H. Kingsley, a certified trichologist (a specialist in hair and scalp) and owner of British Science Corporation, which counsels and treats people with hair and scalp problems, on Staten Island, New York. That said, the elements and poor lifestyle choices overwhelmingly cause dry hair in the rest of us. Overheated offices, poor nutrition, harsh sunlight, improper shampooing and conditioning, chlorine-laden pools, and blow-dryers all conspire to wick the moisture out of our hair, says Kingsley.

▶HOW SERIOUS

Dry hair can be an embarrassment, but it's not too serious, medically speaking. An exception is if you notice a sudden change in the character of your hair, especially if it's accompanied by hot or cold spells, lethargy, irritability, hair loss, or heart palpitations. Then you should get yourself checked by a doctor to make sure that it's not a thyroid

DO THIS NOW

Soak your head. One of the best things you can do for dry hair is to rinse it *extremely* well, says Stephen Moody, assistant general manager of the Vidal Sassoon Academy in Santa Monica, California. "If you leave shampoo products in your hair, that will really promote dryness," he says. "You really can't rinse too much." He suggests shampooing and conditioning first, then going on to wash the rest of your body. Just before you get out of the shower, rinse again. If you take a bath instead of showering, don't just use the grimy tub water for rinsing. Stick your head under the faucet and rinse with clean water.

194

Did You Know?

Dry hair goes back at least to the days of the Romans.

Roman women used recipes for bleaching their hair that they acquired from the conquered Gauls. But because Roman women had finer hair than that of the flaxen Gauls, the bleaches often left their hair dry, damaged, and pretty ugly.

To compensate, conditioning creams were devised to help bring back some semblance of luster to the women's hair. If you think that beer and egg conditioners are bad, you should know that Roman women put pomades made of sheep or bear grease on their heads. Or sometimes marrow extracted from deer bones.

And if that didn't work, the more hearty among them used remedies concocted from hellebore (a poisonous type of buttercup) and pepper mixed with rat heads and excrement.

No wonder the empire fell.

---

abnormality, says Susan P. Detwiler, M.D., a dermatologist in private practice in San Diego.

And, adds Kingsley, if you neglect dry hair indefinitely, it can lead to increased hair loss and breakage—not something you want if you're already getting a little thin up there.

▶SOLUTIONS

Get in peak condition. Use a conditioner every time you shampoo. "It's good for the feel and the consistency of the hair," Dr. Detwiler says.

It's best to avoid the two-in-one combination shampoo/conditioners, says Kingsley, since it's the hair that needs the conditioner, not the scalp. Put the conditioner on your fingertips, run them from the middle through the ends of your hair strands, wait 30 seconds (you can scrub the rest of your body during this time), and rinse very thoroughly. Are you having a tough time deciding which conditioner you should buy? Kingsley says that the one that might already be on your bathtub shelf is a good start. "To save money initially, why not try what your wife or girlfriend is using?" he says. You'll know soon by the feel of your hair if it works.

Protect your pate. Wear a hat in bright sunlight, says Dr. Detwiler. Hair is dead tissue that takes a beating from the sun's ultraviolet-filled rays. A wide-brim hat not only makes you look cool but also provides the best protection from old Sol. "But a baseball cap is better than nothing," says Dr. Detwiler.

Try vinegar for vitality. Apple cider vinegar, to be specific. "A lot of soaps and hair products leave our hair alkaline," explains Steven S. Greenbaum, M.D., director of the Skin and Laser Surgery Center of Pennsylvania in Philadelphia. The hair's natural state is a slightly acidic one, he says. To swing the pH of your locks back to a more normal side of the scale, Dr. Greenbaum suggests a hair rinse of two tablespoons of apple cider vinegar in a quart of warm water. Use the rinse after your regular shampoo and conditioning once or twice a month. Don't worry; you can leave it on your hair without smelling like a dinner table. The scent of vinegar rapidly dissipates.

Shampoo, you. It's a fallacy to think that washing too often will further dry your hair, Kinsgley says. Your hair needs daily (or almost-daily) washing to remove pollutants and salty residue from sweating that can desiccate your 'do. Try using a shampoo for normal hair, Kingsley says. You'll have to experiment here; even baby shampoos may contain ingredients that will be too harsh for your hair. Alternately, you can water down your existing shampoo by filling its container about a quarter full of water, says Kingsley.

▶ALTERNATIVE APPROACHES

Don't hold the mayo. If you're looking for conditioner and your bathroom shelf comes up empty, try your refrigerator. Mayonnaise is ideal for trapping the moisture in your hair. After wetting your hair, use your fingertips to apply a couple spoonfuls of mayo from the middle of your hair strands to their ends, says Kingsley. Don't put it on your scalp, he adds. Leave on for 15 minutes, then rinse out. Follow with a shampoo. Start with a once-a-week treatment. When your hair begins to feel less dry and more smooth, switch to once or twice a month.

Be a purist. Consider getting an air purifier for your home or office to keep gunk out of your hair. "The hair is like a sponge. It picks up all the dirt in the air and the environment but doesn't show it," says Kingsley.

Beat the heat. Central heating systems can really dry your hair. Kingsley suggests using humidifiers in your house. If you have radiators, place bowls of water near them. Just remember to wash out the bowls at least once a week.

▶PREVENTIVE MEASURES

Brush off the brush. Dry hair is damaged hair, says Kingsley. Rough brushing only worsens it by breaking shafts and damaging others. Get a wide-tooth comb, preferably one made of rubber, avoiding any that have sharp edges left on the teeth from the mold. Stay away from steel combs, too, he adds. They can add static to your already dry hair, causing it to be more flyaway than ever.

Take this handy test. Test the temperature of your blow-dryer to see if it could be damaging your hair. Hold your hand about six inches away from the dryer for a couple of seconds. If it's too hot for your hand, then it's too hot for your hair. Use a lower heat setting and dry for a longer time, suggests Kingsley. And don't overdry your hair; stop when it's dry, he adds.

Dry Mouth

▶PROBLEM

You're not necessarily thirsty, but your mouth feels like you just ate a box of saltines. "It feels as if you have cotton mouth all the time," says Phillip Bonner, D.D.S., a dentist and director of the Oral Health Education Foundation in Fairburn, Georgia. "It's often difficult for people who have chronic dry mouth to talk, eat, or swallow."

That's long-term dry mouth, but most of us experience temporary bouts. Perhaps you're about to give a speech or are nervous about saying something important to a close friend or family member. Saliva flow is regulated by the autonomic nervous system, so if you're fearful or anxious, you could dry up a bit. These situations are much easier to remedy and much less serious than chronic xerostomia, or dry mouth.

▶CAUSE

Your mouth is dry because you have less saliva circulating than you need. Doctors used to think that dry mouth was an inevitable consequence of aging, but no more. Now physicians realize that most cases of dry mouth develop as a side effect from medications or because of an underlying illness.

"There are more than 400 prescription and nonprescription medications that can cause dry mouth," Dr. Bonner says. These include drugs for depression, hypertension, allergies, and a host of others. Some autoimmune diseases, such as rheumatoid arthritis and lupus, list dry mouth as a side effect. In these cases, the salivary glands don't produce enough saliva.

▶HOW SERIOUS

Saliva is necessary for healthy mouth function. Without it, bacteria thrive, settling on your teeth and around your gums. It's very important to see a den-

Did You Know?

Saliva. It contains electrolytes, calcium, phosphates, antimicrobials, and even oxygen. So where does all that spit come from and go to? Your salivary glands produce it, and then your body reabsorbs it. When you're healthy, you're always producing a fresh supply. As unbelievable as it may seem, your body produces about a half-quart every day.

tist if you have chronic dry mouth, Dr. Bonner says. In the first place, it could be a sign that something else is wrong and needs to be treated. Second, the problem could damage your teeth. If you think that dry mouth is a side effect of a medication you're taking, by all means, tell your physician (and dentist) because they can help find a different prescription that works better for you.

▶SOLUTIONS

Take small sips of water. You don't need to worry about swallowing enough water to relieve thirst, Dr. Bonner says. You're just trying to moisten the inside of your mouth. Other liquids will work, says Dr. Bonner, but if they have sugar or are highly acidic, you could damage your teeth.

Care for your teeth. Two of the most important things you can do for yourself if you have dry mouth are to lower the amount of sugar you eat and brush your teeth more often. "Tooth decay is a real problem for people with dry mouth," Dr. Bonner says. "Anything that can cause cavities should be avoided." Think twice before eating sugary foods like candy or raisins, or anything highly acidic like lemon drops or citrus juice.

Use an oral moisturizer. These sprays, such as MouthKote and Optimoist, are sold in drugstores. They are sometimes hard to locate, so check with your pharmacist. "They moisten and lubricate the tissues in your mouth," says Dr. Bonner. "Depending on the brand and the severity of your problem, they can last from a half-hour to a couple of hours." Follow label directions and speak to your dentist about possible overuse, since they can irritate tender tissue when used too frequently. Look for products without alcohol or sugar.

Moisten the air. If you're bothered by dry mouth at night, use a humidifier, especially if you sleep with your mouth open. "It won't solve the problem, but it may keep you comfortable through most of the night," Dr. Bonner says.

▶ALTERNATIVE APPROACHES

Get prickly. Prickly ash is foremost among the herbs that promote saliva flow, says Eugene Zampieron, a doctor of naturopathy in Middlebury, Connecticut, and a professional member of the American Herbalists Guild. "Buy tincture of dried prickly ash bark and put five or six drops on your tongue," he suggests. It should produce a good saliva flow within a minute, as long as your salivary glands are still working, he says. It is safe for long-term use, but be sure to see a physician if the problem lasts more than a week or so. You can find this in health food stores.

▶PREVENTIVE MEASURES

Read the label. Look at the fine print on many medications and you'll see the caution: "May cause dry mouth. . . ." Don't take it lightly. It's worth it to your teeth and gums to find a way to keep that saliva flowing. So if it's a prescription medication and dry mouth is a side effect, talk to your doctor about remedies or other alternatives, Dr. Bonner says.

Don't use tobacco. There are more than 30,000 new cases of oral cancer every year, one American dies every hour from oral cancer, and men account for twice as many cases and deaths from oral cancer as women. Using tobacco is a leading cause. Dry mouth is a major side effect of treatment for oral cancer because radiation, chemotherapy, and surgery can damage salivary glands. "If you have a cancer of the throat or neck, it's likely that it will, in some way or another, affect your saliva production," Dr. Bonner says.

Dry Skin

▶PROBLEM

Itchy? Scratching? Red? Uncomfortable? Do people shake your hand and ask if you've been out chopping wood? Are there parts of your skin that look white, hard, and scaly?

You may have xerosis, the 10-cent word for dry skin, which is characterized by skin that has a rough feel, is scaly, and may be itchy but have no accompanying rash.

▶CAUSE

Your skin naturally loses water to the environment through evaporation. "Your skin is a barrier between the water in your cells and the atmosphere. Some people are predisposed to dry skin because they have bad barrier function," explains Robert Schosser, M.D., chief of the division of dermatology at the University of Kentucky A. B. Chandler Medical Center in Lexington. In other words, you can get as wet as you want, but if your skin can't hold the moisture in, it will continue to be dry.

▶HOW SERIOUS

"Skin is like a brick wall," says Yohini Appa, Ph.D., director of research and development for the Neutrogena Corporation in Los Angeles. "The cells are the bricks, and the lipids are the mortar. If the mortar, or barrier layer, is cracking, then you don't have a very strong wall."

In fact, severely dry skin can increase your risk of infection. Chapped, cracking skin won't protect you from viruses and infections as well as plump skin can, so it's worth taking a few seconds each day to moisturize your skin.

> **DO THIS NOW**
>
> Use a moisturizer that contains alpha hydroxy acids, says Robert Schosser, M.D., chief of the division of dermatology at the University of Kentucky A. B. Chandler Medical Center in Lexington. Alpha hydroxy acids—which include glycolic, citric, and lactic acids—hold water in the skin. Dr. Schosser recommends Lac-Hydrin Five or AmLactin, which are both available in drugstores. Use these twice a day, but not immediately after showering. They tend to sting and burn.

Did You Know?

Dry skin doesn't just affect your hands and the middle of your back, where you can't scratch an itch. It's also possible to have dry skin on your penis, one of the more significant spots on your body that doesn't look good with scaly, scratchy skin. "Dry skin on your penis can be made worse by overwashing, or by the friction that comes with masturbation or intercourse," says Vail Reese, M.D., a dermatologist with the Dermatology Medical Group of San Francisco. "All you need is to use a gentle moisturizer." And perhaps a little less friction.

If, however, the skin is extremely red, cracking, or seems to have an infection, then get to a doctor pronto, suggests Dr. Reese.

Dry skin is uncomfortable and somewhat unsightly, but it's also very easy to correct.

▶SOLUTIONS

Oil up. One way to trap moisture in the skin is through the use of oils. And you don't need to get fancy. Plain old mineral oil will do just fine, says Dr. Schosser.

If you'd prefer something that contains natural ingredients that will soothe the skin, look for moisturizers with ginseng, aloe, chamomile, or honey, suggests Joseph W. Rucker Jr., M.D., a plastic and reconstructive surgeon in private practice in Eau Claire, Wisconsin.

Hum along with humectants. Another moisturizing option would be to choose a humectant, which helps the protein component of the skin hold water. Humectants include glycerin and propylene glycol. Many dry-skin products contain oils and humectants.

Glycerin, a natural humectant that Dr. Appa has found helps keep the skin fluid, can be found in the list of ingredients on many moisturizers.

Get wet. The best time to use a moisturizer is just after you shower or bathe, because the skin is hydrated already, and you want to make sure that moisture stays in the skin. "The idea is to train your skin to hold moisture in without too much help," Dr. Appa says.

In fact, truly dry skin can become addicted to moisturizer, so remember that if your skin and moisturizer are working well together, twice a day (once in the morning and once at night) ought to be plenty. If you still feel dry during the day, try a more therapeutic moisturizer, Dr. Appa says.

Use a humidifier. If you live in a dry climate, or it's winter and the heating system in your home or office dries up the air, a humidifier will be a big help, says Dr. Schosser. With the air wet, your skin won't lose so much moisture through evaporation.

▶Alternative Approaches

Eat healthy oils. Although most of us consume far too many saturated fats, few of us actually eat healthy oils, which would contribute to the overall health of our skin. "The oils in your diet are part of every cell membrane in your body," says Eugene Zampieron, a doctor of naturopathy in Middlebury, Connecticut, and a professional member of the American Herbalists Guild. "Try to use flaxseed oil, avocado oil, or walnut oil in your diet. You'll notice a difference in the texture of your skin.

▶Preventive Measures

Bathe in warm water. People with dry skin know that excessive washing can make the problem worse. But water isn't the culprit; water temperature and bathing products that aggressively remove oil are. "Bathing can put water back into your skin, but if the water is too hot, it melts the protective skin lipids, which will then go down the drain," says Dr. Schosser. "So, soak in a tub for 20 to 30 minutes, but make the water warm, not hot. Afterward, put a capful of mineral oil on a wet washcloth and apply this to the areas that tend to be dry such as the arms, legs, and body (avoid the face, underarms, and groin) to keep that added water in. After that, you may also use a moisturizing cream like Eucerin original formula cream to your arms and legs."

Cleanse gently. If you need to use a deodorant soap, try Lever 2000, Dr. Schosser says. This soap has a mild antibacterial in a moisturizing bar base.

Earache

▶PROBLEM

Your ear hurts—on the outside, from your ear canal out, or on the inside, behind your eardrum. The pain is dull and throbbing or so exquisitely sharp that it makes you whimper and fear to move your head. There may or may not be discharge, which can smell quite foul.

▶CAUSE

Have you had a cold or sinus infection lately? You might have a middle-ear infection, caused by a buildup of mucus, pus, and fluid in the middle ear. This purulent brew causes swelling that closes the eustachian tube, a narrow channel about the width of the lead in a pencil that connects the back of the nose with the middle ear. When the tube swells shut, fluid is sucked from the bloodstream into the middle ear and can get infected. Uninfected fluid and pressure cause discomfort but rarely pain.

Or you may be experiencing what's called referred pain (pain that comes from somewhere else) from an infected tooth or sinus, or even arthritis or temporomandibular disorder. Other causes of ear pain include swimmer's ear, caused by bacteria in the ear canal (see Swimmer's Ear on page 519), a sudden change in air pressure during air travel or deep-sea diving that blocks your eustachian tube, or a ruptured eardrum, caused by a middle-ear infection or trauma (like getting hit in the ear or probing too deeply with a cotton swab).

▶HOW SERIOUS

In most cases, ear pain—especially middle-ear infections and pain caused by trauma—requires a doctor's care, says Evany Zirul, D.O., professor of clin-

Did You Know?

Sometimes there's a good reason for your ear to hurt: Something's in there that doesn't belong. Here are some of the objects that have gotten stuck in people's ears.

Roaches	**The backs of earrings**
Moths	**Pieces of twisted-up napkin**
Superglue	**Cotton**
Bullet fragments	**Earplugs**
Bomb fragments	

ical medicine at the University of Health Sciences in Kansas City, Missouri, and assistant professor of clinical medicine at the University of Kansas in Kansas City. If left untreated, ear pain could lead to permanent loss of hearing, so Dr. Zirul recommends that you see a doctor if your pain lasts longer than 24 hours.

▶SOLUTIONS

Heat it up. If you have a middle-ear infection, cover a heating pad (set on low) with a damp towel and place it on the infected ear. A hot-water bottle wrapped in a dish towel will work, too. "Heat matures an ear infection," Dr. Zirul says. The eardrum may eventually rupture. It's very painful, but the relief is almost immediate. Most of the time, this won't happen, Dr. Zirul adds, because antibiotics stop the progression of the infection before the eardrum ruptures.

Don a shower cap. If you have a ruptured eardrum, it's critical to keep your ears dry until the eardrum heals. Water can lead to continued infection. It's best not to swim at all if you have a ruptured eardrum, Dr. Zirul says. When you shower, wear a shower cap or stuff your ears with cotton balls slathered with petroleum jelly, or plastic earplugs, to keep water out of your ears.

Take it like a man. Your prescribed medicine, that is. Middle-ear infections require antibiotics, and you have to take them for the entire time they're prescribed (usually 10 days to two weeks), says Mark K. Mandell-Brown, M.D., an otolaryngologist in private practice in Cincinnati. If you don't, the infection could flare up and be more painful than the first one.

▶ALTERNATIVE APPROACHES

Watch your diet. "I advise people with ear infections to stop consuming dairy products, sugar, and coffee," says Amy Rothenberg, a doctor of naturopathy in Amherst, Massachusetts, and editor of the *New England Journal of Homeopathy.* "These foods all seem to make the body work harder to heal."

Battle back with herbs. The herbs echinacea and goldenseal can help your immune system fight off a middle-ear infection, Dr. Rothenberg says. These herbs are commonly sold as tinctures—liquid herbal preparations typically sold in health food stores. "Take one dropperful of echinacea or goldenseal tincture in a quarter-cup of water every two to three hours," says Dr. Rothenberg. Do not use echinacea for more than eight weeks or goldenseal for more than three weeks in a row.

Supplement with C. During an infection, take 500 to 1,000 milligrams of vitamin C three times a day, Dr. Rothenberg recommends. Just be aware that excess vitamin C (more than 1,200 milligrams) may be enough to cause diarrhea in some people.

Listen to homeopathy. Homeopathic remedies, which you can buy at health food stores, can help relieve ear pain, says Dr. Rothenberg. If your ear pain is accompanied by great irritability and chills, she suggests using *Lepar sulphuricum*. If it's teamed with a stuffy nose, excess saliva, and diarrhea, select *Mercurius vivus*. If the pain has made you really irritable and pain radiates from your teeth to your ear, she recommends *Chamomilla*. With each of these remedies, select a 30X potency and take two or three pellets, advises Dr. Rothenberg. She recommends taking the remedy one time and only repeating it if you get better and then worse again. If it doesn't work, it means that you need a different remedy, Dr. Rothenberg says.

▶PREVENTIVE MEASURES

Take a snort of relief. If your ears become blocked and painful during airplane flights (a condition called eustachian tube dysfunction), take an oral decongestant before takeoff or snort a snoutful of over-the-counter nasal spray about 30 minutes before your plane begins its descent. These preparations shrink the mucous membranes in the nose, allowing the eustachian tube to balance the air pressure on the inside of the eardrum with that on the outside, Dr. Zirul says.

Take a hint from the top guns. Here's a trick that military pilots and veteran civilian fliers alike use to relieve stopped-up ears: When you're told that your plane is about to descend, take a small breath, close your mouth and pinch your nose shut, and try to gently force air through your pinched-off nostrils, Dr. Mandell-Brown says. This forces air into the eustachian tube, helping to equalize middle-ear pressure. Repeat every few minutes throughout the descent.

Blow some bubbles. Another trick from the frequent-flyer crowd is to chew gum during air flights. You swallow more often when you chew gum, and swallowing makes the eustachian tube open and close faster, Dr. Zirul says.

Don't be a blowhard. If you have a cold, blow your nose slowly and gently. Blowing too hard can force bacteria-laden mucus into the middle ear, leading to an ear infection, warns Anne Simons, M.D., assistant clinical professor of family and community medicine at the University of California, San Francisco, and co-author of *Before You Call the Doctor*.

Earwax

▶PROBLEM

You don't hear as well as you used to. Or your ears itch like crazy. Either way, you blame earwax, a loathsome blend of oil, sweat, glandular secretions, and dead skin cells. But don't judge that yellow or orange-brown goo too harshly: Earwax serves an important purpose. In normal amounts, it traps dust, microorganisms, and foreign particles, keeping them from entering and damaging your eardrums. "Earwax is good," says Evany Zirul, D.O., professor of clinical medicine at the University of Health Sciences in Kansas City, Missouri, and assistant professor of clinical medicine at the University of Kansas in Kansas City. "It works as a lubricant and an antibiotic, and bugs hate the taste of it."

It's only when you have too much or too little that it becomes a problem. Too much earwax can cause ear pain, ringing in the ear, and hearing loss. "Impacted earwax can reduce your hearing by 20 to 30 percent," says Mark K. Mandell-Brown, M.D., an otolaryngologist in private practice in Cincinnati.

▶CAUSE

If you're having earwax problems, it's likely that you've been using cotton swabs or other objects as a battering ram to jam wax up against the eardrum. "Since earwax is formed in the outer part of the ear canal, poking and

DO THIS NOW

Over-the-counter earwax softeners, such as Debrox, "change the wax from rock-hard to soft and gooey," says Evany Zirul, D.O., professor of clinical medicine at the University of Health Sciences in Kansas City Missouri, and assistant professor of clinical medicine at the University of Kansas in Kansas City. "Then you wash it out with a bulb syringe."

While these preparations are not as strong as the prescription wax softeners a doctor uses, they do work for some people. Don't use these kits if you know you have or have had a ruptured eardrum, says Mark K. Mandell-Brown, M.D., an otolaryngologist in private practice in Cincinnati. They could start an infection.

prodding just pushes it in deeper," Dr. Zirul says. If your ears itch, on the other hand, you're likely earwax-deficient, she says. So leave your earwax alone; you can't afford to lose any more.

▸How Serious

If earwax collects in the ear canal, it can jam up against the eardrum and cause temporary hearing loss. If home remedies or over-the-counter products don't remove earwax, you'll need to have a doctor do it, says Dr. Mandell-Brown. He or she will wash or suction out the wax or scoop it out with a small instrument called a curet. Ears that make too little earwax are more vulnerable to infections, such as swimmer's ear, and have to be protected.

MEN'S HEALTH INDEX

People use all kinds of things to get the wax out of their ears. The following is a list of items that doctors have seen patients try. Needless to say, don't try any of these at home, kids.

Fingernails
Bobby pins
Safety pins
Matchbook-cover strips
Keys
Paper clips
Pen caps

▸Solutions

Change the oil. Using an eyedropper, place a few drops of room-temperature baby oil or mineral oil in your ear, says Dr. Mandell-Brown. Use the oil twice a day for two or three days. On the third or fourth day, fill a small bulb syringe with warm water and gently squirt the water into your ear. (You should feel pressure, but no pain.) If you have particularly stubborn wax, you may have to repeat the process a few times, Dr. Mandell-Brown says. When the wax oozes out with the water, insert one full eyedropper of rubbing alcohol into your ear canal (to dry the ear canal and help prevent infection).

Don't use this treatment if you have or have had a punctured eardrum, however. If you have a history of perforated eardrums, you need to be careful because there could be areas of weakness in your eardrums, Dr. Mandell-Brown says. Consult your doctor instead, he advises.

Ditch the itch, not the wax. Many people with chronically itchy ears blame earwax, "when many times it's not wax at all," Dr. Zirul says. "What happens is that a lump of wax gets stuck in your ear canal, you get your ears wet, and water sits behind the wax, tickling." Using cotton swabs to relieve the itch can make things worse. Here's a safer way to relieve itchy ears: Mix equal parts of alcohol and white vinegar and wash out your ears with the solution every time you swim or shower. (Use an eyedropper to insert the solution.) "This mixture will dry up the moisture in the ears, which will relieve the itch," says Dr. Zirul.

Soften the wax. Fill an eyedropper with full-strength hydrogen peroxide (available in drugstores) and put a few drops in each ear, suggests David Zwillenberg, M.D., clinical associate professor of otolaryngology at Thomas Jefferson University Hospital in Philadelphia. Repeat about once a week to keep the earwax soft and draining properly, he says.

▶ALTERNATIVE APPROACHES

Flush wax with herbs. Fill an eyedropper with warm garlic oil and place a few drops into the affected ear, suggests Amy Rothenberg, a doctor of naturopathy in Amherst, Massachusetts, and editor of the *New England Journal of Homeopathy*. "This can be done once a week to aid the body's natural manner of clearing earwax," Dr. Rothenberg says.

Wet your feet, dry your ears. "A hot foot bath will help draw congestion away from the head and ears," Dr. Rothenberg says. "Simply place your feet in hot water for 10 to 15 minutes, then splash with cold water, put on warm socks, and go to bed." People with diabetes or others with poor circulation in their feet should ask for help to make sure that they don't burn their feet, she adds.

▶PREVENTIVE MEASURES

Just say no to swabs. Run a damp washcloth around the outside of the ear to remove earwax, Dr. Zirul says. Don't use cotton swabs. They only push the stuff farther into your ear. "Then you have to pay to have someone else dig it out," Dr. Zirul says. Plus, there's less than one inch separating the outer ear canal from the eardrum, which makes it all too easy to puncture your eardrum or scratch the canal while you're rummaging around for wax.

Eczema

▶PROBLEM

Eczema is a general term used to describe various problems related to dry, red, cracking, and thick skin. It can strike almost anywhere on your body, although some people only get it in their body creases, such as inside the elbows or the backs of the knees. It may also be called atopic dermatitis.

▶CAUSE

"I like to think of the skin as a wet sponge with plastic wrap on top," says Gary White, M.D., chief of the department of dermatology at Kaiser Permanente Hospital in San Diego. "The plastic wrap is an oil layer called the stratum corneum, and it serves as the water barrier, which prevents you from evaporating. With eczema, the plastic wrap has holes in it, so the underlying skin dries out and you become a dry, cracked sponge."

A bath or shower feels good to someone with eczema because it moistens the skin, but the moment you get out of the water, it begins to feel worse. That's because the top layer isn't working correctly to keep the moisture in.

▶HOW SERIOUS

Eczema itself is not a serious disease. The intense itching that accompanies the red rash, however, can really interfere with your life. Also, eczema isn't an attractive problem. "Most men come see us when the problem begins to make them self-conscious," Dr. White says.

DO THIS NOW

Take a tepid shower, then use a heavy cream moisturizer within three minutes of getting out of the water. "The best time to use a moisturizer is when your skin is wet," says Gary White, M.D., chief of the department of dermatology at Kaiser Permanente Hospital in San Diego.

Dr. White recommends Cetaphil, Eucerin, or Aquaphor, which you can find in your drugstore. "Don't use a lotion," Dr. White says. "They're 85 percent water and are not as good."

Did You Know?

Itching, some anthropologists suggest, may date back to our primitive past. In those simpler times, our caveman ancestors didn't need a referral from their primary cavedoc to figure out what was wrong. When a caveman itched, he knew it was time to pluck out body lice and other skin parasites. Or, if he was really lucky, maybe he could get his cavemate to do it for him—especially if she looked like the Hollywood cavebabes portrayed by Barbara Bach or Racquel Welch.

Eczema is an inherited condition, and usually shows up in infants or young children, but most people grow out of it. If you're an adult dealing with eczema for the first time, see a doctor if it persists for more than a few weeks, says Dr. White. It may be a symptom of another problem, such as an allergy, or it may not even be eczema.

▶SOLUTIONS

Take short showers. Long, hot showers will melt the lipid barrier of your skin, limiting its ability to keep the moisture in. "Five minutes, no more, of a warm or cool shower," Dr. White says. "And only once a day."

Don't scratch. It will just aggravate an already-aggravating problem and may lead to scarring. "Moisturizing creams, such as Eucerin and Cetaphil should soothe the itch," says Alan Menter, M.D., chief of dermatology at Baylor University Medical Center in Dallas. "If they don't, try hydrocortisone creams. But be careful with the use of over-the-counter anti-itch medications because they often lead to new allergies and aggravation of the eczema."

Take an antihistamine. If you're having trouble sleeping at night because of the itch, try taking Benadryl or another over-the-counter antihistamine, Dr. Menter says. "A humidifier is also helpful, especially in the winter. And don't take hot showers or keep the room too warm."

▶ALTERNATIVE APPROACHES

Incorporate fatty acids. If you're plagued by eczema, your diet may be low in essential fatty acids, called omega-3 and omega-6 oils. They are found most abundantly in salmon, mackerel, and herring; so try eating fish three or four times a week, says Eugene Zampieron, a doctor of naturopathy in Middlebury, Connecticut, and a professional member of the American Herbalists Guild. Or take a supplement of flaxseed oil. Dr. Zampieron recommends 3 to 4 grams every day for a month, then decreasing the intake to 1 gram a day, which you may do indefinitely.

▶PREVENTIVE MEASURES

Get tested. Many cases of eczema are caused by food allergies, Dr. Zampieron says. You could try eliminating the most common food allergens—dairy, wheat, eggs, white sugar, citrus, and yeast—from your diet to see if that helps your skin. Eliminate them all at once from your diet and keep them out for three to four weeks as a "cleansing period." Then reintroduce them one at a time, waiting up to three days to see if there is a reaction. If there is a reaction (your eczema returns), then you have your culprit and should eliminate it from your diet for at least one year before you try eating it again. If you still have a reaction, then it's probably best to keep away from it. Do this with each food until you finish the list, says Dr. Zampieron. The best way to determine if your skin problem is allergy-related, however, is to have a doctor test you for allergies.

Wear gloves. Contact dermatitis is a form of eczema. This happens when your skin (derm) touches (or comes into contact with) something that aggravates it, which causes inflammation (-itis). If eczema regularly strikes your hands and forearms but no other part of your body, try wearing cotton-lined gloves when you wash the dishes, work on your car, or garden. These could prevent your skin from reacting to an allergen, Dr. Menter says. And if you color your hair, be sure to wear the gloves that are provided and test a patch of hair before you cover your head with the product. Hair dye is a leading cause of contact dermatitis, Dr. Menter says.

Envy

▶PROBLEM

You covet your neighbor's goods: his Harley-Davidson, pretty wife, quick wit, or corner office.

▶CAUSE

Envy often comes from an unfulfilled need within the envious person, says Christopher Hershman, doctor of ministry, a Lutheran pastor and licensed psychologist in Allentown, Pennsylvania. You find your life and position lacking, and you dislike people who are where you want to be, says Dr. Hershman.

"You may feel that you deserve all these things, but they do not," Dr. Hershman adds.

Envy also may be that nagging voice in your head saying you haven't done what it takes to reach your goals, says Dr. Hershman. Perhaps you made some mistakes or didn't take risks. You didn't go back to school, didn't go into business for yourself, or walked away from a wonderful opportunity years ago.

▶HOW SERIOUS

Envy may start off as admiration or friendly competition, but eventually, you feel hostile toward the object of your envy. It doesn't have much to do with the other fellow (he may be entirely unaware of it); it's more a personal problem with you, says Albert Ellis, Ph.D., president of the Albert Ellis Institute for Rational

DO THIS NOW

Force yourself to encounter the object of your envy, says Albert Ellis, Ph.D., president of the Albert Ellis Institute for Rational Emotive Behavior Therapy in New York City. Talk to him in the hall or take him to lunch. Don't avoid the person. Envy usually happens when you view someone from afar, says Dr. Ellis. You see only the good side, but not the faults and vulnerabilities of the person.

"Maybe the guy's real intelligent and a hard worker, but he has a crummy marriage and that's why he spends all his time at the office," says Dr. Ellis. "When you see the whole person, there will be aspects that you won't envy. You may have it over him in many respects."

History Lesson

Edward Cope and Othniel Marsh, two eminent fossil collectors in nineteenth-century America, were good friends until they got caught up in the dinosaur craze of the 1870s.

Cope went to dig in Colorado, Marsh in Wyoming. And when the two began shipping East the largest, most abundant dinosaur finds up until that time, the public went wild with speculation about these enormous ancient beasts.

To rack up academic points by shipping and naming more bones than his rival, each scientist began using dynamite to remove large fossils, even though they destroyed lesser finds. They also hired armed thugs to fill in each other's digs and intercept bones being shipped by train. Cope named a new species of dinosaur after one of his spies in Marsh's camp.

Newspapers referred to this envious, bitter rivalry as the "Great Bone War" and "Fossil Feud," but their envy for one another's accomplishments destroyed countless prehistoric fossils—not to mention their friendship.

Emotive Behavior Therapy in New York City. If you've reached a point where the green-eyed monster is causing you to think seriously about harming the object of your envy, it's time to hash these feelings out with a counselor.

▶SOLUTIONS

Make a wish. Sometimes we confuse wants with needs. Perhaps you really think you need a $35,000 Ford Explorer, a fly-fishing trip to Alaska, or an ocean-front house.

"You've decided that if you don't have this stuff, you can't be happy. What you've done is turn desires into imperatives," observes Dr. Ellis. "Reevaluate and ask yourself if these things are really necessary." That doesn't mean that you should give up your dreams, but they shouldn't be all-consuming, he adds.

Just be you. Let's say that you're a car salesman trying to emulate Mr. Flash, a fellow salesman who glad-hands customers and tells such funny jokes that people have to wipe away the tears before they can sign the loan agreement. Now, you could envy him for his easy way with people. But you've also watched customers stalk out of the showroom when they found that Flash didn't know beans about product. You're terrible with one-liners, but when it comes to product, you're a walking encyclopedia. The point is to revel in your own strengths, then build on them, suggests Dr. Hershman.

"Pick a style that works for you, not someone else" suggests Dr. Hershman. "You can't be that other person."

Get out of a jam. Sometimes you're in gridlock because of long-held beliefs. You won't leave a miserable relationship because you're certain that being alone would be worse. You want to change careers but believe that taking a job at lower pay would be foolish.

Reevaluate your assumptions, says Dr. Hershman. Some beliefs formed years ago may be paralyzing you now. "Sometimes you have to change course, break the mold," says Dr. Hershman. "That's what those people you envy are doing. They aren't always playing it safe."

▶ALTERNATIVE APPROACHES

Draw your fears. Maybe you don't understand the source of your envy or can't find words to express it. One way to unearth your feelings is to draw and doodle, says Doris Arrington, Ed.D., an art therapist and psychologist at the College of Notre Dame in Belmont, California.

"Art taps into the subconscious," Dr. Arrington says. "You can say things in pictures or admit things to yourself that you never could in words." Get a small unlined journal and a box of colored pencils, and begin to draw. The subject matter or quality of the work isn't important, says Dr. Arrington. "It's not literal interpretations you're looking for but clues and symbols about the way you are feeling," she adds.

If you draw boxes or confining shapes, you could feel trapped. Expansive free forms might symbolize optimism, says Dr. Arrington. Is there humor, irony, or tragedy in your drawings? Examine also your use of color: Blue could be coldness or loyalty; red, passion or anger; and yellow, curiosity or cowardliness. "Look at the whole continuum. A certain color is neither bad nor good," she says.

▶PREVENTIVE MEASURES

Form a plan. Envious people frequently have high expectations of themselves but no action plan on how to fulfill their desires, says Dr. Hershman. They just assume that it will happen. Avoid that by making out a five-year plan. Where do you want to be? What will it take to get there? Do you have the resources, education, and support you require?

"Just because you wanted to be a millionaire at 40 doesn't mean that you should be devastated because you're not, especially if you haven't done much to get there," Dr. Hershman says. "Planning makes you more realistic about your future."

Eyebrow Issues

▶PROBLEM

The short, coarse hairs above your eyes do have a purpose. Eyebrows help shade the eye from sunlight and prevent sweat from trickling down your forehead and into your eyes. They also give your face a look—one you may not particularly want.

▶CAUSE

Eyebrows frame the face and help create the expression of the eyes, says Maurice Stein, owner and founder of Cinema Secrets, a movie makeup store in Burbank, California, and a makeup consultant to major motion picture studios. A man's eyebrows say a lot about him or even undermine him. If a man's eyebrows are thin, they convey a "weakness," Stein says, whereas having bushy, uncontrollable eyebrows gives a man a sinister look.

▶HOW SERIOUS

Other than looking a bit menacing or weak, not-so-perfect eyebrows pose no health risks. But if you suddenly start to lose eyebrow hair, take note. Losing eyebrow hair as well as other bodily hair could be a sign of several underlying illnesses, including syphilis, says Douglas D. Altchek, M.D., associate professor of dermatology at the Mount Sinai School of Medicine of the City University of New York.

▶SOLUTIONS

Undo the unibrow. If Stein wants to make a movie character look sinister and evil, he adds a small amount of hair between a man's eyebrows and above

DO THIS NOW

Beat back the bush. Trim long, bushy eyebrows with a snip of small, manageable scissors, says Douglas D. Altchek, M.D., associate professor of dermatology at the Mount Sinai School of Medicine of the City University of New York. First, using an eyebrow brush or a comb, brush the eyebrow hairs straight up. Then cut right along the natural upper border of the brows with scissors, he says. Only trim the flyaway hairs above the natural margins.

his nose. Unless this scares your co-workers and family members into complete obedience, you probably don't want this look working for you. To tame the hair growing between your eyes, you have to pluck, Stein says. Use tweezers with an angled tip, as opposed to flat and pointed tips. Your local drugstore should carry these. The angled tip allows you to see the hair as you pull it out, giving you more control. Before

MEN'S HEALTH INDEX

Some men are as famous for their eyebrows as they are their accomplishments. Here's a brief list of a few of the best and bushiest.

1. Bert (Ernie's buddy from *Sesame Street*)
2. Jack Nicholson
3. Andy Rooney
4. Leonid Brezhnev
5. Mr. Spock

and after plucking, wipe both the tweezers and the plucked area with an antiseptic such as alcohol to prevent infection.

Derail the droop. Many men have eyebrows that reach too far down their face, almost past their eyes. "If they go down too much, they add age to a person's face. It makes them look like they are drooping," Stein says. Pluck those runaway hairs as well. The outer sides of the eyebrows should not reach the eye itself.

Bottoms up. If you pluck to thin out your eyebrows, pluck from the bottom up, Stein advises. Starting from the bottom creates more distance between the brow and the eyelid, making for a cleaner appearance. Also, pluck slowly. Too many mis-plucks throws your eyebrows off kilter. "Think about each hair you are plucking," Stein says.

Keep it to your beard. If you prefer to shave the area between your eyebrows, don't use your handy everyday beard shaver. "These razors are not made for this purpose," Dr. Altchek says. Use a mustache shaver instead. This light, mini safety razor with interchangeable blades is nonelectric and cuts out less of your eyebrows. You can find them at beauty supply stores.

▶ALTERNATIVE APPROACHES

Pencil it in. A few minutes with an eyebrow pencil replenishes thin or patchy eyebrows. Draw several fine strokes in the thinner areas of your eyebrows, Stein says. Draw the stroke in the natural direction of your eyebrow hair. "Done properly, it will look completely natural," Stein says. Choose a color that closely matches your own eyebrow hair. Unfortunately, you'll have to buy a women's eyebrow pencil. (Just tell the cashier that it's for your wife, or ask your wife to buy it for you.) Buy waterproof and smearproof pencils, Stein advises.

▶PREVENTIVE MEASURES

Avoid electronics. Electric shavers and trimmers may seem like a quick and easy way to control your eyebrows, but one wrong move can mark you, Dr.

Altchek says. Despite the fact that it may seem to grow endlessly and quickly, eyebrow hair takes a lot longer to grow than hair on the rest of your body. If you mistakenly remove a section of your eyebrows, they may take months to grow back, or may not grow back at all.

Take a lesson. If you're a little hesitant about using sharp objects around your eyes, take your brows to a professional the first time, Stein says. Some salons in large metropolitan areas may offer grooming classes for men that touch on eyebrow care. Or you can have a licensed aesthetician do it for you while you take mental notes. "If you see it done properly once, you can probably do it yourself," Stein says.

Give them a wax job. To keep eyebrows tame throughout the day, apply mustache wax to them. Brush the mustache wax into the hairs, then mold the eyebrows into the shape you want. "Mustache wax keeps those hairs in place all day," Dr. Altchek says.

Eye Irritation

▶PROBLEM

An irritant—some pollen, chlorine, smoke, bacteria or virus—gets into your eye area, leading to swollen, reddened, puffy, scratchy, bloodshot eyes.

▶CAUSE

Besides irritants, eye diseases like dry eye syndrome, conjunctivitis, contact lenses over-wear, and blepharitis (an inflammation of the eyelid margin) all can cause sore eyes.

▶HOW SERIOUS

Eye irritation is usually not a very serious problem. However, this depends on the cause. If your vision is affected, if you have a discharge coming from your eye, if you look at lights and see a haze around them, or if you have extreme sharp pain, see an ophthalmologist.

▶SOLUTIONS

Ponder the problem. Since relieving this pesky irritation is linked to the cause, you should "think over what you've done in the last day or so and see if there is any obvious cause for it," says Jeffrey Anshel, O.D., an optometrist in Carlsbad, California, and author of *Healthy Eyes—Better Vision*. If you're allergic to cats and you played with your girlfriend's kitty all afternoon, then it's a no-brainer where your puffy red eyes came from. Ditto for sleeping with your daily-wear contact lenses in. Once you have an idea of the cause, it's usually easy to pick the appropriate remedy.

Fight allergies. If you think your sore eyes are caused by allergies, try some

DO THIS NOW

Try to wash away whatever's irritating the eye by using a preservative-free artificial tears product. A drop or two—as directed—of a solution like Refresh or Hypo Tears PF (available at your local drugstore) can often provide immediate relief. Do not use tap water to rinse out sore eyes, says Carol L. Karp, M.D., assistant professor of ophthalmology at the Bascom Palmer Eye Institute/University of Miami School of Medicine. Tap water is teeming with organisms that can cause a terrible infection in the eye.

Did You Know?

Through the centuries, there have been many strange remedies for sore eyes. Here are a few. Needless to say, don't try these at home, kids.

- Two teaspoonfuls of sea salt in a pint of water is an ancient eyewash used by Cornish sailors.
- Mesquite leaves, nowadays used for smoking foods, were part of a Native American salve for the eyes.
- A drop or two of honey in the eye is an old eye remedy from Vermont.
- Wearing golden earrings and bathing the eye in a solution of baking powder and water is a Spanish gypsy cure for blepharitis (when the thin edge of skin between your eyeball and eyelids swells).

antihistamine or anti-inflammatory drops. There are a number of these drops available without a prescription, including Naphcon A, says Carol L. Karp, M.D., assistant professor of ophthalmology at the Bascom Palmer Eye Institute/University of Miami School of Medicine. Follow the directions on the label.

Be like Fonzie. No, we don't mean parade around in a leather jacket snapping your fingers at women that pass by. Instead, think cool—as in cool compresses. Just run fresh, cold water over a washcloth, says Dr. Anshel. Put the washcloth over your eyes for 5 to 10 minutes; this should help relieve the itchiness and swelling that often accompany allergy-caused eye irritation.

Scrub-a-dub-dub. Since irritated eyes are often caused by blepharitis, a disease where your eyelid margins (the thin edge of skin between your eyeball and eyelashes) are swollen due to an excess of oils produced there, lid scrubs often ease the problem. Dip a cotton swab into a solution made up of two or three drops of baby shampoo and three ounces (about ⅓ cup) of water, then gently rub the bottom eyelid margin with the eye open. For the top eyelid margin, close your eyes and hit the same margin right where the bottom of the lid runs into the eyelashes. If some of the baby shampoo gets into your eye, it may burn, so use a "no tears" formula, says Dr. Karp. She says to try this once or twice a day to relieve blepharitis-induced irritation. "Since blepharitis is a chronic problem due to your skin type, you should incorporate this regimen into your daily routine," Dr. Karp says.

▶ALTERNATIVE APPROACHES

Extinguish your eyes. The Indian medical discipline of Ayurveda is based on the idea that sickness is an imbalance of one of the five elements that make us up: space, air, fire, water, and earth. According to Pratima Raichur, a doctor of naturopathy, an Ayurvedic practitioner, and author of *Absolute Beauty*, eye irritation means that the fire element is unbalanced in your body. To restore the balance, soak cotton pads in rose water, cold milk, fennel tea, or coriander tea; squeeze out the excess liquid; and then place them over your closed eyes for about 5 minutes once a day until your eyes feel better.

Don't play with fire. Dr. Raichur stresses the importance of prevention when it comes to maintaining fire balance in your body, and that means reducing the amount of hot and sour foods and drinks you consume. She recommends cutting down on alcohol, spices, coffee, and tobacco.

▶PREVENTIVE MEASURES

Cover up. If you go swimming in a pool, protect your eyes with goggles. This will prevent the chlorine from reddening your eyes, says Dr. Karp.

Imitate Jake and Elwood. While the black hats and suits may not be a look for you unless you're a Blues Brother, the shades sported by these guys will certainly help your look by preventing eye irritation. Dr. Karp says that sunglasses can help shield your eyes from pollen and dust, two prime irritants. They also protect your eyes from ultraviolet light damage.

Drop the drops. Think twice before you use eyedrops for your bloodshot eyes. They reduce redness by constricting the swollen blood vessels that cause the bloodshot eyes. But Dr. Anshel says that your eyes can get addicted to the stuff and may cause the blood vessels in your eyes to actually get bigger over time. "So it actually makes the eye redder, requiring you to use more drops," he says. Pretty soon your eyes will be hooked, but you'll still have the problem.

Keep your hands off. No matter how much your eyes itch or water, don't rub them. If you happen to rub your irritated eyes with dirty hands, for instance, that introduces a whole new set of bacteria into an irritated area. Also, Dr. Karp says that constantly rubbing your eyes can deform the shape of the cornea and possibly contribute to a condition called keratoconus (a protrusion of part of the cornea).

Check your contacts. Often your eye will be red because a speck of pollen or dust is attached to your contact lens. Pop them out and make sure, says Dr. Anshel. Also, as contacts get older, they don't get oxygen to the eye as well as they used to, which forces your body to send over more blood. This, in turn, leads to red, puffy eyes. This could be a sign that you need a new pair, so see your optometrist or ophthalmologist.

Eyestrain

▶PROBLEM

Eyestrain answers to the medical name of asthenopia, which covers any symptoms related to fatigue in using your eyes. There are many different kinds of eyestrain, but the symptoms are similar for all. They include headaches, blurred vision, dryness, and overall discomfort.

▶CAUSE

Most often, you have eyestrain from doing a lot of close work, like reading or staring at a computer screen. This type of work requires two sets of muscles in your eye to work together. One set turns your two eyes toward each other to make one image, and the other set focuses on the object. Sometimes there's a lack of coordination between the two, and this results in eyestrain. Also, you might have presbyopia, a focusing problem that hits people in their late thirties or early forties and will require you to wear glasses for close work.

▶HOW SERIOUS

"This one is not going to cause any blindness; it's not going to cause anything bad except a little discomfort. But if it's persistent, then you should be evaluated by an ophthalmologist," says Carol L. Karp, M.D., assistant professor of ophthalmology at the Bascom Palmer Eye Institute/University of Miami School of Medicine.

If you have dizziness and double vision along with eyestrain, you should see your optometrist or opthalmologist, advises Jeffrey Anshel, O.D., an optometrist in Carlsbad, California, and author of *Healthy Eyes—Better Vision*.

Did You Know?

Here's a list of weird eye facts you can use next time you're stuck next to Cliff Clavin at the bar. Cheers.

- The whites of Napoleon's eyes were not actually white but lemon yellow.
- When Teddy Roosevelt rode up San Juan Hill during the Spanish-American War in 1898, he stuffed 12 pairs of glasses in his pockets in case the pair he was wearing got shot off.
- When Abraham Lincoln gazed upon Old Glory, he saw the dark gray, white, and light gray instead of the red, white, and blue. Lincoln was almost completely color-blind.
- Saint Lucy plucked out both of her eyes to punish herself for looking lustfully at a man. After she got a replacement pair of peepers from God, she was elevated to the patron saint of ophthalmology.

▶SOLUTIONS

Cry fake tears. Often while you're staring at something up close, the surface of your eyes can dry out and cause burning, Dr. Karp says. A preservative-free artificial tears solution like Refresh or Hypo Tears PF (available at your local drugstore) will lubricate your eyes and also help break up the spasm behind the eyestrain, relaxing the eyes, she says.

Get called for palming. Rub your hands together and get them a bit warm, then gently cover your closed eyes with your palms, Dr. Anshel says. "That'll let all the muscles around your eyes relax and keep your eyes from having to work," says Dr. Anshel. Breathe easily as you palm your eyes. Do this for about five minutes, and this should rest your eyes quite nicely, he says.

Take a deep wink. Take a deep breath while raising your shoulders and scrunching your eyes and fists closed as tightly as you can, then exhale and relax all of the muscles at once, recommends Anne Barber, O.D., an optometrist and director of program services at the Optometric Extension Program Foundation in Santa Ana, California. This technique is called a deep wink. She says that by "tightening up the voluntary muscles (like your fists and shoulders) and letting them go, we frequently can trick the involuntary focus muscles to let go at the same time." This should help relax those overworked eye muscles.

▶ALTERNATIVE APPROACHES

Cool the fire. According to the principles of Ayurveda, a 5,000-year-old traditional form of medicine from India, your body is governed by five elements—space, air, earth, fire, and water. When one of these elements is not balanced, you get sick. The eyes are the seat of *pitta*, or fire, in the body, so eyestrain suggests a fire imbalance in the body. One thing that helps cool this fire is sandalwood essential oil, available in health food stores, says Pratima Raichur, a doctor of naturopathy, an Ayurvedic practitioner, and author of *Absolute Beauty*.

Add a drop of the oil to an ounce (two tablespoons) of water and stir. Soak two cotton pads in the diluted oil, squeeze out all the excess liquid, and put them over your closed eyes for about five minutes, Dr. Raichur says. This helps rebalance the heat element and alleviate the eyestrain.

Calm your mind, calm your eyes. You can relax your eyes through meditation anywhere, even in your office, by "sitting and closing your eyes, paying attention to your breath and how you're breathing," Dr. Raichur says. "And as we start paying attention, the breath starts slowing down. It relaxes by itself." This signals your mind to relax. "And when the mind is relaxed, the eyes become relaxed," she says.

▶PREVENTIVE MEASURES

Make the light right. "Lighting is probably the most overlooked and underemphasized aspect of office work," says Dr. Anshel. "The lighting is very critical because it causes glare. If it's not directed properly, it can cause poor vision, which can cause strain in itself. And without light, there's no sight." So turn off your computer monitor and check to see if there are any reflections of lightbulbs on the blank screen. If so, that could be causing your problem. Move the light or the computer so that there is no glare on the screen, he says.

Distance yourself. Keep at least 20 inches between yourself and the computer screen and ideally 26 inches or more, Dr. Anshel says. This "reduces the amount of focusing that people have to do on the screen." The closer you are, the more you need to focus, which is part of the problem with eyestrain.

Brighten up. Pay attention to the contrast between your office lighting and the computer screen, Dr. Anshel says. It's like when Mom told you not to watch TV in the dark because it was bad for your eyes. You shouldn't look at a dim computer screen in a brightly lit office. Your eyes will have to readjust from the room light to the monitor light, causing fatigue and strain, Dr. Anshel says. To remedy this, adjust the brightness control on your monitor if the screen seems dark, he says.

Fatigue

▶PROBLEM

You often are so tired that you can barely get through the day at work, and you have little or no energy for your partner, your children, running errands, and the like. Men don't complain as often as women about fatigue, but they may suffer from it equally, says Mack Ruffin IV, M.D., associate professor in the department of family medicine at the University of Michigan Medical Center in Ann Arbor. Some estimates say that one in four Americans is so tired on a daily basis that getting through the ordinary routines of the day seems overwhelming.

▶CAUSE

There are lots of reasons that you might be fatigued. Depression, stress, overwork, lack of exercise, sleep disorders, side effects of medication, and dietary habits are among them. With men, job burnout is often the main reason, says Dr. Ruffin.

▶HOW SERIOUS

Fatigue can be a symptom of many different serious illnesses, but most often it is not. If you're eating well and getting plenty of rest yet are still constantly tired for more than six months even with vacations, then you should consult your family doctor, says Dr. Ruffin.

Fatigue from sleep deprivation also can be serious because it makes you more likely to have an accident, says Claire Etaugh, Ph.D., professor of psychology and dean of the College of Liberal Arts and Sciences at Bradley University in Peoria, Illinois. "You're less alert. Your reflexes are slower."

Sleeplessness could cost U.S. employers more than $18 billion a year in lost productivity, the National Sleep Foundation estimates. Some guys may suffer from chronic fatigue syndrome, a mysterious ailment characterized by lethargy, sore throat, headaches, muscle pain, and other symptoms. Only about 1 out of 1,000 adults, however, is thought to have this condition.

▶SOLUTIONS

Walk, man. When your brain feels like mush and you need toothpicks to pry your eyes open, take a walk, advises Dr. Etaugh. Even a few minutes of brisk walking can make you more alert, she says. If this isn't possible, stretch a bit or go to the men's room and splash cold water on your face. Breaks are especially valuable for people who do repetitive work, such as word processing and sorting, she says.

Be active. "One of the most successful methods to eliminate fatigue is exercising on a regular basis, or being physically active," says Dr. Ruffin. "With regular physical activity, you'll be able to tolerate more stress and you'll feel better." You should aim for three to five 30- to 45-minute exercise sessions a week, he says. Try incorporating more physical activity into your daily routine by taking the stairs instead of the elevator and parking farther from your destination instead of setting aside time to just exercise. "I am always amused at the fighting over parking places next to the door of my favorite gym," says Dr. Ruffin.

If you're about to start an exercise regimen, try to do it in the morning because you will be more likely to stick with it, says Amy Rothenberg, a doctor of naturopathy in Amherst, Massachusetts, and editor of the *New England Journal of Homeopathy*. Exercise also may help you sleep better. One study found that physically fit older men awaken less often during the night than their couch potato counterparts. Check with your doctor before starting a new exercise program.

Take it slow. Too much exercise can also be a cause of fatigue, says William Fink, assistant to the director of the Human Performance Laboratory at Ball State University in Muncie, Indiana. Fink, who has been studying the connection between nutrition and exercise for more than 20 years, says that guys who are just beginning an exercise program are especially ripe for fatigue and sore muscles. "Build up stamina slowly. You want to start by walking, not running. Not with an hour, but with 15 minutes," he says.

Make time for meals. Don't miss meals, advises Dr. Ruffin. "A lot of men skip breakfast, don't eat much for lunch, and wonder why they feel miserable by the time they get home," he says.

Be a grazer. Eating a big meal diverts blood to your digestive system and away from your brain, making you sleepy, Dr. Etaugh says. So it's no surprise that after you down a plate of pasta, a salad, and dessert at lunch, you hit an afternoon slump when you return to work. Instead, learn to graze by eating several small meals or healthy snacks during the day, Dr. Etaugh suggests.

Did You Know?

It's probably a safe bet that at least some of our fellow mammals don't often suffer from fatigue. Certain armadillos, opossums, and sloths, for example, spend up to 80 percent of their lives snoozing or dozing. Arctic ground squirrels are well-rested, too. These residents of Alaska and Canada hibernate nine months of the year.

Eat a balanced diet. "You need to have a diet that is diverse, that you like, and that is high in fruits and vegetables and low in fat and animal products," says Dr. Ruffin. He suggests following the 5 a Day—for Better Health! program from the National Institutes of Health. The focus is on eating five or more servings of fruits or vegetables each day. This diet was developed by the National Cancer Institute and the Produce for Better Health Foundation, a nonprofit consumer education foundation representing the fruit and vegetable industry. It emphasizes adding, not restricting, to give you more energy and also help combat man-killers such as heart disease and colon cancer, Dr. Ruffin says.

Say good night to nightcaps. Don't drink caffeine or alcoholic beverages close to bedtime, advises Dr. Etaugh. "A lot of people think that alcohol makes you drowsy, so that's good to have before you go to bed. But actually, it interrupts sleep because, while you may feel drowsy and you may drift off initially, you'll wake up." Even moderate amounts of alcohol can disrupt normal sleeping patterns, she says, because alcohol interferes with the brain's ability to produce an adequate amount of the dreaming periods of sleep, called rapid-eye-movement sleep, or REM sleep.

Take a nap. If you're tired a lot because you suffer from a sleep disturbance such as sleep apnea or insomnia, a 20- to 30-minute nap after lunch but before 3:00 P.M. can recharge your mental batteries, says Dr. Ruffin. Any longer or later than that, however, can make sleeping at night more difficult, he cautions.

Stuff the puff. Smoking contributes to fatigue because it decreases lung capacity and one's ability to exercise, says Dr. Ruffin.

▶ALTERNATIVE APPROACHES

Try a supplement. A good, high-potency multivitamin every day can help give you an energy boost, says Dr. Rothenberg. "People are often eating on the go. It covers all the bases," she says. Be sure to pick up one made specifically for men, without extra iron.

Don't worry, be happy. If your fatigue seems to be mood-related, take 300 milligrams of Saint-John's-wort three times a day, says Dr. Rothenberg. She stresses, however, that it seems to help people who are fatigued and have mild depression rather than those dealing with profound depression. Saint-John's-wort can be taken for years with no side effects, she says. But don't try Saint-John's-wort without checking with your doctor if you are taking prescription drugs for depression.

Unwind. A relaxation technique—whether it be yoga, meditation, visualization, or some combination of methods—is helpful because men tend to worry about things they can't control, bringing on self-induced stress and fatigue, says Dr. Ruffin. One such technique, he says, consists of tightening, then relaxing, one group of muscles, then another and another, and so on. You should try this for 5 to 10 minutes a day for from three times a week to daily.

Put it in writing. Write down issues that bother you before going to bed, Dr. Ruffin says. For men, this seems to be a useful technique to transfer the problem out of the mind and onto paper, especially if you are a "list-maker," he says.

Shock yourself. End every hot bath or shower with a 15-second blast of cold water, advises Dr. Rothenberg. If standing under a cold shower sounds unbearable, soak a washcloth in cold water and vigorously rub it for three to four minutes over your chest, arms, legs, and so forth, she says. "It's very invigorating."

▶PREVENTIVE MEASURES

Junk the sweets. Sugar-laden junk food will give you a quick boost by driving up blood sugar levels, but those levels come crashing down rapidly, causing fatigue and a generally crummy feeling, says Dr. Ruffin. So when the breakfast cart rolls around, choose the bagel over the jelly doughnut. The junk-food blues are compounded if you are consuming a lot of caffeine to get you through the day, every day, Dr. Ruffin adds.

Get some supplemental help. You know that high-sugar snacks are only a temporary fix and do more harm than good in the long run. But you just can't lay off them. Here's something that will help: Take 200 micrograms of chromium daily to lessen sweet tooth cravings, Dr. Rothenberg recommends.

Fear

▶PROBLEM

You sense danger—it makes no difference whether it's physical or emotional, real or imagined—and your body's instinctive fight-or-flight response takes over. Your muscles tense. Your blood pressure skyrockets. Your breath quickens. Your palms sweat. You feel sick to your stomach. You tremble. All of these are your body's way of saying, "Let's get outta here."

▶CAUSE

Fear is a perfectly natural and even positive reaction to dangerous events such as car accidents, house fires, and muggings. In such moments, the fight-or-flight response can keep you alive by giving you extra energy and strength, says Thomas D. Borkovec, Ph.D., professor of psychology at Pennsylvania State University in University Park. Other times, though, we feel fear even when there is no physical danger. It's all in our head. For instance, you may fear public speaking or a confrontation with your wife. Neither event is life threatening, but your fearful thoughts cause your body to react as if you were in harm's way. And in those cases, your fear hampers you much more than it helps.

▶HOW SERIOUS

Whether your fear is in response to an actual or imagined threat, the sensation can hamper your ability to think clearly. Also, the hormones and chemicals released during a fight-or-flight response can, over time, hinder your im-

DO THIS NOW

To stop your mind from racing, concentrate on your breath as it comes in and out of your nose. You'll feel a slight coolness as the breath comes in and a slight warmth as the air leaves. "This will stop your mind chatter," says Phil Nuernberger, Ph.D., president of Mind Resource Technologies in Honesdale, Pennsylvania, and author of *The Quest for Personal Power.* "You'll still be able to see, hear, and react to danger. You are simply bypassing the emotional process and trusting your deeper mind to guide you."

Did You Know?

Quiz time: 84 percent of the things we worry about turn out better than expected or much better than expected, says Thomas D. Borkovec, Ph.D., professor of psychology at Pennsylvania State University in University Park. This means that only 16 percent turn out as bad as we expected, or worse. Of those, Dr. Borkovec says, we cope better or much better than expected 80 percent of the time. So, how often do our fears actually come true, and how often do we wind up coping with them as badly as we feared?

Time's up. The answer: 3 percent of the time. It's no wonder that Franklin D. Roosevelt said, "The only thing we have to fear is fear itself."

mune system, causing health problems. If you find yourself constantly agitated and none of the tips in this chapter bring you relief, you should seek professional help from a mental health practitioner, Dr. Borkovec says.

▶SOLUTIONS

Practice breathing. Fear usually makes us breathe shallowly, which actually makes us more fearful. Instead, concentrate on bringing your breath deep into your abdomen, says Phil Nuernberger, Ph.D., president of Mind Resource Technologies in Honesdale, Pennsylvania, and author of *The Quest for Personal Power*. You'll need to use your diaphragm—a large sheet of muscle that separates your chest from your abdomen. When you use your diaphragm to pull air into your lungs, your belly will expand and look round. Of course, drinking lots of beer will get the same result. But with deep breathing, when you exhale, your belly will flatten.

Practice diaphragmatic breathing when you're calm. That way, you'll teach yourself to continue to breathe deeply when frightened. To do so, Dr. Nuernberger recommends the following technique: Lie down on the floor on your back. Put your right hand on your belly and the left on your chest. As you breathe in, imagine your breath filling a small balloon in your stomach. Your right hand will rise with the inhalation and fall with the exhalation. The hand on your chest should remain still.

Talk to yourself. Often, we fear things that aren't truly threats. We worry that we've made someone angry. Or we get anxious over a high-profile assignment at work. When you're frightened even though you're not in any immediate danger (your house isn't burning down), take a moment to examine your perceptions, Dr. Borkovec says. Ask yourself the following questions.

- What are the thoughts, beliefs, images, or predictions running through my mind?

- Are they accurate? For instance, if you worry that the flight you are about to take is going to blow up, look at crash statistics.

- If your fears are unfounded, what's another less fearful and more accurate way of seeing the situation? For instance, if the thought of getting on an airplane makes you feel sick to your stomach, tell yourself that you have very little chance of dying in a plane. You'll often need to repeat such accurate thoughts each time you notice the inaccurate negative thoughts occurring, Dr. Borkovec says.

Rate your worries. Take some time during the day to list what you fear. Then keep track of whether your fears come true. If they do, rate whether each situation turned out better than you expected, as bad as you expected, or worse than you expected. Then rate how you coped.

"Our biggest fear is that bad things will happen and that we won't be able to cope," says Dr. Borkovec. In reality, however, most of our fears never materialize. And when they do, we handle them better than expected.

▶ALTERNATIVE APPROACHES

Let your mind do the tightrope walking. Or airplane riding. Or first date going. Or any other activity you fear. You see, the more you confront your fears, the less fear you'll feel. But you don't physically have to do the confronting. You can simply imagine the whole experience, says Dr. Borkovec. To do so, first relax by breathing slowly and deeply. Then, visualize yourself in the situation you fear. See yourself act calmly or courageously. Then, return to your deep breathing. Visualize the same scene over and over until you feel ready to confront the fear in real life, he says.

▶PREVENTIVE MEASURES

Concentrate. When you focus your attention on a point—your breath, your heartbeat, or a repetitive sound—you're meditating. "That leads you to the deepest levels of your mind where strength lies," says Dr. Nuernberger. The more often you meditate, the more easily you can call up the calm, focused feeling when danger arises. Your breath is one of the easiest and most effective points of concentration. Pay attention to breathing in and out. Listen to the air. Feel it enter your lungs. When you notice yourself losing concentration—and you will—refocus on your breath.

"Don't struggle with the mind. Gently train it to be one-pointed," Dr. Nuernberger says. He recommends doing this meditation exercise once or twice a day for 15 minutes.

Make a scene. Picture a relaxing image—lying on a warm beach, watching a waterfall, lounging on the recliner, says Dr. Borkovec. Try relaxing with your favorite scene for 10 to 15 minutes twice a day. Once you get in the habit, you'll be able to picture this scene to ease your anxiety in a fearful situation.

Fever

▶PROBLEM

Your head feels like a blast furnace. And when you aren't sweating buckets, you might have chills.

▶CAUSE

A fever develops when your internal thermostat, the hypothalamus gland, goes on the fritz. What causes this to happen? Inflammation, infection, or both. Normal body temperature at rest is around 98.6°F (oral). This varies from person to person and from hour to hour. A fever exists when you have a consistently elevated temperature. A low-grade fever is between 99.5° and 101°F, and a high-grade fever occurs at more than 101°F. In either case, the body releases substances called pyrogens that reset the body's thermostat to a higher temperature, in an attempt to burn off whatever's causing the infection. Chills and shivering may then result from muscular activity and an increase in the metabolic rate as the body attempts to raise its temperature. Your pulse will go up, and you'll get thirsty.

▶HOW SERIOUS

"A fever is a clinical sign, like a rash or a cough," says Thomas E. Young, M.D., a doctor of internal medicine in private practice in Emmaus, Pennsylvania. Temperature alone may not be a barometer of how sick you are. "At 103°F, it could be a cold. At 101°F, it could be something more serious," he says.

DO THIS NOW

To lower fever, take ibuprofen or acetaminophen per the instructions on the bottle, advises Thomas E. Young, M.D., a doctor of internal medicine in private practice in Emmaus, Pennsylvania. Avoid aspirin. Physicians tend not to recommend aspirin any longer because of the remote possibility that a person could contract Reye's syndrome—a reaction between the drug and viral illnesses that can lead to swelling of the brain and other organ damage. Although Reye's normally afflicts children, says Dr. Young, there is a very slim chance that it could affect adults.

Did You Know?

Whether it's sung by Peggy Lee or Little Willie John, "Fever" is one of the great blues tunes, evoking images of raging, unbridled, heat-producing passion. But can feelings of love and lust actually give us a fever?

Nope—it just feels that ways, says Thomas E. Young, M.D., a doctor of internal medicine in private practice in Emmaus, Pennsylvania. Our bodies regulate the temperature, not our emotions, he says. Dr. Young thinks that there's an innocent explanation for the perception that we can be "hot" for somebody—that they can give us fever. When we get excited or aroused, blood starts rushing to various places, including our faces. Thus, lovers become flushed with emotion, "and that might be mistaken for a fever," he says.

The key is to put your fever in context. If you have flu symptoms and others in your family have been stricken, it's probably just a normal part of the illness. But if you are also coughing up gunk and can hardly breathe, it's a good idea to see a doctor, says Dr. Young.

Children tend to have higher fevers than adults, but if yours tops 104.5°F and is not responding to at-home treatment, get to a doctor. Regardless of your symptoms, always see a doctor if you have a fever above 101°F for more than two days, Dr. Young says.

▶SOLUTIONS

Sweat it out. "There is no need to treat mild fevers (below 101°F) with fever-lowering drugs or natural remedies for lowering temperatures," says Dr. Young. Remember, an elevated temperature is the body's solution to fighting infection, he adds. But if you are too uncomfortable, or if your fever is high-grade, try the tips that follow.

Cool it. A cool compress to your forehead will feel good and can help lower a fever, says Dr. Young.

Drink all day. Not alcohol, which will only make you feel worse, but clear liquids such as water, ginger ale and apple juice, says Dr. Young. "You tend to get dehydrated because you burn up extra water when you have a fever. You tend to sweat. You need to replace that water by drinking more than you usually do." Since it's imperative to drink, alert your doctor if you cannot hold down your fluids, he adds. (Drink extra liquid regardless of whether you are treating your temperature.)

Bathe the heat away. Take a bath or shower for 20 minutes in water slightly cooler than what you normally use, advises Dr. Young. "It brings the fever down about 1.5°F," he says.

▶ALTERNATIVE APPROACHES

Schedule a tea time. You can make a tea with one to two teaspoons of dried willow bark steeped in a cup of boiling water for about 20 minutes and have an effective fever-fighter, says James A. Duke, Ph.D., the world's foremost authority on healing herbs and author of *The Green Pharmacy*. Loose, dried willow bark may be difficult to find, so look for it in already-prepared tea bags at health food stores. It has a bitter taste that can be made more palatable by adding flavorful herbs such as cinnamon or chamomile.

The active compound salicin was isolated in willow bark and became the key component in aspirin. Willow bark should not be taken with aspirin, and don't take it if you are allergic to aspirin. Also, since willow bark has similar compounds to aspirin, don't take it if you need to avoid aspirin because of ulcers, asthma, diabetes, gout, hemophilia, hypothrombinemia, or kidney or liver disease. Mixing willow bark with alcohol can irritate your stomach. It may also interact with barbiturates such as aprobarbital (Amytal Sodium) or sedatives such as alprazolam (Xanax).

Try flower power. Like willow bark, meadowsweet flowers are an excellent source of salicin, says Dr. Duke. He suggests drinking up to three cups a day of a tea made with one to two teaspoons of the flowers.

▶PREVENTIVE MEASURES

Don't get wrapped too tightly. When your fever is giving you a bad case of the chills, don't go overboard to keep yourself warm, says Dr. Young. "You don't want to be naked, but you don't want to put five blankets on. The heat needs to get out. Keep yourself appropriately clothed."

Five o'Clock Shadow

▶PROBLEM

You shave. You go to work. By the time your late afternoon meeting rolls around, you have a chin that looks like Fred Flintstone's.

▶CAUSE

It's a family thing. If you come from a background of heavily bearded men with dark hair, chances are very good that you'll have five o'clock shadow. Men with blond hair or those who grow scant beards rarely have to worry about it.

▶HOW SERIOUS

Medically speaking, it rates about a zero in seriousness, says Jerald L. Sklar, M.D., attending dermatologist at Baylor University Medical Center in Dallas. Professionally and socially, it's another matter. A haze of whiskers can make you look unkempt at work, and your favorite lady may not appreciate snuggling up to Mr. Sandpaper.

▶SOLUTIONS

Soften up. Before you grab your razor, wrap your face in a hot, moist towel for two to three minutes or wait until just after you shower to shave, says Larry Fila Jr., director of the Maryland Barber School in Brooklyn Park. Both techniques soften the whiskers.

Lube your face. After you've moistened your skin, apply a base oil to your

History Lesson

A cover-up cost President Richard M. Nixon the White House in 1974. But a decision not to cover up may have cost him his first attempt at the nation's highest office 14 years earlier.

Nixon, vice president at the time, and then-Massachusetts Senator John F. Kennedy squared off in the first televised presidential debate in history during the 1960 campaign. What the public saw was the handsome, stylish Kennedy verbally duking it out with a sweating Nixon, who was sporting a bad case of five o'clock shadow. Both men had been offered makeup before going on air. But when Kennedy decided to go bare-faced, Nixon also declined.

Although it's unlikely that Kennedy shrugged off makeup as a strategic move, some feel that Nixon's poor television image in those debates helped give Kennedy his razor-thin presidential victory.

---

cheeks and chin. This can be any oil designed for application to the skin, such as the ones you can find at specialty bath and body shops. The oil will keep your razor lubricated and your skin supple.

Get foamy. Lather up with shaving cream. If you're applying the base oil first, save some money on your shaving cream. Any brand will work just as well as a premium one; all it's doing is holding up your whiskers while you shave.

Do the deed. Dig out a good double-blade razor, disposable or cartridge. If your skin isn't too sensitive, pull it taut in front of the blade, Fila advises. This pops the whiskers farther out of their follicles, plus it helps eliminate nicks. When you've finished shaving, go back over your face a second time. Shaving against the grain gives you a closer shave. But if your skin is sensitive or easily irritated then be sure to shave with the grain only, never against, and pass on the second shave.

End with a splash. Splash your newly shaved skin with cold water and, if you like, slap on some witch hazel lotion. This astringent also has an antiseptic property but doesn't burn or dry like alcohol-based aftershaves. It's available at most drugstores. Apply a light moisturizer; your closely scraped skin will appreciate the extra protection, especially in the winter. Fila recommends avoiding those heavily scented moisturizers that not only have a high alcohol content but also contain strong fragrance, which may irritate the skin.

Be electrifying. Sometimes there's no way around it, says Dr. Sklar: If you have an exceptionally heavy beard, you'll just have to shave twice. "You can use your blade in the morning, and later you can take an electric or rechargeable razor in the car or office and do a little touch-up," he says.

▶ALTERNATIVE APPROACHES

Scorch it. A chemical depilatory (like Neet or Nair) acts by dissolving the hair at or just below the skin's surface. There are depilatories on the market specially formulated for facial skin. While they may provide a closer shave, they are too caustic to be used every day, cautions Fredric S. Brandt, M.D., clinical associate professor of dermatology at the University of Miami School of Medicine. Use them on clean skin and follow label directions carefully. It is a good idea to do a patch skin test on the inside of your elbow to make sure that you do not have a reaction to the chemicals.

▶PREVENTIVE MEASURES

Don't fight it. There is one guaranteed way to make sure that you'll never worry about five o'clock shadow again: Grow a beard. "I think that certain types of beards are back in style, even among professionals," Dr. Brandt says. He suggests that a close-cropped, neatly groomed beard might be the way to go for someone tired of shaving all the time.

Flatulence

▶PROBLEM

Flatulence—also known as passing gas, breaking wind, and farting—is how the body gets rid of excess gas in the intestinal tract. Breaking wind is certainly a useful activity, but it's not particularly pleasant for anyone else in the room. The average person passes 1,500 milliliters of gas daily (about the amount of air in a half-inflated party balloon), released about 30 to 120 milliliters at a time. Flatus, the gas we pass via the rectum, is made of nitrogen, oxygen, carbon dioxide, hydrogen, methane, and trace amounts of other gases. Interestingly, the embarrassing odor that most of us can quickly identify as a fart is related to strong-smelling sulfur compounds that make up only 1 percent of flatus. Apart from its odor and embarrassing social consequences, flatulence itself is harmless and completely normal.

▶CAUSE

One common cause of flatulence is swallowed air, says Harris Clearfield, M.D., professor of medicine and section chief of the division of gastroenterology at Allegheny University of the Health Sciences MCP–Hahnemann School of Medicine in Philadelphia. Men who chew gum or eat too quickly tend to gulp down a lot of air, which, of course, is made of gases. Most beers and sodas are as well; the gas carbon dioxide is what accounts for their fizziness—and yours, too. Whatever the cause, gas builds up in the digestive tract. Your body has to get rid of it either by belching or by passing it out the rectum.

The foods we eat, however, are often the more likely cause of flatulence—in particular, fiber-rich foods like broccoli, bran, and beans. Because these com-

History Lesson

Joseph Pujol of nineteenth-century France was a musical genius of an altogether different stripe. Pujol had the extraordinary talent of sucking air through his anus and then releasing it to make birdcalls and blow out candles from a distance of about 18 inches. Nicknamed "le Petomane" (the Fartomaniac), Pujol was also highly regarded for his ability to fart out a variety of tunes and do an anal imitation of a violin tremolo and a solo falsetto. Talk about classical gas.

plex carbohydrates aren't fully digested in the small intestine, undigested bits travel to the colon where they're fermented by bacteria, causing gas. For men who are lactose-intolerant, dairy products cause gas. Lactose intolerance is caused by a deficiency of lactase, an enzyme needed to break down the milk sugar lactose in the small intestine. Lactose is happily broken down by the bacteria that live in your colon, but gas is the unfortunate by-product. (See Lactose Intolerance on page 352 for more tips on how to deal with this condition.)

▶HOW SERIOUS

Flatulence is simply your body's way of ridding itself of gas; its presence doesn't usually signal a problem. Sometimes a problem with flatulence could simply be a "functional disorder," meaning that your intestinal tract may not always function properly, leaving you uncomfortable but not at risk for serious disease. But some people are very sensitive to normal amounts of gas in their system and suffer from bloating, cramping, and pain. If these troublesome symptoms persist, see your doctor to rule out more serious conditions such as diverticulitis, peptic ulcer disease, or a hiatal hernia, says Dr. Clearfield.

▶SOLUTIONS

Get a little culture. The active culture *Lactobacillus acidophilus* found in some yogurts—look for it on the label—not only digests the lactose in the yogurt but also may help to digest the lactose in other dairy products. To get the benefit, you need to eat them at the same meal, says Roger Gebhard, M.D., professor of medicine at the University of Minnesota Medical School in Minneapolis and staff physician at the Minneapolis Veterans Administration Medical Center.

Lose the lactose. If cheese or milk products are chief offenders (and they are for some men), don't give up the pizza yet. Try over-the-counter digestive aids like Lactaid or Lactinex. They'll help digest the milk sugar lactose before it reaches the colon (where it ferments and causes gas), says Dr. Gebhard.

Eliminate with enzymes. Beans, of course, are a gas giant among foods, but there's over-the-counter help for that, too. By dashing your food with the enzyme alpha-galactosidase (Beano), you can break down the offending sugars in beans before they make you break wind.

▶ALTERNATIVE APPROACHES

Tame it with tea. Brew a tea with one to two teaspoons of anise or fennel seeds per cup of boiling water and steep for 10 minutes, suggests William Keller, Ph.D., chairman of the department of pharmaceutical sciences at the McWhorter School of Pharmacy at Samford University in Birmingham, Alabama. Drink as much as you want of this brew between meals, whenever you want relief, says Dr. Keller. Other gas-relieving teas, available premade in many supermarkets, include peppermint, ginger, and chamomile.

▶PREVENTIVE MEASURES

Swallow slowly. Wolfing down your lunch may leave you howling later, so to speak. To avoid swallowing the excess air that could turn you into a gas giant, try to be more conscious of the need to slow down while you eat. You may be able to avoid flatulence in the first place, says Dr. Gebhard.

Cut the cheese. Avoid it, that is. Some adults who are lactose-intolerant experience some trouble digesting dairy products like milk and cheese, says Dr. Clearfield. If you think you might be one of them, try limiting the amount of dairy products you consume, says Dr. Gebhard. That might stop the music.

Quit chewing the cud. Avid gum chewing can also translate into too much swallowed air and gastrointestinal distress, says Dr. Gebhard. The same goes for sucking on hard candies and the like. Cut back on these candies and save your teeth at the same time that you avoid flatulence.

Beware of bubbly. Since drinking carbonated beverages can also increase the amount of gas in your stomach, cut back on the amount of soda and beer you drink, says Dr. Clearfield.

Food Poisoning

▶PROBLEM

You have flulike symptoms that may include any of the following: vomiting, severe abdominal cramps, diarrhea, chills, fever, and occasionally, headache and a generally achy feeling.

▶CAUSE

Food poisoning is caused by bacteria, such as *Escherichia coli* and *Salmonella*, and viruses, which may taint raw or undercooked meats, poultry, raw eggs or foods made with them, unpasteurized dairy or juice products, and seafood. It typically occurs when one of the three Cs—clean, cooked, or cold—is lacking, says Margy Woodburn, Ph.D., professor emeritus of nutrition and food management at Oregon State University in Corvallis. "Men have poorer food safety habits than women, and younger men have poorer habits than older men," she says.

> ### DO THIS NOW
>
> Mix a half-teaspoon of salt and three tablespoons of sugar in a quart of water, recommends Margy Woodburn, Ph.D., professor emeritus of nutrition and food management at Oregon State University in Corvallis. Drink a half-cup to a cup of the stuff after each episode of diarrhea, or 10 minutes after vomiting, if possible.

▶HOW SERIOUS

The Centers for Disease Control and Prevention (CDC) in Atlanta estimates that between 50 million and 80 million people a year come down with food-borne illnesses. Often their symptoms are mild, but the CDC estimates that 9,000 people die annually from food poisoning. Only about 1 person in 18 who has contracted food poisoning sees his doctor about it, says Penny Adcock, M.D., a medical epidemiologist in the food-borne and diarrheal diseases branch of the CDC. You need to see a doctor if you have severe vomiting and diarrhea that lead to dehydration, if you have bloody diarrhea, or if you have diarrhea that lasts more than four days, says Dr. Adcock.

Some guys are definitely more at risk of getting food poisoning than others,

Dr. Woodburn adds. Older men, men who drink excessively (and thus, may have cirrhosis of the liver), and those who've had organ transplants or are taking chemotherapy are all in the higher-risk group, she says. Taking antacids puts men in a more moderate-risk group, Dr. Woodburn says, because the antacids neutralize stomach acid, which might have otherwise killed the bacteria or virus causing the food poisoning.

▶SOLUTIONS

Play detective. If you think you have food poisoning, talk to someone who ate the same thing you did to see if he or she is sick (although it's possible that one person could get food poisoning while another one eating the same food does not). If you suspect that you picked up the bug at a public eatery, report it to the local health department, Dr. Adcock says.

Drink lots of fluids. Long bouts of vomiting or diarrhea will dehydrate you, so drink plenty of water, advises Dr. Adcock. Gatorade or other liquids are fine, too, if you can tolerate them. Dr. Adcock also recommends this homemade electrolyte solution: Mix one teaspoon of salt, one teaspoon of baking soda, four teaspoons of sugar, and a small amount of flavored gelatin (just enough to make the solution taste okay) in a quart of water.

As your symptoms improve, you can have broth and then bland foods like cooked cereal, eggs, or gelatin, Dr. Adcock says. How much do you need to drink? The general rule of thumb is to estimate how much fluid you think you've lost and replace it by sipping small amounts of liquid frequently, Dr. Adcock says.

Rest. Your body is trying to rid itself of poison, so accept that you have to ride this unpleasantness out and make yourself as comfortable as possible, Dr. Adcock says. And make sure that you pick a resting place that has quick and easy access to the bathroom.

Let loose. Over-the-counter medications aimed at ending diarrhea can make food poisoning symptoms linger longer, says Dr. Adcock. That's because diarrhea flushes bacteria out of your intestines. By not having the runs, you run the risk of the bacteria hanging around longer. So don't take these medications if you think you might have food poisoning, Dr. Adcock says.

▶ALTERNATIVE APPROACHES

Seek homeopathic relief. If you suspect that you have food poisoning and you feel anxious, restless, and chilly and have simultaneous nausea, vomiting, and diarrhea, try taking three to five pellets of *Arsenicum album* in 12C or 30C potency every two to three hours until you feel better, says Mitchell Fleisher, M.D., a family practitioner and homeopath in private practice in Nellysford, Virginia. If you have similar symptoms, but also have cold sweats and crave ice-cold beverages, Dr. Fleisher recommends trying three to five pellets of a 12C or 30C potency of *Veratrum album* every two to three hours.

History Lesson

The Alfred Hitchcock film *The Birds* may have been inspired, in part, by birds behaving bizarrely as a result of food poisoning. Hordes of seabirds flew into light poles and cars, chased people, and vomited bits of anchovies near Santa Cruz, California, in 1961. The theory at the time was that they became disoriented in foggy weather.

The local newspaper reported that Hitchcock phoned and asked for a copy of its story on the wayward birds. Two years later, the movie—based on a short story by Daphne Du Maurier—was released.

David Garrison, Ph.D., a research marine scientist at the Institute of Marine Sciences at the University of California at Santa Cruz, believes that the birds' behavior was caused by eating anchovies that had consumed algae with a toxin called domoic acid. Domoic acid's effects were unknown until an outbreak in Canada in 1987. Other incidents of domoic acid illness in birds and humans occurred in California, Oregon, and Washington in 1991, Dr. Garrison says.

"I think that's what explains the birds' behavior in 1961, but we have no way to prove that," Dr. Garrison says.

If you are experiencing intense abdominal cramping that makes you double over in pain, but you aren't vomiting, Dr. Fleisher says that you can sit on the edge of your bed or on a chair and bend forward over a pillow, putting pressure on your stomach, for 5 to 10 minutes at a time. You can also try placing a hot compress against your stomach, he says, although the pressure is what brings the most relief. Dr. Fleisher also suggests taking three to five pellets of Colocynthis in 12C or 30C potency every two to four hours. Homeopathic remedies are available at many health food stores.

Caution: If you don't have any improvement in your symptoms after taking one dose of a homeopathic remedy, go to the hospital, Dr. Fleisher says.

▶PREVENTIVE MEASURES

Keep your fridge cold. Your refrigerator should be kept at 40°F or colder, Dr. Woodburn says. She recommends buying a refrigerator thermometer and placing it in the back of the fridge for an accurate temperature reading. You should be able to find these at most discount department stores or possibly at your grocery store.

Keep a cooler in the car. On warm days when you're running a couple of errands after buying groceries, place perishable items in a cooler, suggests Dr. Woodburn.

Thaw carefully. If you remove meat from the freezer to be cooked, the best way to thaw it is in the refrigerator, says Dr. Woodburn. If you don't have time, then place it in a waterproof bag in cold water. If you must cook it immediately, zap it in the microwave.

The least desirable way to thaw meat is to leave it on a counter at room temperature, Dr. Woodburn says. It is important to thaw frozen meat—especially burgers, meat loaf, and cube steaks—and poultry before cooking so that it will cook evenly to the center, where some harmful organisms may otherwise survive.

Don't dally after dinner. Put leftovers in the refrigerator within two hours of finishing a meal, Dr. Woodburn advises. If the food is still hot, place it in a shallow container that will enable it to cool more quickly. Food left on the table can get bacteria from people, flies, and other sources. Bacteria already present in the food also begin to multiply. "After two hours, the bacteria can reach dangerous numbers," Dr. Woodburn says.

Avoid the pink. Don't eat hamburgers cooked rare, or in which the meat remains pink in the center, says Dr. Woodburn. They can carry the *E. coli* or *Salmonella* bacteria. "Many men are saying they know the risk but that they like a rare hamburger," she says. It's not worth the risk.

Resist the raw. Eating raw oysters and clams is risky, Dr. Woodburn says. "Even if they're harvested from water that meets the quality standards, there may still be pathogenic bacteria and viruses present for hepatitis A," she says.

Sushi is generally safe, however, as long as you don't have a compromised immune system, Dr. Adcock adds.

Cook eggs carefully. Forget what you saw in *Rocky*. Raw eggs can make you sick, says Dr. Woodburn. They should be thoroughly cooked—no runny whites and thick yolks. And guys should be aware of foods that might contain raw eggs, such as chiffon pie, homemade mayonnaise, cookie dough, cake batter, and certain salad dressings, Dr. Woodburn says. So avoid these, too. She also suggests that rather than making your own eggnog over the holidays, buy a commercial one that has used pasteurized eggs.

Cook stuffing separately. Don't stuff stuffing inside your holiday turkey when you cook it. Instead, cook it separately, Dr. Adcock says. Pathogens are more likely to lurk inside the bird where the temperature does not always get adequately high, she says.

Stop the drips. Don't let meat or poultry stored in your refrigerator drip on other foods below, advises Dr. Woodburn. Place meats in waterproof bags, or on a tray or plate below other foods.

Keep utensils clean. Don't allow plates, knives, spatulas, and the like that have touched raw meat to come into contact with any other food. They can contaminate it, Dr. Woodburn says. "All utensils should be cleaned very thoroughly immediately after you have cut up or used them with any raw meat, fish, or poultry," she says.

Foot Odor

▶PROBLEM

Everything is fine when your shoes are on. But take them off and, man, something smells. And that stench is pungent, acrid, fetid—in short, just plain offensive.

And it's not just your feet that smell. Your shoes and socks are also quite odoriferous. "Foot odor is actually a combination of odors emanating from your shoe, foot, and sock," says Herbert Lapidus, Ph.D., vice president and technical director of research and development for Combe of White Plains, New York. And Dr. Lapidus knows his foot odor. He's the guy who invented Odor-Eaters.

▶CAUSE

"The perspiration from your foot doesn't smell on its own," Dr. Lapidus explains. "When the bacteria on the foot grow as a result of the moisture of perspiration, it produces odor. One of the compounds that is part of foot odor is isovaleric acid. This is volatile, and when it wafts up to your nose, it is perceived as odor."

To fight foot odor, you need to fight bacteria. Because bacteria thrive in moist and dark places, they just love your feet and the inside of your shoes, says John Venson, D.P.M., chairman of the department of medicine and surgery at the Dr. William M. Scholl College of Podiatric Medicine in Chicago. So you need to make your feet and shoes inhospitable to bacteria. Think dry, airy, and light.

▶HOW SERIOUS

Well, listen, no one's going to literally die from smelly feet, but you could die of embarrassment. We all know someone whose feet smell, which means that sometimes, smelly feet are a guy's most obvious attribute. Do you want to be known as Stinky, Cheesy, or "What-the-Hell-Died-in-Here?" There are, however, times when foot odor should be taken seriously.

"If you try to get rid of foot odor on your own and fail, then you probably should see a doctor," says Dr. Venson. "You may have an infection that isn't healing or another problem that can only be helped by professional care." You should also see a doctor if the skin on your foot is extremely dry and is cracking.

▶SOLUTIONS

Fire up the charcoal. Here's a new vocabulary word for you: adsorption. "Activated charcoal adsorbs odor," says Dr. Lapidus. "In other words, its surface area attracts the odor molecules, so they don't reach your nose."

Simply cut a pair of one-size-fits-all activated charcoal shoe inserts down to size, put them in your shoes, and use for a few months. Replace them every three to six months, depending on how often you wear each pair of shoes. Look for charcoal shoe inserts at drugstores.

Roll on the deodorant. You can use an underarm deodorant on the bottom of your feet, says Marjorie Menacker, D.P.M., a podiatrist with Chesterfield Podiatry Associates in Midlothian, Virginia. Deodorants fight bacterial odor, whether it's under your arm or on your foot. Deodorants do not control wetness, however.

If your feet also perspire too much, then try an antiperspirant made specifically for feet. Called Certain-Dri, it's available in most drugstores. And both the deodorant and the antiperspirant can be used daily, says Dr. Menacker.

Lick it with Lysol. Spraying Lysol in your shoes will help get rid of the smelly bacteria that are living in them, says Dr. Venson. Open your shoes and lift the tongue to let them dry out. If the odor in the shoe persists, you can spray them very lightly with Lysol. Then let them dry for 24 hours before wearing them.

Soak safely. It seems that a guy with foot odor will stick his poor doggies in a lot of suspicious substances to try to get rid of the smell. So here's a good rule of thumb, courtesy of Dr. Menacker: "If you soak your foot in anything you'd be willing to drink, then it's probably okay."

Some good choices include tea, vinegar, and table salt. An exception to the drinking rule is Epsom salts, which you definitely would *not* want to drink. "Vinegar, tea, and Epsom salts can all draw some of the excess moisture out of your foot," Dr. Menacker says.

The next time you need to give odor the boot, try soaking in one of the following solutions for 15 to 20 minutes, once or twice a day. You can soak as often as every day as long as you do not develop a rash, dry skin, or some other skin problem, says Dr. Menacker.

Vinegar: Add a half-cup of white vinegar to a quart of warm water.

Did You Know?

Mosquitoes have a decided preference for certain odors, namely, those that come from the feet. How did scientists test this hypothesis?

A researcher, wearing only "close-fitting" underwear, and having not bathed for nine hours previously, sat in a room with 200 5- to 10-day old female malaria mosquitoes. The little nippers, who had been "starved the night before," were released individually into the test site. The bloodsuckers went straight for the stinky feet (and smelly breath) of the tester.

In fact, when the researcher washed his feet, the little buggers didn't head for the guy's feet at all but, instead, went looking for other odoriferous parts of his body. You don't even want to think about where they chose to dine.

Tea: Make a cup of tea with hot water, but use a few regular black tea bags. Add that to some cool water. "Black tea has tannin in it that will help absorb moisture," Dr. Menacker explains.

Epsom salts: Add a half-cup of Epsom salts to a quart of warm water.

Test the water you soak your feet in with your fingers, not your toe, and be sure that the water is lukewarm, not hot, says Dr. Menacker. Men who have diabetes, lots of calluses, or other serious foot problems are sometimes unable to detect extreme heat with their feet quickly enough to prevent burning, she warns.

▶ALTERNATIVE APPROACHES

Detoxify with tea. "Foot odor may be a sign that your kidneys and colon need to detox," says Christopher Trahan, a doctor of Oriental medicine and licensed acupuncturist in private practice in New York City. "Get some dry burdock root or burdock seed from a health food store and simmer a half-tablespoon of the dry root or a half-tablespoon of the seeds in three cups of water for 15 minutes," says Dr. Trahan. "Then strain. Drink in three doses throughout the day, reheating the tea and drinking it warm." After the first three days, up the amount used to one tablespoon of the root or seed taken in three doses throughout the day. Take at this dosage for three to four weeks. If your foot odor has improved, you may repeat the three- to four-week course. But if you're not happy with the results after the initial three to four weeks, you should consult a professional, advises Dr. Trahan.

Massage with essential oils. Lavender, bitter orange, and tea tree oils smell great and are also potent antimicrobials, says Nancy Dunne-Boggs, a doctor of naturopathy at Bitterroot Natural Medicine in Missoula, Montana. In other words, they'll help kill the bacteria that's causing the odor. "Rub enough of the oil into your foot to coat the skin, and give yourself a nice massage with it," suggests Dr. Dunne-Boggs. "Make your feet pink and warm. Then put socks on to protect your sheets, and sleep with the oil for four or five consecutive nights at least."

Lavender and tea tree oils are available at health food stores, and bitter orange oil can be ordered through the Essential Oil Company, 1719 Southeast Umapilla, Portland, OR 97202. Do not use bitter orange oil on an area of the skin that will be exposed to the sun. If you have sensitive skin, you should talk to your doctor before using tea tree oil.

▶PREVENTIVE MEASURES

Care for your shoes. If you take proper care of your shoes, there's a good chance that foot odor will bid you goodbye. "Prevention is the best treatment when it comes to foot odor," says Dr. Venson. Here are his tips.

- Buy shoes that are all leather since they "breathe" more than synthetic shoes.
- Alternate your shoes on a day-to-day basis. On off-days, let them air-dry as thoroughly as possible by spreading apart the laces and pulling the tongue back.
- Don't keep your shoes in a closed, dark closet or locker.
- If you exercise every day, get two pairs of athletic shoes.

Sock odor away. Wear synthetic socks that wick moisture away from your foot, Dr. Venson suggests. Also, wash your socks in hot water, not cold or warm. Use bleach, if possible, in a sockload of laundry.

Just forget about the notion some guys have that it's okay to soak your feet in bleach. It's not safe. "Bleach is clearly too caustic to be good for your skin or the inside of your body," Dr. Menacker says.

Wash your feet well. Finally, it's time to really clean between your toes. Use soap and a washcloth on your feet. Then be sure to thoroughly dry them when you get out of the tub or shower. Once again, be sure to dry between your toes, Dr. Venson says.

Foot Pain

▶PROBLEM

Are your dogs tired and aching at the end of the day? It could be fallen arches. Do you have sudden pain in the back of your heel (rather than at the bottom)? Uh-oh. You may have injured your Achilles tendon (for more information, see Bursitis/Tendinitis on page 119). Most foot pain, however, is either plantar fasciitis or fallen arches. Fascia is fibrous tissue that lies beneath the skin but over bone and muscle. *Plantar* means "under your foot." And *itis* means "inflammation." Put it all together and you get inflammation in the tissue on the underside of your foot that supports you when you stand (which is why you don't feel any pain when you're sitting down). It's the most common culprit of foot pain for men and strikes most often in the mornings, the first time your feet touch the ground.

Fallen arches, as the name implies, is a change in the depth of the arch in your foot. "The 'fall' occurs not overnight but over time as we age, if the foot isn't properly supported by the shoes you wear," says Richard Braver, D.P.M., a sports podiatrist and head of the Active Foot and Ankle Care Centers in Englewood and Fair Lawn, New Jersey. A high arch can become a moderate arch, while a moderate arch can become flatter. Flat feet can bring on their own set of problems, as the arch stretches out more, causing strain (and pain) of the foot.

DO THIS NOW

Stretch and massage your feet before getting out of bed, says Marjorie Menacker, D.P.M., a podiatrist with Chesterfield Podiatry Associates in Midlothian, Virginia. This will ease the pain of plantar fasciitis, a pain felt in the arch and heel of the foot. A general rule of thumb for stretching is to hold each stretch for 10 seconds and repeat each stretch 10 times.

"While lying on your back in bed, move your ankles back and forth to stretch out your calf. Next, put the heel of one foot under the toes of the other and pull your toes back with your heel," explains Dr. Menacker. "Finally, rub each foot with your hands to warm it up, if needed."

▶CAUSE

Think "increase" when trying to figure out what has caused the sudden onset of plantar fasciitis, says Dr. Braver. You've probably either gained weight or increased the amount you exercise (especially walking or running). Or you haven't been wearing good supportive shoes, and that has weakened your arches. Wearing poorly fitted shoes can lead to multiple foot problems, including plantar fasciitis and fallen arches.

▶HOW SERIOUS

Plantar fasciitis and fallen arches can take a long time to heal or remedy, so it's best to start fixing the problem as soon as your symptoms develop, says Marjorie Menacker, D.P.M., a podiatrist with Chesterfield Podiatry Associates in Midlothian, Virginia.

But you still have a few more questions to ask yourself to determine if you should even attempt to heal yourself because some instances of foot pain are serious, says Andrea Cracchiolo III, M.D., an orthopedic surgeon and director of the University of California, Los Angeles, Adult Foot and Ankle Clinic.

Do you feel nauseated? Nausea signifies a deep injury, such as a tendon or ligament tear. Make an appointment with your doctor. Is your foot black and blue anywhere? If so, you also should see a doctor. "If there's enough strain or energy to cause a rupture of small blood vessels, then there may have been enough pressure or strain to fracture a bone or tear a ligament," Dr. Cracchiolo says.

And forget about "if you can move it, it's not broken," Dr. Cracchiolo adds. "You can't move some of the bones in your foot even when they're healthy, so that's not the way to figure out if something's broken."

▶SOLUTIONS

Insert relief. An orthotic is a molded insert for your shoe that helps to support your foot. They're available at medical supply stores or through a podiatrist.

"An orthotic should be your first line of defense against foot pain," says Dr. Braver. "If you have a flat foot or falling arches, look for a firm arch support. On the other hand, if you have a high arch or plantar fasciitis, find a more cushiony, yet supportive orthotic."

You might need to trim an orthotic down to size. "Stand on it to see if the arch in the orthotic matches up with the arch in your foot," instructs Dr. Braver. "Also, make sure that your shoe is deep enough to withstand the extra height of the orthotic. If it causes blisters, then you shouldn't use it."

A guy who is very heavy (and therefore putting more weight on his feet) may need to use two inserts together or go to a podiatrist for a "custom" orthotic. The right orthotic will make the pain go away, Dr. Braver says.

Get called for icing. Put some ice on your feet for 15 to 20 minutes at a

History Lesson

Back in the good old days, when men were gods and women were sea nymphs, a young mother (and nymph) named Thetis dipped her son, Achilles, into the waters of the River Styx. Holding him by the heel of his foot, she created an injury-proof child, except, of course, for the one spot on his body that didn't get wet.

Achilles grew up to be the "bravest, handsomest, and greatest warrior" in Agamemnon's army during the Trojan War. He overcame being sent away by his father, dressing like a woman for awhile in order to hide, and fathering a son to fight glorious battles all over the Mediterranean. Alas, a well-aimed arrow to the heel finally brought him down, an event remembered to this day every time a fatal weakness is referred to as an Achilles' heel.

---

time, once or twice a day, advises Dr. Menacker. Do this for two or three days in a row to decrease any inflammation in your foot.

If you use an ice bag, wrap it in a dish towel so that it does not come in direct contact with your skin. Or you can freeze water in a small paper cup and peel off the top edge to make a ½-inch ice cup. Then massage in circles over the painful area for 10 minutes, recommends Dr. Menacker. If your feet feel no better after a few days to a week of trying a combination of ice, stretches, and wearing shoes with good arch support, you should see a doctor, advises Dr. Menacker.

Change exercises. If you're a runner, get on a stationary bicycle to rev up your heart. Or start swimming, at least for awhile, says Dr. Cracchiolo. It might be best to give your feet a break for a few weeks and then start running a little bit at a time to see how much stress your feet can take, he says.

▶ALTERNATIVE APPROACHES

Stretch your Achilles tendon. A tight Achilles tendon can force the fascia and tendons underneath your foot to work harder to support you. To stretch and strengthen your Achilles, try a wall stretch.

"Stand an arm's length away from a wall, with your toes pointed toward it," Dr. Menacker says. "Keep your palms against the wall. Your arms should be straight to start, then bend them as you lean into the wall with your chest. Your heels should remain on the ground as you lean into the wall. Hold for 10 seconds and repeat for one to two minutes."

You should always warm up before you do any sort of stretch, Dr. Menacker adds. A good way to warm up your feet and legs is by rotating your ankles around a few times.

▶PREVENTIVE MEASURES

Make a footprint. To determine what kind of arch you have, put your foot in water, then step on a piece of paper. This should give you a footprint. "If you can see a full footprint, then you have flat feet," explains Dr. Menacker. "If your print has two distinct areas at the toes and the heel, but no print in the middle, then you have a high arch. If, on the other hand, you can see your whole foot, but there's an indention for the arch in the print, then you have a moderate arch."

Knowing the shape of your foot will help you choose orthotics and, most important, is a good piece of information to give shoe salespeople, who will, hopefully, steer you to the right type of shoe and lacing technique for your foot shape.

Frequent Urination

▶PROBLEM

You gotta go a lot, pure and simple. Worse, the urge often strikes in the middle of the night. You may have an urgent and sudden desire to urinate that is hard to delay, yet you might feel like you haven't completely emptied your bladder when you finish. You may also have trouble starting and stopping your stream.

▶CAUSE

Frequent urination is often caused by benign prostatic hyperplasia (BPH)—an enlarged prostate gland in plain English. As the prostate grows, it may compress the urethra, the tube through which a man passes urine, making it more difficult to urinate. And when you do go, you don't completely empty your bladder, so it fills up more quickly and you need to relieve yourself more often. Half of all men have BPH after age 60, and by age 85, 9 out of 10 men do. Luckily, an enlarged prostate is not the same thing as prostate cancer, nor does it cause cancer. Some men also have to urinate frequently because they lose some kidney function as they age, causing them to have to go more often, says Robert Cowles, M.D., a urologist in private practice in Atlanta. Others keep heading to the head during the night because their legs don't return fluid back to their central system as efficiently as when they were younger, he says. This sometimes causes legs to swell when fluid accumulates there. When you lie down at night, says Dr. Cowles, that fluid is released in the form of urine.

▶HOW SERIOUS

Having to make more pit stops than a rookie race car driver is usually more of a nuisance than anything, but it still warrants getting checked out by your

DO THIS NOW

If you have to urinate frequently because of prostate problems, try to limit the use of antihistamines and over-the-counter cold remedies, advises Robert Cowles, M.D., a urologist in private practice in Atlanta. They can cause a tightening of the bladder neck and the prostate and make it more difficult to urinate. This, in turn, makes you have to go more often.

Did You Know?

What's a nuisance for one man may be a tonic for another. Some people swear that urine has medicinal value. Urine therapy advocates say that gargling it can soothe a sore throat or tame a toothache and that it is effective in treating an earache when used as eardrops. Diluted with water, it can even be used as eyedrops, they contend.

Not having much luck restoring your dwindling hair with Rogaine? Urine therapy enthusiasts claim that urine sometimes stimulates hair growth when massaged into the scalp. Some tout it as an aftershave. As bizarre as all this may sound, there has even been a world conference on urine therapy. And a German woman has written three books on the subject.

The poster boy of urine therapy is former Indian prime minister Morarji Desai, who disclosed while in office that he (gulp!) drank a glass of his own urine every day. He died in 1995—at age 99.

But that's certainly not to say that you should start drinking a urine cocktail before dinner every night. "The scientific validity of this kind of therapy has not been proven," says Robert Cowles, M.D., a urologist in private practice in Atlanta. "Any recommendations for this therapy should be viewed with great discretion, and valid medical opinions should be sought before considering this therapy." That is, don't even think about trying this at home.

---

doctor. If it is due to an enlarged prostate, it probably requires no treatment unless it's creating a lot of discomfort or it has gotten to the point that you are having difficulty urinating at all, says George Ibrahim, M.D., assistant clinical professor of urology for Duke University School of Medicine at the Asheville Veterans Affairs Medical Center in North Carolina.

Prostate or bladder cancer, however, can also cause a guy to have to urinate more often, and only a test done by a doctor can determine whether the cause is an enlarged prostate, prostate cancer, or something else. And just because you don't have symptoms doesn't mean that you don't have prostate cancer, says Dr. Ibrahim You can have frequent urination without having prostate cancer, but you can also have prostate cancer without having frequent urination or any symptoms at all, he says. That's why men need to have an annual blood test and a digital rectal exam after age 40 to be sure that this second most deadly cancer among men is not present, he says.

▶SOLUTIONS

Elevate your legs. If you notice your feet or legs swelling up during the afternoon or early evening, lie down for 45 minutes with your feet atop a couple of pillows, advises Dr. Cowles. By raising your feet above your heart like this, you rid yourself of some of that fluid in your legs that you might otherwise eliminate as urine after going to bed.

Supplement with vitamin E. Preliminary indications are that this popular antioxidant helps protect against prostate disease, says Dr. Cowles. He recommends 1,000 international units a day. If you are considering taking large amounts of vitamin E, discuss it with your doctor first.

Select selenium. Like vitamin E, the mineral selenium may help stave off prostate disease, says Dr. Cowles. It, too, is still being studied in this regard. Dr. Cowles recommends 100 micrograms a day. "I take vitamin E and selenium," he says. "I tell my patients to take them."

▶ALTERNATIVE APPROACHES

Try saw palmetto. Take 80 to 160 milligrams of saw palmetto standardized extract daily, recommends Thomas Kruzel, doctor of naturopathy, professor of urology at the National College of Naturopathic Medicine in Portland, Oregon. Several studies show that the seeds from this palm tree are effective in treating BPH and its symptoms by blocking the conversion of testosterone into harmful dihydrotestosterone, Dr. Kruzel says. You should consult with your doctor regularly when using saw palmetto for treatment of enlarged prostate. In rare cases, people taking this herb have experienced stomach problems.

▶PREVENTIVE MEASURES

Cut off the source. If you're getting up a lot during the night to urinate, don't drink beverages with alcohol or caffeine after 8:00 P.M., advises Dr. Cowles. Both can act initially as a diuretic, causing you to produce more urine than usual.

Getting Up in the Morning

▶PROBLEM

An alarm clock with an annoying buzzer and a clock radio tuned to the even more annoying Howard Stern still can't drive you out of bed on time. Then, when you do finally get up, all you can think about is going back to sleep. You're tired, you're cranky . . . and you just woke up.

▶CAUSE

It seems simple, and it is: You aren't getting enough sleep. "By definition, people who wake up to an alarm are not getting enough sleep," says Mark Chambers, Ph.D., clinical director of the Sleep Clinic of Nevada in Las Vegas. "Natural awakening is more likely to indicate that you've had a good night's rest."

▶HOW SERIOUS

It ranges from the aggravating—because you start all your days in a huff and a rush—to the symptomatic. "Consistently feeling as if you haven't gotten enough sleep can be a sign that you suffer from sleep apnea," Dr. Chambers says. *Apnea* means "without breath," and that's precisely what happens to men with this condition. The airways

DO THIS NOW

Part of the reason your brain knows that it's time to wake up is because it perceives light. "You need 45 minutes of good strong sunlight to affect your internal clock," says Mark Chambers, Ph.D., clinical director of the Sleep Clinic of Nevada in Las Vegas. "But having said that, there's still a lot of benefit to simply turning on all the lights in your bedroom or even just looking out the window for a few minutes."

may close so completely that they can't breathe. During the night, they may stop breathing dozens or even hundreds of times, awakening briefly—though they may not know it—each time as they struggle for air.

If you try the solutions below but still find yourself tired during the day, then it's time to see a sleep specialist. "I would go to a sleep doctor as well as seeing your primary care physician," Dr. Chambers says. "A physician could easily prescribe sleeping pills, which can be very dangerous to someone who has sleep apnea. You won't know you have sleep apnea without seeing a sleep specialist." (For more on sleep apnea, see Snoring on page 488.)

MEN'S HEALTH INDEX

Percentage of night workers in the utility, manufacturing, petroleum, and chemical industries who admitted to falling asleep on the job at least once a week: 52 to 63

Percentage of train drivers who fell asleep on most or all of their night shifts: 11

Percentage of train drivers who reported falling asleep on most or all early-morning shifts: 5

▶SOLUTIONS

Have it your way. If it takes 15 minutes between the time when you first open your eyes and when you can put your feet on the floor, factor that in to your daily schedule. Set your alarm for 15 minutes before you actually have to roll out of bed instead of for the last minute. "It takes a few minutes for most people to adjust to being awake, so give yourself some time to wake up," Dr. Chambers says. Don't spend every morning of your life trying to rush yourself out of bed.

Face the music. Carefully choosing the music you hear when your clock radio goes off may help you not only rise but also shine.

"You should listen to what you like in the morning," says Don Campbell, a music researcher, director of the Mozart Effect Resource Center in St. Louis, and author of *The Mozart Effect*. "But make sure that it will suit your needs. If you need to get up early, then I wouldn't advise listening to a Mahler symphony or slow New Age music. It will put you right back to sleep." Here are Campbell's suggestions for selected mornings.

When you have to get up and at 'em . . . A Sousa march, Bach's Brandenburg Concertos, or Mozart's violin concertos.

On a nonrushed day . . . Mozart's string quartets, which are organized and stimulating but not impulsive, or your favorite folk or light rock album.

On the weekend . . . Natural, environmental sounds; soundtracks to movies (Campbell says that he has clients who love to wake up to *Star Wars*); or *Music for the Mozart Effect, Volume II, Rest and Relaxation*.

Eat light. People with hiatal hernias and acid reflux often have disturbed sleeping patterns, says Dr. Chambers, so it's a good idea to avoid foods that are known to exacerbate those problems. They include acidic foods such as tomato-based products, fatty foods, and alcohol.

It's also a good idea to give your stomach a head start when it comes to resting. In other words, to help make sure that your sleep won't be disturbed by indigestion, don't go to bed with a full stomach. A light snack immediately before bed probably won't bother most people, but a heavy meal within two or three hours of bedtime could be a problem for some. Each person needs to learn what works best for him, adds Dr. Chambers.

▶ALTERNATIVE APPROACHES

Set the coffee alarm clock. Your body will respond to a change in the environment's smell, just as it responds to a change in the environment's sound (as in an alarm clock), explains Beverly Cowart, Ph.D., director of the Taste and Smell Clinic, Monell Chemical Senses Center, in Philadelphia. So set the coffeemaker for 6:00 A.M.—or whenever you need to arise—and let the aroma of java wake you up.

Other sensory changes that can help include sight (which is why light can wake you up) and touch (which is why having your hand stuck in a bowl of Jell-O would help wake you up, but we won't suggest that).

Set the light alarm clock. If a loud alarm clock is too much in the morning, try a more gentle way to wake up. There are now a number of alarm clocks on the market that will begin to glow and slowly brighten over the course of a half-hour.

Color your world. As time goes on, we realize just what it means to use color as a tool to help wake up in the morning.

"People think of taxicab yellow as a wake-up color, but really it helps to wake up to the warmer colors of the spectrum," says Leatrice Eiseman, director of the Pantone Color Institute near Seattle and author of *Coloring Your Every Mood*. "That means that it's a good idea to have more subdued yellows in your bedroom, along with light wood stains."

The dark, woodsy colors that some men gravitate toward evoke connected and rooted feelings. They won't make you feel as happy and rarin' to go as bright colors will, but then again, we're not expecting you to paint the walls bright yellow either. It will help, however, to have pale colors and bright accents in your room to help you wake up in the morning.

▶PREVENTIVE MEASURES

Be a regular guy. Start getting up at the same time every morning, even on the weekends, Dr. Chambers advises. What doesn't work is trying to go to bed earlier at night. "You don't have any control over what time you'll actually fall asleep," Dr. Chambers explains. "But if you get into a pattern of waking up at the same time every morning, then you will likely begin to fall asleep at the appropriate time at night, which will make getting up in the morning easier."

Gout

▶PROBLEM

You have inflammation, swelling, and severe pain in a joint. About half of all gout cases flare up in the big toe. Other joints that gout frequents include the instep, ankle, and knee. It may be accompanied by chills, shivers, and a little fever.

▶CAUSE

Uric acid, a by-product of the waste that your kidneys usually flush out of the body, builds up in your system and settles into the lining surrounding a joint.

▶HOW SERIOUS

"The pain is excruciating," says Richard Brasington, M.D., director of clinical services in the division of rheumatology at Washington University School of Medicine in St. Louis.

More than one million Americans have gout, and it's much more likely to affect men than women. In fact, three-quarters of those with gout are men, ages 45 to 50, says Doyt Conn, M.D., senior vice president of medical affairs for the Arthritis Foundation in Atlanta. "A gout sufferer is usually an overweight, hypertensive male who drinks too much," he adds.

For reasons that aren't completely clear to doctors yet, there are a few other things that can lead to gout attacks. "A person in the hospital who may have suffered from an attack of gout

---

DO THIS NOW

Take a prescription-strength amount of ibuprofen, says Richard Brasington, M.D., director of clinical services in the division of rheumatology at Washington University School of Medicine in St. Louis. "That means 800 milligrams four times a day," Dr. Brasington says. You can try this for up to a week. "The pain and redness should ease within a few hours, and you'll be completely better in a couple of days." Some people should not take such high doses of ibuprofen, so check with your doctor first. If you are currently taking blood thinners or have a heart condition or kidney disease, avoid high doses of ibuprofen, Dr. Brasington cautions.

Did You Know?

Although gout is often mistakenly considered the "rich man's disease," generations of Appalachian moonshiners have also had this illness. "Aside from the fact that drinking a lot can cause gout, moonshiners often use lead pipes or containers in their stills," says Doyt Conn, M.D., senior vice president of medical affairs for the Arthritis Foundation in Atlanta. "We know that lead contributes to the development of gout by damaging the kidneys."

While Benjamin Franklin and other aristocratic gout sufferers could blame any number of lifestyle choices—high meat intake, drinking lots of liquor, and leading sedentary lives—the real culprit might have been lead contamination, Dr. Conn speculates.

in the past or is prone to gout is likely to suddenly suffer from a gout attack when admitted to the hospital for treatment or surgery," Dr. Conn says. "We think that the injury or surgery causes uric acid crystals to build up in the joint and then the stress of surgery somehow mobilizes the uric acid crystals in a painful way."

Gout attacks are acute (meaning that they come on suddenly and strongly and then the symptoms disappear), explains Dr. Brasington. But most people who have one episode will continue to get them over time. If there are more and more attacks, the pain will become chronic, he says.

"Even though gout has recognizable symptoms, only a doctor can diagnosis it," says Dr. Conn. "He'll take some liquid out of the joint, then put it under a microscope to see if there are uric crystals in it."

▶SOLUTIONS

Try a different anti-inflammatory. If ibuprofen doesn't do the trick for you, try naproxen sodium (Aleve). It also helps relieve the pain and swelling. Take up to five regular-strength tablets a day for up to a week, Dr. Brasington says. You should only take these higher doses if your doctor says that it's okay, he adds.

Apply ice. Wrap ice in a towel and place it on the painful joint for 20 minutes three times a day for several days, says Dr. Conn.

Drink water. Drink at least eight, eight-ounce glasses of water a day to help flush the uric acid out of the kidneys, says Dr. Conn.

▶ALTERNATIVE APPROACHES

Double up. Bromelain, an enzyme found in pineapples, and quercetin, a bioflavonoid (a pigment in plants), are two natural remedies available in pill form at health food stores. "You should take 125 to 250 milligrams of each three times a day between meals when you experience a flare-up," says Devra Krassner, a doctor of naturopathic medicine and homeopathy in private practice in Portland, Maine. "You can also add 1.8 grams of eicosapentaenoic acid (EPA) to this every day." EPA is a fatty acid found in foods.

Scientists have discovered that oils like flaxseed oil and fish oils are rich in EPA (also known as omega-3 fatty acid), which is valued for its anti-inflammatory effects. Foods rich in EPA include green leafy vegetables, seeds (especially flaxseed), nuts, and grains. Some of the best seafood sources of EPA are anchovies, bluefin tuna, herring, mackerel, sardines, and all types of salmon except smoked. EPA is also available in pill and liquid form at health food stores.

Call on colchicum. "Colchicum is the homeopathic equivalent of colchicine, the prescription medicine that many Western doctors prescribe," Dr. Krassner says. "It may alleviate the acute pain of gout. Take two or three pellets of the 12C or 30X potency two times a day until the pain subsides." If the pain continues for more than a week, a professional homeopath should be consulted. You can find this homeopathic remedy, which is specific to gout, in a well-stocked health food store.

Sting like a bee. Apis, a homeopathic remedy made from bee venom, also is available at many health food stores. "Apis helps in conditions that mimic the symptoms of a bee sting, like swelling, stinging pain, and heat," Dr. Krassner explains. Take two or three pellets of a low potency, such as 12C or 30X, two or three times a day. If symptoms do not resolve in a week, a professional homeopath should be consulted, she adds.

Get juiced. Drinking a quart a day of sour cherry or bing cherry juice can help prevent attacks of gout, says Dr. Krassner. "The flavonoids in dark cherry juices are useful in the treatment of gout," Dr. Krassner adds. "You can also eat a half-pound of fresh or canned cherries to accomplish the same effect."

▶PREVENTIVE MEASURES

Cut your meat. Foods that are high in a compound called purine lead to high uric acid levels in the body. "Most people with gout eat a lot of meat, which is high in purines," Dr. Conn says

Quit drinking. "Alcohol reduces the body's ability to get rid of uric acid," Dr. Conn says. "It's very important to cut it out of your life to possibly get rid of gout long-term."

Slim slowly. Carrying too much weight can cause uric acid levels to build up, Dr. Conn says. "However, you don't want to go on a crash diet," he says. "Slow and steady weight loss will not only be more effective but also will help keep your gout from flaring."

Avoid aspirin. Low doses of aspirin may increase blood uric acid. "If you're on low-dose aspirin therapy for heart disease, talk to your doctor about your risk of gout," advises Dr. Conn. "It isn't an automatic cause-and-effect relationship, but it's a possible side effect to keep in mind."

Groin Pull

▶PROBLEM

Groin pull is a catchall term for a strain injury involving the muscles of the upper thigh in front of the hip joint.

▶CAUSE

A groin pull is frequently due to a muscle hyperextension. You're practicing field goals, and your buddy thinks that it would be funny to pull the ball away at the last moment, transforming you into Charlie Brown. You're playing soccer, and instead of kicking the ball, your foot slams into the ground. Or maybe you're trying to accelerate suddenly to outrun a slow grounder to first base.

▶HOW SERIOUS

A groin pull is like any muscle pull with the accompanying inflammation and microtearing of the muscle. But because you need these muscles to walk, a groin pull takes a long time to heal—at least six weeks, says Richard M. Bachrach, D.O., medical director at the Center for Sports and Osteopathic Medicine in New York City. If normal walking hurts, see your doctor, he says.

▶SOLUTIONS

Keep off your feet. Depending on the severity of the injury, you probably won't want to use those muscles vigorously for a time. That

DO THIS NOW

Following an acute injury like a groin muscle pull, apply ice wrapped in a towel for 20 to 30 minutes at a time, three to four times a day, along with a compression wrap (elastic bandage or thigh sleeve), says Duane Iverson, a physical therapist, certified athletic trainer, and director of the sports medicine department at the University of Oregon Student Health Center in Eugene. The immediate application of cold can help limit the damage to the tissues. In addition, the anesthetic affects of cold make the pain more tolerable, Iverson says.

While heat may feel good on the area, delay the warming urge for two to three days or until the acute inflammation subsides.

Did You Know?

European physicians are better-versed in dealing with groin pulls than their counterparts across the Atlantic. The reason is soccer. As the popularity of soccer grows in the United States, sports medicine physicians expect to see more patients complaining of groin pain. And that doesn't even count the hooligans.

means no running and probably limited walking, says Duane Iverson, a physical therapist, certified athletic trainer, and director of the sports medicine department at the University of Oregon Student Health Center in Eugene. "If you can't walk without a limp, you may want to get yourself a pair of crutches. Resting the area may be one of the best things you can do for a few days," he suggests.

Wrap it. Maybe you don't need crutches, but your muscles sure could use some support. Encase your aching leg with an elastic bandage or elastic thigh sleeve, available at most sporting good stores, Dr. Bachrach says.

Hail a stretch limo. If your soreness still lingers weeks later, perhaps you're re-injuring yourself while stretching, says James Waslaski, sports massage therapist at the Center for Pain Management and Clinical Sports Massage in Tampa, Florida, and author of *International Advancements in Event and Clinical Sports Massage*.

"Some folks concentrate too much on stretching the groin, and they overwork the muscles," Waslaski says. "Or they stretch too vigorously."

Here's a groin stretch that Waslaski developed while working with the New York Yankees and some professional hockey players: While sitting on the floor with your legs out in front and with the knees straight, move the injured leg out to the side as far as you can without pain. Using a towel or a rope looped around the foot for resistance, try to pull the leg inward while pulling outward with the towel for 10 seconds with no pain. (No movement occurs; this is an isometric contraction, says Waslaski.) Relax for about 2 seconds and then actively bring the leg out a little farther than the first time, repeating the 10-second contraction—again with no pain. Try to avoid bending the knees; it twists the muscles you're trying to stretch and may cause re-injury to the area. Repeat several times. If you feel increasing pain in a muscle you're stretching, stop immediately, warns Waslaski. And do not exercise if the injury is acute, he adds.

▶ALTERNATIVE APPROACHES

Take a powder. You can make a very effective herbal treatment for inflammation from the powdered turmeric in your spice rack, says Alison Lee, M.D., a pain-management specialist and acupuncturist with Barefoot Doctors, an acupuncture and natural-medicine resource center in Ann Arbor, Michigan. Simply pour the turmeric into a bowl, add a little water, and stir until it forms a sticky paste that you rub on your injured thigh. Using petroleum jelly instead of water may make it blend better and provide a consistency that's easier to use. You'll feel some burning or stinging sensations, but that means that it's working, explains Dr. Lee.

"Unless it's uncomfortable, leave it on for 30 minutes and repeat three or four times daily during the first few days of the injury," Dr. Lee says. Wrap plastic over the paste; it stains everything it touches yellow, she warns. Skin staining will decrease over several days.

Join the resistance. While sitting on the floor, have a partner hold your foot or put your foot against an immovable object and push, Waslaski says. When you contract the injured muscle against resistance, you can then put your index finger directly on the involved fibers. By gently massaging the injured fibers in all directions, you can soften and lengthen the muscle, says Waslaski. You will then have an expanded range of motion, he adds.

It may be a bit uncomfortable at first, but you'll eventually get some relief from the soreness. And the massage will bring fresh blood to the area to flush out toxins and waste products from the injured muscles, Waslaski says.

Bring out a stretcher. When you're well on your way to recovery, the modified lunge stretch builds up and loosens the injured muscles around the hip, says Dr. Bachrach.

While standing up, extend one leg behind you, and then slowly lean or lunge forward, raising the heel of your back leg off the floor. You should feel the stretch in front of the hip of your back leg, says Dr. Bachrach. Keep your knee and your back straight, and hold for 10 to 30 seconds. Start with your right leg back; return to standing. Repeat with the left leg back, then the right leg again, and so on.

"You can do this up to 20 times a day and always before and after you exercise," Dr. Bachrach says.

▶PREVENTIVE MEASURES

Ease into exercise. Many groin pulls happen because you ask your body to do something—sprint to first base, play full-court basketball—that it's not ready for or accustomed to, says Iverson. Even if you're in great shape, perhaps jogging daily, you're not ready for sprints and sudden direction changes that many team sports require, he cautions.

Before your first softball game of the year, try to warm up for the demands of the activity. This might include a progression of gradually faster strides and sprints and backward running. Stretching the calves, quadriceps, hamstrings, and groin muscles may be helpful.

"The key to injury prevention is to first practice the activity in a controlled way," Iverson says. "Then when it's time to sprint in a game, hopefully your body will be ready."

Gum Ailments

▶PROBLEM

Your gums are red or reddish purple, puffy, swollen, bleeding (or bleed easily), receded, and sore, especially when you brush your teeth.

▶CAUSE

You either have gingivitis or gum abrasion, says Eric Spieler, D.M.D., a dentist and lecturer in dental medicine at the University of Pennsylvania School of Dental Medicine in Philadelphia. If the problem is abrasion, you're probably brushing your teeth so hard that the gum tissue is being damaged.

More likely, the problem is gingivitis, which means that tiny bugs have taken up residence in your mouth and are trashing the place. The culprits are bacteria that feed on the leftover bits of food in your mouth. As these oral freeloaders reproduce, eliminate wastes, and die, they form a filmy layer called plaque. (Yes, we're talking bacteria poop and bacteria corpses.) If the plaque in your mouth isn't removed by brushing and flossing, it accumulates and begins to irritate the sensitive tissues of your gums, especially when the plaque hardens into tartar.

"When you don't clean your teeth and gums properly, the bacteria population in your mouth gets out of control," Dr. Spieler says. "You have to cull the herd."

▶HOW SERIOUS

Gingivitis, which basically means inflamed gums, is bad enough. But left unchecked, it can deteriorate into periodontitis, the greatest cause of tooth loss in adults, says James Kohner, D.D.S., a periodontist in private practice in Scottsdale, Arizona. Irritated gum tissue starts pulling back from the teeth, and even-

---

DO THIS NOW

Mix a teaspoon of salt in one cup of warm water, swish the mixture between your teeth, and then spit. That will help soothe your irritated gums, giving you a measure of temporary relief until you reach your dentist and can be examined, says Judith Post, D.M.D., a dentist in private practice in Montclair, New Jersey.

Did You Know?

One reason that gum disease is so common in the United States—three out of four Americans over age 35 have some form of it—is that a lot of people aren't thrilled by the idea of having sharp instruments stuck in their mouths. A 1994 survey by the American Dental Association found that 19 percent of Americans were "very apprehensive" about going to the dentist; another 32 percent said that they were "somewhat apprehensive."

tually, the bone structure beneath the gums dissolves. In the end, your teeth simply fall out or have to be pulled because of recurring infection.

Be aware that gum disease usually progresses for a long time before you notice it. If your gums are sore and bleeding, a visit to the dentist is definitely in order.

▶SOLUTIONS

Ease up. To avoid gum abrasion, brush your teeth gently, for a longer period of time. "Most people are impatient to get it over with, so they compensate by brushing too hard," Dr. Spieler says. "That does remove plaque, but it also removes skin."

Dr. Spieler recommends brushing for at least two minutes, or however long it takes to cover all the surfaces of your teeth. One sign that you're brushing too aggressively, he adds, is if the bristles on your brush are splaying outward. Using a soft-bristle brush is also a good idea, according to the American Dental Association.

Fetch the floss. Brushing helps remove plaque, but flossing launches a direct assault on the bacteria's home base in your mouth: between the teeth. To keep gingivitis at bay, floss at least once a day, says Robert Rioseco, D.M.D., a dentist in White Plains, New York. You might blanch at the prospect of putting any foreign object near your aching gums, but Dr. Rioseco says that a gentle flossing will bring relief, not pain. "Don't be afraid that your gums are bleeding," he says. "They're bleeding because the tissue is inflamed, and it's inflamed because you have irritants there. The key is to get rid of the irritants."

Nuke bacteria with a hydrogen bomb. Gargling once or twice a day with hydrogen peroxide can help disinfect irritated gums, Dr. Spieler says. Brush your teeth first to break up the plaque, then use the peroxide (just as it comes from the bottle; no dilution is necessary) to wash it away. Rinse a lot afterward, and be careful not to swallow.

Numb the pain. Gums that ache painfully can be soothed by applying an over-the-counter numbing gel such as Anbesol, suggests Dr. Spieler.

▶ALTERNATIVE APPROACHES

Hit a C note. A regimen of vitamin C can help your gum tissues resist the bacterial onslaught. Gary Bachman, a naturopathic physician in private practice in Mount Vernon, Washington, recommends taking 500 milligrams three times a day. Be aware that excess vitamin C may cause diarrhea in some people

Take a Q. Another supplement that helps promote healthy gum tissue is coenzyme Q_{10}. Andrew Weil, M.D. director of the Program in Integrative Medicine at the University of Arizona College of Medicine in Tucson, suggests taking between 60 and 100 milligrams a day.

Play with paste. Mix a little hydrogen peroxide in with some baking soda, Dr. Weil says, so that it forms a sticky paste. Use your toothbrush to gently rub this mixture onto your gums. Leave it on a few minutes, then rinse.

Swallow some gold. Goldenseal is an herb well known for its antibacterial powers. Dr. Bachman recommends mixing 5 to 10 drops of non-alcohol-based goldenseal into a cup of warm salt water. Rinsing with such a mixture daily will help disinfect the gums and promote healing, Dr. Bachman says, although the taste may be somewhat bitter. And don't forget to spit. Be careful, too, as it may irritate your mouth.

▶PREVENTIVE MEASURES

Make a habit of good habits. If you'd enjoy keeping your teeth as you get older, practicing good dental hygiene consistently is a necessity. That means brushing at least twice a day with a soft toothbrush, flossing at least once a day, and visiting your dentist for regular checkups and cleanings. For most people, regular means twice a year, although patients who are prone to gum problems may need more frequent visits, says Judith Post, D.M.D., a dentist in private practice in Montclair, New Jersey.

Apply appliances. Anything that encourages people to spend more time cleaning their teeth is a plus, Dr. Post says. So it helps to maintain a well-stocked arsenal in the battle against plaque. Among her other weapons of choice beside soft toothbrushes and floss are dental irrigators (WaterPik is probably the best-known brand); rubber gum stimulators, which allow you to clean at the gum line; and interproximal brushes, which get in between the teeth and under bridges where there are larger spaces. Interproximal brushes are miniature-size toothbrushes with tiny bristles covering the round-headed brush. You can usually find them in drugstores next to the regular toothbrushes. All take aim at those spots between the teeth where bacteria love to hide—the spots brushes often miss. Dr. Post is also enthusiastic about the electric toothbrush, which she says has helped many of her patients improve the health of their gums.

Hangover

▶PROBLEM

Last night, you proclaimed yourself the King of Quaff, the Sultan of Sip; and this morning, you feel like the Duke of Puke. Your head feels like a floor with 100 fiendish flamenco dancers stomping on it furiously. Your mouth is as dry as Utah on a Sunday morning. And your stomach hasn't been this queasy since you read *The Bridges of Madison County*.

▶CAUSE

Surprisingly, little is known about hangover—either what causes it or what makes it feel better. "It has not been well-studied, considering how common it is," says Alan Wartenberg, M.D., assistant professor of medicine at Tufts University School of Medicine and director of the addiction-recovery program at Faulkner Hospital, both in Boston. It appears, however, that alcohol makes the blood vessels swell, causing headache pain and perhaps some sweating. Alcohol also can act as a diuretic, leading to dehydration.

▶HOW SERIOUS

"An awful lot of people end up not going to work, not going to school, and not taking care of responsibilities when they're hung over," says Dr. Wartenberg. "I'm sure that it has an economic impact. But it's not lethal. It's a nuisance."

▶SOLUTIONS

Slurp some broth. Drink fluids that contain minerals and salts that provide relief from dehydration. A cup of bouillon, for example, will replace fluid and is easy on your churning stomach, says Frederick G. Freitag, D.O., a spokesperson for the National Headache Foundation.

> **DO THIS NOW**
>
> Before or after drinking, eat a cracker or a piece of toast with honey, says Frederick G. Freitag, D.O., a spokesperson for the National Headache Foundation. Honey supplies fructose, which helps the body metabolize the alcohol ingested and reduces any hangover symptoms.

History Lesson

The late New York Yankee slugger Mickey Mantle's off-field drinking exploits were reputedly as prodigious as his feats on the diamond. Veteran baseball writer Roger Kahn, however, says he only knows of one occasion when a hangover affected Mantle's performance. Even then, Mantle—ever the great athlete—rose to the occasion. According to Kahn's book, *Memories of Summer*, Mantle felt so terrible that afternoon that he couldn't get to the ballpark until the fifth inning. Casey Stengel, the Yankees' manager, greeted him with fury. "Yer late. Get in and pinch-hit fer me right now."

Trembling under a high, bright sky, Mantle took one swing and hit a 425-foot home run. He trotted around the base paths, returned to the dugout, and said to Stengel, "You'll never know how hard that was." Then he retreated to the clubhouse to lie down.

Drink some java. A cup of coffee might provide some relief in helping headache symptoms and decreasing the duration of the pain, according Dr. Freitag. The caffeine constricts blood vessels. But coffee also can make you feel more edgy than you already do. Trial and error is the best course here.

Get a gentle analgesic. Take some acetaminophen (Tylenol) on the morning after. It's the over-the-counter painkiller that is most gentle on your stomach, which already is inflamed from your overindulgence, says Dr. Wartenberg. He cautions, however, that habitual drinkers who take multiple doses of Tylenol can damage their livers. Acetaminophen should not be taken regularly in people drinking three or more standard drinks a day. A standard drink is one shot of 80-proof distilled spirits, 12 ounces of beer, or 6 ounces of wine. But the guy who seldom drinks excessively should have no such trouble, he says.

▶ALTERNATIVE APPROACHES

Swallow some vitamins. Some hangover symptoms may be due to the loss of B vitamins that occurs when drinking, Dr. Wartenberg says.

Andrew Weil, M.D., director of the Program in Integrative Medicine at the University of Arizona College of Medicine in Tucson and author of several books, including *Eight Weeks to Optimum Health*, recommends taking a B-complex vitamin supplement plus an extra 100 milligrams of thiamin.

▶PREVENTIVE MEASURES

Fill 'er up. Before you drink, eat a good meal. "Alcohol levels go up much faster on an empty stomach," Dr. Wartenberg says. "Food slows alcohol's absorption. The faster your level rises, the drunker you get." And the drunker you get, the worse you will feel in the morning.

Avoid the dark. There is anecdotal evidence suggesting that drinking darker colored alcoholic drinks the night before is more likely to bring you brain pain the next day, Dr. Wartenberg says. These drinks contain congeners, chemicals that add color and flavor, which may promote a headache. Red wine also appears to be a high-risk drink for the hangover-prone. Clear liquors like vodka and gin are better bets, although they too can produce hangovers if abused.

Drink water. It's a good idea to drink a lot of water while you're drinking alcohol to avoid the next-day dehydration that can make hangovers even worse, says Dr. Weil.

Spit out the hair of the dog. You've probably heard of this hangover cure: the "hair of the dog"—drink in the morning whatever got you drunk the night before. Your stomach is already inflamed by imbibing too much, so drinking more of the same makes no sense, says Dr. Wartenberg. The hair-of-the-dog remedy may have a calming effect on drinkers who are physically dependent on alcohol and suffering through withdrawal, but it only feeds their dependency, says Dr. Wartenberg. The best solution for hangovers, of course, is to not drink alcohol, or only do so in moderation.

Headache, Migraine

▶PROBLEM

You have head pain so blinding it could bring Superman to his knees. Some migraines are preceded by an aura or warning. Nausea, vomiting, and sensitivity to light and sounds often are symptoms accompanying these pounding headaches, which can wipe a guy out for four hours to three days.

▶CAUSE

Blood vessels surrounding the brain initially constrict, then dilate and swell, becoming inflamed during a migraine. Why this happens isn't really known, but about 70 to 80 percent of migraine sufferers have a hereditary link. The headaches also can be triggered by a host of things, including change in sleep cycle, missing or postponing a meal, medications that cause a swelling of the blood vessels, excessive use of medications for migraine and other headaches, bright lights, sunlight, fluorescent lights, television and movie viewing, loud noise, and certain foods.

DO THIS NOW

When you experience auras before a headache—a warning such as seeing flashing lights, squiggly lines, or feeling a tingling in the arms and hands—immediately stick your face in a paper bag. By breathing for a few minutes into a bag, you re-breathe some of the air you exhaled, building up the carbon dioxide concentration in your blood, says Egilius Spierings, M.D., Ph.D., a neurologist and headache specialist in private practice in Wellesley Hills, Massachusetts. This, in turn, helps fend off migraines.

▶HOW SERIOUS

"Probably two-thirds of people, when they have a migraine, cannot function at a normal level," says Glen Solomon, M.D., a headache expert and consultant to the Cleveland Clinic Foundation. "Men, on average, miss a little over a week of work a year, either in lost productivity or in absence due to migraine. It's pretty serious.

"Migraine sufferers should see a doctor if they are finding that headaches interfere with their work or family life, if their headaches are getting worse, or if they take medication on a daily basis or almost daily basis for headache," says Dr. Solomon.

▶**SOLUTIONS**

Pull the shades. Since light aggravates migraine symptoms, lie down in a dark room, advises Dr. Solomon.

Buck it with ice. When you lie down, put an ice pack wrapped in a towel or a cold compress on your throbbing head to soothe swollen, pulsing blood vessels until the pain subsides, says Dr. Solomon.

Dip your hands. If for some reason you don't want to put a cold compress on your head to relieve the pain, soak one or both of your hands in ice water for only as long as you can tolerate it, advises Egilius Spierings, M.D., Ph.D., a neurologist and headache specialist in private practice in Wellesley Hills, Massachusetts. While your hands are in the water, ball them into fists and open and close them repeatedly. It can have the same effect as a compress on your head. "The cold water stimulates the cold pressor response, causing your blood vessels (including those in your head) to narrow," explains Dr. Spierings.

Have some caffeine. It's a paradox of headaches: Ingest too much caffeine and you may get a headache; take a little bit and it can help make the pain disappear. Studies have shown that aspirin and ibuprofen are more effective when combined with caffeine, says Dr. Solomon. So if you take aspirin or ibuprofen at the onset of a migraine, wash it down with a cup of java.

Sleep well. "Changes in sleep patterns, changing shifts, jet lag—any of those can trigger migraines," says Dr. Solomon. It's best to maintain a regular schedule and get up and go to bed at the same time every day, he adds.

Eat well. Skipping meals is a common trigger of migraines, says Dr. Solomon. "One way to avoid this trigger is to eat smaller meals throughout the day or be sure to eat three meals," says Dr. Solomon.

Make note of what you eat. Certain foods prompt migraines in about 10 percent of migraine sufferers, says Dr. Solomon. It can take from 30 minutes to

MEN'S HEALTH INDEX

Here's a list of foods most likely to trigger a migraine headache.

- **Ripened cheeses such as Cheddar, Swiss, Stilton, Brie, and Camembert**
- **Chocolate**
- **Sour cream—no more than a half-cup daily**
- **Nuts and peanut butter**
- **Foods containing monosodium glutamate (MSG) and soy sauce, meat tenderizers, and seasoned salt**
- **Citrus fruits—no more than a half-cup daily**
- **A lot of tea, coffee, or colas—no more than two cups daily**
- **Pizza**
- **Cured meats such as sausage, bologna, pepperoni, salami, summer sausage, and hot dogs**
- **Alcoholic beverages**

12 hours for a food to cause a reaction. If you get a migraine, think back to what you ate in that time frame and try eliminating some of those foods from your diet.

▶ALTERNATIVE APPROACHES

Raise your riboflavin. Studies have shown that taking 400 milligrams a day of riboflavin, can help thwart migraines, says Dr. Solomon.

Try some red pepper. The hot ingredient in red pepper, capsaicin, is a terrific painkiller, writes James A. Duke, Ph.D., the world's foremost authority on healing herbs, in *The Green Pharmacy*. He thinks it can help those who have migraines feel better once they are in the throes of a headache. There's no need to start including red peppers on your cereal in the morning. You can buy cayenne pepper capsules in health food stores. "Take three 450-milligram doses a day (maximum 1,350 milligrams) as an analgesic until the pain subsides," says Dr. Duke. "Or read the label for the manufacturer's recommendation."

▶PREVENTIVE MEASURES

Beware being a slugabed. "Don't sleep late on weekends," advises Dr. Solomon. After a week of daily stresses, it might seem like a reward to relax and sleep in. But giving yourself that letdown after stress is a common trigger. Awaking late can also trigger a migraine for two other reasons, Dr. Solomon says. It is a change in your normal sleep pattern and may cause you to miss a meal—breakfast—which can both trigger a migraine.

Headache, Tension

▶PROBLEM

"It's almost impossible to find someone who has never had a headache," says John Arena, Ph.D., professor of psychology at the Medical College of Georgia School of Medicine and director of the Pain Evaluation and Intervention Program at the Department of Veterans Affairs Medical Center, both in Augusta. By far the most prevalent is the tension headache. Also called a muscle contraction headache, it can leave a dull, steady aching in your head, with feelings of tightness or pressure. Sometimes it creates a feeling of a constriction about the head, as if you are wearing a hat that is much too small.

▶CAUSE

As the name suggests, tension headaches are often caused by tension, or as a result of other emotional states, such as anxiety, anger, and repressed hostility. "Headaches aren't merely a function of stress, however," says Joseph P. Primavera III, Ph.D., a psychologist at the Jefferson Headache Center in Philadelphia. "People have certain genetic loadings that make them susceptible to headaches. It's not an emotional problem but a biological problem." Other causes include being confined to one uncomfortable position for a prolonged period, such as cramped driving or riding in a car, or doing the same repetitive task over and over again on a job. Eyestrain, fasting, and even fun things like eating ice cream and having sex can trigger a hurt in the head.

▶HOW SERIOUS

A simple tension headache is merely bothersome. But headache symptoms can also be a harbinger of something serious, such as a brain tumor. Dr. Arena says that you should see a doctor if:

> **DO THIS NOW**
>
> Feel behind your earlobes for the ridge of bone there and rub—on both sides of your head—for 10 minutes, says Fred Sheftell, M.D., director of the New England Center for Headache in Stamford, Connecticut. Then do the same with your temples, then the back of the neck. These are major tension spots where muscles tighten and cause headaches.

1. Your headache problem is new.
2. The intensity, frequency, or duration has changed markedly within the last three months.
3. Numbness or weakness in any part of the body accompanies the headache.
4. The headache began after some trauma to the head.
5. You are older than age 60 and just started having headaches.
6. You have other medical conditions, such as high blood pressure, cancer, or a history of cerebral aneurysm in your family.

▶Solutions

Take the obvious action. When headache strikes, taking aspirin, ibuprofen, or another over-the-counter analgesic is one of the most effective things you can do when you feel the onset of a mild everyday headache, says Dr. Arena. Just follow the dosage directions on the label, he adds.

Get off your duff. Some guys find that exercising when they get a headache makes it disappear. Others say that it makes things worse. But if you work out regularly, you may get fewer headaches, says Dr. Primavera. There are several reasons for this. If you're in shape, you have less muscle fatigue and less of the headache-causing tightness in the neck and shoulders that accompanies it. Exercise builds up your cardiovascular system, which tends to slow your pulse. This, in turn, makes your body more resistant against stress, says Dr. Primavera. And being active has a positive effect on levels of serotonin, a neurotransmitter that improves your mood and helps you manage headaches, he says.

Cut the caffeine. Too much caffeine gives some guys a pain in the head. Cutting back on your caffeine consumption can help, but it is something that should be done gradually, says W. Marvin Davis, Ph.D., professor of pharmacology at the University of Mississippi in Oxford. Going cold turkey can give you the very thing you're trying to prevent—a headache. "You're actually undergoing a caffeine withdrawal," Dr. Davis says. He recommends tapering off over a period of two to three weeks.

Sit up straight. "Make sure that you're not hunched over a keyboard or reading in a funny position that would put a lot of pressure on your neck or shoulders," advises Dr. Primavera.

▶Alternative Approaches

Keep a diary. Maybe a diary conjures up visions of prepubescent girls jotting down conversations they had with their dolls that day. Okay, call it a journal or whatever you want, but keep a record of what you did before the onset of a headache that may have triggered it and what you did afterward that might have made it go away. Dr. Primavera says that it took awhile before it dawned on him that he was getting fairly frequent headaches simply because he

Did You Know?

They are two of the most chilling words in the English language: *brain freeze*—that piercing pain that penetrates your skull like a dagger when you're scarfing down your favorite ice cream or cold food.

It's a matter of such grave international importance that Joseph Hulihan, M.D., assistant professor of neurology at Temple University Health Sciences Center in Philadelphia, deemed it worthy of an article in *British Medical Journal*. He discloses that brain-freeze victims seem to be stricken randomly. One study found that migraine sufferers are crippled by brain freeze far more often than other folks, but a later study concluded the opposite.

Dr. Hulihan writes that chilling the back of the palate is most likely to produce an ice cream headache. So next time you're savoring that triple-scoop ice cream sundae with extra jimmies, do so in the front portion of your mouth.

"Ice cream abstinence is not indicated," writes Dr. Hulihan, tongue planted firmly in cheek.

---

wasn't wearing sunglasses when he drove. "Sometimes the really obvious things can be very helpful," he says. "Common sense isn't that common."

Take a mental trip. Guided imagery—imagining that you are in a pleasant place—has been used as a relaxation technique for more than 2,000 years, says Dr. Arena. "For most people, it's going to be a beach scene, either at sunset or sunrise," he says. Whatever image calms you, fix that in your mind. Think about how peaceful it makes you feel. Your muscles will unclench, and you'll start to feel better.

Say a little prayer. "Prayer is certainly the oldest form of relaxation," says Dr. Arena. "It has extremely beneficial physiological as well as psychological effects." If you're not the praying type, just sitting quietly and letting your mind clear of worrisome thoughts can be wonderfully relaxing.

Talk to yourself. Repeat a relaxing phrase over and over in your head. No, you needn't move your lips. "My favorite one is, 'My mind is quiet,'" says Dr. Arena. "My whole body is relaxed and warm," could be another. "You have to say them anywhere from 15 to 50 times," Dr. Arena says. "You have to try to experience the sensations that the phrase is trying to convey."

Get loose. Try muscle-relaxation therapy, in which you repeatedly tense a group of muscles then let them go. You can do anywhere from 4 to 18 muscle groups, Dr. Arena says. "At the time you do that, you focus in on the difference between the tense state and the relaxed state." Some people eventually advance to the point where they can reach this relaxed state by simply recalling the feeling they got from this exercise rather than actually doing it, making it a technique that can be employed anytime, anywhere, says Dr. Arena.

▶PREVENTIVE MEASURES

Avoid a pain-pill plethora. Taking too many over-the-counter pain medications for headaches can cause "rebound" headaches. Even if you don't exceed the number of tablets or capsules on the label, the headaches can occur after repeated doses, says Dr. Primavera. He says that three pills a day for a month—100 in all—can trigger rebound headaches. "If you find that you're taking daily analgesics and you're having a daily headache, you may want to check with your doctor as to whether you're heading in the right direction," says Dr. Primavera. That guideline includes any combination of pain relievers, he stresses. "Having aspirin one day, Advil another day, and Tylenol another is only fooling yourself," he says.

Head off food sensitivity. Sometimes, what you eat can cause a headache. Many people are sensitive to ingredients in food, like monosodium glutamate (MSG), which you'll find in many processed foods. Other offenders include the nitrates in lunchmeat and hot dogs, and the sugar substitutes in diet sodas. Pay attention. If headaches strike after something you've eaten or drunk, you might be sensitive to that foodstuff, says Dr. Primavera.

Heartburn

▶**PROBLEM**

This painful burning sensation behind the breastbone strikes more than 60 million Americans a month, usually an hour or two after eating. It can be felt as high up as in the jaws and the back of the throat, resulting in hoarseness, and can even radiate into the arms and back.

▶**CAUSE**

The flame to blame is stomach acid, which enters into the esophagus via the lower esophageal sphincter at the top of the stomach. When things go awry, this muscular valve—which normally opens and shuts to let food pass—can reopen, allowing acid to shoot upward. Some contributing factors are high-fat and spicy foods, including chocolate, peppermint, and garlic; certain medications, such as aspirin; smoking; beverages that contain carbonation, caffeine, or alcohol; and hiatal hernia.

▶**HOW SERIOUS**

Occasional heartburn is not serious. However, chronic, severe heartburn is a symptom of a reflux problem, meaning that stomach acid is regularly flowing upward, often due to a faulty esophageal sphincter. Reflux can result in complications such as bleeding, shortness of breath, difficulty swallowing, and even weight loss. Self-treating this condition long-term also can mask

DO THIS NOW

Chewing gum can provide quick, temporary relief of heartburn, says Norman J. Goldberg, M.D., clinical professor of medicine in the division of gastroenterology at the University of California, San Diego, School of Medicine in La Jolla. Chewing gum causes you to create saliva. And saliva is alkaline-based, which neutralizes acid. In addition, saliva contains a hormone called epidermal growth factor, which helps heal the esophageal lining. Just steer clear of peppermint-flavored gum. Peppermint will make heartburn worse because it lowers the pressure in the lower esophageal sphincter and allows acid reflux into the esophagus, explains Dr. Goldberg.

more serious problems, namely, cancer of the esophagus, says Norman J. Goldberg, M.D., clinical professor of medicine in the division of gastroenterology at the University of California, San Diego, School of Medicine in La Jolla. Between the early 1970s and the early 1990s, the death rate for esophageal cancer in men increased by 24 percent, according to the American Cancer Society. Since this cancer is far more common in males, Dr. Goldberg recommends seeing a physician if your heartburn occurs three or four times a week for weeks at a time.

▶SOLUTIONS

Pop an antacid. Yes, it's painfully obvious, but taking an antacid makes sense because it contains chemicals that neutralize acid instantaneously, says Edwin J. Zarling, M.D., associate professor of medicine at Loyola University Medical Center in Maywood, Illinois. Chilled liquid antacids are best for a soothing, throat-coating result.

Be aware, however, that the four types of antacids (grouped by active ingredients) have their own unique side effects, says Dr. Goldberg. Magnesium salts are more likely to cause diarrhea and should not be taken by people with kidney disease. Aluminum salts can trigger constipation and can weaken bones with overuse. Calcium salts such as Tums can lead to kidney stones if taken long-term. And some sodium salts, such as those Alka-Seltzer products that contain aspirin, can cause stomach irritation.

Many of the antacids out there are a combination of these ingredients. Maalox and Mylanta, for example, contain both magnesium and aluminum. And Rolaids contains magnesium and calcium. So, which antacid works best? Well, it's no exact science, but Dr. Goldberg recommends the antacids that contain a combination of magnesium and aluminum such as Maalox, which he says is best taken one hour and three hours after a meal and at bedtime in a dose of about two to three teaspoons at a time. You can use these for your heartburn pain unless you have kidney disease, adds Dr. Goldberg. And if you're taking a prescription drug, you should check with your doctor before taking any antacid.

Quench the fire. Drinking an eight-ounce glass of water may bring temporary relief, Dr. Goldberg says. "Water can wash acid back down the esophagus and dilute the acid in the stomach," he explains. But since water absorbs quickly in the stomach, don't expect this relief to last long. This is best used to buy yourself some time until the antacid kicks in.

Don't be fooled by milk. The worst thing you can do for heartburn is drink a glass of milk before bedtime, Dr. Goldberg says. Sure, milk neutralizes acid when you take it, but during the night, it produces more acid. "So you wake up two to three hours after you go to bed with intense heartburn from that glass of milk," he says.

Outsmart gravity. If you must lie down within several hours of eating, raise the head of your bed. Prop six-inch blocks under the headboard bed legs or place a foam, triangular-shape wedge under your shoulders, says Philip Katz, M.D., associate professor of medicine and director of the Comprehensive Chest

History Lesson

In 1997, at age 80, Joe Redington hopped on his dogsled down the 1,150-mile icy path that leads to Nome, Alaska. Thrilled to be racing again, the founder of the Iditarod Sled Dog Race earned his third-fastest time in his 19-race career—after four years off. Why, you ask, did he quit in the first place? Well, it wasn't the cracked ribs, collapsed lung, or pneumonia from previous races. It was the heartburn.

Redington's heartburn compromised even his sleep. Forced to spend his nights leaning upright against a tree, sled, or cabin wall, he became known by some as the man who "could sleep on a coat hanger"—a title he happily relinquished after he started taking the "miracle drug" omeprazole (Prilosec). With heartburn now under control, Redington continues to race mushers 40 to 50 years his junior.

Pain and Swallowing Center at Allegheny University Hospitals, Graduate, in Philadelphia. But don't use pillows to prop yourself up. "Often, people end up with the pillows under their heads, not their shoulders. So they don't get the elevation they need," Dr. Katz says. If sleeping in chairs has become a habit to get relief at night, he warns, it's time to see your doctor.

▶ALTERNATIVE APPROACHES

Sip soy. Unlike cow's milk, soy milk can soothe heartburn without making it worse hours later, says Steven Bailey, a naturopathic doctor at the Northwest Naturopathic Clinic in Portland, Oregon, and a member of the American Association of Naturopathic Physicians. Mix 2 tablespoons chlorophyll (found at health food stores) with ½ cup soy milk, and drink it slowly. You can do this two to four times a day for up to two weeks, says Dr. Bailey. If you haven't gotten relief from your heartburn after those two weeks, you should see a doctor, he advises. And if you're allergic to soy, you should not try this remedy, he adds.

Mix a vinegar cocktail. As unpleasant as it sounds, apple cider vinegar aids digestion and eases heartburn by neutralizing excess acid, says Dr. Bailey. "And since the pH in the cider is not the same as antacids', it's more natural and doesn't damage the stomach like antacids can," he says. Mix 1 teaspoon apple cider vinegar with 8 ounces water and ½ to 1 teaspoon honey. Take this once in the morning and once at night, as needed. You can also drink this mixture after a meal if you are having digestive problems.

Position your belly. A common heartburn cause, hiatal hernia can keep food from going down the esophagus, says Arlo Gordin, D.C., nutritionist and health programs director for acupuncture, chiropractic, and naturopathic medicine at University City Medical Group in Los Angeles. To bring quick relief, press the fingers of both of your hands just snug underneath the "V" in the center of your rib cage and push the top of your stomach downward. You can do one swift push or several different pushes. "This is not a dangerous procedure, though a chiropractor trained to do this will tend to do it more effectively and faster," Dr. Gordin says.

Heat things up. Putting a heating pad on a certain spot in your back can help bring relief from heartburn, says Lino Zarrillo, D.C., a chiropractor in private practice in Trexlertown, Pennsylvania. The spine is related to the digestive organs, he says. In particular, the area just below your shoulder blades has nerves that supply the upper gastrointestinal tract, which includes the esophageal sphincter—a major player in heartburn.

Lie on your back with a heating pad under the spot between your shoulder blades for 20 minutes and put your feet up on a pillow or two. Just make sure that you wear a shirt to prevent getting burned. "Lying in this position and applying heat helps you to relax. Since tension and stress often cause heartburn, alleviating that stress can also alleviate your heartburn," Dr. Zarrillo says.

▶PREVENTIVE MEASURES

Eat light. A very full stomach increases incidence of heartburn, probably by forcing the lower esophageal sphincter open, Dr. Katz says. So keep portions small. In fact, you shouldn't eat anything within two to three hours of going to sleep.

Plan and prevent. When anticipating a fattening or spicy meal, it makes sense to take an over-the-counter H_2 receptor antagonist (such as Zantac or Pepcid AC) 20 to 40 minutes beforehand, says Jack A. DiPalma, M.D., professor of medicine and director of the division of gastroenterology at the University of South Alabama College of Medicine in Mobile. Unlike antacids, which neutralize acid, H_2 receptors block acid production, preventing heartburn.

H_2 receptors also work when taken after meals. But remember that, unlike the immediate relief of antacids, they take 20 to 40 minutes to kick in. The effects, however, last hours longer, Dr. Zarling says.

Eat your enzymes. With age, our bodies produce fewer enzymes, and we rarely eat enough enzyme-supplying fruits and vegetables. So it's a good idea to supplement, Dr. Bailey says. If you're eating primarily proteins and fats, you're not getting enough enzymes in your food and your body has to use its own supply. For these concerns, Dr. Bailey recommends taking one digestive food enzyme capsule about 15 minutes before meals to help digestion. Some men may have to take an enzyme capsule every day before every meal, while others may only need to take it occasionally. You can buy digestive food enzymes (such as Nature's Plus and Enzymatic Therapy) at most health food stores.

Tune out stress. So many people eat in front of the TV or discuss problems at the dinner table, creating a nervous stomach and, as a result, heartburn, says Dr. Bailey. To control your postmeal outcome, declare dinnertime a stress-free zone by eating slowly in a pleasant atmosphere and listening to relaxing music, he suggests.

Heart Disease

▶PROBLEM

The number one killer of men, heart disease claims more lives each year than the next eight leading causes of death combined. The disease progresses as clogged, narrowed arteries fail to deliver enough blood to the heart, slowly suffocating the muscle. Though chest pain alerts some men early, nearly half of the men who die suddenly of heart disease have no previous symptoms.

▶CAUSE

Heart disease is the end result of a long chain of events. The chain starts with a diet high in fatty, protein-rich foods, low in fruits and vegetables, and low in vitamins. Eating this way raises the levels of the fats low-density-lipoprotein (LDL, or "bad") cholesterol and triglycerides (fatty substances that can irritate the lining of artery walls) circulating in the blood. It also increases levels of a molecule called homocysteine, which can damage arteries, encourage plaque growth, and promote clotting. Though researchers are still unraveling exactly how LDL, triglycerides, and homocysteine interact, they suspect that the substances embed themselves in your artery walls, irritating and injuring them. Your immune system then tries to repair the damage by pasting over the injured sections. Such repair work results in hardened plaque along your artery wall. The plaque grows in size over time, narrowing your artery and restricting blood

> ### DO THIS NOW
>
> Drinking one 12-ounce glass of purple grape juice will slow the level of platelet activity in your blood within a few hours. So, if you consume something that slows down platelet activity, this should reduce your risk of a heart attack, says John D. Folts, Ph.D., professor of medicine and director of the coronary thrombosis laboratory at the University of Wisconsin Medical School in Madison. Other grape products such as red wine do the same. Daily intake of grape juice would probably be best, says Dr. Folts. He adds, "It is too early to know how much consuming grape juice would reduce the risk of heart attacks. More research is needed."

flow. Sometimes sections of the plaque completely block blood flow, causing a heart attack.

▶HOW SERIOUS

It's very serious. Heart disease kills. If you suspect that you have heart disease, consult a physician. If you feel any symptoms of a heart attack—chest pain, nausea, radiating pain to the jaw or arm—go immediately to the emergency room, advises Kilmer McCully, M.D., pathologist at the Department of Veterans' Affairs Medical Center in Providence, Rhode Island.

▶SOLUTIONS

Drink Guinness daily. Two bottles of dark beer a day will give you the amount of anticlotting, vitamin-like flavonoids that may help keep your arteries clear, research suggests. Flavonoids are found in hops—the ingredient that gives beer a bitter taste. So some paler, hoppy beers such as India Pale Ale may have just as many flavonoids as darker beers. But no one has tested them to find out, says John D. Folts, Ph.D., professor of medicine and director of the coronary thrombosis laboratory at the University of Wisconsin Medical School in Madison.

India Pale Ale aside, the brewing process usually filters much of the flavonoids from paler-color beers. So you'd have to drink much more Budweiser to get the same effect as a Guinness. The problem is that drinking too much beer or other types of alcohol can raise your blood pressure. So, if you want to drink for your heart, stick to two dark 12-ouncers a day, Dr. Folts says.

Mind your peas and carrots. Fruits and vegetables contain numerous substances that fight off the artery-clogging process. Scientists have yet to isolate all of the anticlogging fruits and vegetables, though they suspect that grapes, apples, and onions may top the list. Produce is naturally high in fiber, a substance that may block cholesterol and triglycerides from making their way into your arteries. Aim for five to seven servings of produce every day, Dr. Folts says. Any whole fruit or vegetable, a half-cup of chopped produce, an eight-ounce glass of fruit juice, or a cup of leafy greens all count as one serving.

Stop tailgating. Stress damages your arteries, makes your blood clot, and may even raise blood pressure. You probably can't eliminate stress. But you can change your reaction to it. For instance, take the typical commute. "Certainly, you need to be alert and aware so that you don't have an accident," says Michael Babyak, Ph.D., assistant clinical professor of medical psychology at Duke University Medical Center in Durham, North Carolina. "But you can learn to expect what happens during your commute. Sometimes people are going to cut you off. Sometimes you are going to sit in traffic. Sitting behind the steering wheel clenching your fists and stewing isn't going to change anything."

Instead, try focusing your mind on something else—like what you feel like eating for lunch. "Pay attention to breathing and muscle tension," Dr. Babyak adds. "Slow breathing down and relax your muscles."

History Lesson

We all know what happened to those wise guys in history who challenged common knowledge, such as "the world is flat" and "the Earth is the center of the universe." People ridiculed them—and worse.

But few of us have heard of the man who dared to challenge the accepted wisdom that "the heart is too fragile and important to even think about operating on it." His name was **Werner Forssmann, M.D.** In the 1920s, he knew he would never get permission to experiment on a real person. So like many of our great scientists, he chose to experiment on himself. When just a German intern, Dr. Forssmann took a metal tube and inserted it into a vein near his elbow and directed it toward his heart. Once he got close enough, he walked into another room and took an x-ray of himself. Then he removed the tube.

Dr. Forssmann reported his findings to his boss, intending to show how such a device could be used to navigate the arteries near the heart. Instead of a pat on the back, his boss fired him, calling the stunt "a circus trick." Dr. Forssmann then abandoned research and became a urologist.

In 1956, the rest of the world finally caught up with Dr. Forssmann when the doctor was awarded the Nobel Prize for his work. His discovery in cardiac catheterization paved the way for artery-clearing work such as angioplasty.

Fish for better health. Eating a lot of fish may reverse and prevent heart disease by inhibiting clotting and lowering levels of triglycerides, says William S. Harris, Ph.D., professor of medicine at the University of Missouri—Kansas City School of Medicine and director of the Lipid Research Laboratory at St. Luke's Hospital of Kansas City.

Fish's heart-healing properties probably come from high amounts of omega-3 fatty acids, an oil mostly found in fattier fish such as mackerel, salmon, and herring. Studies have yet to determine how much fish oil does the trick, Dr. Harris says. But you'd probably do your heart a favor by eating at least three, three-ounce fish servings a week, Dr. Harris says. Remember that shellfish and whitefish are not good sources. You need fatty fish to do an artery good.

Move. Regular exercise can help keep your arteries clear and decrease your risk of heart disease. And you don't have to spend thousands of dollars on a posh health club membership to get the benefits. Taking a quick walk for 20 minutes a day can make a huge difference, experts say. Stairclimbing, moderate sports, or even gardening activities are good ways to get regular exercise. "Diet is the most important factor in reducing the risk of heart disease, but exercise complements it by controlling weight gain, lowering homocysteine levels, and raising high-density-lipoprotein (HDL, or "good") cholesterol levels," says Dr. McCully.

▶Alternative Approaches

Switch from coffee to tea. Drinking a lot of coffee—nine or more cups a day—can raise levels of homocysteine. On the other hand, drinking any kind of tea can lower homocysteine levels because tea contains folate, says Dr. McCully.

In addition to lowering homocysteine levels, drinking four to five cups of green or black tea a day can provide your arteries with protective flavonoids to help keep cholesterol from sticking to the sides of your arteries, Dr. Folts says. Tea has approximately half the caffeine content of coffee. So if you usually drink two cups of coffee a day, four cups of tea will keep you just as alert.

Lose the fat. The American Heart Association recommends keeping your fat intake to less than 30 percent of your daily calories. Some evidence, however, suggests the less fat—particularly animal fat—the better. For the past 20 years, Dean Ornish, M.D., president and director of the nonprofit Preventive Medicine Research Institute in Sausalito, California, has studied how fat and heart disease interact. He recommends holding fat intake to 10 percent of your calories.

"Several studies have shown that the majority of people with coronary heart disease who only make moderate changes in their diet and lifestyle (including lowering their fat content to 30 percent) show worsening of their coronary artery disease. They get worse more slowly than if they made no changes, but they still get worse. On the other hand, our studies indicate that if you reduce fat and cholesterol much further, when combined with other lifestyle changes, you are likely to see a reversal in the progression of coronary artery disease," says Dr. Ornish, author of *Dr. Dean Ornish's Program for Reversing Heart Disease*.

▶Preventive Measures

Let your kids win. Pushy men—guys who talk fast, interrupt others, and incessantly play to win (even when it's a game of Uno with a six-year-old)—die earlier than laid-back men, especially from heart attacks, according to one study. "We are pretty sure that pushy men are more stressed than other folks. And we know that stress damages blood vessels, raises cholesterol levels, makes blood thicker and clot more easily, impairs immunity, and probably even makes blood pressure rise," says Dr. Babyak.

To pinpoint your pushiness quotient, ask your children if they've ever beaten you at a board game. If they shake their heads no, you're too pushy. (By the way, a lot of guys *let* their kids win.) Next time you find yourself competing, whether it's to get the last word or the last free sample at the deli counter, ask yourself if it's worth ruffling your feathers. Some situations are. Most are not, Dr. Babyak says.

Forget about world peace. Guys who worry excessively about possible war, the economy, or the future of the country—things that psychologists call social conditions—are 2½ times more likely to have a heart attack as guys who don't, according to Laura Kubzansky, Ph.D., research fellow at Harvard School of Public Health. "Those are all issues that people have very little control over. Some studies suggest that when people have less control, they develop heart disease," says Dr. Kubzansky.

Of course, some worry is constructive. Worry can alert you to a problem that needs solving, Dr. Kubzansky says. But if you find yourself in a worry cycle, constantly fretting over something that you can't possibly do anything about, you are putting your heart to the test.

Go nuts. Here's some news you'll like. Peanut butter may actually be good for your heart. Here's why. Peanuts are rich in vitamin E, a powerful antioxidant that prevents LDL cholesterol from embedding in the walls of your arteries. "LDL particles carry cholesterol around your arteries," explains Lawrence Kushi, Sc.D., associate professor of public health, nutrition, and epidemiology at the University of Minnesota School of Public Health in Minneapolis. "If LDL particles get oxidized, they can damage the arteries a lot easier. Vitamin E helps prevent oxidation."

Eating more nuts and vegetable oils will boost your vitamin E levels, Dr. Kushi says. True, both sources also contain a bunch of fat. But the fat found in nuts and vegetable oils does not clog arteries like the type of fat found in animal products, he says.

Though Dr. Kushi doesn't usually advocate supplements, vitamin E ranks as an exception. The average guy would find it tough to get more than about 10 to 20 international units (IU) of vitamin E a day from food. With the Daily Value at 30 IU, and some experts recommending up to 400 IU, most men should probably supplement, he says. Dr. Kushi recommends 200 IU taken daily, "which will get you in the range of getting the vitamin E that you need," he says.

Make a B-line. Your body needs three B vitamins—folate, B_6, and B_{12}—to activate important enzymes responsible for breaking down and disposing of excessive levels of homocysteine. Without those vitamins, the homocysteine levels rise, damaging the arteries and causing plaque growth and clotting.

You probably get plenty of B_{12} from your diet. But folate and B_6 are another story. Men should be sure to get the Daily Value of 400 micrograms of folate, says Dr. McCully. And they should shoot for 3.5 milligrams of B_6 daily, almost double the Daily Value. Good sources of folate include green leafy vegetables, orange juice, and beans. Good sources of B_6 include bananas, nuts, grains, and fish.

Be kinder to animals. Animal protein is rich in an amino acid called methionine, which can raise blood levels of the artery-clogging molecule homocysteine. So reducing or eliminating animal protein from your diet can help keep your arteries healthier, says Dr. Kushi.

Heart Palpitations

▶PROBLEM

Your heart usually has a steady rhythm, so steady that you don't notice it. Sometimes, however, your heart skips a beat or beats too quickly—a problem called arrhythmia, a Greek word that means "lack of rhythm." Some physicians also refer to palpitations as dysrhythmia, meaning "bad rhythm."

▶CAUSE

Your heart is powered by electricity. Life-threatening palpitations are caused by a disturbance in the electrical flow to the heart. A lack of blood flow to the heart or a malfunction of the heart muscle can also cause palpitations. Fatigue, caffeine, and stress can bring on more palpitations.

▶HOW SERIOUS

Many palpitations rank more as nuisances than as a true threat. If you feel faint with your palpitations, however, you probably have a serious problem and should go to the emergency room, says Peter M. Abel, M.D., director of cardiovascular disease and prevention at the Cardiovascular Institute of the South in Morgan City, Louisiana. If you feel your heart skip a beat and then you pass out, get to the emergency room as soon as you come to. If you feel short of breath coupled with a tightness in your chest, sweating, and nausea, you need to go to the hospital immediately, Dr. Abel says. If you feel dizzy when you have palpitations, your problem probably isn't as severe, but you should consult your doctor.

Heart disease is a major killer in America. Dr. Abel stresses the importance of not trying to self-diagnose a heart problem; a mistake can prove disastrous.

DO THIS NOW

Breathe deeply. Palpitations can be caused by fear and anxiety. Often, when scared, we hold our breath. And the added anxiety will only make matters worse, says Stephen T. Sinatra, M.D., director of the New England Heart Center in Manchester, Connecticut, and author of *Optimum Health* and *Heartbreak and Heart Disease*. Breathe deeply and slowly, drawing the air down to your abdomen.

Did You Know?

Great works of art can make your heart skip a beat—literally. At least that's the finding of Dr. Graziella Magherini, chief specialist at Santa Maria Nuevo Hospital in Florence, Italy, and author of *The Stendhal Syndrome*. Dr. Magherini examined more than 100 tourists in Florence who experienced heart palpitations when they looked at art. Other than palpitations, the tourists also felt dizziness and stomach pain. Most likely caused by jet lag, travel stress, and shock, art-induced palpitations are more likely in people ages 26 to 40 who rarely leave home, Dr. Magherini concluded. For such people the great, old works of art remind them of the huge passage of time before their own birth. They feel overwhelmed, and they worry about their own mortality.

And if you feel no other symptoms with the heart flutter, although you probably have nothing to worry about and can refer to the following tips for relief, it is still a good idea to let your doctor know.

▶SOLUTIONS

Check your emotional barometer. Your heart may be telling you what your mind is trying to conceal, says Stephen T. Sinatra, M.D., director of the New England Heart Center in Manchester, Connecticut, and author of *Optimum Health* and *Heartbreak and Heart Disease*. Anxiety, stress, depression, and other negative emotions can cause palpitations. So when you feel your heart skip a beat, stop and pay attention to your feelings, he says. They may surprise you.

Talk to yourself. Tell yourself: I'm healthy. This is no big deal. My heart's as strong as ever. The comments will help you relax until the palpitations subside. "A third of the people who have heart palpitations are totally normal," Dr. Sinatra says. "They just need reassurance." In fact, many patients who take medication for palpitations don't need the prescriptions to counter physical symptoms. Physicians prescribe drugs to relieve the patient of the symptom of a palpitation much like a person will take acetaminophen to ease a headache, says Dr. Abel.

Watch what you drink. Caffeine can make your heart race, causing palpitations, Dr. Abel warns. Different amounts of caffeine may cause problems in different people. If you're drinking more than two cups of coffee a day, chain-drinking soda, and living off chocolate bars, you're probably getting too much. Some decongestants also stimulate the heart. Try cutting back slowly until your fluttering attacks go away.

▶ALTERNATIVE APPROACHES

Find emotional release. The mind-body therapy can help you relieve stress, a common cause of palpitations, Dr. Sinatra says. There's really no one way to meditate. As long as you take 5 to 15 minutes every day to sit or lie quietly, you'll do your heart some good. Just let your mind relax. Don't focus on your heart or the palpitations specifically.

▶PREVENTIVE MEASURES

Get a good night's sleep. Lack of sleep can set the stage for palpitations by causing fatigue. Get on a schedule where you go to sleep and wake up at the same time most days. Give yourself seven to eight hours of rest a night, Dr. Abel says.

Cut back on sugar. High amounts of sugar or artificial sweeteners will put your body on a blood sugar roller coaster, setting you up for palpitations. Try cutting back on sweets and artificially sweetened items until the palpitations stop bothering you, says Dr. Sinatra.

Hemorrhoids

▶PROBLEM

You've seen people with varicose veins before—those bulging, ugly ropes snaking along their legs. Hemorrhoids are similar, only in a less visible place—around your anus and lower rectum. "Everyone has hemorrhoids," says James Surrell, M.D., a colorectal surgeon at the Ferguson Clinic in Grand Rapids, Michigan. "They're a normal part of the human anatomy. More than 75 percent of people will have problems with hemorrhoids sometime in their life. There are two types: internal and external. Internal hemorrhoids are inside the anus. Symptoms typically are blood covering a stool, on toilet paper, or in the toilet bowl. You can't see or feel them except in the case of a protruding or prolapsed hemorrhoid, which can push through the anal opening and cause a dull ache, itch, or bleed. External hemorrhoids may include painful swelling or a hard lump around the anus that occurs when a blood clot forms. If irritated, they can itch and bleed.

▶CAUSE

Constipation, excessive straining, rubbing, or cleaning around the anus; obesity; lifting heavy objects; and standing or sitting for long periods can cause flare-ups. There may also be a hereditary factor.

▶HOW SERIOUS

"Hemorrhoids never turn to cancer," says Dr. Surrell. "They're more of a nuisance." Dr. Surrell emphasizes, however, that whenever there is rectal

History Lesson

Most guys wouldn't want it announced to the world that they have hemor-rhoids from hell, but that's what happened to retired major-league all-star George Brett. It was October 1980, and Brett's Kansas City Royals were playing the Philadelphia Phillies in the World Series. The problem was that Brett's butt was causing him more grief than any pitcher was.

The condition became so bad that Brett had to come out of Game 2 of the series after five innings. His hemorrhoids made headlines, and he was the butt of jokes. "Everybody's laughing about it, but it's not funny," he com-plained at the time.

After the Phillies won the first two games of the series, the teams had a day off. Brett underwent a 20-minute operation, in which a proctologist lanced a blood clot in his external hemorrhoid. The next night, Brett played again. In his first at bat, he dragged his tender tush to the plate and hit a home run. The Royals won the game, but the Phillies took the series, even though Brett hit .375.

bleeding, it should be evaluated by a doctor. Rectal bleeding is always abnormal, he says; it could be a symptom of colorectal cancer or other serious problems.

▶SOLUTIONS

Try cortisone cream. Over-the-counter topical steroid creams containing cortisone can help relieve itching but should only be used for a few weeks, says Lester Rosen, M.D., professor of clinical surgery at the Milton S. Hershey Med-ical Center of the Pennsylvania State University in Hershey, Pennsylvania, and a colorectal surgeon at Lehigh Valley Hospital in Allentown, Pennsylvania. You can go back to using them several months to years later. They can thin the skin, making it more susceptible to cracking and bleeding if used excessively, he cautions.

Consume fiber supplements. Over-the-counter fiber supplements and stool softeners containing psyllium and methylcellulose can be effective when taken with a meal, Dr. Rosen says. Two examples would be Metamucil, which con-tains psyllium, and Citrucel, which contains methylcellulose. Dr. Rosen recom-mends taking them with breakfast or lunch to relieve constipation and exces-sive straining, which can lead to hemorrhoids. Taking these kinds of supplements every day would be a good habit for anyone who has experienced constipation problems in the past, he advises.

Drink more. Fluids help move what you've eaten through the digestive tract and soften stools, says Eric G. Weiss, M.D., staff colorectal surgeon and director of surgical endoscopy at Cleveland Clinic Florida in Fort Lauderdale. He rec-ommends drinking eight to ten 10-ounce glasses of any alcohol-free and caffeine-free fluids a day to help you stay regular and avoid painful hemorrhoids. Beverages containing alcohol and caffeine act as diuretics, causing you to lose fluids.

Become more active. Regular exercise helps make for regular guys, Dr. Rosen says. So guys with hemorrhoids should walk a mile or two, bike, or do some kind of aerobic activity every day. "Walking and exercise will help tone the abdominal muscles," he says. "That usually makes for more regular people."

Don't count. "People believe the fallacy that you need to have a bowel movement every day," says Dr. Weiss. "It's not true. Normal is three times per day to three times per week." You should determine what is normal for you, and only be concerned if there is deviation from it.

▶ALTERNATIVE SOLUTIONS

Summon witch hazel. Soaking a piece of toilet paper or cotton in witch hazel and applying it to the affected area works for some people, Dr. Rosen says. "Some people say that it burns; others say that it's soothing," he says. "If they have very irritated hemorrhoids that are open and bleeding, witch hazel doesn't usually work well. With hemorrhoids that are pushing out and are a little irritated and itching, witch hazel works." As long as it soothes, you can apply it several times a day.

Say 'ello to aloe. Applying an aloe gel can supply hemorrhoid relief, says Andrew Weil, M.D., director of the Program in Integrative Medicine at the University of Arizona College of Medicine in Tucson and author of several books, including *Eight Weeks to Optimum Health*. Use a pure gel, with no additives. These can be found in most drugstores. You can apply a small amount several times a day.

▶PREVENTIVE MEASURES

Put down *War and Peace*. If you're in the habit of reading for long periods on the can, stop. With your legs open and knees up, this position can cause slippage of hemorrhoids, says David Beck, M.D., chairman of the department of colorectal surgery at the Ochsner Clinic in New Orleans.

That's not all. "People who sit on the hopper and strain a lot and push and just can't go are better off getting off," says Dr. Rosen. "I think if you don't go within 10 minutes, you probably should leave and try again later."

Eat more fiber. Fiber-rich foods such as fruits, vegetables, seeds, nuts, and legumes can soften stools and make them easier to pass, says Dr. Rosen. He recommends at least 20 grams of fiber a day. You'll get about 2 grams of fiber per serving from each of the above food groups, and an all-bran type cereal would account for another 5 to 10 grams, he says. Check the nutrients listing on the food package to get the exact amounts. Dr. Rosen suggests slowly building up your fiber intake. Too much too fast can cause bloating and cramps.

Be wary of dairy. Dairy products such as cheese, chocolate, ice cream, and milk can make you constipated, causing the straining on the toilet that aggravates hemorrhoids, says Dr. Rosen.

Hiccups

▶PROBLEM

It's the big one—the sales presentation that will make or break your career—when suddenly *hic . . . cup! hic . . . cup!* You continue. But that squeaky *hic* returns, this time louder. You wonder, "Why now? And what the heck are hiccups anyway?" Hiccups are a result of your diaphragm throwing a spastic fit. That's the muscle separating your chest from your abdomen. The irksome *hic* sound comes from the air you quickly suck in, which gets cut off suddenly by your closing vocal cords. And that jerky head-and-neck action? That's just a by-product of your trembling diaphragm.

DO THIS NOW

Grab a tall glass of cold water and take several quick sips without stopping, says Steven Shay, M.D., a gastroenterologist at the Cleveland Clinic Foundation. If your hiccups persist, repeat four or five times.

It sounds scary, but hiccups are basically harmless. They serve no purpose except to make you look and sound ridiculous. More men than women suffer from them for unknown reasons. Most guys will hiccup less than 7 times or more than 63 times in a single bout, usually at a rate of 4 to 60 per minute. Then the hiccups disappear.

▶CAUSE

Just about anything can set them off. Drinking alcohol, chugging carbonated beverages, wolfing down too much food, emotional stress, sudden excitement, indigestion, or a sudden change in body temperature can trigger spasms.

▶HOW SERIOUS

In extremely rare cases, hiccups can persist for hours or days at a time and recur over many weeks, months, and even years, causing insomnia, fatigue, depression, dehydration, and weight loss. So if your hiccups linger for more than 48 hours or recur for a month or more, see your doctor, advises Steven Shay, M.D., a gastroenterologist at the Cleveland Clinic Foundation. Chronic hiccups indicate that you may have a more serious medical problem such as diabetes or

History Lesson

While slaughtering a hog one day in 1922, Charles Osborne of Anthon, Iowa, developed a case of the hiccups. This is kind of like saying that Bill Gates developed a taste for money. For the next 67 years and five months until February 1990, Osborne hiccuped every 1½ seconds. He passed away, presumably hiccup-free at last, in 1991.

kidney disease. Once your illness is treated, your hiccups should cease, says Dr. Shay. But if an underlying disease is not the problem, your doctor can prescribe medications to control them, he says.

▶SOLUTIONS

Hear no evil. Stick an index finger in each ear. The theory is that you'll stimulate the branch of your vagus nerve that goes to the middle ear. The vagus nerve is believed to be a major player in the hiccup cycle and, if stimulated, the hiccups may cease, says James H. Lewis, M.D., associate professor of medicine in the division of gastroenterology at Georgetown University Medical Center in Washington, D.C. This is one of many "cures" that have come down through the ages and are still used today, Dr. Lewis says.

Open a jar of Jif. Another way to stop a hiccup attack is to try swallowing a teaspoon of peanut butter, which stimulates the vagus nerve fibers in the throat, says Dr. Lewis.

Use a scare tactic. A longtime favorite is to get someone to scare the living daylights out of you when you least expect it. So how does it work? "If you gasp when you're startled, it disrupts your respiratory rhythm and the hiccups may cease," explains Dr. Lewis.

Raid the candy dish. Try sucking on a piece of hard candy. The effect is similar to swallowing a spoonful of sugar, which stimulates the vagus nerve fibers in the throat, explains Dr. Lewis.

Brown-bag it. Place one hand around the opening of a paper bag. Then deeply inhale and exhale into the small opening for 60 seconds. "Breathing in your own breath increases the carbon dioxide level in your blood, which may break the hiccup cycle," says Dr. Shay.

Get waterlogged. Drink a tall (12-ounce) glass of cold water without stopping. The combination of gulping without breathing should interrupt those spastic rhythms, Dr. Shay says. Or you can try to drink upside down from the far side of the glass. "The mental wrangling that goes into figuring this out is enough to give your hiccups the boot," adds Dr. Lewis.

Play a gag. If none of the above remedies work, stick your finger down your throat and gag. "I find this retching maneuver to be the best. It's a strong-enough stimulus to short-circuit the hiccup reflex," Dr. Shay says. Stop short of actually throwing up, however.

▶ALTERNATIVE APPROACHES

Press your pinkie. Firmly squeeze the middle joint of your pinkie finger while exhaling for five seconds. Let off the pressure while inhaling for five seconds. Repeat for about two minutes or until your hiccups go away. "This acupressure technique will help relax your stomach nerves to the point where your hiccups can disappear," says David J. Nickel, a doctor of Oriental medicine and a licensed acupuncturist in Santa Monica, California, and author of *Acupressure for Athletes.*

Get hot and bothered. Put a teaspoon of grated fresh ginger and a teaspoon of sugar into a four-ounce cup of boiling water. Squeeze the juice of half a lemon into the cup, let it cool, and drink slowly. "The tangy taste will more than likely jolt you out of the hiccups," says James A. Duke, Ph.D., the world's foremost authority on healing herbs and author of *The Green Pharmacy.* You can also eat a cracker spread with hot mustard to send your hiccups packing.

Eat some gentian. Gentian is a bitter herb that you can buy in many health food stores. It's also known as *Gentiana lutea.* Dribble a few drops of the gentian tincture (the alcoholic extract of the root) on a lemon wedge and suck. "The bitter taste stimulates gastric juices in your stomach, which will improve digestion. So your hiccups will likely take a hike," Dr. Duke says.

Caution: Taking more than four milliliters of gentian tincture a day may cause nausea and vomiting. Gentian is not recommended for people who have high blood pressure, a gastric or duodenal ulcer, or gastric irritation and inflammation.

▶PREVENTIVE MEASURES

Swig less booze. Chugging beer or slinging shots with your buddies can trigger hiccups faster than you can catch a buzz. The reason is that "alcohol depletes zinc and other nutrients essential for proper digestion," Dr. Nickel says. "Zinc is a mineral that also calms your nerves. So without it, your digestive system won't work properly and the nerves responsible for fueling hiccups will become irritated."

Don't gorge yourself. Stop eating when you feel full. "Overloading your stomach can irritate your phrenic and vagus nerves that lead to your diaphragm," Dr. Nickel says. And the end result? *Hic . . . cup!*

High Blood Pressure

▶PROBLEM

One in three American men has high blood pressure. Specifically a health concern of men, African-Americans, and Southerners, high blood pressure can prematurely tire out your heart as well as damage artery walls. When your blood surges through your vessels, it erodes material from your artery walls, much the same way a river slowly erodes its bed. Your immune cells rush in to repair the damage, leaving a thick, hard paste behind. This clogs your arteries (as can high-fat foods), making your heart beat harder to squeeze blood through a narrower opening, further damaging your arteries.

Blood pressure is measured with two numbers: the systolic (the high number) and the diastolic (the low number). The systolic measures how hard your heart must beat to pump blood through your body. The diastolic measures the pressure when your heart relaxes between contractions. A pressure reading of 120/80 is considered optimal, and 140/90 is viewed as high.

▶CAUSE

Blame your age and your narrowed arteries. As you get older, your arteries naturally get more ridged, making your heart beat harder. Also, years of high-fat foods have upped levels of blood cholesterol, which irritate your artery lining, resulting in plaque buildup. Drugs such as nicotine can also constrict arteries. The less room blood has to flow through, the more the

DO THIS NOW

Take a hike. Exercise relaxes and dilates your blood vessels, creating less resistance for the heart to push against. "After exercise, your blood vessels are wide open. If you want some low blood pressure numbers, take your blood pressure right after you exercise," says Peter M. Abel, M.D., director of cardiovascular disease and prevention at the Cardiovascular Institute of the South in Morgan City, Louisiana. Consistent exercise can also permanently lower your blood pressure. Be sure to get your heart pumping for a half-hour to an hour three to five times a week, says Dr. Abel.

heart has to push to move the blood along. "If your heart has to pump through pipes the size of the Hudson River, it doesn't have to push much to get the blood out. But if your heart has to push blood through something the size of the lead in a pencil, it's going to push pretty hard," says Peter M. Abel, M.D., director of cardiovascular disease and prevention at the Cardiovascular Institute of the South in Morgan City, Louisiana. Stress also can make blood pressure soar by dumping heart-stimulating hormones into your system.

▶HOW SERIOUS

Though do-it-yourself machines at drugstores can give you a ballpark look at your blood pressure, the only way to get an accurate reading is to see a health professional. Because high blood pressure can cause stroke and heart attack, you should consult a doctor. Once you hit 140/90, serious health problems such as stroke or heart attack become likely, Dr. Abel says.

▶SOLUTIONS

Lose weight. Think of your heart as a pump that's designed to keep a medium-size home stocked with liquid. Now imagine that you've hooked that poor little pump up to a condominium complex instead of a medium-size home. "Fat is alive. Fat is very vascular. It needs blood. So having extra fat makes the heart do extra work," Dr. Abel says. To quickly get a rough estimate of your healthy weight, grab a calculator. Multiply your weight in pounds by 700, divide that number by your height in inches, then divide again by your height. If the answer is 25 or above, you're overweight. Dropping just 10 percent of those pounds will do your blood pressure some serious good.

Fill up on fruits and vegetables. Researchers have long suspected that nutrients found in both fruits and vegetables—such as magnesium, fiber, and potassium—could lower blood pressure. The problem is that supplement pills that provided the nutrients typically did not reduce blood pressure. The only exception is potassium supplements. Then they tried a different approach. In one study, instead of supplements, researchers fed people foods naturally high in those nutrients. In the people with high blood pressure, systolic blood pressure dropped 7.2 points and diastolic 2.8. "We don't know if it is the potassium, magnesium, or fiber. What we can say is that fruits and vegetables can be beneficial even in persons with lower levels of blood pressure," says Lawrence Appel, M.D., a study co-author and associate professor of medicine and epidemiology at Johns Hopkins University School of Medicine in Baltimore.

To get the same benefit, you'll need to work 8 to 10 daily servings of fruits and vegetables into your diet, says Dr. Appel—more than double the national average and three servings more than the minimum government recommendation. Any whole fruit or vegetable, a half-cup of chopped produce, an eight-ounce glass of fruit juice, or a cup of leafy greens all count as one serving.

Be a dairy king. People who ate 8 to 10 daily servings of vegetables saw

History Lesson

The warning signs were certainly there. Just before the invasion of Normandy, President Franklin D. Roosevelt's (FDR's) blood pressure was recorded as 226/118. And before the Yalta conference, it was measured at 260/150, according to the personal notes of Howard G. Bruenn, M.D., the cardiologist who cared for FDR during the last year of his life.

But back in the 1940s, not all doctors considered high blood pressure a health risk. In fact, up until the day of his death, FDR's personal physician, Vice-Admiral Ross T. McIntire, declared the president to be in excellent health. In reality, the president's blood pressure was eroding his artery walls and enlarging his heart, according to British physician and author Richard Gordon, in his book *An Alarming History of Famous (and Difficult!) Patients.*

What FDR's personal doctors and the rest of America couldn't see, doctors in other parts of the world could, according to Gordon. When Roosevelt went to Yalta in January 1945, Lord Moran, Winston Churchill's physician, took one look at the president, realized what a sick man he was, and predicted that he would not live longer than a few months.

He was correct. On April 12, 1945, the president complained of a severe headache and lost consciousness immediately afterward. His blood pressure was 300/190 when Dr. Bruenn took it 15 minutes later. Roosevelt died at 3:35 P.M. of a cerebral hemorrhage. No autopsy was done to chronicle the extent of FDR's disease. But during the embalming process, FDR's arteries were so clogged that the formaldehyde pump strained and stopped numerous times.

Since the 1940s, modern medicine has made fatal hypertension, as observed in FDR, a rare occurrence.

---

even larger blood pressure drops when they improved their diet in other ways. This diet provided two to three servings of low-fat dairy products a day. (A cup of skim milk or yogurt equals one serving.) A diet this low in fat and rich in dairy products further reduced blood pressure by an additional 4.1 points systolic and 2.6 points diastolic. Dr. Appel suggests that you stick with low-fat foods and that you eat and drink dairy products rather than calcium supplements.

Watch what you stick up your nose. Chronic use of some over-the-counter nasal sprays can constrict blood vessels all over your body, making your heart pump faster to get the blood through, Dr. Abel says. Nasal sprays can provide temporary relief from allergies and colds by constricting the blood vessels in the nose, thus opening up passageways. But many people get addicted to the sprays, eventually squirting much more up their noses than they should. The nasal spray vasoconstriction is so powerful that their use can render prescription blood pressure–lowering medication ineffective, says Dr. Abel. If you are addicted to the sprays and can't quit cold turkey, give prescription nasal sprays a try, Dr. Abel advises. They won't make your blood pressure rise.

Cut back on salt. You probably have read about various conflicting studies on sodium restriction. The truth is that some people are salt-sensitive. Some are not. African-Americans usually are more salt-sensitive than Whites, Dr. Abel says. Other than race, doctors have no way of figuring out who's who. So stay on the safe side and ban the shaker from the table and cut back on high-salt foods such as canned soups, Dr. Abel says.

▶ALTERNATIVE APPROACHES

Ban aspartame from your diet. The artificial sweetener can cause mood swings, which can raise blood pressure. Also, each time you drink a diet soda laced with aspartame, the amino acids phenylamine and aspartic acid are dumped into the blood. This is what causes the fluctuations in your blood sugar levels. If you abuse aspartame (drinking six to eight diet sodas a day), you can eventually become prone to insulin resistance, a condition that can further result in higher blood pressure, says Stephen T. Sinatra, M.D., director of the New England Heart Center in Manchester, Connecticut, and author of *Optimum Health*. In addition, these blood sugar fluctuations may cause nausea and diarrhea and may even lead to bowel cancer, Dr. Sinatra warns.

Close your eyes. The Transcendental Meditation technique can lower systolic blood pressure by as much as 11 points and diastolic by 6, say studies conducted on older African-Americans in the inner city. Two related studies show these reductions occurring within three months of beginning the practice of this simple meditation technique. "The technique works by promoting a special state of 'restful alertness' in mind and body that is beneficial to physiological systems affected by the wear and tear of stress," says Charles Alexander, Ph.D., professor of psychology and co-director of the Center for Health and Aging Studies at the Maharishi University of Management in Fairfield, Iowa, who has done many investigations into meditation's health benefits.

Various forms of meditation exist, but not all are equally effective at reducing high blood pressure or other effects of stress. In some, you focus on your breath, on an image, or on a word. In the Transcendental Meditation technique, you sit comfortably with your eyes closed and, using a special procedure received from your instructor, attend to an individually assigned sound or "mantra," which is known from long tradition to produce the restful alertness or transcendental consciousness state, says Dr. Alexander. This simple, natural technique gently moves your attention from the things going on around you to the thinking process inside, he says. Eventually, the mind transcends even this internal thinking process and is left in a rare state of silence. Research has found that this procedure, when practiced twice a day for 15 to 20 minutes, produces a spectrum of health benefits, including reducing the symptoms of heart disease and increasing the longevity and quality of life of older persons in nursing homes. You can learn more about the Transcendental Meditation program by calling the Maharishi Vedic University school nearest you (they are found in many cities across the United States). Or check out the book *Transcendental Meditation* by Robert Roth, suggests Dr. Alexander.

▶PREVENTIVE MEASURES

Divide your six-pack into thirds. Some alcohol can protect your blood vessels. Too much, however, can raise blood pressure, says Dr. Abel. Stick to two drinks or fewer a day. (A drink, incidentally, is defined as 12 ounces of regular beer, 5 ounces of wine, or a cocktail made with 1½ ounces of 80-proof distilled spirits.)

Hang up the habit. The nicotine from cigarette smoke can constrict blood vessels, boosting blood pressure, says Dr. Abel. Kick the habit now.

High Cholesterol

▶PROBLEM

A fatlike substance that circulates in the blood, cholesterol is deposited in and irritates artery walls, causing plaque buildup. Once enough plaque accumulates, clots form more easily, blocking blood flow and potentially causing heart attack or stroke. Not all cholesterol is created equal. Low-density lipoprotein (LDL) is the villain responsible for artery damage. High-density lipoprotein (HDL) is considered good cholesterol because it carries cholesterol from the different organs to the liver for disposal from the body. The lower your LDL and higher your HDL, the better.

▶CAUSE

Our bodies are capable of making all the cholesterol we need. (Yes, some cholesterol is needed to manufacture hormones.) So when we eat cholesterol-raising foods and live a cholesterol-raising lifestyle, we end up with far more cholesterol in our blood than our bodies could ever use, says James Cleeman, M.D., coordinator of the National Cholesterol Education Program in Bethesda, Maryland. The excess builds up in the arteries. Among the factors we can control, saturated fat is the worst cholesterol-raiser, closely followed by dietary cholesterol, inactivity, and being overweight.

Your genetic makeup may predispose you to high blood cholesterol. Some people are born with fewer or less-efficient LDL receptors than others. That means that their bodies can't remove excess LDL from their blood systems as well as they should. Some of these people can still lower their levels with diet

DO THIS NOW

It doesn't matter whether it's raw, pickled, fried, sautéed, or made into a pill; garlic's organosulfur compounds lower cholesterol levels, says Stephen Warshafsky, M.D., assistant professor of medicine at New York Medical College in Valhalla, New York. The more garlic you eat, the better. Eating a half-clove to a whole clove a day can lower your cholesterol levels 5 to 10 percent in just three months. And eating 10 cloves a day can lower levels 21 percent over the same period.

and lifestyle changes, but they must wage a more vigilant battle, Dr. Cleeman says. Others have to add medication to their diet and lifestyle regimens to sufficiently lower cholesterol levels.

▶How Serious

"If you have high blood cholesterol in your teens and early twenties, you will have a higher risk of heart attack 30 to 40 years later," Dr. Cleeman says. "You want to lower your levels as soon as possible. Otherwise, you'll wind up in middle age where, although cholesterol lowering is still worthwhile, it won't reduce your risk as much or, at worst, it may literally be too late." So get your cholesterol levels checked at least once every 5 years.

Look to the diet and lifestyle tips in this chapter as your first resort to lowering cholesterol levels. But if your LDL levels stay above 190 milligrams per deciliter despite your best efforts, you should talk to your doctor about cholesterol-lowering medication, even if you have no other heart disease risk factors, says Dr. Cleeman. If you have two or more risk factors, consider medication if your levels stay above the 160 mark. And if you have heart disease or artery blockages, consider medication whenever your LDL levels are at the 130 mark or above. If you are younger than 35, your LDL levels should be 220 or higher before taking medication to reduce the risk of long-term side effects, he says.

▶Solutions

Fill up on fiber. In the body, soluble fiber forms a protective gel that keeps cholesterol from getting absorbed in the intestine, Dr. Cleeman explains. Eating 10 grams of soluble fiber a day (a cup of cooked oat bran, one orange, a cup of navy beans, and one baked potato) can lower blood cholesterol levels by 5 to 10 percent, he says.

Go for soy, boy. Eating 20 to 25 grams of soy protein each day can lower blood cholesterol levels by up to 10 percent, according to one study. To get soy's cholesterol-lowering effect, you don't have to choke down plain tofu, says Carla Green, R.D., a research dietitian at the University of Kentucky in Lexington. "I really emphasize that tofu is not something you take a bite of," says Green. Instead, try the following soy-boosting methods.

- Experiment with various types of soy milk (some taste better than others).
- Substitute half of the white flour in baked goods with soy flour.
- Mix textured soy protein into spaghetti sauce.
- Hide tofu in other recipes, such as stir-fries, soups, and pasta casseroles. For instance, make a tofu mousse by pureeing a box of tofu with ¾ cup chocolate chips and ½ teaspoon vanilla.

For 20 to 25 grams, you'll need to drink a cup of soy milk, have a couple of soy muffins, and eat some tofu stir-fry for dinner, says Green.

Spice up your life. Hot peppers contain the oil capsaicin, which can keep

LDL cholesterol from sticking to the sides of your arteries, says Stephen T. Sinatra, M.D., director of the New England Heart Center in Manchester, Connecticut, and author of *Optimum Health*. "A little goes a long way," warns Dr. Sinatra. You don't need to stick so many hot peppers in your chili that you burn your tongue off. Just experiment by adding some ground red pepper and other pepper spices to your favorite foods and watch the cholesterol numbers fall.

Work up a sweat. Exercise raises levels of the good HDL cholesterol, which shuttles artery-clogging LDL cholesterol out of your arteries, says Peter Wilson, M.D., director of laboratories at the Framingham Heart Study in Massachusetts. There's some controversy about the level of exercise intensity you should undertake.

The best data come from runners. In a large study at Georgetown University in Washington, D.C., men who jogged between 11 and 14 miles a week had higher levels of HDL (11 percent) than those who didn't exercise. If jogging's not for you, try walking 2 miles or more a day, suggests Dr. Sinatra.

MEN'S HEALTH INDEX

High blood cholesterol is just one of many heart attack risk factors. In descending order, here's how much you'll lower your risk of heart attack by lowering cholesterol and making other dietary and lifestyle changes, according to Peter M. Abel, M.D., director of cardiovascular disease and prevention at the Cardiovascular Institute of the South in Morgan City, Louisiana.

- **Stop smoking: Risk drops 50 to 70 percent**
- **Exercise: Risk drops 45 percent**
- **Maintain an ideal weight: Risk drops 35 to 55 percent**
- **Take an aspirin a day: Risk drops 33 percent**
- **Consume one alcoholic drink a day: Risk drops 25 to 45 percent (Excessive alcohol consumption, however, increases your heart disease risk, says Dr. Abel.)**
- **Lower cholesterol levels 1 percent: Risk drops 2 to 3 percent**
- **Lower blood pressure 1 point: Risk drops 2 to 3 percent**

▶ALTERNATIVE APPROACHES

Take up heavy petting. Petting a dog, cat, or some other domestic furry creature can quickly lower your cholesterol levels, says Dr. Sinatra. Petting probably works because the animal almost always returns your gesture with love and affection, making you feel good and melting away artery-clogging stress.

▶PREVENTIVE MEASURES

Cut back on fat. While saturated fats found in meat and whole-milk dairy products raise cholesterol levels, other types of fat (such as the unsaturated fats of olive oil, soybean oil, corn oil, and nuts) don't seem to clog the arteries, Dr.

Cleeman says. But such fats are still high in calories. So if you are overweight, which also contributes to high blood cholesterol, you'll want to use them moderately, too. Aim to keep your saturated fat intake to 8 to 10 percent of your daily calories. If you already have heart disease, keep it below 7 percent.

You can cut your saturated fat levels by opting for leaner cuts of meat and dairy products made from skim or low-fat (1%) milk. Also, limit your intake of meat, poultry and fish to six ounces or less a day—roughly the size of two decks of cards. And watch out for coconut, palm, and palm kernel oils in commercially baked products; they're extremely high in saturated fat, says Dr. Cleeman.

Collar dietary cholesterol. The cholesterol you eat can raise the level of cholesterol in your blood, says Dr. Cleeman. Keep your daily intake to less than 300 milligrams a day. If you have heart disease, keep it to less than 200 milligrams a day. So put down the breakfast croissant with egg, cheese, and sausage and back away slowly. That one tasty treat is loaded with a whopping 216 milligrams of cholesterol.

Impotence

▶PROBLEM

Ten million to 30 million men in America are believed to have a total inability to have an erection, an inconsistent ability to do so, or an ability to maintain only brief erections. The condition is often called erectile dysfunction.

▶CAUSE

About 10 to 20 percent of cases are due to psychological factors such as stress, anxiety, guilt, low self-esteem, depression, and fear of sexual failure. Between ages 20 and 40, psychological causes are more common, says Neil Baum, M.D., associate clinical professor of urology at Tulane University Medical School and Louisiana State University School of Medicine, and director of the Impotence Foundation, all in New Orleans, and author of *Impotence*.

After age 50, it's most often a physical problem. Diseases and disorders—including diabetes, kidney disease, chronic alcoholism, vascular disease, and especially atherosclerosis (hardening of the arteries)—account for about 70 percent of cases of impotence. Other causes include prostate, bladder, and rectal surgery; pelvic and spinal cord injuries; drugs to treat high blood pressure; antihistamines, antidepressants, tranquilizers, and appetite suppressants; and chronic use of alcohol, marijuana, and other intoxicants. Excessive tobacco use can also block penile arteries.

▶PROBLEM

While impotence may be a symptom of a serious disease such as diabetes, its psychological impact also is significant. A guy's manhood is defined in part

DO THIS NOW
If your efforts at intercourse have been limited to the evening, try making whoopee first thing in the morning, says Neil Baum, M.D., associate clinical professor of urology at Tulane University Medical School and Louisiana State University School of Medicine, and director of the Impotence Foundation, all in New Orleans, and author of *Impotence*. A man's testosterone level is higher in the morning than at night, and chances are that you'll be less fatigued, he says.

by his, well, manhood. If he can't get an erection, he often feels like less than a whole man, says Dr. Baum. He may well become discouraged and depressed. His wife also is affected, says Dr. Baum. She isn't sexually fulfilled and may wonder if her husband is cuckolding her. "She thinks that he's giving at the office," says Dr. Baum. "It creates a lot of anxiety and tension and marital discord." For men who find that they are failing in the bedroom more than they are succeeding, Dr. Baum suggests that they visit a physician. One or two doctor visits can often identify if it is a physical or psychological problem, he says. For psychological impotence, a referral is then made to a therapist who meets with the man and his partner to resolve any emotional or marital conflict, Dr. Baum explains.

▶SOLUTIONS

Do not enter. Rather than focusing on vaginal penetration, allow yourself to have leisurely, gentle foreplay with your partner, advises Dr. Baum. This promotes intimacy while removing the pressure to perform, and if you get and sustain an erection, you may want to try and have intercourse next time, he says.

Don't smoke. Smoking can narrow blood vessels, preventing sufficient blood from surging into your penis when you're aroused and denying you an erection, says Dr. Baum.

Get fit. Obesity can impair a man's ability to get erections, says Dr. Baum. A healthy lifestyle helps maintain healthy erections. Obesity often is a precursor of that erection-killer diabetes—yet another reason to watch your weight, says Dr. Baum. He adds that regular exercise will also maintain the general health of the blood vessels.

Relax more. "A lot of guys don't realize it, but they get a lot of stress from work and elsewhere," says David Schwartz, M.D., a urologist in private practice in Alexandria, Virginia, who treats men with impotence. "If you get stressed out enough, that will turn off your erections."

Use a splint. There is at least one penile splint on the market whose maker says it enables a man to have intercourse with or without an erection. Makers of the rubber gadget, called Rejoyn, call it a penile support sleeve. Little more than two inches long, it fits over a flaccid penis. The wearer places a lubricated latex condomlike gizmo over it called a comfort cover for his partner's benefit. Since the end and bottom of the Rejoyn is not enclosed, it can accommodate an erection, should that happy event occur. It's yet the latest variation of a penile splint, says Robert Birch, Ph.D., a sex therapist in private practice in Columbus, Ohio.

Saddle up safely. There is some evidence that riding a bicycle—especially on long journeys—can create impotence problems as the saddle presses against your perineum, the area between the back of the scrotum and the bottom of the rectum, in which arteries and nerves that feed the penis are located, says Dr. Baum. You needn't scrap your two-wheeler, however. Instead, buy a bike with

Did You Know?

We are not, repeat not, recommending that you try this at home. But martial arts expert Master Tze Tan Chan lifts more than 100 pounds of weights attached to ropes with his testicles two or three times a week—a practice that he contends has made him more potent. It doesn't seem to have hurt; the twice-married Chan is a father of five.

More incredibly, Chan—in his early fifties—has hoisted as much as 350 pounds with his testicles, which he maintains are the strongest part of a man's body. He doesn't do so to show off. It's all part of his Daoist religion, which includes the Qi Gong, or lifting of weights this most unconventional way. The regimen gives a man more energy, according to Chan. There seems to be no arguing that Chan has that. And he has never injured himself.

an amply padded, wide saddle that puts the pressure on your buttocks rather than your genital area, says Dr. Baum.

▶ALTERNATIVE APPROACHES

Put the E in erection. A study done by Suresh Sikka, Ph.D., associate professor of urology and director of urology research at the Tulane University School of Medicine in New Orleans, found that impotent men with diabetes had significantly lower levels of vitamin E in their plasma than either men with diabetes who were potent or a control group. Vitamin E is an antioxidant that can help stave off damage to red blood cells that is common in men with diabetes, says Dr. Sikka. He recommends 400 to 800 international units of vitamin E combined with 500 milligrams of vitamin C daily as a preventive measure. If you are considering taking this amount of vitamin E, discuss it with your doctor first.

Get some Siberian ginseng. "Ginseng definitely works if you use it over a long period of time," says Thomas Kruzel, doctor of naturopathy, professor of urology at the National College of Naturopathic Medicine in Portland, Oregon. He recommends 500 milligrams once a day of Siberian ginseng (*Eleutheroccus senticosus*). It can be taken over a long period of time but should probably be stopped periodically. "I recommend that you either take the dosage every other day or take the dosage every day, taking one to two weeks off every two to three months," says Dr. Kruzel. Those with elevated blood pressure, fever, or insomnia should not take ginseng. Also, to avoid irritability, do not consume caffeine and other stimulants while using ginseng.

Go ginkgo. Another useful herb for erection problems, especially those due to circulatory problems such as with diabetes, is ginkgo, says Dr. Kruzel. Ginkgo comes in different strengths and forms, explains Dr. Kruzel. He recommends the whole-herb powder, suggesting that you take two 250-milligram capsules two times a day. "Periodically, I will have a patient who complains of excess gas from this dose and form," he says. "Then I prescribe an extract at 80 milligrams two times a day with meals." Taking too much concentrated ginkgo extract (more than 240 milligrams) can cause dermatitis, diarrhea, and vomiting. The herb may increase the action of monoamine oxidase (MAO) inhibitors such as Nardil, so avoid ginkgo if you are taking these medications. People with hypotension should avoid high doses (above 1,000 milligrams) of ginkgo.

Add a pinch of powder. For men who have erection difficulties, Dr. Kruzel recommends a teaspoon a day of a nonprotein substance found in health food stores called creatine monohydrate. Popular with weight lifters, it provides quick muscle energy, he says. "It has worked quite well for a lot of my elderly patients." Dr. Kruzel cautions that creatine monohydrate should not be used indefinitely. Rather, take one teaspoon a day in a little juice or water for four to six weeks or until your energy level increases, he says. Then discontinue use for two to three months and start again, if needed. Higher doses than described here should be monitored by a physician, especially in the elderly, he adds.

▶PREVENTIVE MEASURES

Close the bar. Alcohol is a sedative that actually makes getting an erection more difficult, says Dr. Baum. "Alcohol stimulates the desire but inhibits the performance," he says.

Indecision

▶PROBLEM

Racked by fear of rejection and self-doubt, you hemmed and hawed for an hour or more before calling a girl for a date when you were in high school. Sometimes you wimped out and never did make the call.

Now that you're older, your indecisiveness rears its timid head in other ways: You might hold up work while you endlessly contemplate the merits of a project. Or you have an opportunity to make a career change, and you can't decide what to do.

Maybe your ambivalence is evident in more prosaic ways: You agonize over what video to rent or which tie to buy. Regardless of what it is, you make decisions with glacierlike speed.

▶CAUSE

Conflict is often at the root of indecisiveness, says Seymour Epstein, Ph.D., professor of psychology at the University of Massachusetts in Amherst and author of *Constructive Thinking: The Key to Emotional Intelligence*. This conflict arises most often when your head tells you to do one thing but your heart yearns for another option.

In your heart, you may want to buy a sleek, sporty car; but your head tells you that it often needs repairs. "If there is no conflict, you just have a motive and you act on it," Dr. Epstein says.

▶HOW SERIOUS

Usually, indecision is not serious. "But for some people, it's a major pathology," says Dr. Epstein.

History Lesson

Perhaps nobody epitomizes indecisiveness more than Civil War Union General George B. McClellan. His excessive preparation and penchant for over-estimating the strength of rebel forces led McClellan to shamelessly shirk the battlefield. His inertia was a constant source of irritation to President Abraham Lincoln.

Wrote James M. McPherson in *Battle Cry of Freedom*: "He lacked the mental and moral courage required of great generals—the will to *act*, to confront the terrible moment of truth on the battlefield. Having experienced nothing but success in his career, he was afraid to risk failure."

President Lincoln became so frustrated with McClellan that he wrote him the following note: "If you don't want to use the army, I should like to borrow it for awhile." McClellan blamed his inaction on others, complaining falsely that he was outmanned and outgunned and that Lincoln was "an idiot" and "a well-meaning baboon."

▶SOLUTIONS

Trust your gut. If you think that your instincts are good, then trust your gut feeling and act on it, says Peter Wylie, Ph.D., a psychologist and management consultant in Washington, D.C. Behavioral scientists at the University of Iowa concluded that unconscious emotional signals—gut feelings—have a biological basis and can help most people make good decisions.

Imagine the worst. Imagine the worst-case scenario if your decision goes awry and how you would cope with it, suggests Rebecca Curtis, Ph.D., professor of psychology at Adelphi University in Garden City, New York, and a psychologist in Manhattan. Do this in writing, if you think that it will help. Having a plan to deal with potential adversity can give you the confidence to then make a decision, she says.

Learn from your mistakes. When you make a decision that turns out badly, learn from it rather than becoming fearful of the next decision you must make, says Dr. Wylie. He uses a broken romance to illustrate the point. You can put all the blame on the woman and approach another relationship like a guy walking through a minefield. Or you can try to grow wiser from the experience and figure out how to avoid repeating it.

Take small steps. A large, undefined task can be daunting, so plan to do it in small, doable steps that make decision making easier, advises Dr. Epstein.

See the big picture. When faced with a decision, don't think in absolute terms of the best choice or the right choice, advises Dr. Curtis. Think of all the choices as having advantages and drawbacks, and weigh them accordingly.

Identify your conflict. Maybe a teacher once embarrassed you in front of the entire class, or a parent ridiculed something you did. If you can identify why you feel conflicted when you have to make a decision, it can make the decision-making process easier, says Dr. Curtis.

Diminish importance. The strongest predictor of everyday stress is the degree of significance that people attribute to the events in their lives, Dr. Epstein says. "Don't sweat the little stuff, whether in the choices you make or otherwise."

▶ALTERNATIVE APPROACHES

See what it's like. If you don't have a prior experience to draw upon when faced with a decision, try visualizing the outcome, says Dr. Epstein. Let's say you're thinking about marrying a woman but are feeling ambivalent at the prospect. Vividly imagine yourself coming home to this woman, having dinner with her, sharing a life with her. "Don't try to reason it out, but try to get a feeling. See what it feels like—what your body is telling you," says Dr. Epstein.

▶PREVENTIVE MEASURES

Get real. Of course you want any decision to turn out perfectly, but this isn't realistic, says Dr. Wylie. "That's why they put erasers on pencils," he says. "We all screw up. It's part and parcel of being human." Being a perfectionist paralyzes some men from taking any action at all, Dr. Wylie says.

Don't take it so hard. If you do fail, don't take it personally, says Dr. Epstein. People are often highly critical of themselves but more tolerant of others, he says. So if a decision you make turns out badly, others may not be as judgmental of you as you are with yourself.

Dare to fail. There's powerful wisdom in the old saying, "Nothing ventured, nothing gained." And that's not just at the Friday night poker game. "Failure is an important part of success," Dr. Epstein says. "If you're afraid of failure and won't risk it, then you're not going to succeed."

Inflammatory Bowel Disease

▶PROBLEM

Inflammatory bowel disease usually takes the form of ulcerative colitis or Crohn's disease. The first is an inflammation of the inner lining of the colon and rectum, while the latter is an inflammation that goes into the deeper layers of the intestinal wall.

People with Crohn's disease may also have inflammation of the mouth, esophagus, stomach or upper section of the small intestine. Both ailments can also cause fever, weight loss, bloody stools, diarrhea, and a tenderness around the abdomen.

▶CAUSE

It's a mystery why some people get inflammatory bowel disease. There is a familial link; 10 to 25 percent of those with the disease have a relative with Crohn's disease or ulcerative colitis.

Some researchers think that a virus or bacterium interacts with the body's immune system to trigger an inflammatory reaction in the intestinal wall of people susceptible to the disease.

DO THIS NOW

People with inflammatory bowel disease often feel worst after a meal. If your symptoms are severe, skip a meal and drink Gatorade instead, says William B. Ruderman, M.D., a practicing physician at Gastroenterology Associates of Central Florida in Orlando. This way, you will still get some electrolytes and calories without forcing any roughage through your sensitive digestive tract. "You should do this no more than once every few months. More often means that you need to be under a doctor's close supervision," he says.

History Lesson

San Diego Chargers placekicker Rolf Benirschke was not about to let ulcerative colitis end his distinguished NFL career. During the 1978 season, Benirschke began having symptoms of his condition, eventually spending weekdays in the hospital before being released on weekends to join the team for games. Four games into the 1979 season, after Benirschke was admitted to a hospital for his condition, he almost died from complications surrounding two surgical procedures. His weight dropped to 123 pounds.

The following season, Benirschke, now wearing an external bag for waste, resumed his career by making 37 of his next 41 field goal attempts. He was voted to the Pro Bowl after the 1982 season and received the NFL Man of the Year Award in 1983. In 1997, he became the 20th member of the San Diego Chargers Hall of Fame.

After he retired from football, Benirschke was the daytime host of *Wheel of Fortune* for awhile. Today, he is a businessman and a motivational speaker.

▶HOW SERIOUS

Inflammatory bowel disease is serious enough that you should be seeing a doctor periodically, says Bret Lashner, M.D., director of the Inflammatory Bowel Disease Center at the Cleveland Clinic Foundation. People with widespread ulcerative colitis have a much higher risk of colon cancer. About 25 percent of them undergo surgery in which the entire large intestine is removed and an internal pouch is created to act as a reservoir until bowel movements are socially convenient, explains Dr. Lashner. About 80 percent of people with Crohn's disease eventually undergo surgery to treat complications or to relieve symptoms that have not responded to other remedies, says Dr. Lashner. The surgery is not curative, as the disease often recurs in the bowel, he adds.

▶SOLUTIONS

Eat less fiber. You've heard repeatedly about the benefits of adding fiber to your diet. But when inflammatory bowel disease flares up, you should reduce your fiber intake by half, says Dr. Lashner. This will cut down on gas and bloating. When you are feeling all right, you can go back to eating a normal or high-fiber diet every day, he adds.

Eat fewer fatty foods. This is always a good idea, and it's especially true if you have inflammatory bowel disease. Forgo fatty, greasy foods, or at least cut back on them, advises Dr. Lashner. The same goes for spicy foods. They can make symptoms such as diarrhea and bleeding worse.

Lay off lactose. People with Crohn's disease are four times as likely to be lactose-intolerant as other folks, Dr. Lashner says. If dairy products make your symptoms worse, avoid them. (For more tips on dealing with lactose intolerance, see page 352.)

Take a vitamin. If you have chronic diarrhea because of inflammatory bowel disease, you probably are losing vitamins and minerals. A multivitamin every day can help restore what you lose, says Dr. Lashner.

Use aspirin or ibuprofen with caution. This applies only to those guys with Crohn's disease. Aspirin and ibuprofen sometimes cause flare-ups of symptoms, says James Cerda, M.D., professor of medicine and chief of nutrition support at the University of Florida in Gainesville. If they do, try acetaminophen instead if you need a painkiller.

Eat sparingly. Diarrhea and cramps make it hard to tolerate any food at all when you are having an inflammatory bowel disease attack, says Sheila Crowe, M.D., gastroenterologist and assistant professor of medicine in the department of internal medicine in the division of gastroenterology at the University of Texas Medical Branch at Galveston. To keep pain to a minimum, "eat very plain food, such as applesauce or boiled, skinless chicken or soft, cooked carrots—and not much of them," says Dr. Crowe.

Drink deeply. If you have diarrhea (and with inflammatory bowel disease you probably do), you may get dehydrated. To replace lost fluid, try to drink at least 10 eight-ounce glasses of water or juice a day during an attack, says Dr. Crowe.

▶ALTERNATIVE SOLUTIONS

Add folic acid. People with inflammatory bowel disease often are deficient in folic acid, says Dr. Lashner. "It should be replaced. There are some studies that show if you replace it, you can lower your cancer risk," he says. He suggests taking a multivitamin with 400 micrograms of folic acid, or a folic acid supplement.

Eat more onions. The top compound with anti-inflammatory bowel disease effects is quercetin; the best source of this compound is onion skins, according to James A. Duke, Ph.D., the world's foremost authority on healing herbs and author of *The Green Pharmacy*. Since we don't eat onion skins, put the whole onion, skin and all, into soups and stews while they're cooking. Just remember to remove the parchmentlike skin just before serving. You could also take a 400-milligram supplement of quercetin (available at health food stores) about 20 minutes before each meal, to ease the symptoms of inflammatory bowel disease.

▶PREVENTIVE MEASURES

Relax. Tension and stress don't cause inflammatory bowel disease, but they can make symptoms worse, Dr. Lashner says. Learning stress-management or relaxation techniques can make symptoms less severe.

Ingrown Toenails

▶PROBLEM

Pain in the corner of a toenail and, possibly, some redness and swelling usually mean an ingrown toenail, says John Scanlon, D.P.M., chief of podiatric services at Chestnut Hill Hospital in Philadelphia.

You should start to treat an ingrown toenail as soon as possible to prevent Stage One ingrown toenails (pain and swelling) from turning into Stage Two (drainage and infection) or, even worse, Stage Three, when the nail thickens and the skin overgrows it to the point that the only option is to remove the toenail.

▶CAUSE

It's most likely that one of two things caused your ingrown toenail. First, your shoes are too tight. They are squeezing your toes together, which is forcing your toenail into the surrounding skin of the toe. Second, you might have trimmed or picked your toenails incorrectly, and that may have started the nail growing into the skin of your toe.

▶HOW SERIOUS

"An ingrown toenail can actually become a very serious problem," says Marjorie Menacker, D.P.M., a podiatrist with Chesterfield Podiatry Associates in Midlothian, Virginia. "If it's not handled properly, it can easily become infected." Signs of infection include pus, redness, swelling, and extreme tenderness. If infection occurs, see your physician or podiatrist, says Dr. Menacker.

DO THIS NOW

Soak your foot in warm salt water, advises Marjorie Menacker, D.P.M., a podiatrist with Chesterfield Podiatry Associates in Midlothian, Virginia. "This will help soften the piece of nail and the skin around it, maybe enough for you to clear the two pieces away from each other," she says. "Even if that doesn't happen, the salt water will help fight any infection that might occur."

Add one to two tablespoons of salt to a quart of lukewarm water. Before putting your feet in, test the temperature with your fingers to make sure that it's not too hot for you. Soak for 15 to 20 minutes.

History Lesson

Ingrown toenails accomplished what countless NBA opponents couldn't: They shut down Michael Jordan and Grant Hill. Jordan missed three pre-season games in 1997 because of surgery on two ingrown toenails. Hill also missed several games because of surgery to remove a toenail.

Why are toes the Achilles' heel of basketball players? All those fast stops and turns mean lots of toe jabbing in tight sneakers. If the nails are cut incorrectly or not cared for properly, then it's only a matter of time before they start making their way into the skin of the toes. And when ingrown toenails become chronic, surgery is just about the only way to solve the problem, says Edward Beckett, D.P.M., a podiatrist in private practice in Lehighton, Pennsylvania.

Many people can't see well enough to take care of their feet after a certain age, says Andrea Cracchiolo III, M.D., an orthopedic surgeon and director of the University of California, Los Angeles, Adult Foot and Ankle Clinic. "If you put a newspaper down by your feet and can't read the type, then you need someone else to take care of your feet. You shouldn't approach your toes with a thing like scissors if you can't see what you're doing." Anyone with diabetes should also have a doctor take care of his toes because that illness affects both your eyesight and your feet.

▶SOLUTIONS

Separate with cotton. To fix an ingrown toenail, you need to find a way to separate the nail from the skin. "Sometimes you can fit a little piece of cotton between the piece of nail and the bit of skin that it's growing into," Dr. Scanlon says. "That will cushion the flesh against the nail trying to come in." Not everyone with an ingrown toenail will be able to do this, by the way. It's not always easy to even find a small bit of space in which to put the cotton.

Open up. Resist the urge to bandage your toe. "People have a tendency to wrap bandages really tightly," warns Edward Beckett, D.P.M., a podiatrist in private practice in Lehighton, Pennsylvania. "That's going to push the nail more severely into the toe."

In fact, you should try to keep your foot uncovered as much as possible. Wear sandals, for example, or at least take your shoes off in your house, to give your toe some room.

Medicate, medicate, medicate. The danger with an ingrown toenail is infection because the nail is puncturing the skin and, as Dr. Scanlon diplomatically says, "the foot isn't the cleanest part of the body." So it's important to keep the toe as clean as possible. Fresh socks, lots of warm water, and antibiotic ointment applied regularly will help prevent the toenail from getting infected.

Antibiotic ointments are available in most drugstores. They include Polysporin and Neosporin, among others. Follow label directions when using these products.

▶ALTERNATIVE APPROACHES

Wear shoes that fit. Shoes can make all the difference when it comes to the comfort of your toes, say podiatrists. It's worth the time it takes to become a discriminating shoe shopper.

"Don't buy shoes by size; buy by fit," advises John Venson, D.P.M., chairman of the department of medicine and surgery at the Dr. William M. Scholl College of Podiatric Medicine in Chicago. "I wear a size 10 dress shoe and a size 11½ gym shoe by Nike, but my New Balance pair is a size 11. You need to try shoes in various sizes to see which one feels best." You're looking for adequate room in the toe box so that even if you slide your foot forward as you walk and your foot spreads, your toes don't hit the front of the shoe. Stick with name brands, says Dr. Venson, and be willing to spend some money.

Lace 'em up. How you lace your shoes can help relieve the pressure from and even prevent ingrown toenails, says Carol Frey, M.D., associate clinical professor of orthopedic surgery at the University of Southern California School of Medicine in Los Angeles. Here's how.

Start by poking the shoelace through one of the top eyelets (those closest to your ankle) and down through the opposite bottom eyelet; leave enough of the lace not threaded through to tie the shoe when you're finished. Next, lace across to the other bottom eyelet, then diagonally up to the next eyelet. Then go through the eyelet directly across and then diagonal again and so on; repeating diagonal and across until the shoe is fully laced. Remember to always lace over the section of lace running from the top of the shoe to the bottom.

▶PREVENTIVE MEASURES

Cut your nails right. Even toenail experts (also known as podiatrists) can't agree on proper toenail shape. Straight across? Slightly rounded edges?

"The best thing to do is know your own feet," says Dr. Scanlon. "You need to follow the normal anatomy of your toe, and for most people, that means curving the nail a little bit at the edges." You absolutely do not want to cut the nail very much below the top of your toe, because that will give it the opportunity to grow into the skin. Smooth any rough edges with an emery board. But don't use the file on a nail clipper, as it is too rough and will likely cause jagged edges.

Don't pick. Aside from being a disgusting habit, picking your toenails makes for really unattractive feet. Plus, it's unhealthy.

"The danger in picking your toenails is that you'll also pick off some of the cuticle," says Dr. Scanlon. "If you do that, you can break the membrane of the skin, which allows bacteria and fungus to get in." Bits of nail, too, are more likely to dig into your toe when you pick rather than cut and file.

Ingrown Whiskers

▶PROBLEM

Ingrown whiskers, or pseudofolliculitis barbae, is a common dermatologic condition that affects men with curly whiskers who shave on a regular basis. Because of the nature of their whiskers, up to 80 percent of black men have ingrown whiskers. It's also called razor bumps or shaving bumps.

▶CAUSE

When you shave on a regular basis, those curly whiskers don't have a chance to straighten out. Instead, they exit the hair follicle and almost immediately curve back into the surrounding skin, producing a foreign-body reaction and bump. To make it worse, razor blades can form the whisker into a perfect spear for the purpose. "When you look at it under a microscope, the tip of the hair is like a little stiletto. It's very sharp," says Victor Newcomer, M.D., clinical professor of dermatology at the University of California, Los Angeles, UCLA School of Medicine. The same condition is often seen in men and women who shave their pubic region, another area of particularly curly hair.

▶HOW SERIOUS

Aside from being prone to ingrown whiskers, black men are also more susceptible to the associated scarring that can accompany the problem. Untreated, or treated improperly, ingrown whiskers can leave big, thick, elevated scars along a man's beard area, Dr. Newcomer says. And because a man has ingrown hairs penetrating the skin and hair follicle walls, those sores can lead to infection. "The bug of the day can move in, and now you have a bacterial infection as well as a foreign-body reaction, at which point you should seek medical attention," adds Dr. Newcomer.

> ## DO THIS NOW
>
> **Sheath the blade, Zorro. "Stop shaving. Give your face a little bit of a rest,"** says Nicholas V. Perricone, M.D., associate clinical professor of dermatology at Yale University School of Medicine. Since shaving is the cause of ingrown whiskers, back off from razors for a couple of days.

Did You Know?

If you're a lean, mean, fighting machine with ingrown whiskers, you may just be out of a job, Marine. Not by the hair of your chinny-chin-chin, you say? It's true: Ingrown whiskers can be a cause for release from the Marine Corps.

In severe cases of pseudofolliculitis barbae (the 10-cent name for ingrown whiskers) where military doctors determine the only course of treatment is to grow a beard, it doesn't matter if you're Chuck Norris himself. You're outta there.

Marine Corps order 6310.1B says that since Marine Corps regulations do not permit the wearing of a beard, those ingrown whiskers and the person they're attached to have to go. Semper Fi and *sayonara*.

▶SOLUTIONS

Drop acid. Not that kind. A few years ago, Nicholas V. Perricone, M.D., associate clinical professor of dermatology at Yale University School of Medicine, came across a way of treating ingrown whiskers that he says surpasses all others. The key, he says, is glycolic acid, one of the alpha hydroxy acids often found in anti-aging creams and other skin treatments. The effectiveness of the acid was proven in a study he conducted for Yale University School of Medicine. Find a cream or lotion with 10 to 12 percent glycolic acid, such as Alpha Hydrox's AHA Enhanced Creme, at your local drugstore. Apply it twice every day, morning and night, as part of your daily routine, says Dr. Perricone. In the morning, make sure that you apply it right after shaving. It may sting a bit, but the sting will go away in a few minutes, he adds.

"Within a very short period of time, you'll start getting relief from the bumps," Dr. Perricone says. Most men, he says, experience a 60 to 70 percent reduction in bumps. "It's not perfect, but it works better than anything else, short of growing a beard," says Dr. Perricone. Also look for an anti-razor bump lotion, shaving cream, and toner in the cosmetic section of Nordstrom's department stores. The products, developed by Dr. Perricone, are under the brand name N. V. Perricone, M.D., Cosmeceuticals.

Go slow but sure. If you're suffering from ingrown whiskers, soak your skin in warm water or wrap your face in a wet towel to soften the beard hairs, advises Richard G. Glogau, M.D., clinical professor of dermatology at the University of California, San Francisco/Stamford Medical Center. The water or wet towel should be as hot as you usually tolerate in a shower. Soak your skin or leave the wet towel on for four to five minutes to adequately soften the beard hair. Then find a pair of fine tweezers and, one by one, gently tease the loose end of the ingrown hair back out of the bump. Don't use a pin or toothpick to do this or you may end up piercing the skin and causing yourself some of the problems you're trying to avoid. Take a small pair of scissors (which leave less of a sharp cutting edge on the hair shaft than does a razor blade) and trim the hair back close to the skin's surface. But don't trim it too close or else the problem starts all over again, says Dr. Glogau. Be sure not to trim the hair so close to the skin that the curl of the hair allows the hair shaft to dig back into the skin. And above all, you don't want to yank that ingrown hair out, adds Dr. Glogau. By pulling that whisker out by its little roots, it doesn't even have a chance to exit the hair follicle before it curves back into the follicle wall.

Try a special razor. The closer your whisker tip is to your skin, the greater the chances of it becoming ingrown. Following that premise, a host of different razors are on the market, designed specifically for the man with ingrown whiskers. Among them are the PFB Bumpfighter by the American Safety Razor Company, a foil-wrapped, single-edge blade. Electric razors designed for in-grown whiskers have also met with some success. No matter which type of razor you choose, the key is to keep from cutting your beard too close to the skin. You can still have a clean-shaven appearance without a baby-smooth shave, especially if you have dark skin, Dr. Newcomer says.

Watch for pus. If you see pus or increasing inflammation around your razor bumps, it means that you have a secondary infection, says Dr. Glogau. He recommends a topical antibiotic such as Polysporin or Neosporin to fight it off. Apply the topical antibiotic ointment two or three times daily until there are no whiteheads or pus. The inflammation won't go away until the hair shaft is able to grow out above the skin surface, adds Dr. Glogau.

▶ALTERNATIVE APPROACHES

Dissolve your problem. Chemical depilatories such as Neet, Nair, or Magic Shaving Powder can be useful, if used appropriately, says Dr. Newcomer. One note of caution: Make sure that you read the directions. Failure to follow the product's directions can leave you with some nasty chemical burns on your chin. "The line between dissolving the hair and irritating the skin is very fine," Dr. Newcomer warns. He recommends using chemicals no more than once or twice a week, depending on the thickness of your beard and your skin sensitivity.

▶PREVENTIVE MEASURES

Give your skin some slack. Many men, in order to get a closer shave, pull their skin tight to get at the lowest part of the whisker. Don't. "Pulling your skin pops the hair out of the follicle," says Dr. Newcomer. When the skin snaps back, the hair lodges in the wall of the follicle.

Go with the grain. Always shave with the grain of your beard, says Dr. Glogau. That is, the way your whiskers grow. If they grow down, shave down. On the neck, they can grow in several directions, so pay attention. And avoid double-bladed razors. The lift and cut action gives too close a shave.

Inhibited Sexual Desire

▶PROBLEM

Your rocket is capable of liftoff; it just needs a spark to ignite it. Simply put, you're in the mood a lot less often than you wish you were.

▶CAUSE

There can be several reasons why you don't much feel like having sex anymore. Among them are depression, illness, side effects of medications, a childhood trauma such as being a victim of sexual abuse, fatigue from work or family responsibilities, hormonal changes, or boredom with one's partner.

▶HOW SERIOUS

"It can be a major problem if the desire for sexual activity from one partner is significantly greater than the desire of the other partner," says Robert Hawkins Jr., Ph.D., professor emeritus of health sciences in the School of Health Technology and Management at the State University of New York at Stony Brook. "A lot of us males feel like we're expected to be ready to go anytime, anywhere. When we're not, we run a risk of some self-esteem damage." On the other hand, if a guy only feels like having sex once a month and so does his partner, he doesn't have a problem.

DO THIS NOW

Get out of your rut. Add some new elements to your lovemaking repertoire, such as fantasizing more, watching an adult video with your partner, or playing sexual games together, suggests Robert Hawkins Jr., Ph.D., professor emeritus of health sciences in the School of Health Technology and Management at the State University of New York at Stony Brook.

Did You Know?

When the authors of *Sex in America* took the sexual pulse of the nation, one of the findings that surprised them was how infrequently most of us are doing the horizontal bop.

Roughly 2 out of 10 men said they had sex only a few times in the previous year, and 14 percent reported none at all. Another 37 percent of men said they had sex a few times a month, while 26 percent reported getting intimate two or three times a week. A mere 8 percent said they had sex four or more times a week.

Apparently, it is feast or famine for guys between ages 18 and 24. They were the most likely to have had no sex at all, but they also were the age group most often having sex four or more times a week. And contrary to the stereotypes about swinging bachelors, married guys and those living with women were getting more action than the men who did not live with women.

▶SOLUTIONS

Make an appointment. It doesn't sound too romantic, but couples frazzled by the demands of careers and children should schedule private time together, says Dr. Hawkins. If they don't, they may discover two or three weeks have whisked by without their having been alone, he says. That time to themselves doesn't necessarily have to culminate in intercourse. "What you do in that interaction has to be determined by the needs of the couple," Dr. Hawkins says.

Make it a priority. A lot of men with a low sex drive are workaholics, says Martin Goldberg, M.D., clinical professor of psychiatry at the University of Pennsylvania School of Medicine in Philadelphia. They spend so many hours at the office that they have little or no energy left for sex. An active and fulfilling sex life should be in the top three or four priorities of a man, he says. If it's not, he needs to ask himself why that is.

Use it or lose it. Some research indicates that being sexually active increases a man's testosterone level. "In other words, there is some basis to 'the more you get, the more you want,'" says Dr. Hawkins.

Learn why you're inhibited. If you've always had inhibited sexual desire, think about what may have caused this or talk to somebody about it, advises Dr. Goldberg. "It helps to know," he says. "Knowing is part of the cure."

▶ALTERNATIVE APPROACHES

Get a whiff. Certain smells have been found to increase blood flow to the penis, says Alan R. Hirsch, M.D., a psychiatrist and neurological director of the

Smell and Taste Treatment and Research Foundation in Chicago. In one study, Dr. Hirsch found that a combination of pumpkin pie and lavender elicited a 40 percent increase in penile blood flow. Second place went to a cross between black licorice and doughnuts. The reason may be a combination of nostalgia and instinct. So try to recall the scent of a particularly fond experience you shared with your partner and re-create it with scented candles, incense, or potpourri.

Stay positive. Don't view sex as an obligation, a relationship requirement, or something that is work, advises Dr. Goldberg. "That's about the most self-defeating and negative thing that can happen," he says. "It does happen an awful lot." He suggests that we should view sex as part of loving someone, having fun, and as a chance to be physically expressive and creative.

▶PREVENTIVE MEASURES

Exercise. Generally, the more fit you are, the better you feel about yourself. The better you feel about yourself, the more sexually aroused you are apt to feel, says Dr. Hawkins.

Eat right. A guy who eats healthy foods and keeps in shape is going to benefit physically, emotionally, and sexually, says Dr. Goldberg.

Insect Bites and Stings

▶PROBLEM

Biting insects are usually just annoying, but in hordes, these gossamer beasts turn picnics and hikes into maddening sessions of slapping and self-flagellation.

▶CAUSE

Your main nemeses are chiggers, spiders, ticks, mosquitoes, bees, wasps, and critters with descriptive names like no-see-ums. They all want a piece of you. Mosquitoes and ticks drink your blood. Chiggers shove mouth parts down your hair follicles, pump in digestive fluids, and then slurp up your disintegrated cells. Bees only sting when irked but make certain that you get the message by leaving behind a venom sac that pushes poison in for several minutes.

▶HOW SERIOUS

Most bites redden, itch, swell, and go away after a few days. Tick bites can be serious if the tick is infected with Lyme disease or Rocky Mountain Spotted Fever, diseases that should be treated with antibiotics. The most dangerous insects are members of the hymenoptera family—

DO THIS NOW

If the insect left a stinger behind, scrape it out. The sooner the better, says Mark Rosoff, an emergency medical technician and director of the Front Range Institute of Safety in Fort Collins, Colorado. "Use the edge of a credit card, a knife, or your fingernail to scrape out or flick away the stinger," he explains. Then you can put an ice pack wrapped in a thin towel on for 15 to 20 minutes to soothe the pain and keep down the swelling, he adds.

History Lesson

If it weren't for mosquitoes, the United States may never have gotten the land deal of all time.

In 1802, French emperor Napoleon Bonaparte sent an army to Haiti to put down a native revolt. The Haitian uprising failed, but a yellow fever epidemic nearly destroyed the victorious army. No one knew then that mosquitoes carried the disease, believing instead that it arose from miasma (poisoned air), or "heat acting on moist animals and vegetables producing putrid exhalations." Each summer in French New Orleans, nearly half the population left the city to avoid getting the "Yellow Jack."

After his army's experience, Napoleon decided to unload some of his disease-ridden New World lands to the Americans, who were eager to buy. In 1803, President Thomas Jefferson bought Louisiana and its holdings north to Canada and west to the Rockies for just $15 million, doubling the size of country.

---

bees, wasps, and fire ants—because you could be allergic to their venom, says Howard Backer, M.D., a physician who practices emergency sports and wilderness medicine for Kaiser Permanente Medical Centers in the San Francisco Bay area and teaches wilderness medicine through the Wilderness Medical Society. About 50 people die of bee stings in the United States each year. Most deaths are preventable if the victim gets to a hospital or injects himself with a form of adrenaline called epinephrine, available by prescription, says Dr. Backer.

▶SOLUTIONS

Resist the itch. Most bites and stings heal themselves after a few days. If you scratch open a bite, it has a good chance of getting infected, especially in warm, moist climates, says Dr. Backer. Leave it be.

Go over the counter. To soothe the savage sting, apply some over-the-counter lotion, such as After Bite, says Dr. Backer. For the itching that comes later, apply an over-the-counter cortisone cream.

Kill the pain. To further relieve pain and itching, take an over-the-counter analgesic such as aspirin or acetaminophen, says Mark Rosoff, an emergency medical technician and director of the Front Range Institute of Safety in Fort Collins, Colorado. Take as directed on the label.

React to reactions. The typical reactions to bee and wasp stings are itching, a hot feeling, and a red welt. Some people develop large local reactions: Their entire forearm may swell up from a bite on the wrist. If you develop hives, a drippy nose, a swollen mouth or tongue, and difficulty breathing, you're having a serious allergic reaction called anaphylaxis, says Rosoff.

"The sooner the symptoms develop, the quicker the reaction can become life-threatening," says Rosoff. "If you're wheezing and having difficulty breathing a few minutes after being stung, you should get yourself to an emergency room immediately where you can get a shot of epinephrine. Remember to observe for symptoms of allergic reaction for up to 60 minutes after a sting. Sometimes someone will look fine for the first 15 minutes or so and then develop a life-threatening reaction. If you know you're allergic to bees, get a prescription for an epinephrine kit from your doctor and always have it handy," he suggests.

▶ALTERNATIVE APPROACHES

Slap on the soda. A paste of baking soda and water takes away the sting of most bites, especially bee stings. "The baking soda neutralizes the acidity of the bee sting," says Rosoff.

Neutralize the bite. Unlike bee stings, however, wasp bites are alkaline, so you'll need something acidic to neutralize them. Rosoff suggests applying some lemon juice or vinegar to soothe those stings.

Make a poultice. Poultices ease stings, help heal wounds, and reduce swelling, says Susun S. Weed, an herbalist and herbal educator from Woodstock, New York, and author of the *Wise Woman* series of herbal health books. The simplest poultice for treating insect bites is a dab of mud. Or if you want to be more hygenic about it, you can buy powdered clay at a health food store and mix it with a little water.

▶PREVENTIVE MEASURES

Shield your skin. If a bug can't light, a bug can't bite. Wear a long-sleeve shirt and long pants, suggests Dr. Backer. Insects like bright colors and floral patterns, so choose white, green, tan, and khaki hues.

Tell bugs to bug off. Always apply bug repellent when you're out, says Dr. Backer. On clothing, use a repellent containing permethrin (such as Permanone), the synthetic version of a natural insecticide found in chrysanthemums. Permethrin repels bugs even after several washings. On your skin, you can try a natural product that contains citronella, such as Natrapel, which provides short-term protection from bugs, says Dr. Backer. These products are available at most health food stores.

Spray on protection. "To repel ticks, mosquitoes, and black flies, I spray diluted tincture of fresh flowers of yarrow (*Achillea millefolium*) on my skin," says Weed. Use it either full-strength or diluted with the same amount of water. Respray yourself every hour or two as needed.

Insomnia

▶PROBLEM

There are three types of insomnia: you can't fall asleep, you wake up several times a night, or you get up too early in the morning.

▶CAUSE

What makes sleep elusive? Everything from job stress, grief, traffic noise, alcohol, medications, jet lag, shift work, a hard bed, or a soft bed to an off-kilter biological clock.

"Usually, there's a real identifiable cause. You're worried about something, or you're just not physically relaxed in your surroundings," says Sam Krachman, D.O., director of the Sleep Disorders Center at the Temple University Hospital in Philadelphia.

▶HOW SERIOUS

Most insomnia lasts only a few nights or a couple of weeks until the situation causing the sleep loss resolves itself, says Dr. Krachman. "Meanwhile, you're probably tired, irritable, and out of sorts. But you recover as soon as you start sleeping better," he explains. Any sleeplessness that lasts three weeks or more, however, isn't normal and could be a warning sign to see your doctor, says Dr. Krachman.

▶SOLUTIONS

Make a ritual of it. Many men have poor sleep hygiene, meaning that they don't have good habits for bedtime, says John Harsh, Ph.D., professor of psychology at the University of Southern Mississippi in Hattiesburg. "Create a ritual around sleep so as to prepare the body and mind that it's time to rest,"

DO THIS NOW

Naps aren't bad if they allow you to recharge your batteries when you're feeling tired during the day, but too much daytime napping often interferes with nighttime sleep, says Peter Hauri, Ph.D., administrative director of the insomnia program at the Mayo Clinic and co-director of the Mayo Clinic Sleep Disorders Clinic, both in Rochester, Minnesota. "Either eliminate napping altogether or keep your naps short, to a half-hour or less," he suggests.

Did You Know?

W. C. Fields was a man of many odd habits, including sleep. Having insomnia, he sometimes found sleep by sprawling out on pool tables or, because he enjoyed haircuts, seated in a barber's chair wrapped in warm towels. On his worst nights, he could only reach the Land of Nod by lying under a beach umbrella while a garden hose sprayed the canvas with water, imitating the soothing sound of falling rain.

---

suggests Dr. Harsh. Put out the cat, use the half-hour before bed for light reading or watching TV, or do some light stretching or relaxation exercises.

Lie down when you like. If you're not sleepy, don't force yourself to go to bed; you'll just lie awake thrashing. Instead, go to bed only when you feel tired, says Dr. Harsh.

Get up, get out. No matter how little or how much sleep you've had during the night, always get out of bed at the same time every day. This includes weekends, says Peter Hauri, Ph.D., administrative director of the insomnia program at the Mayo Clinic and co-director of the Mayo Clinic Sleep Disorders Clinic, both in Rochester, Minnesota. "When sleep doesn't come easily, you have to be more regular in your habits," he says. "You can't expect your body to do one thing on the weekdays and another on the weekends."

Have a bite. Hunger pangs, even slight ones, sometimes interfere with sleep. A glass of milk, crackers, or an apple before bed takes the edge off and allows sleep to come, says Dr. Hauri. "Have just a small snack. You don't want to eat a meal before bed," he cautions.

▶ALTERNATIVE APPROACHES

Get heavy. Falling asleep is all about letting go, says Dr. Harsh. Try this simple self-hypnosis technique. While breathing slowly through your nose, concentrate on relaxing the muscles in your feet. Imagine your feet, your bones becoming heavier, sinking into bed, and losing feeling. After a few minutes, move to your calves, your knees, and eventually further up the body. You'll probably be asleep by the time you reach your head.

"All some people need to do is let go of their thoughts and concentrate on relaxing the body," says Dr. Harsh.

Take an herbal sedative. Drink some valerian tea before turning in for the night, recommends John Crellin, M.D., Ph.D., John Clinch professor of the history of medicine at Memorial University of Newfoundland Faculty of Medicine in St. John's. "There's plenty of clinical and historical evidence that it has a sedative effect," he adds. And for some, valerian is balm for anxiety as well, says Dr.

Crellin. Steep one tablespoon of the dried herb in a pint of water, and brew it for three to four minutes. Drink it before bed as needed.

Get lit. Maybe you're a night owl who can't sleep before 2:00 A.M. or a lark who is in bed by early evening and up at 4:00 A.M. Either way, you're out of phase with the rest of humanity. Your problem could be a biological clock that runs too slow or too fast, says Dr. Hauri.

"Light tells your brain when you should be awake or asleep. By exposing yourself to bright light, you may be able to reset your clock where it needs to be," says Dr. Hauri. Getting outdoors more may be all that you need, he says.

Bright light in the morning "phase advances" night owls so that they can get moving in the morning and be ready for sleep earlier in the evening. Larks can delay sleep by exposing themselves to bright light in late afternoon or early evening, says Dr. Hauri. You should be outside 45 to 60 minutes every day, he recommends. Since you know that you'll be outside for a good length of time, be sure to break out the sunscreen—and make sure that it has an SPF (sun protection factor) of at least 15.

▶PREVENTIVE MEASURES

Work out before supper. Vigorous exercise—fast walking or bike riding for 20 to 30 minutes—revs up the metabolism and body temperature for four to five hours. If you exercise about five to six hours before bedtime, your metabolism will slowly decline at the same time your body is naturally winding down for sleep, says Dr. Hauri. But if you exercise too late in the evening, you may be too charged up to get to sleep.

"Exercise is great for sleep if you do it at the right time. It can reinforce your body's natural rhythms, and the exertion makes you physically tired as well," says Dr. Hauri.

Internet Addiction

▶PROBLEM

You're officially addicted if you log on to the Internet more than 38 hours a week for nonacademic or nonemployment reasons. Other addictive signs include a psychological rush or a feeling of well-being when using the Net, craving more time with your computer, neglecting family and friends because of the Internet, feeling depressed or irritable when not using your computer, and lying to family and employers about your usage.

▶CAUSE

The Internet allows a bored, lonely, depressed, shy, or underconfident guy to forget his problems. "People who have low self-esteem or low self-worth or who are very shy and withdrawn can become anyone they want once they are introduced to the Internet. Their esteem and self-worth are magnified and multiplied a hundred times, and that rush of self worth—even though it is very cosmetic—is so exhilarating and intoxicating that the adrenaline and the endorphins present for chemical addictions can be present with the interaction with the computer," says Randee McGraw, certified addictions specialist and manager of the Illinois Institute for Addiction Recovery at Proctor Hospital in Peoria.

Also, like gambling, "the odds are set against winning," says Maressa Hecht Orzack, Ph.D., founder and coordinator of McLean Hospital's computer-

DO THIS NOW

The next time you look up at the clock and realize that 10 hours slipped past while you were chatting with those charming cybervixens at the exhibitionism chat room, ask yourself, "Why am I here? What void is this filling?" Are you bored with your marriage? Do you hate your job?

Now, what else could you do, other than use the computer, that could fill that same need? Once you find some alternatives, your computer will become less enticing, says Maressa Hecht Orzack, Ph.D., founder and coordinator of McLean Hospital's computer-addiction services in Belmont, Massachusetts.

addiction services in Belmont, Massachusetts. Whether surfing for a good Internet site, looking for a cyberdate, or trying to beat other online players of Quake or Astra or other interactive games, you'll find intermittent rewards. One Web site may pay off, but the next 20 will be duds. "There have to be losses in order for there to be successes. That's what keeps people hanging on," Dr. Orzack says.

> **MEN'S HEALTH INDEX**
>
> Percentage of people who on an on-line survey agreed that "if it weren't for my computer, I wouldn't have any fun at all": 13
>
> Percentage of people who on the same survey said that they had gotten less than four hours sleep because they were too busy surfing the Net: 40

▶How Serious

Internet addiction could cause you or your kid to flunk out of college, can get you fired or divorced, and can even harm your health. (Many addicts forget to eat because they are so consumed by their computers.) If your time with your computer is threatening your work or home life, make an appointment with an addictions specialist experienced in computer and Internet addiction, McGraw advises.

▶Solutions

Set an alarm. Unlike some other addictions, quitting your computer cold turkey probably isn't an option. Most likely, you need to use the computer to get your job done. Take an alarm clock to your office and set the buzzer to go off a half-hour to an hour once you log on for "work" purposes, suggests Dr. Orzack. The time limit should keep you focused enough that you'll complete that presentation in Microsoft PowerPoint before straying to the Kathy Ireland home page.

Don't play that game. To nonaddicts, the following rule is common sense. Perhaps you should write it down and tack it to your cubicle wall: Never download a game off the Internet onto your computer at work, Dr. Orzack says. Never. Got that? Never. And, nowadays, most computers are being monitored at work by employers seeking to crack down on Internet misuse. Be aware that computer games do not have to be on the Net to be addicting, Dr. Orzack says. Watch out for Solitaire, Minesweeper, and their kind. If you must play, set a timer for a reasonable amount of time, say 20 minutes, and quit when it goes off. Do not always insist on winning, she advises.

Go slow. If you don't own a modem, or have one that's so slow it takes hours for your computer to download a page, you won't feel tempted to dial into the Internet from home, Dr. Orzack says. Without a modem, you'll only use your home computer for good: word processing and checkbook balancing.

▶ALTERNATIVE APPROACHES

Join Gamblers Anonymous. Few support groups exist specifically for Internet addicts. Since Internet addiction and gambling are so closely linked, however, you could gain some needed camaraderie and motivation from attending Gamblers Anonymous meetings, says Dr. Orzack. You'll also meet a few friends IRL (that's "in real life" for you nonaddicts who are reading this entry just to pass time). Or start your own support group—definitely not online, though.

▶PREVENTIVE MEASURES

Get a life. Start exercising. Call a friend. Join a group. Talk to your kids. Take part in anything except using your computer, Dr. Orzack says.

Irritable Bowel Syndrome

▶PROBLEM

This colon disorder causes changes in bowel habits that leave you feeling gassy and bloated. You may have cramps and an urge to move your bowels, but you cannot do so. Some people have constipation, while others experience diarrhea. Some guys have both.

▶CAUSE

There are no definitive answers as to why some people have irritable bowel syndrome. They may have a more sensitive colon that reacts more strongly to stimuli. Certain foods, medicines, and stress may trigger these spasms.

▶HOW SERIOUS

Irritable bowel syndrome is a nuisance to some people, debilitating to others. It is not curable. It does not, however, cause permanent damage to the intestines, nor does it lead to more serious diseases such as cancer. It is important, however, to make sure that what you are experiencing *is* irritable bowel syndrome. If you first experience these symptoms and they don't clear up after a day or so, it is a good idea to have a doctor evaluate your condition, says Gerard Guillory, M.D., assistant

History Lesson

In the name of medical research, 25 employees of a Veterans Affairs Medical Center in Minnesota kept a detailed record of the number and fullness of their farts. Researchers wanted to know what connection, if any, there is between feelings of abdominal bloating and excessive gas.

The 13 women and 12 men recorded each fart, their impression of its volume (0 for none and 5 for severe), and their sensations of bloating. Those who were given a supplement of a nonabsorbable sugar tooted an average of 19 times per day. Participants who swallowed a supplement of the fiber supplement Metamucil passed gas only 12 times a day, while those who had another fiber supplement, Citrucel, let loose an average of 11 times a day. Without any supplements, the group passed gas an average of 10 times per day. In case you're counting, more than 20 farts per day indicates excessive gas, researchers said.

The researchers concluded that people who complain of abdominal bloating probably are not producing excessive gas but may be experiencing symptoms of irritable bowel syndrome.

---

clinical professor of medicine at the University of Colorado Health Science Center in Aurora, Colorado, and author of *IBS: A Doctor's Plan for Chronic Digestive Troubles*. If you have already been diagnosed with irritable bowel syndrome, the following home remedies should help ease your discomfort. But check with your physician if any of your symptoms seem to suddenly change, Dr. Guillory adds.

▶SOLUTIONS

Eat small, eat often. "Eat small amounts of food frequently," Dr. Guillory advises. "You can overwhelm your digestive tract at any one time." When that happens, you may get that bloated feeling of which people with irritable bowel syndrome often complain.

Diminish the dairy. "Dairy products are probably the most common trigger for irritable bowel symptoms," Dr. Guillory says. Eat them in moderation, if at all.

Can the beans. Go easy on—or eliminate from your diet—beans, nuts, and other foods that produce flatulence if gas is a real problem as a part of your irritable bowel syndrome, advises James Cerda, M.D., professor of medicine and chief of nutrition support at the University of Florida in Gainesville. "They just add to the nagging problem," he says.

Reduce your fat. Fatty, fried foods also seem to spark symptoms in people with irritable bowel syndrome, says Dr. Guillory. So does chocolate. Go easy with these foods.

Eat more fiber. Most people with irritable bowel syndrome should eat more fiber, such as that found in fruits, vegetables, and grains, Dr. Guillory says. Aim for 20 to 40 grams of fiber a day if you have irritable bowel syndrome, says Dr. Guillory.

Monitor your meals. What sparks a flare-up of symptoms varies from one person to the next, so the best way to determine what foods are causing you problems is to keep track of what you eat, says Dr. Guillory. If you have sporadic symptoms, keep a food diary, he suggests. Every time you feel crummy, write down what you ate recently. See if a pattern emerges. If your symptoms are more persistent, try an elimination diet. Stick to foods you are confident cause symptoms rarely, if ever. Then reintroduce, one by one, food groups you have been avoiding until your symptoms strike again. Chances are that you've found what caused them.

Move your body, move your bowels. "Exercise seems to help people with chronic constipation, which is part of the syndrome," Dr. Cerda says.

It also helps relieve stress, one of the triggers of irritable bowel syndrome, adds Dr. Guillory. He recommends walking as the perfect exercise and suggests 30 minutes every day.

▶ALTERNATIVE APPROACHES

Sip some tea. A cup of peppermint tea can make you feel better once your symptoms have struck, Dr. Guillory says. "Peppermint is a natural antispasmodic," he says. A cup of chamomile tea also can soothe a roiling digestive tract, he says.

▶PREVENTIVE MEASURES

Swear off sweeteners. Sugars and artificial sweeteners are hard to digest, and some people with irritable bowel syndrome have adverse reactions to them, Dr. Guillory says. Limit your use of both. If you use a commercial fiber product that contains ground psyllium seeds with sugar or aspartame added, it may cause your irritable bowel syndrome to act up. Look instead for one that has pure psyllium seeds and no added sugar or artificial sweeteners, Dr. Guillory suggests.

Learn to relax. Irritable bowel syndrome seems to be triggered, at least in part, by stress, says Dr. Cerda. Learning a stress-management technique such as meditation or yoga can help.

Jet Lag

▶PROBLEM

As a plane whisks you across time zones, you pick up some unwanted travel companions: fatigue, insomnia, nausea, muscle aches, and a general feeling of malaise.

▶CAUSE

Your body operates on a 24-hour cycle called circadian rhythms. These rhythms tell you when to wake up, when to sleep, and even influence bodily functions such as when to eat and go to the bathroom.

The circadian rhythms base themselves on your usual day-and-night routine. And when you fly across time zones, it's much harder to reset your internal body clock than your traveling alarm clock. Your body tells you it's time to sleep when it's time to be awake, and vice versa.

"We change our internal time zone so quickly that the body doesn't have the time to adapt," says Karl Doghramji, M.D., director of the sleep disorders center at Jefferson Medical College of Thomas Jefferson University in Philadelphia.

DO THIS NOW

Drink like a fish. Sorry, guy, but we're talking about water here. That recycled airplane air sucks the water right out of you, especially during a long flight. And dehydration can make the effects of jet lag even more pronounced.

So drink an eight-ounce glass of water each hour during your flight, says Karl Doghramji, M.D., director of the sleep disorders center at Jefferson Medical College of Thomas Jefferson University in Philadelphia.

▶HOW SERIOUS

Jet lag is rarely serious, although it may have been the cause of a bad business decision or two. It can knock you out of your peak performance level for a day or two. Other side effects include altered appetite, fatigue, nausea, constipation, diarrhea, or just having to go to the bathroom at inconvenient times, Dr. Doghramji says.

▶SOLUTIONS

Act like a local. The best way to get acclimated to your new time zone is to get right into the swing of things. As soon as you get off the plane, switch your watch to the time of your destination. "On the plane, you should be thinking, 'What would I be doing at this time of day?'" says Jeffrey G. Jones, M.D., medical director of the St. Francis Traveler's Health Center in Indianapolis. Once you arrive, get out into the town and do whatever the locals do—eat, walk, sightsee, or play.

Take a day off. If you can manage it, don't do any business or make major decisions within 24 hours of your arrival when you've crossed more than three time zones. "You may be making an important move when your brain is saying it's 3:00 A.M. That's not a time of high intellectual performance," says Dr. Doghramji.

Snooze a little. Many flights leave in the evening your time, but when you arrive, it's morning or early afternoon. And you probably did not get much sleep—or at least good sleep—on the plane. But no matter how tired you are when you arrive, fight the urge to go to sleep after stepping off the plane. By falling asleep immediately, your body will continue to function on its old time. It will take you longer to get up to speed with your new schedule. But if by afternoon you need a little shut-eye, go ahead. "A small nap, about 20 minutes, will help repay your sleep debt," Dr. Doghramji says. But keep it short, or you'll confuse your body even more, he warns. Some people sleep too long and wake up feeling more groggy, he says. If it is nighttime when you arrive, then by all means, hit the sack.

Lay off the hotel buffet. After hours of eating or avoiding airplane food, you may be ready to dive into the hotel kitchen and eat everything in sight. But unless it's dinnertime, hold off on the big meal. Eating a huge meal can make you tired. But it can also send a signal to your body that it's almost time to go to bed. You usually eat a big meal at dinner only a few hours before bedtime. Your body gets that meal and thinks it should start winding down, preparing for a night's rest. If you eat that big meal soon after you arrive but it is still early in the day, your body may start to go into sleep mode—even in the afternoon, Dr. Jones says. Stick to light meals and snacks when you arrive.

▶ALTERNATIVE APPROACHES

Mellow out with melatonin. Take a three-milligram melatonin tablet for every two time zones you go through, says Terence Collins, M.D., director of Healthy Journeys, the University of Kentucky A. B. Chandler Medical Center's International Travel Clinic in Lexington. Melatonin is a hormone your body produces that regulates your internal clock. Melatonin supplements have been shown to fight jet lag symptoms, especially those related to being thrown off your normal sleep cycle, such as fatigue.

Start taking the supplement on the plane if it is a night flight. If you are only

Did You Know?

Most college football teams struggle with how to perform efficiently in the red zone. But the University of Hawaii at Manoa squad has a bigger problem: performing in the red-eye zone. The Rainbow Warriors are members of the Western Athletic Conference, which means that they play teams in California, Wyoming, Nevada, Colorado, New Mexico, Utah, and Texas.

"We're closer to Tokyo than Texas," says Andrew Nichols, M.D., associate professor in the departments of family practice and orthopedic surgery and head athletic teams physician at the University of Hawaii at Manoa in Honolulu. The team plays at least four or five away games a year—as in far, far away. Most flights are at least five hours long, during which the team jumps anywhere from two to five time zones ahead. The only break they get from the schedule-makers is that they rarely have to play back-to-back away games.

---

crossing two time zones, take one pill on the flight. If you cross four time zones, take one pill on the night flight, then take the second pill the next night, about two hours before bedtime. If you cross six zones, take one pill on the flight , and one pill each night for two nights after that.

If you're crossing an odd number of time zones (five, for example), take the dosage for the previous even number (in this case, four—which would be two pills over two nights). For a day flight, start taking the supplement (one pill) the night before, Dr. Collins says. Short-term use of melatonin seems benign so far, although some people report odd dreams. Regular, long-term use, however, is not recommended.

Get out. If the sun is shining when you arrive at your destination, get out and enjoy it, says Dr. Collins. Sunlight tells your body that it's daytime and that you should be doing all the things you normally do in the daytime. If you lock yourself in your dark hotel room right after your flight, your body will never get the message to change direction.

Take a walk. Strolling outside provides a double whammy against jet lag, says Andrew Nichols, M.D., associate professor in the departments of family practice and orthopedic surgery and head athletic teams physician at the University of Hawaii at Manoa in Honolulu.

First off, it gets you into the sunlight, which helps readjust your internal clock. Second, it's a quick and easy form of exercise. Exercise seems to lessen jet lag symptoms and helps you get a more restful night's sleep. Take a walk right after you check in. Then start each day at your new destination with a morning stroll to get you going, Dr. Nichols says.

▶PREVENTIVE MEASURES

Be prepared. A lot of the problems blamed on jet lag have nothing to do with jet lag at all. People wait until the last minute to pack. Travelers often feel stressed or at least anxious about a big trip. Last-minute details take up your time the night before you leave. By the time most people get on the plane, they are already exhausted, Dr. Doghramji says. Plan out the last few days before your trip, he suggests.

Pack a day or two ahead of time, and make a checklist to ensure that you brought everything you need. Make another list going over what you have to get done. "Plan for your trip so that it's not so hellish before you even get to the airport," Dr. Jones says.

Stay on your time. If it's a very short trip or you're only traveling across one or two time zones, stay on your natural time, if possible. This means eating, sleeping, working, and exercising during the same time you would in your own time zone. When the University of Hawaii has a late-afternoon or evening football game on the mainland, they keep the student athletes on Hawaii time, Dr. Nichols says. Staying on your natural time limits the chaos your body goes through. And it eliminates having to readjust when you come back home.

Work the night shift. About three days before a long trip, start changing your schedule to fit your destination time. If traveling east, go to bed and get up an hour earlier the first night. The next day, eat meals an hour earlier than usual. Then jump back another hour the next night, and then again the next. By doing that, your body gets a head start in catching up to your new time, Dr. Doghramji says. Go to bed an hour later a night (again for three nights before the trip) if you're going westward.

Jock Itch

▶PROBLEM

The skin in the vicinity of your private parts is moist, itching, chafing, and red. That means that you have one of the following conditions: irritated skin, a fungus (tinea cruris), a yeast infection, or a bacterial infection. "The symptoms are all very similar, and you can treat them all," says Debra Wattenberg, M.D., a dermatologist in private practice in New York City.

▶CAUSE

When you exercise, the area around the family jewels grows hot, sticky, and sweaty—a perfect breeding ground for a not-so-friendly fungus. Then your thighs rub up against each other, and that makes the already-irritated skin even more aggravated. It's also possible that you used a towel on your feet and then dried the rest of your body with it, causing your tinea pedis (athlete's foot) to become tinea cruris (jock itch).

Fungal infections and yeast infections also can be transmitted from person to person, so if your partner has a rash, chronic itchiness, or dry, flaky skin she should see her doctor and use an over-the-counter product such as Lotrimin AF cream, says Dr. Wattenberg.

▶HOW SERIOUS

Jock itch is no big deal health-wise, but it's uncomfortable and awkward, to say the least. Fortunately, it's fairly easy to treat. The key is to recognize when the symptoms you have need to be examined by a professional. "If you have blisters or a rash with sharp borders, see a doctor," says Dr. Wattenberg, "because it may not be jock itch."

You also should see a doctor if the itch doesn't clear up in a couple of

DO THIS NOW

"I find the single best treatment for jock itch is Zeasorb, which is a superabsorbent powder, or Zeasorb AF, which adds an antifungal to the product," says Gary White, M.D., chief of the department of dermatology at Kaiser Permanente Hospital in San Diego. Both products are available in drugstores. Just dust it on after your shower and at nighttime.

Did You Know?

So, which came first: the jock or the jockstrap? Actually, it was the word *jock*, which was first used in 1790 as a slang term for the genitals (male, of course). Logically, this was followed by the invention of the jockstrap, a word whose meaning is explained by its name. The first recorded reference to jockstrap was 1963.

weeks, Dr. Wattenberg says. Again, that may be a sign that you have something other than jock itch.

▶SOLUTIONS

Cream it. Put an over-the-counter antifungal such as Lotrimin AF cream on the rash, Dr. Wattenberg says. "Follow the directions, and don't use it more than twice a day for a week or two," she advises. "If your condition doesn't improve, go see a doctor."

Stay loose. Wear boxers and leave tight jeans in the closet. "You want to stay cool and dry," says Gary White, M.D., chief of the department of dermatology at Kaiser Permanente Hospital in San Diego. If you find yourself in hot clothes during the day, at least try to stay, uh, loose in the evening, he recommends.

Hit the showers. Washing with an antibacterial soap, such as Lever 2000, helps kill the germs that are flourishing in the first place. "There's no need to overdo it," says Dr. Wattenberg. "Just once or twice a day in the shower, especially after you exercise." Make sure to rinse and dry well with a clean, dry towel.

Beware, buyer. Don't use any cream containing hydrocortisone without a doctor's approval. If you have a fungal infection, it will get worse by using hydrocortisone improperly, says Dr. Wattenberg.

▶ALTERNATIVE APPROACHES

Try other powders. Look for over-the-counter powders that contain bentonite clay, but not cornstarch, says Eugene Zampieron, a doctor of naturopathy in Middlebury, Connecticut, and a professional member of the American Herbalists Guild. And don't, we repeat *don't*, use anything made for the feet and not for the groin. It may be the same infection, but, in case you haven't noticed, one of those areas is slightly more sensitive than the other.

Touch yourself with thyme. The herb thyme is a natural antifungal, and if your jock itch keeps coming back, you might want to enlist thyme on your side. "Brew up a tea with fresh or dried organic thyme, which you can get at a health food store," Dr. Zampieron says. "Use two to three teaspoons of the herb in a cup of hot water. Steep it, covered, for 20 minutes. After it has cooled, dab it on your skin with a cotton ball. Dry the area with bentonite powder." Do this once or twice a day for two weeks.

▶PREVENTIVE MEASURES

Stay out of the dirty laundry pile. If it's going to be next to your boys, make sure it's clean. That goes for towels, underwear, and jockstraps, says Dr. White.

Put your socks on first. Athlete's foot is extremely contagious, which is why it can travel—easily and without a map—from your toes to your crotch. Take care of your feet (wash and dry them well), then put your socks on before your underwear. That way you won't get the fungus into your boxers, says Dr. White.

Kicking Bad Habits

▶PROBLEM

Maybe you play with pens, pull on your beard, chomp on toothpicks, tap your feet—the list can go on and on. While relatively minor, these habits are usually nerve-racking, distracting, and sometimes even downright disgusting. And they say things about you that you certainly wouldn't want anyone else to say—that you're nervous, scared, or ill-mannered.

▶CAUSE

We develop these subtle habits over the years when we need to soothe ourselves. We turn to them in times of stress, anxiety, and sometimes even boredom. "Those kinds of habits distract you from the thing at hand," says Philip Levendusky, Ph.D., clinical psychologist at McLean Hospital in Belmont, Massachusetts.

▶HOW SERIOUS

If your foot tapping and ring clinking don't bother you, they probably annoy the heck out of those around you, which can be really problematic if that person is your wife or your boss. "It's hard to have a lot of confidence in a man whose nails are bitten all the way down," says Dr. Levendusky. In some situations, bad habits can leave physical scars, like when your hair-pulling tendency turns into pulling out chunks of your beard.

If your habit is severely impairing your daily functioning, consult your doctor, advises John C. Norcross, Ph.D., professor of psychology at the University of Scranton in Pennsylvania and co-author of *Changing for Good*.

DO THIS NOW

Take out the calendar and set a target date. Kicking bad habits isn't much different than giving up smoking, says John C. Norcross, Ph.D., professor of psychology at the University of Scranton in Pennsylvania and co-author of *Changing for Good*. "Most men say, 'I'm going to stop tomorrow.' But we want to work smart, not quick," he says. Set a date between a week and a month from now. Use the remaining time to prepare for what you'll do in situations where you'd normally seek comfort from the habit you're trying to kick, Dr. Norcross says.

Did You Know?

What's the most common nasty habit? It may be as plain as the nose on your face, say researchers at the Dean Foundation for Health, Research, and Education in Madison, Wisconsin. Of the 254 residents of Dane County, Wisconsin, who responded to a questionnaire, 91 percent confessed to being current nose-pickers. Yet only 75 percent felt that "almost everyone does it." Of course, there are nose-pickers and then there are *nose-pickers*. Two residents admitted to spending between 15 and 30 minutes a day picking their respective schnozzes. And one person fessed up to more than two hours of daily nose picking.

Isn't it great having this kind of information at your fingertips?

And, Dr. Levendusky adds, "if your habit actually entails harming yourself, if you receive chronic complaints from others regarding your habit, or if your habit is jeopardizing your personal or professional life, seek professional help."

▶SOLUTIONS

Start collecting data. The first step in stopping your behavior is to become aware of it, Dr. Norcross says. Write down how often you do it, when you do it, where you do it, and why you do it. That's the information you'll need to stop. If you feel comfortable, ask someone to tell you when you engage in the habit. Ask your wife (if she doesn't already nag you about it) or a trusted friend or co-worker.

Be honest about the consequences. So you have a few chewed-down nails. So what if your pens don't have tops? And who cares if you have a few bald spots on your chin because you pull on your beard? But stop and really think about what these habits say about you, Dr. Norcross says. "Does it make you look weak? Does it make you feel more anxious? Do you look nervous and unconfident to others?" Unless you don't mind conveying these images about yourself, you probably want to eliminate these messages. Write down all the negative consequences of your habit, and keep the list in your wallet or post it on your computer. It'll give you more incentive to stop, Dr. Norcross says.

Fill the gap. You can't just say to yourself this morning, "I am not going to constantly tap my fingers on the desk anymore." You'll be tapping away furiously by noon, Dr. Norcross promises. "You have to prepare. Men are just so eager to change that they don't prepare for the change," he says. Think of activities that you can do in place of your habit. For instance, every time you get the urge to bite your fingernails, clasp your hands underneath your desk or do some strenuous exercises. Or when you feel the need to pull out your hair during times of stress, take a few deep breaths to calm down. Have it all thought out and practiced before you implement your change, Dr. Norcross says.

Buy a lot of sticky notes. Invest in sticky notes because you're going to be using them by the hundreds if you really want to kick your habit, Dr. Norcross says. "People who post reminders to themselves do better than those who don't," Dr. Norcross adds. Post yourself notes everywhere—in your office, on the refrigerator, in the car—reminding you of your habit. You can also post how many times a day you fall prey to your habit, charting your progress. The little yellow notes also will serve as an incentive as you see your numbers go down, Dr. Norcross says.

Get a cheerleader. Now *there's* the advice you've been waiting for since high school. But it's not what you think. You'll need an energetic and sympathetic supporter to get you through your bad habit withdrawal. "You'll need a cheerleader, a positive person who will be on your side and support you," Dr. Norcross says. This person must be willing to be completely honest, to tell you when you're doing well and when you're not doing so well. Your cheerleader should be someone you can call if you need to talk because of a stressful or upsetting situation instead of reverting back to your habit for comfort.

▶ALTERNATIVE APPROACHES

Get isometric. You can do these tension-releasing exercises without leaving your office or getting out of your chair, Dr. Norcross says. In an isometric exercise, you apply pressure on a muscle by pressing against a stable resistance such as a wall, the floor, or even your own hand. Only the muscles contract; the joints don't move. When you feel the need to engage in your habit, simply press your hand against a wall or press your hands together while keeping your arms straight. You can also press your feet into the floor.

Escape with your mind. When things seem out of control and you want to pull your hair out, try quick relaxation techniques such as imagery or deep breathing, Dr. Norcross says. Take a deep breath and picture yourself on a tropical island without a care in the world. Imagine the view, the sounds, and the smells. Or take deep, relaxing breaths for a few minutes. Both exercises will calm you down and make you less likely to revert to your habit, he says.

▶PREVENTIVE MEASURES

Give it time. It takes at least three months to a year to really break a habit, Dr. Norcross says. And you can expect to have a few setbacks during the trip, he says. According to a study by Dr. Norcross, 62 percent of people who make New Year's resolutions break their resolution at least once, even though they end up keeping the resolution in the long run. Most people slip at least six times before they actually kick the habit, Dr. Norcross adds. So don't get discouraged if you stray off course. Maybe it's just a sign that your plan needs tinkering, Dr. Norcross says. Try different diversion tactics or give yourself more rewards to keep going.

Kidney Stones

▶PROBLEM

Suddenly, you have pain so excruciating in your lower back or abdomen that you'd even give away your prized 1961 Eli Grba Topps baseball card to make it go away. You may also have nausea and vomiting. There may be blood in your urine, a feeling that you need to urinate more often, or a burning sensation when you do go. It's an agony that some say is only equaled by childbirth. Since men get kidney stones much more often than women, maybe it's nature's way of evening the score in the pain arena. "By age 70, approximately 10 percent of men will have had a kidney stone, particularly those who live in arid climates, since they tend to get dehydrated more often," says E. Douglas Whitehead, M.D., associate clinical professor of urology at the Albert Einstein College of Medicine of Yeshiva University and director of the Association for Male Sexual Dysfunction, both in New York City.

In a particularly cruel twist, men who get one stone stand a good chance of forming another within five years. Men between the ages of 20 and 40 are most susceptible to forming their first stone, as are those with a family history and who are White.

▶CAUSE

A kidney stone is formed from crystals that separate from urine and build up in the inner

DO THIS NOW

Drink at least eight, eight-ounce glasses of water spread out over the course of the day, every day, not just when you're having a kidney stone attack. "That's about twice as much as most people drink," says Linda Massey, R.D., Ph.D., professor in the department of food science and human nutrition at Washington State University in Spokane. All that water dilutes the chemicals in your urine so that calcium and oxalate—the two main components of most kidney stones—can't get together, Dr. Massey says. "It works," she says. "People say, 'It's inconvenient because I have to go to the bathroom so often.' Well, which is worse: the pain or going to the bathroom?"

surfaces of the kidney. If the crystals remain small enough, they will travel through the urinary tract, and you will pee them out without being aware that they existed. But for the unlucky among us, the sharp-edged crystals may aggregate and grow and scrape like a dagger against the lining of a kidney or the ureter, the tube connecting the bladder with a kidney, causing mind-boggling pain. Stones can also cause an obstruction in the kidney or the ureter, which may be painful.

Seventy to 80 percent of stones are composed primarily of calcium oxalate. Oxalate is an acid that all people make and also is found in plants, says Linda Massey, R.D., Ph.D., professor in the department of food science and human nutrition at Washington State University in Spokane.

▶HOW SERIOUS

A kidney stone may produce such severe pain that it causes significant loss of work, Dr. Whitehead says. In addition, kidney stones also can cause infections and bleeding; if untreated, irreparable damage may be caused to the kidneys, Dr. Whitehead says. If you have had two or more stones or if you are feeling the awful pain associated with kidney stones, you ought to see a urologist for tests that can determine why you are forming stones and what sorts of changes in diet or lifestyle you can make or medications you may take that may prevent future episodes, says Dr. Whitehead.

▶SOLUTIONS

Consume calcium. It wasn't too long ago that doctors were telling people with kidney stones to restrict their calcium intake. Since then, they've learned that calcium binds to oxalate, preventing it from forming stones, says Dr.

MEN'S HEALTH INDEX

Certain foods may promote kidney stone formation in people who are susceptible, but researchers don't think that eating any particular food causes stones to develop in people who are not susceptible. If you're among those who are prone to calcium oxalate stones, Linda Massey, R.D., Ph.D., professor in the department of food science and human nutrition at Washington State University in Spokane, says to avoid or limit the following eight foods that are rich in oxalates.

1. **Black tea**
2. **Spinach**
3. **Rhubarb**
4. **Beets—the roots and the leaves**
5. **Chocolate, especially concentrated chocolate, such as that in a candy bar (flavoring isn't too bad)**
6. **Wheat bran, particularly the concentrated form used to enrich food, such as in bran muffins**
7. **Nuts, especially peanuts**
8. **Berries, including strawberries, raspberries, and gooseberries**

Massey. She recommends including a high-calcium food, such as a glass of milk, with every meal. Or add a slice of cheese to your sandwich or other sources of calcium with each meal, every day.

Cheer for citrus. Beverages rich in citric acid, such as orange juice and lemonade, act as inhibitors of calcium stone formation, says Dr. Massey. A 6-ounce glass of orange juice with each meal, or a 10-ounce serving of lemonade a couple of times a day, every day, should be effective, she says. An extra benefit is that some orange juices are fortified with calcium.

Cut down on caffeine. Keep caffeine use, especially coffee, at moderate levels, advises Dr. Massey. Caffeine increases urinary calcium, which ups the risk of having a calcium-containing kidney stone. She suggests no more than two cups of coffee a day.

Pass the salt. Salt consumption should be watched for the same reason as caffeine, says Dr. Massey. It's harder to do so, she says, because salt, which consumers may be unaware of unless they read food labels, is included in many processed foods. Dr. Massey recommends keeping your salt intake under 2,400 milligrams per day.

▶ALTERNATIVE APPROACHES

Switch to herbal teas. If you drink tea regularly, try sipping herbal teas instead, suggests Dr. Massey. Regular tea is high in oxalates, but herbal teas have only small amounts, she says.

▶PREVENTIVE MEASURES

Stay fluid. Men who are what doctors call stone-formers need to be especially diligent about drinking plenty of fluids when they exercise, be it tennis, weight lifting, or anything else, says Dr. Whitehead. He recommends drinking fluids before, during, and after exercise, and drinking past the point at which your thirst is quenched.

Knee Pain

▶PROBLEM

After a day on the trail, an afternoon of kneeling in the garden, or a game of pickup basketball, your knees are sore and stiff, and you're wondering, "Do I have a knee problem?" If you do, you have lots of company. Almost 5 million people visit orthopedic surgeons each year with knee problems, and another 1.4 million go to hospital emergency rooms.

▶CAUSE

Most soreness and stiffness in the knee are probably just symptoms of tight muscles, strained ligaments, or inflamed tendons, says Charles Bush-Joseph, M.D., associate professor of orthopedic surgery at Rush–Presbyterian–St. Luke's Medical Center in Chicago. "You just overdid it. You ran five miles instead of your usual two or jumped onto the bike after a long layoff," he says. "It's a classic overuse injury."

But if the pain doesn't subside in a few days or you wince climbing stairs and squatting down, you may have patellofemoral syndrome. Your patella (kneecap) isn't tracking correctly on your femur (thighbone), explains David Alvarez, D.O., clinical instructor in the department of family medicine at the University of Michigan Medical Center in Ann Arbor.

"The kneecap migrates laterally instead of staying midline. The kneecap is out of alignment," Dr. Alvarez says. "That usually comes from having weak muscles in the thigh."

DO THIS NOW

When your knee is in flames, your first line of defense is ice. Put a bag of frozen vegetables or bag of crushed ice wrapped in a towel on the hurt. Or you can soak the towel in ice water and wrap that around your leg, suggests Charles Bush-Joseph, M.D., associate professor of orthopedic surgery at Rush–Presbyterian–St. Luke's Medical Center in Chicago.

Apply for 15 to 20 minutes at a time with a half-hour break in between in the first 24 hours after the injury. "Ice helps with the pain, but it also keeps down swelling and inflammation. It can limit the extent of the injury," Dr. Bush-Joseph says.

▶HOW SERIOUS

Usually, rest and strengthening/stretching exercises will take care of most knee pain. But if you're still hurting after a few weeks, go to a doctor, says Dr. Bush-Joseph. And see a physician immediately if you can't bear weight on your knee, bend it, or extend it fully.

If it swells up dramatically and feels "squishy" to the touch, you may have more seriously injured your knee, Dr. Bush-Joseph says. You may have torn cartilage, fluid in the joint, or other mechanical problems that may require treatment or even surgery, he adds.

▶SOLUTIONS

Stretch that sheath. If the pain is on the outside of your knee, it may be caused by a tight iliotibial band, a sheath of muscle and connective tissue that runs from the hip to the knee, Dr. Alvarez says. "We see this problem in weight lifters, runners, and others who have strong muscles but haven't done much flexibility work," he says.

To loosen up the right iliotibial band, stand up, put your right foot behind the left, and raise your hands over your head, Dr. Alvarez says. Then slowly bend to the left until you "feel" the stretch along the outside of your right thigh. Hold the stretch for at least 10 seconds, repeat 10 times, and then switch positions to stretch your left leg.

"You should do one set in the morning, another at night, and always before an activity," Dr. Alvarez says.

Keep your kneecap in line. If a wandering kneecap is your problem, you need to strengthen the quadriceps muscles, especially the vastus medialis, the muscle most important to the proper mechanics of the patella, Dr. Alvarez says.

Lie on your back with your legs straight. Start with your right leg and point your right foot out. Keeping your leg straight, lift your right leg approximately eight inches off the floor and immediately return it back toward the starting position until it almost touches the floor. Repeat this motion 50 to 100 times. Repeat the same exercise with the opposite leg.

The vastus medialis muscle is isolated during this exercise by keeping the toes pointed in an outward direction, Dr. Alvarez says. Pointing your toes straight up works the lateral muscles of the thigh more, he adds.

"It will take about three weeks or so before the muscles start getting stronger," Dr. Alvarez says.

Squelch that swelling. Anti-inflammatories can be very helpful after an injury for controlling pain and reducing swelling, says Dr. Bush-Joseph. Ibuprofen and naproxen (Aleve) are the most commonly used. Patients with sensitive stomachs or a history of ulcer disease should avoid anti-inflammatories, he cautions. They should use acetaminophen instead, he advises. Acetaminophen may not reduce swelling, but it is at least equal to anti-inflammatories in relieving pain. "Follow the directions on the package label," Dr. Bush-Joseph adds.

Did You Know?

Your knees, the largest and most complex joints in the body, can absorb a vertical force nearly seven times your body weight. But they crumple under horizontal blows and hard twisting movements. It's no surprise, then, that 50 percent of all professional football players suffer a serious knee injury during their careers.

Change the surface. Sore knees need a break. You probably should cut back on the impact activity for awhile, Dr. Bush-Joseph says. If road running is your thing, jog on grass or a treadmill for a time. Or take the load off completely and go swimming or ride a stationary bike, Dr. Bush-Joseph suggests.

"Rest doesn't have to be total rest, but you shouldn't keep on doing what caused the pain in the first place—not until you've had some time to heal," Dr. Bush-Joseph says.

Wrap it up. To keep down swelling, wrap an elastic bandage with firm even tension around your knee or slip on a neoprene or elastic knee sleeve, Dr. Bush-Joseph suggests. "If you do it early on, you'll limit swelling and have a faster recovery," he says. "Compression, as long as it's not unduly tight, also gives you added support." If the wrap or sleeve is too tight, swelling will occur below the knee and pain will increase. If that occurs, immediately rewrap the bandage or switch to a larger-size knee sleeve.

▶ALTERNATIVE APPROACHES

Learn yoga. If you have recurring knee pain, you may want to take up yoga and concentrate on basic, simple positions that stretch out the muscles of the leg, especially the hamstrings and quadriceps, says Glenn Terry, M.D., orthopedic surgeon and fellowship director of sports medicine at Hughston Sports Medicine Hospital in Columbus, Georgia.

Yoga is especially good for breaking through the "stretch receptor response" of muscles, Dr. Terry says. "Whenever you stretch a muscle, it naturally resists by contracting slightly. The only way to get past that response is to hold the stretch for at least 10 seconds. It's even better if you can do it for much longer," he says. "Yoga makes you do that. It puts you into a stretched position that you have to sustain for some time."

▶PREVENTIVE MEASURES

Milk the joint. The synovial fold is a membrane that lines the knee joint and helps supply synovial fluid—the oil that makes a joint move smoothly and supplies nutrition—to your cartilage. As you age or as a consequence of injury, the membrane thickens and becomes less elastic, and more prone to swelling and irritation, Dr. Terry says.

Quadriceps "muscle sets" are an effective way to keep the membrane loose, draw out fluid built up after exercise, and provide nutrition to the cartilage in the knee, Dr. Terry says. Sit down on the floor with your legs out straight. Using only your quadriceps muscles, push the underside of your knee flat against the floor until your heel comes off the ground. Hold for 5 to 10 seconds. Relax the muscle and repeat. Begin by doing 50 muscle sets a day per leg, and eventually work up to about 200, suggests Dr. Terry.

"By engaging the muscles on both ends of that synovial membrane, you're milking out any excessive fluid from the knee, making the synovial membrane more supple and improving the nutrition to articular cartilages," Dr. Terry says. "It's a good thing to do if you're having recurring soreness after an activity."

Lactose Intolerance

▶PROBLEM

Thirty minutes to two hours after consuming dairy products, you are one miserable guy. You may have gas, diarrhea, bloating, cramps, or nausea.

▶CAUSE

Your body's dislike of dairy foods is caused by an inability to digest sufficient amounts of lactose, the primary sugar of milk. This occurs when there is a shortage of the enzyme lactase, which normally is produced by the cells that line the small intestine. Lactase breaks down milk sugar into simpler forms that can then be absorbed into the bloodstream. Certain digestive diseases and injuries to the small intestine can create a lactase shortage, but for most people, it is a condition that develops naturally over time.

Our bodies actually begin producing less lactase when we are still toddlers, but many folks don't notice symptoms until they are much older. The condition has a strong hereditary factor and is especially prevalent among many ethnic groups. As many as 75 percent of African-Americans and Native Americans, and 90 percent of Asian-Americans are lactose-intolerant. Jewish people also have a high incidence of the condition.

▶HOW SERIOUS

It can be pretty embarrassing if you're sitting in a quiet, crowded room like a library or a church, and your lactose-laden innards are rumbling like a Montserrat volcano. But odds are that you won't be the only one. An estimated 30 million to 50 million Americans are believed to be lactose-intolerant, al-

> **DO THIS NOW**
>
> Experiment. Through trial and error, learn what your limits are with dairy products. "People have varying degrees of lactose intolerance," says Naresh Jain, M.D., a gastroenterologist in private practice in Niagara Falls, New York. "Some people may have symptoms only if they consume a lot of dairy products, while others may have severe intolerance where even putting milk in their coffee will give them symptoms."

though some experts think that the scope of the condition has been exaggerated. The condition is not curable, but it is treatable.

▶SOLUTIONS

Eat yogurt. "People who are lactose-intolerant generally can tolerate yogurt," says Naresh Jain, M.D., a gastroenterologist in private practice in Niagara Falls, New York. "The lactose in yogurt is already digested by the bacteria in the yogurt, so yogurt is much better tolerated than milk."

This is not true, however, of frozen yogurt. The beneficial bacteria in it are killed in the pasteurization process, explains Steven Hertzler, R.D., Ph.D., assistant professor of nutrition at Kent State University in Kent, Ohio.

Say cheese. Hard or aged cheeses, such as Cheddar or Swiss, have little lactose and usually can be eaten by lactose-intolerant people, Dr. Hertzler says.

MEN'S HEALTH INDEX

Milk and foods made from milk are the only natural sources for lactose, but often it is added to prepared foods. Here are some foods containing "hidden lactose," according to the National Institute of Diabetes and Digestive and Kidney Diseases.

- **Bread and other baked goods**
- **Processed breakfast cereals**
- **Instant potatoes, soups, and breakfast drinks**
- **Margarine**
- **Lunch meats, other than kosher**
- **Salad dressings**
- **Candies and other snacks**
- **Mixes for pancakes, biscuits, and cookies**
- **Some nondairy products, such as powdered coffee creamer and whipped toppings**
- **Food items whose labels state that they contain whey, curds, milk by-products, dry milk solids, and nonfat dry milk powder**

Do without dairy. If lactose intolerance is making your life miserable, just give up milk, cheese, frozen yogurt, and other dairy products. "When you get right down to it, there aren't many people who have lots of this intestinal lactase past the weaning period, which raises the question of whether we were intended to drink milk," says Douglas McGill, M.D., consultant in medicine and gastroenterology at the Mayo Medical School and Mayo Clinic in Rochester, Minnesota. Just be sure to get enough calcium in your diet, which we explain how to do in the following tips.

Eat other calcium-rich foods. If you can't ingest many dairy products, eat other foods high in calcium, says Dr. Jain. After dairy products, sardines with the bones still in them and tofu are among the best food sources of calcium.

Take a supplement. If your lactose intolerance is severe enough that you barely touch calcium-rich dairy products, a calcium supplement may be advisable, says Dr. Jain. He recommends that men take no more than 500 milligrams a day in supplement form. Men should get a total of 1,000 milligrams a day of calcium through food and supplements.

Drink milk light. Supermarkets usually stock lactose-reduced milk, enabling you to get the calcium and other nutrients of milk without the side effects, says Dr. Jain. It's not for everybody, however. "It tastes very sweet," says Dr. Jain. "Many people don't like the taste."

▶ALTERNATIVE APPROACHES

Be a soy boy. "There are some calcium-fortified soy milks that will work just fine" for lactose-intolerant folks, Dr. Hertzler says. Try a health food store if you don't find soy milk in your supermarket.

Take a hike. Going for a walk may make it easier for you to release residual gas, Dr. Hertzler says. It's helpful to walk any time, not just after eating dairy products, he says.

▶PREVENTIVE MEASURES

Don't drink on an empty stomach. Most people who are lactose-intolerant can drink at least small amounts of milk, especially if they don't do so on an empty stomach, says Dr. McGill. "Most Asians, for example, who have very little lactase, are perfectly able to drink milk in their coffee and put some milk on their cereal. It's when they get into a half glass of milk on an empty stomach and drink it right down that they get some symptoms, such as gas and bloating," he says.

Use an additive. Tablets you take with dairy products, such as Lactaid, can be purchased without a prescription, Dr. Jain says. They basically predigest for you. Follow the package directions.

Laryngitis

▶PROBLEM

When your larynx or throat becomes swollen, it can prevent your vocal cords from vibrating correctly, often resulting in raspy, low-pitched speech. The same thing would happen if you stuck a puffy blanket under some guitar strings. The blanket would choke off the sound.

▶CAUSE

Shouting your favorite football team on to victory can tax your throat and vocal cords. But on its own, it probably won't rob you of your voice. Usually, it takes a combination of factors to do that. For example, shout while eating scorching-hot chicken wings and watching Monday Night Football at your favorite smoke-filled bar, and you're begging for trouble. You abuse your throat by yelling, you irritate your larynx by breathing in secondhand smoke, and those wings will probably send your stomach acid into super churn, burning its way up your esophagus and into your already-tender throat while you sleep.

The common cold can also zap your voice as tissues swell to isolate an infection. Tumors from throat cancer can cause long-term bouts with laryngitis.

▶HOW SERIOUS

Usually, laryngitis is not very serious. "If it persists for a few weeks or longer, a doctor should take a look at your vocal cords," says Jonas T. Johnson, M.D., professor of otolaryngology at the University of Pittsburgh School of Medicine. The procedure is simple. Your family physician or otolaryngologist—a fancy term for a doctor who specializes in ears, noses, and throats—will ask you to open your mouth and say "a-a-ah." Then he'll easily be able to see any

DO THIS NOW

Warm, moist air soothes the vocal cords. So turn on your shower as hot as possible and wait for your bathroom to turn into a steam room. Hang around outside the shower in the bathroom for five minutes a few times a day as you inhale the steam, says Jonas T. Johnson, M.D., professor of otolaryngology at the University of Pittsburgh School of Medicine. And use a humidifier when sleeping at night.

History Lesson

In 1799, the father of our country came down with the mother of all laryngitis cases. When President George Washington contracted laryngitis while horseback riding in the cold, winter snow, the presidential doctors knew just what to do. They bled the president four times. Then they rubbed a concoction of dried cantharide beetles or Spanish flies onto his throat to blister his skin. (The doctors thought the blisters would cleanse President Washington's body of impurities.) They then asked Washington to gargle some molasses mixed with vinegar and butter. The president nearly choked to death on the gargle. After that, the doctors gave Washington a violent laxative called calomel, the same stuff that killed Napoleon. Finally, they stuck some hot-mustard poultice on his chest, bringing on even more blisters.

After a long day of such miserable medical care, Washington asked his physicians to let him die in peace. He did so only a few hours later on December 14, 1799.

possible tumors in your throat. "If that approach was used by everyone in the country, no one would ever die of larynx cancer because we would catch them all early," says Dr. Johnson.

▶SOLUTIONS

Shut up already. Keep talking to an absolute minimum. "I know when I tell people, 'Don't talk,' they can't do it. You have to talk a little," Dr. Johnson says. To give your throat and vocal cords the R and R they need to recuperate, rely on alternative forms of communication. For instance, at work, use e-mail instead of the phone. Send written memos instead of making presentations. And leave sticky notes for co-workers and family members.

Eat early and often. Severe heartburn involving acid reflux—stomach acid that creeps up into the esophagus and throat—can cause persistent laryngitis. You can reduce reflux by eating smaller, more frequent meals instead of a few larger meals; by waiting three hours after eating before laying down; and by raising the head of your bed about six inches higher than the foot, says Dr. Johnson. (For more tips on avoiding acid reflux, see Heartburn on page 277.)

Watch what you inhale. Any form of smoke will irritate your throat. So steer clear of smoke-filled bars, diners, and clubs, says Dr. Johnson. Obviously, if you're the one smoking, now is a good time to kick your cigarette habit.

Drown the frog in your throat. Drink at least eight, eight-ounce glasses of water a day to keep the lining of your throat moist and to thin your mucus, says Susan Miller, Ph.D., assistant professor of otolaryngology and director of the

Center for the Voice at Georgetown University Medical Center in Washington, D.C. Some people prefer the water to be cool or warm rather than ice-cold.

▶ALTERNATIVE APPROACHES

Soothe with herbs. Teas of horehound, mullein, and English plantain can help with laryngitis, according to James A. Duke, Ph.D., the world's foremost authority on healing herbs and author of *The Green Pharmacy*. To make horehound tea, put one to two teaspoons of the dried herb in one cup of boiling water and let it steep for 10 minutes, or until cool. For mullein tea, steep one to two teaspoons of the dry herb in a cup of boiling water for 10 minutes; and for a plantain tea, steep one teaspoon of the dry herb in one cup of boiling water until cool. Dr. Duke suggests drinking one to three cups of tea a day. You can find these in health food stores.

Resonate like Pavarotti. If you have to talk, don't try to project a whisper or yell. You'll eventually lose your voice entirely. Instead, speak the same way professionals learn to sing. Stand up straight, breathe into the small of your back, and speak as you exhale. Don't talk too fast or try to fit in too many words in one breath, says Dr. Miller.

Play charades. If you have lost your voice completely, take a tip from the deaf community. Sign languages differ around the world just like spoken languages. So when a deaf person from the United States needs to communicate with a deaf person from Russia, the two must spontaneously create a brand-new language, something called gestuno. You can easily do the same, says Jennifer Olson, a specialist for PEPNet, a national consortium that educates postsecondary schools on serving deaf students. For instance, if you look inquisitively at someone while pointing to the top of your wrist where you normally would wear a watch, people will know that you want to know the time.

▶PREVENTIVE MEASURES

Sing in the shower. Humming and singing in the shower focus your voice away from your throat and assure correct breathing. So humming and singing train you to put the least amount of stress on your larynx when talking, saving your voice in the long run, says Dr. Miller. Doing so in the shower makes you breathe in lots of warm, moist air, which also thins out mucus.

Avoid milk, chocolate, and nuts. All three can thicken mucus, making you clear your throat more often, which closes the vocal folds forcefully. This can eventually make you hoarse, says Dr. Miller. If you notice yourself clearing your throat often, perform a personal experiment. Start cutting back on those foods and increase water to see if your mucus thins out.

Leave the grunting to your ancestors. Grunting while straining to bench-press your weight or whack a hard-to-reach tennis ball can strain your throat and vocal cords, making your voice hoarse. More important, women list it as a major turn-off. Instead, breathe out slowly and steadily, says Dr. Miller.

Loneliness

▶PROBLEM

Ten to 30 percent of the population—that's 25 to 75 million people—suffer from pervasive loneliness, the feeling of being emotionally cut off from others, says William Brassell, Ph.D., a psychologist in Lenoir, North Carolina, and author of *Belonging: A Guide to Overcoming Loneliness.* There are actually two kinds of loneliness. *Transient* loneliness is short-lived and has a specific cause. For example, you'd feel lonely if your company transferred you to another state and you had to leave friends and family behind. Eventually, though, you'd make new friends and the loneliness would recede. *Chronic* loneliness drags on and on, like a cold you can't shake. The worst kind of chronic loneliness, called emotional loneliness, results from an ongoing lack of warmth and affection. Its usual cause is low self-esteem.

▶CAUSE

Men may be more prone to chronic loneliness than women because it's harder for them to open up, says Frank J. Bruno, Ph.D., professor of psychology at San Bernadino Valley College in California and author of *Conquer Loneliness.* "Women form close emotional bonds because they can talk about their feelings," he says. Most men can't—or don't think they should.

What's more, a man's best friend is often his spouse or girlfriend, so those without partners or in unhappy couplings are most likely to be lonely, says Frank Pittman III, M.D., a psychiatrist in Atlanta and author of *Man Enough*

> ### DO THIS NOW
>
> Join a club or take a class that will attract people who share your interests or passions. "It's one of the most effective ways to meet people," says Frank J. Bruno, Ph.D., professor of psychology at San Bernadino Valley College in California and author of *Conquer Loneliness.* Join a softball league or take a swimming class at the YMCA. Check out that book club for mystery buffs. Hell, join Mensa if you can get in. Again, the more people you talk to, the better the odds that you'll meet someone you actually like. "All you have to do is find one or two people who share your interests," says Dr. Bruno.

and *Private Lies: Infidelity and the Betrayal of Intimacy.*

▶How Serious

Transient loneliness is painful but temporary. Chronic loneliness is serious because it deprives you of emotional sustenance. "You need affection the way you need food and water," says Dr. Bruno. In a classic experiment, infant monkeys deprived of parental love failed to thrive, a condition called hospitalism. You might say that chronically lonely people also "fail to thrive," says Dr. Bruno. It's like they've been sentenced to solitary confinement—forever.

▶Solutions

Get the look. If you want to make a friend or meet a woman, you have to convey that you're an open, friendly guy that anyone would be delighted to know. A first step to broadcasting this likableness is to make eye contact when you speak with someone, says Dr. Bruno. "Eye contact is a psychological reward," Dr. Bruno says. "It's a way of saying, 'I'm interested in you.'" There's actually a formula, based on studies of eye contact behavior: Look directly into the other person's eyes for about 15 to 20 seconds. (Any longer, and you'll make them uncomfortable.) Then, look away for about 5 seconds. Continue this pattern of looking at them and looking away. This eventually becomes habitual. But if you are a person who tends to look away too long and too often when others speak to you, you should re-examine your eye contact behavior. If you make poor eye contact when another person is talking, it will be interpreted as a lack of interest on your part and is often perceived as mildly insulting, according to Dr. Bruno.

Turn the double play. If you belong to more than three organizations, scale back to two, advises Dr. Bruno. While joining clubs can help you meet new people, belonging to too many can leave you too pressed for time to find meaningful friendships. "A lot of superficial backslapping is not the answer to loneliness," Dr. Bruno says. So concentrate your efforts on the clubs or organizations you truly enjoy.

Learn to listen. Another key to breaking through to other people is to give them your rapt attention, also known as active listening. Say you meet an at-

---

MEN'S HEALTH INDEX

Loneliness is not the same as being alone. Throughout history, many men have preferred their own company to that of others, for various reasons and periods of time. Here are three who left a lasting legacy by choosing to go it alone.

1. **Admiral Richard E. Byrd (1888–1957), first man to fly over the North Pole; spent five months alone in Antarctica and enjoyed it**
2. **Thomas Merton (1915–1968), Trappist monk and author who celebrated solitude**
3. **Henry David Thoreau (1817–1862), champion of individualism, author of *Walden, or Life in the Woods* (1854), poster boy for the simple life**

tractive woman at a business function. As she talks, you look her in the eye, nod your head, and say, "Uh-huh," from time to time (a phrase that has been shown to encourage talking). You occasionally ask probing questions based on the conversation; this shows that you are listening and being receptive, says Dr. Bruno.

Try "decoding the message," Dr. Bruno suggests. If you are talking to someone who is upset emotionally, listen and perhaps make a comment like, "I can see how upsetting that experience was for you." With that one remark, you have succinctly summarized the conversation, actively listened, decoded the message and responded in an empathetic manner, he says. Active listening may feel phony, but it works. Besides, "when you find someone with interests and values that are similar to yours, all that head-nodding and eye contact won't be phony," says Dr. Bruno. "It will be genuine."

Ease up. Very driven or aggressive men are often lonely because their need to control other people overrides their need for affection and companionship, Dr. Bruno says. If this sounds like you, resist the urge to control or manipulate the people in your life. Realize that your need to be top dog may be pushing people away.

▶ALTERNATIVE APPROACHES

Heal it with flowers. This may sound strange (it did to us), but an alternative treatment called flower essence therapy can help reduce loneliness, says Patricia Kaminski, co-director of the Flower Essence Society in Nevada City, California, and author of *Healing with Flower Essences* and co-author of *Flower Essence Repertory*. Flower essences are liquid preparations distilled from plants and are used exclusively for emotional healing, explains Kaminski. She recommends the flower essence mallow (*Sidalcea glauscens*) to help overcome social discomfort and develop trust and warmth. You can buy flower essences in health food stores, and many are available directly through mail order. The recommended dose is four drops (placed under the tongue) four times a day. Flower essences contain only minute traces of actual physical substance. This means that they are nontoxic and that one cannot overdose on them, unless you were to drink a huge quantity of them and be affected by the alcohol, which is used as a preservative.

▶PREVENTIVE MEASURES

Be a listener. "Being self-centered is one of the primary psychological factors in loneliness," says Dr. Bruno. "Having the ability to take an interest in the people around you is one of the hallmarks of mental health." So make an effort to focus on the other guy—his thoughts, his feelings, his life. If you're truly interested in other people, you're more likely to have friends who will be interested in you.

Work at your relationships. It takes as much work to keep friends as it does to make them, Dr. Brassell says. "If friendships are taken for granted, they will disintegrate until there's nothing left," he says.

Low Self-Esteem

▶PROBLEM

Low self-esteem can mean much more than just having a poor opinion of yourself. People tend to walk all over you, you stay away from chances or opportunities that can improve your home life and career, and it impacts every personal relationship you develop.

▶CAUSE

Men tend to base their self-worth on a set of criteria that stresses money, power, possessions, and tangible accomplishments. "At some point early in life, an equation is made between your worth as a human being and what you are accomplishing out in the world," says Robert Motta, Ph.D., director of the psychology doctoral program at Hofstra University in Hempstead, New York. Many times men feel that they can't measure up to these high and mainly artificial standards, so they view themselves as failures, Dr. Motta says.

And the negative opinions of others—parents, wives, siblings, teachers, schoolmates, bosses, co-workers—can erode self-esteem. If all a man has ever heard is how worthless he is, he believes it, says Bruce Ogilvie, Ph.D., professor emeritus of sports psychology at San Jose State University in California.

DO THIS NOW

Men with high self-esteem often possess a strong sense of purpose. If you find yourself wandering through life without a clue why you're here, volunteer at a local soup kitchen, homeless shelter, or some other cause you believe in, says Bruce Ogilvie, Ph.D., professor emeritus of sports psychology at San Jose State University in California. By working for a cause, you give yourself a positive sense of purpose. This is one of life's true win-win situations: You gain self-esteem while helping others.

▶HOW SERIOUS

Low self-esteem severely affects your quality of life. You can't thoroughly enjoy life if you don't have a high opinion of yourself. But low self-esteem can

Did You Know?

Some men who seem to have it all—money, power, position—want nothing more than to be taken across a woman's knees and given a spanking. Why? They want to escape from their identities, according to Roy F. Baumeister, Ph.D., professor of psychology at Case Western Reserve University in Cleveland. It's not, as has long been thought, that they have low self-esteem. If anything, it's just the opposite. Dr. Baumeister reviewed various studies and theories about those who practice sadomasochistic sex and proposed that sadomasochism partners enjoy humiliation during sex because it signifies the abandonment of the pursuit of self-esteem. Some findings, he noted, show that people who take part in sadomasochism are successful and highly educated but submit to the will of another just to shed all the autonomy and responsibility of being that successful.

---

also be a springboard to more severe problems such as depression, alcoholism, and other self-destructive behavior, Dr. Ogilvie says. If you feel desolate and can't find a way to truly feel good about yourself, you should probably seek out a therapist, he says.

▶SOLUTIONS

Become your own Knute Rockne. Say something positive about yourself right now and on a regular basis. Men with high self-esteem give themselves internal pep talks reminding them of their positive traits and accomplishments, Dr. Ogilvie says.

Set specific goals. Many people with low self-esteem mutter about their lack of accomplishment. But do you even know what you want to accomplish in the first place? Without a goal in sight, you probably won't achieve anything, says Michael W. Mercer, Ph.D., an industrial psychologist with the Mercer Group in Barrington, Illinois, and author of *Spontaneous Optimism*. Visualize what kind of life you want to live. Think about your desired career, money, relationships, and body image, Dr. Mercer says. Write those goals down or even make a poster with magazine pictures that represent your goals. Look at your poster or goal list every day, and work toward meeting those goals.

Stay grounded. While you want to aspire to something, deciding that you will be Arnold Schwarzenegger, Donald Trump, and Bill Gates all wrapped up in one dooms you to perpetual low self-esteem. "Some people have these extreme standards. You can almost guarantee failure," Dr. Motta says. Set reasonable, attainable goals so that when you achieve them, you'll enhance your self-esteem.

Go for a jog. Steady exercise obviously raises your self-esteem by improving your health. But it also can improve your mood through brain chemicals that are released during a workout. "I've worked on a number of studies on exercise and mood states, and regardless of the type of exercise, it enhances one's self-esteem," Dr. Motta says. Do something you enjoy, he advises. It can be as simple as taking a walk. Then do it at least three times a week, for approximately 30 minutes each time, to get the maximum benefit, he adds.

Join the club. Exercising with others, whether it's playing basketball or joining a karate club, gives your self-image an added boost. "A very important part of a karate club or team sport is building interpersonal relationships. You build camaraderie and receive team support," says Charles Richman, Ph.D., professor of psychology at Wake Forest University in Winston-Salem, North Carolina. By interacting with teammates in an atmosphere of constructive encouragement, you'll feel better about yourself, Dr. Richman adds.

▶ALTERNATIVE APPROACHES

Take the higher road. Men tend to base their self-esteem on measurable markers such as career status, financial worth, and the women they can attract, Dr. Motta says. Why not take a different path? Strive to be the nicest guy, a better husband and father, a great gardener. "These people feel quite good about themselves without using the artificial criteria most people use," Dr. Motta notes.

Knock out that voice. The source of many men's self-esteem problems lies in the past—the criticizing voice of a father, a mother, or a nagging wife. For example: You're not good enough. You always mess up. Even in times of success, these comments can keep a man's self-esteem in the cellar, Dr. Ogilvie says. Drown out those voices using visualization, he advises. Dr. Ogilvie tells clients to imagine the comments as balls or any kind of object. Then visualize swatting or hitting the comments away with your hand or a baseball bat. "After awhile, you feel some sense of mastery over the comments and the people," he says.

▶PREVENTIVE MEASURES

Find some real friends. When you and your friends hang out together, do they find your troubles and failures the source of entertainment? Chuck this group of buddies. "Quit hanging around people who keep putting you down, even if they just pseudo-joke about it," Dr. Mercer says. "Friends should raise your self-esteem and help you achieve your goals, not bring you down."

List your finer attributes. Take a piece of paper or even a tape recorder and list good things about yourself. Record your accomplishments, your activities, what makes you a good friend. Give yourself credit for such obvious qualities as loving your mother or appreciating art. "You'll find things out about yourself that you didn't realize," Dr. Ogilvie says. Look at the list or play the tape when you feel down on yourself. Keep adding to your positives as well.

Making a Commitment

▶PROBLEM

She wants to get married (or live together). You don't. Or you want to get married (or live together), but thinking about it gives you the cold sweats.

▶CAUSE

Fear of the emotional (and financial) consequences of divorce, or memories of his parents' less-than-perfect marriage, can cause a man to be uncomfortable with the idea of a committed relationship, says Alvin Baraff, Ph.D., a clinical psychologist and founder and director of Men-Center Counseling in Washington, D.C. He may also have the irrational idea that settling down means relinquishing control. In a healthful relationship, the couple would share responsibilities and control, says Dr. Baraff.

"Whatever the joys of a relationship with a woman, there's the fear that they'll become engulfed, that they'll lose some big part of themselves," says Frank Pittman III, M.D., a psychiatrist in Atlanta and author of *Man Enough* and *Private Lies: Infidelity and the Betrayal of Intimacy.*

▶HOW SERIOUS

"Men who don't commit because they want to keep their options open end up with nothing," warns Scott Stanley, Ph.D., co-director of the Center for Marital and Family Studies at the University of Denver, author of *The Heart of Commitment*, and co-author of *Fighting for Your Marriage.* "They may be with

DO THIS NOW

It helps to remember that some of the riskiest things in life are often the most rewarding. "Marriage is like playing the stocks," says Scott Stanley, Ph.D., co-director of the Center for Marital and Family Studies at the University of Denver, author of *The Heart of Commitment,* and co-author of *Fighting for Your Marriage.* "There are lots of risks, and sometimes you do take losses. But over the long term, the people who do well are the people who hang in there and keep investing. The people who are actually taking the greatest risk long-term are those who never get in the game."

Did You Know?

Happily married men live an average of six years longer than single men. They also have more sex than their single brethren, says Scott Stanley, Ph.D., co-director of the Center for Marital and Family Studies at the University of Denver, author of *The Heart of Commitment*, and co-author of *Fighting for Your Marriage*.

somebody or a series of somebodies, but they won't ever have that rich, satisfying sense of family and community."

The answer may be therapy, Dr. Pittman says. "If a man truly fears commitment, a woman screaming at him about it won't get him to change his point of view," he says. But exploring the issue with a therapist—specifically, a male therapist—might. "Therapy may be able to help him to see the situation differently," Dr. Pittman says. "In a way, a therapist is like a golf coach, pointing out what's wrong with your swing."

If you're in a serious relationship, the question is: Do you go into therapy together or alone? Dr. Stanley says that the odds of breaking up increase if you go separately, or if only one of you goes.

▶SOLUTIONS

Face your fear. Force yourself to really reflect on why you may be reluctant to commit, Dr. Baraff says. This soul searching can help reveal whether your reason is sound. One client of Dr. Baraff's was afraid that getting married would erase his individuality. "He felt like, 'If I get married, then I've given in,'" says Dr. Baraff. "He'd be a statistic. He wouldn't be able to do his own thing. He'd lose his creativity. This was a man who had lived with his partner for nine years. And the thing he dreaded most was running into people he hadn't seen in awhile and having to tell them he was married." After he had worked out those fears, he was able to marry. That's because marriage should allow each partner to maintain some individual interests. And it certainly requires some creativity for a couple to work together to resolve the curveballs life is sure to throw at them. Couples who lose their individuality are usually in an unhealthy, codependent relationship, Dr. Baraff explains.

Go with your gut. Maybe it's not a fear of commitment that's stopping you from taking the plunge into matrimony. "Some men who look commitment-phobic really aren't," says Dr. Stanley. He suggests asking yourself whether it's settling down that scares you or whether you're having doubts about this particular woman. "You may find that your anxiety is legitimate," he says.

Don't get steamrollered. Some men panic when faced with an ultimatum—

"marry me or we're through." If your partner threatens to walk, try to stay calm. "Don't jump into the commitment because of the fear of immediate loss," advises Dr. Stanley. You need time to consider her position and your own before you respond.

▶ALTERNATIVE APPROACHES

Put it in writing. Writing about your reluctance to settle down may help you to understand and eventually overcome it, says James Pennebaker, Ph.D., professor of psychology at the University of Texas at Austin, who has studied the role of writing as a therapeutic tool. He recommends writing for 20 minutes a day for four straight days about any topic that runs through your mind. This is a general translation exercise that allows you to write down your deepest thoughts and feelings when dealing with any subject. Then use it to release your feelings about commitment, he suggests. Write down all your fears and emotions regarding settling down. Really let go. Don't edit yourself, and don't worry about grammar, punctuation, or lousy handwriting. The point is to clarify your feelings and write your way to a resolution.

Stop and taste the flowers. According to some alternative healers, flower essences—liquid preparations distilled from plants—can help treat emotional issues, including a fear of commitment. The flower essence sticky monkeyflower (don't ask *us*) can improve the ability to express feelings of love and connectedness, write Patricia Kaminski and Richard Katz in *Flower Essence Repertory*. The recommended dose is four drops (placed under the tongue) four times a day, says Kaminski, co-director of the Flower Essence Society in Nevada City, California, and author of *Healing with Flower Essences*.

Flower essences are sold in some health food stores, and many are available directly through mail order. Flower essences contain only minute traces of actual physical substance. This means that they are nontoxic and that you cannot overdose on them, unless you were to drink a huge quantity of them and be affected by the alcohol, which is used as a preservative.

▶PREVENTIVE MEASURES

Quit holding out for a fantasy. Some men resist commitment because they believe that there's a "perfect woman" out there for them—they just haven't met her yet. "They have this naive belief that there's somebody who will punch every part of their ticket, so to speak. And it ain't gonna happen," says Dr. Stanley. So ditch this illusion, recommends Dr. Stanley. It may prevent you from finding happiness with the partner you already have.

Midlife Crisis

▶ PROBLEM

You have a loss of direction in life and an uncertainty and fearfulness about the future.

▶ CAUSE

Midlife crisis is typically triggered by a birthday, death of a parent, divorce, illness, children leaving home, or being denied a promotion at work.

"The event puts you in touch with your limitations and, sometimes, your mortality," explains Gerald DeSobe, Ph.D., a psychologist and pastoral counselor at the Samaritan Center for Counseling and Education in Houston. "It's a bit of reality setting in. You realize that you're not going to achieve everything you once thought you might."

▶ HOW SERIOUS

How you cope with your situation determines whether it is a transition lasting a few months or a full-blown crisis, says Mara Julius, Sc.D., a psychosocial epidemiologist (emeritus) at the University of Michigan School of Public Health in Ann Arbor. Some men clam up, drink too much, or fall into clinical depression. Others take a new direction in their lives and change careers. A few men decide that their boss, family, or friends are the problem, says Dr. Julius.

Some of these guys leave their wives, get a

Did You Know?

Carl G. Jung, the eminent Swiss psychiatrist, called age 40 the "noon of life," the beginning of a period when there was a resurgence of "individuation." Individuation, a developmental process where a person becomes more uniquely individual, also occurs during childhood and adolescence. Jung felt that it was sorely needed at midlife so that a man could throw off societal demands, pursue his own aims, and lead a more balanced life.

hair transplant, buy a red convertible, and find a young woman with a flowing mane to ride along at their side.

"We all know guys like this, and the fact is that they look foolish," says Dr. DeSobe. "You can't turn back the clock." If your feelings of discouragement or depression last for more than a month, you may want to seek professional help from a psychiatrist, psychologist, pastoral counselor, or social worker sensitive to men's issues, suggests Dr. DeSobe. Ask a friend, your family physician, or a member of the clergy for a recommendation.

▶SOLUTIONS

Negotiate a new life. Recognize that you're entering a new stage of life where there are new rules, expectations, and, yes, limitations, says Dr. Julius. "You're going through a renegotiation with life. What may have previously been important in your life may no longer be," she says. "It's not time to be rigid and clinging to old ways. You must accept that the rules have changed."

Exult in your experience. At first, it may shock you that the suits in the executive suite no longer view you as the eager beaver and the bright-and-rising star. Rather, you're the tried-and-true, the dependable, the old warhorse who has reached his plateau.

If you can accept this position, you may actually find it liberating to no longer worry about your rise on the organizational chart. And as a man of experience, you may have much to offer those who are still struggling up the ladder, says Peter Frazier-Koontz, Ph.D., a pastoral counselor and certified professional counselor at the Community Mental Health Center of Lancaster County in Lincoln, Nebraska.

"Maybe you can informally become a mentor and find your satisfaction in other ways, like helping others," Dr. Frazier-Koontz suggests. "As you think back, remember how you once looked up to those people who had something to teach you."

Join up. Get active in a service organization like the Rotary Club, Big

Brothers of America, the Sierra Club, or your church, suggests Dr. Frazier-Koontz. If you feel a need to connect with other men, join a men's group for discussion, support, or volunteerism, he says.

"Some men need affirmation and connections with people outside the family and the job," Dr. Frazier-Koontz says. "A volunteer group enables you to use your experience and wisdom to help others."

Find your faith. Is yours a midlife spiritual crisis? You're at the top of the heap and wondering, "Is this it?" Or perhaps you've had that sobering realization that you aren't going to live forever.

These questions and concerns may need religious or spiritual answers, says Dr. DeSobe. "I think men often lose touch with their spiritual lives in their quest for career and being providers," he says. "And it can be a very positive experience to reconnect with that side of yourself. It may help you put your life into perspective."

▶ALTERNATIVE APPROACHES

Draw your feelings. Drawing or coloring with crayons is something most of us gave up by age 12, deciding that it was kids' stuff, says Doris Arrington, Ed.D., an art therapist and psychologist at the College of Notre Dame in Belmont, California. Men in crisis would do well to take up the drawing pad and crayons again, says Dr. Arrington. Art is a way to get in touch with your feelings, relax, and explore a side of yourself that you may have completely forgotten about.

Dr. Arrington suggests that you get a blank pad, colored pencils, and just begin to draw: doodles, cartoons, landscapes, people. It doesn't matter. "I think a lot of adults are enormously surprised at how expressive they can be with drawing," she says. "And as a therapy, art can give you a pretty accurate internal picture of yourself."

▶PREVENTIVE MEASURES

Take some risks. That doesn't mean that you should give the boss the "Take This Job and Shove It" speech or cash in your 401(k) and sink your retirement into a gold mine in Saskatchewan. But the source of your frustration could be that you've spent most of your life playing it safe, says Christopher Hershman, doctor of ministry, a Lutheran pastor and licensed psychologist in Allentown, Pennsylvania.

"Safe isn't always bad; there is something to be said for security. But safe doesn't always put you where you want to be. Perhaps you feel stagnated and bored in your job and life," says Dr. Hershman. "Maybe it's time to start something new, to break the old mold.

"The big thing is to take some action, and not just whine or fret about the position you find yourself in. Doing something relieves a lot of the frustration," says Dr. Hershman.

Motion Sickness

▶PROBLEM

Motion sickness may be an offshoot of a survival reaction from ancient times. When cavemen and women ate something poisonous, it induced a feeling of dizziness and confusion. The brain learned that whenever it experienced vertigo, it should expel the offending food—in other words, throw it up. Through the years, we developed another way to create the same feeling: fast travel. When the motion brought on by planes, boats, and cars reaches your brain, it triggers those vertigo feelings. The brain reaches back to prehistoric times and does what comes naturally, telling your stomach to bring whatever poison is down there back up, says Jonathan Clark, M.D., a neurologist and a flight surgeon for the NASA space and life sciences directorate in the medical sciences division at the Johnson Space Center in Houston.

▶CAUSE

Motion sickness is really just a fight between your senses. Your inner ear and your eyes disagree about whether you're moving. The sensors in your ears tell your brain, "Hey, we're moving here." But because you're sitting still inside a car, a boat, or a plane, your eyes tell your brain, "Excuse me, but we're not going anywhere." The stuck-in-the-middle brain reacts by sending out mixed messages, triggering nausea and dizziness.

▶HOW SERIOUS

Although you may feel like dying during a bout of motion sickness, it won't kill you or even seriously harm you. The signs of motion sickness will go away as soon as the motion stops. If after the trip you still feel nauseated and dizzy, take a trip to the doctor's office. You may have a painful condition called barotitis, where air gets trapped in the inner ear and can cause vertigo, says Jeffrey G. Jones, M.D., medical director of the St. Francis Traveler's Health Center in Indianapolis.

▶SOLUTIONS

Look into the distance. Once you have your ideal seat, search for a far-off object about 45 degrees above the horizon. Then keep your gaze on that object for as long as you can, says Terence Collins, M.D., director of Healthy Journeys, the University of Kentucky A. B. Chandler Medical Center's International Travel Clinic in Lexington. Keeping your eyes fixed on something in the distance limits the "disagreement" between your inner ear and your eyes.

Keep your eyes wide open. Closing your eyes in the hopes that motion sickness will go away only makes it worse, Dr. Jones cautions. By closing your eyes, you actually feel the movement even more. Instead, focus on the horizon.

Take the wheel. When you drive, your brain already knows where you're headed. "When you can predict the motion, it reduces the motion sickness," Dr. Clark says. Being behind the wheel also allows you to control the speed and the range of movement.

Get some air. Open the car window or get out on the boat deck. For some reason, fresh air keeps a lot of people from turning green. "I've seen people in unbelievably rough weather stay okay if they are on deck but get really sick when they stick their head inside the cabin," Dr. Collins says.

Put the book down. Reading may seem like a great way to pass the time on a long car ride. But reading further confuses your senses and makes you even more sick, Dr. Jones says. Keep your eyes on the road and save the reading material for later.

Run a counter play. Over-the-counter products such as dimenhydrinate (Dramamine) work fine if you want to take them, Dr. Jones says. But many work by making you drowsy, he warns. If you decide to use medication, take the dosage recommended on the package at least 30 to 60 minutes before you start your travels. If you can't find Dramamine, you can take a dose of diphenhydramine (Benadryl). The antihistamine also makes you drowsy and less susceptible to the ills of motion sickness. These are not to be used with other tranquilizers or sedatives.

▶ALTERNATIVE APPROACHES

Go gingerly. The ancient spice ginger calms the symptoms of motion sickness. Buy ginger in the capsule form, Dr. Collins recommends. Take two 550-milligram capsules two hours before your trip. Take another two 550-milligram capsules four to six hours into your ride. "People have been using this for ages; it has to be worth something," Dr. Collins says.

Did You Know?

NASA calls it pre-adaptation, which is a fancy way of saying that they repeatedly expose you to conditions that will make you green around the gills until you finally get used to it. It's like anything else that you want to get good at. Practice helps make you better.

That's what some **NASA** astronauts do to prepare for space travel. In a virtual-reality setting, **NASA** simulates the type of motion and the visual surroundings (the shuttle or space station) that the astronaut would face in space. The astronaut repeats the motion until his brain and stomach become accustomed to it. The motion along with the surroundings make the process of pre-adaptation work.

"You get to experience what it might be like to float, to be free, to move in ways you normally wouldn't on the ground," says Millard Reschke, Ph.D., **NASA**'s senior neuroscientist and director of the neuroscience laboratory at Johnson Space Center in Houston. "By practicing that which bothers you, you get over it and adapt to it. It's uncomfortable, but it helps." It is not necessary to make people very ill for the process to work, Dr. Reschke says. Short exposures seem to work better than daily practice, and often a single exposure is enough to add some critical protection and reduce symptoms while the astronauts are aloft.

Not all space travelers take this route, Dr. Reschke adds. Although it has been going on for more than 10 years, pre-adaptation is still considered experimental and astronauts must volunteer for the program. Those who don't volunteer fight motion sickness like many of us—with anti-motion sickness medication.

You can also use ginger ale, ginger snaps, or fresh ginger. Persons with gallstones should consult a qualified health-care practitioner before using the dried root. But for serious motion sickness, these products should be used in addition to, not in place of, the ginger supplement, Dr. Collins says.

Press the point. According to the practice of acupressure, applying pressure at the wrists prevents the nausea and dizziness of motion sickness. Based on this concept, a product called Sea-Band is out on the market. You wear these bands around both of your wrists, where they apply continued pressure throughout your trip. Although studies haven't been conclusive, Dr. Collins says that many of his patients have found dramatic relief from car sickness using the bands.

"A lot of people swear by them. If it works for you, then use it," Dr. Jones advises.

You can find them in travel stores, drugstores, or health food stores, Dr. Collins says.

You can always apply your own pressure. Press down with your thumb or finger on the crease of your wrist, Dr. Collins says. You should press just behind the large crease on the inside of the wrist (the soft part of the wrist, below the palm). Press fairly hard for about 10 minutes at a time. The pressure can't be too soft, or it won't work. But it shouldn't be painful either, Dr. Collins says.

Amuse yourself. If you're, worried about getting motion sickness on a long car or boat ride, then do something that will make a long trip seem like a cake-walk. A day at an amusement park is a great way to get used to all kinds of different motion, says Donald E. Parker, Ph.D., professor of otolaryngology at the University of Washington School of Medicine in Seattle. "You can take rides on different devices—roller coasters, Tilt-a-Whirls, and the like. Get used to a variety of motion experiences," Dr. Parker says. But stop once you feel sick, he adds.

▶PREVENTIVE MEASURES

Eat light. Chowing down on a heavy meal before your travels almost guarantees that it'll come right back up. Stick to simple carbohydrate snacks such as crackers or pretzels, Dr. Jones says.

Try the spin cycle. Your office chair is good for more than just sitting and playing roller football. Try this exercise to see if you can build up your motion tolerance: While sitting on a rotating chair, push off with your feet so that it goes round and round. As it moves, close your eyes. Then move your head slowly forward, then slowly back to the upward position. Five seconds later, move your head to the left, then back. Then move your head to the right side and back. Keep repeating the head movements every two to three seconds, Dr. Clark says. The variety of movements can help you adapt to motion and may help keep you from getting sick. And even if they don't, it beats working.

Don't think about it. Just because you've had bouts of motion sickness before doesn't mean that you'll have them again, Dr. Jones says. Many people outgrow the malady (usually during adolescence). But some people worry so much about getting sick that it becomes a self-fulfilling prophecy, Dr. Jones says. Before a trip, tell yourself that you're just as likely not to get sick. And if you do, you'll deal with it. "Try to view it more as a nuisance than as a big deal," Dr. Jones suggests.

Muscle Cramps

▶PROBLEM

You have a sharp, painful contraction or spasm of a muscle or group of muscles, which markedly limits use of a body part. It comes on suddenly and lasts from a few seconds to several hours.

▶CAUSE

Muscle cramps normally occur during hot weather, intense exercise when you're really perspiring, or both. The number one cause is dehydration, says Mary Kintz, an orthopedic physical therapist at Raleigh Community Sports Medicine and Physical Therapy in Raleigh, North Carolina. Your body needs fluids and electrolytes, substances that enable cells to communicate with one another, to carry out its biochemical reactions. When that communication breaks down, your muscles can become spastic—in other words, go into contraction and not let go, explains Kintz.

Muscles may also cramp when they are extremely fatigued from being overworked, says Kintz. These cramps, which include the dreaded charley horse, often occur hours after an activity, when you're relaxing in front of the TV or falling off to sleep in bed.

▶HOW SERIOUS

A muscle cramp is pretty painful and uncomfortable as anyone knows who has had to leap from bed and stumble about the room imitating old Captain

> ### DO THIS NOW
>
> If the cramp is in the calf, contract the opposite muscle—in this case the tibialis anterior, located in the front of the lower leg—against resistance, advises James Waslaski, sports massage therapist at the Center for Pain Management and Clinical Sports Massage in Tampa, Florida, and author of *International Advancements in Event and Clinical Sports Massage*. Actively pull the toes toward your shin, which sends a message to your brain telling the opposing muscle to relax. Once the cramp stops, you should stretch the muscle that was cramping. Always choose stretches that work the opposite muscles as well, he says.

Did You Know?

The term *charley horse* is sports slang for an old racehorse, especially one afflicted with stiffness and ailments.

Peg Leg. Typically, it's temporary, lasting no more than a few minutes, sometimes just seconds, says Kintz.

If the contraction lasts for more than a day, makes it impossible to assume a normal posture or to walk, or occurs as often as two or three times per week, you should see your family doctor, Kintz advises. "Ask the doctor to check your electrolyte balance. You may have a biochemical problem or something else going," says Kintz.

▶SOLUTIONS

Eat better. If electrolytes are the problem, it may be due to a poor diet or inadequate fluid intake, says Karlis Ullis, M.D., assistant clinical professor at the University of California, Los Angeles, UCLA School of Medicine. Make sure that you're getting adequate calcium, potassium, and magnesium in your diet. Dairy products, such as milk, yogurt, and cheese, are good sources of calcium. Magnesium is abundant in nuts and seeds, and you can get your potassium in vegetables and fruit, especially bananas, Dr. Ullis says.

"Usually, you can get what you need if you are conscientious about your diet and water/fluid intake, rather than taking a supplement," Dr. Ullis says.

Smother inflammation. If you get charley horses at night after exercise, you may have inflammation of your muscles and tendons. Make sure that your diet is rich in antioxidants (brilliantly colored fruits and vegetables) and try taking one of the nonsteroidal anti-inflammatory drugs, like ibuprofen, a couple of hours before bedtime, recommends Dr. Ullis. "About 200 milligrams should be enough to decrease the inflammatory response," he says.

Apply ice. If you get a cramp during exercise, it may be related to trauma and small tears in the muscle. Stop exercising immediately and apply ice wrapped in a towel, gently compressing the cramped area to keep down the swelling from injury, says Dr. Ullis.

Put the ice on for 10 to 12 minutes, remove when the area feels cold to touch but is not painfully cold, and repeat as needed, Dr. Ullis says. "You can also wet an elastic bandage with cold water and wrap that around the area," he says. "The quicker you can get the area cold, the better."

Kick the horse. If you get roused from bed by a calf cramp, sit up, straighten your leg, and flex your toes toward your head, says Alison Lee, M.D., a pain-management specialist and acupuncturist with Barefoot Doctors, an acupuncture and natural-medicine resource center in Ann Arbor, Michigan.

"Push your heel away and pull your toes up and toward your shin," explains Dr. Lee. "Usually, it has to be done very gradually, which isn't easy when you're in the grip of a cramp."

▶ALTERNATIVE APPROACHES

Have a kava. An effective herbal remedy for cramps and spasms is kava (*Piper methysticum*), available at most health food stores as a ground-up herb in capsule form, says David Winston, professional and founding member of the American Herbalists Guild and a clinical herbalist in Washington, New Jersey. "It's a powerful antispasmodic, especially good for people who get cramps at night in their feet and lower legs," says Winston.

Look for kava in a standardized extract (capsule) or a tincture. For the capsules, follow the directions on the bottle. he says. If you prefer a tincture, take 4 milliliters (or about 80 drops) three times a day. If you're sensitive to sedative-type drugs, however, be careful with kava. Because of the herb's anti-anxiety, mellowing actions, don't drive, operate heavy equipment, or drink alcoholic beverages when taking kava, warns Winston. And avoid kava if you're taking benzodiazepines (like Valium), he adds.

Supplement your minerals. The mineral deficiencies most often related to muscle cramping are magnesium and calcium. Both are important for proper muscle metabolism, Dr. Lee says.

If you're eating a healthy balanced diet and still cramping at night, try taking a calcium-magnesium supplement. Given typical dietary practices, you're probably not getting the entire 1,000 milligrams of calcium per day that your body requires. Dr. Lee recommends filling in the gap with the proper dose of a supplement. Evaluate your diet, she says, and estimate how much calcium you're lacking. If you have thyroid problems or cancer, ask your doctor before taking calcium supplements, Dr. Lee says. Take most of the dose before bed, says Dr. Lee. Look for a supplement that comes in a ratio of two parts calcium to one part magnesium.

▶PREVENTIVE MEASURES

Drink up. Lack of hydration is easy to correct. Drink plenty of water and sports drinks before and during exercise, Kintz says.

"Water is okay if the exercise lasts less than 60 minutes. But if you're working out longer or working out in the heat, you may need to replace some electrolytes. That's when you want to switch to some of the sports drinks like Gatorade," Kintz says.

Sleep loose. If you've been exercising during the day, make sure that you stretch before you go to bed at night, Dr. Lee says. A slow, light, full-body stretch routine that takes 10 minutes or so is usually sufficient, she says.

Muscle Soreness

▶PROBLEM

You have a localized achiness that occurs soon after exercise and may intensify the following day. It's more discomfort than real pain.

▶CAUSE

Your muscle fibers sustain microtears during exercise, and if you haven't used a muscle for some time or really overwork it, the muscle can't quickly flush out all the waste products. What you get from these tears and toxins is soreness, says Mary Kintz, an orthopedic physical therapist at Raleigh Community Sports Medicine and Physical Therapy in Raleigh, North Carolina. "Even if you are in excellent shape, muscles get very accustomed to a particular pattern of movement," she says. "When you introduce a new activity, you often end up with soreness."

▶HOW SERIOUS

The soreness should go away within a few days as the muscle heals and gets stronger. If you have pain for more than a week, pain that seems centered in your joints, or pain that limits your range of motion, you may have an injured tendon (tendinitis) or inflamed bursa (bursitis), says Kintz. That requires more time to heal, and it may be a good idea to see your doctor for a more accurate diagnosis.

▶SOLUTIONS

Move it. So you overdid it by stacking two truckloads of firewood yesterday, but that doesn't mean that you should sit around all day today, says

DO THIS NOW

A painful muscle often has its trigger points that, when stimulated, can cause the muscle to relax, says Alison Lee, M.D., a pain-management specialist and acupuncturist with Barefoot Doctors, an acupuncture and natural-medicine resource center in Ann Arbor, Michigan. These points may respond well to acupressure, Dr. Lee says. "To find a trigger point, feel around the muscle until you come across a particularly tender area. Then press or knead the point for about a minute or more," Dr. Lee advises.

Did You Know?

Early scientists thought that the action of flexing or rippling muscles resembled little mice scurrying beneath the skin. They named these body structures muscles, which comes from the Latin word *mus*, meaning "little mouse."

Duane Iverson, a physical therapist, certified athletic trainer, and director of the sports medicine department at the University of Oregon Student Health Center in Eugene.

What you need is fresh blood moving through those sore muscles to flush out the waste products and speed healing, Iverson says. Do some walking, light stretching, or low-intensity exercise to warm and loosen the muscles, he suggests.

Freeze, sucker. Ice makes nearly any soft-tissue injury feel better, especially when you combine the cold with a massage, Kintz says. Fill a paper cup with water, freeze it, peel off some paper to expose a bit of the ice, and massage the ice up and down the muscle for 10 minutes, she says. Wait an hour and repeat as needed over the next couple of days, says Kintz.

"Often the pain is fairly localized, so you don't need to put an ice pack over a big area. This way you get the cold right on the hurt," Kintz explains.

Roll that joint. A sore or tight muscle group near a joint can cause you to favor a joint, says Kintz. "That's not good because if you overprotect the joint, you can lose function," she says.

At least three times per day, you should gently put your joint through its normal range of motion, advises Kintz. "It's just commonsense stuff. We all know how our joints normally move," she says. "You may feel a stretch, but it should not be painful. If you have pain, back off the motion."

▶ALTERNATIVE APPROACHES

Give yourself a hand. You can try Korean hand massage, a form of reflexology, to relieve muscle soreness anywhere in the body, says Alison Lee, M.D., a pain-management specialist and acupuncturist with Barefoot Doctors, an acupuncture and natural-medicine resource center in Ann Arbor, Michigan. This medicinal practice looks at the hand as representative of the entire body: the top of the middle finger being your head; the ring and forefinger representing the arms; thumb and pinkie, the legs; the palm, the remainder of your body; and the front and back of the hand representing the front or back of the body, respectively.

Pick out the place on your hand that roughly corresponds to the painful area on your body, and then stimulate that portion with a toothpick, suggests Dr. Lee. You hone in by probing the area for an especially tender spot, she says. "That corresponds to where your pain is ," she says. "When you have the spot, press on it gently for a few minutes."

Arm yourself with arnica. A popular remedy for relieving muscle soreness is homeopathic arnica pills, available from most health food stores, says David Winston, professional and founding member of the American Herbalists Guild and a clinical herbalist in Washington, New Jersey. Winston recommends taking 30X strength at the recommended dosage on the bottle for a few days or until the soreness dissipates.

"If you know that you're going to be exerting yourself and you anticipate soreness, you can begin taking arnica a few days ahead of time," Winston says.

Combine for relief. Two herbs—black cohosh and kava—taken in combination are quite successful in combating muscle pain and reducing muscle-related cramps, says Winston. Both come in pill form or tincture.

"You want to take kava and black cohosh in a one-to-one ratio, meaning equal parts of each," he explains. "The strength of the pills can vary quite a bit, so I would just follow the recommendations on the bottle and take as needed to relieve pain and spasm." If you opt for the tinctures, the same one-to-one ratio applies, but you'll measure equal parts of each in milliliters. If you're sensitive to sedative-type drugs, be careful with kava. Because of the herb's anti-anxiety, mellowing action, don't drive, operate heavy equipment, or drink alcoholic beverages when taking kava, warns Winston. And avoid kava if you're taking benzodiazepines (like Valium), he adds. Occasional gastrointestinal discomfort may occur when taking black cohosh, and you should not take it for more than six months.

▶PREVENTIVE MEASURES

Chill gradually. When you exercise, your muscles, tendons, and fascia—connecting fibrous tissue—warm and loosen up very much like gelatin, says James Waslaski, sports massage therapist at the Center for Pain Management and Clinical Sports Massage in Tampa, Florida, and author of *International Advancements in Event and Clinical Sports Massage.* "If you suddenly stop the workout, meaning you don't cool down slowly, your muscles and tendons may get stuck in a contracted state, held in place by the fascia," he says.

After you exercise, spend a few minutes stretching out your muscles, moving about, and allowing the fascia to cool slowly, Waslaski suggests. "When you do that, the muscles relax and lengthen. Fresh blood gets in, and waste products go out," he says.

Nausea

▶ PROBLEM

An unsettling sensation that can start with a tight throat, increased salivation, and sweating, nausea surfaces as a woozy/dizzy or churning-stomach feeling, often right before your lunch reappears semidigested. The culprit could be as obvious as last night's tequila or helping yourself to thirds at the table. But a number of other triggers exist that are more difficult to finger: peptic ulcers, reactions to medications, gastroesophageal reflux, food poisoning, viruses, and gallbladder or liver disease, just to name a few.

▶ CAUSE

The physiological phenomenon called nausea can happen several ways, depending on the trigger. If it's set off by a stomach irritant, like spoiled food, then the stomach becomes inflamed, sending nerve impulses to the part of the brain responsible for sensation there. The message that something's wrong is then interpreted by you as nausea. Other triggers, however, such as certain medications, do not actually damage the stomach. Instead, they seep into the bloodstream where they are then perceived by the highly sensitive chemoreceptor center in the brain. The brain creates the sensation of nausea as a warning to the intestinal tract that you should not take more of the substance.

▶ HOW SERIOUS

Simply put, the cause determines the seriousness. If it's clearly linked to something you ate or drank, like alcohol, then time and lots of water will make

DO THIS NOW
Sipping a flat, cold, caffeine-free soda may ease your stomach, says Cynthia M. Yoshida, M.D., assistant professor of gastroenterology and hepatology at the University of Virginia Digestive Health Center in Charlottesville. It's an old folk remedy that no one's really sure of why it works, she says.

Your soda should also be clear, like a ginger ale, since the colored ones tend to have a higher acid content, says Edwin J. Zarling, M.D., associate professor of medicine at Loyola University Medical Center in Maywood, Illinois.

it pass. If, however, you experience nausea often and can't determine a cause, you should see your doctor, says Norman J. Goldberg, M.D., clinical professor of medicine in the division of gastroenterology at the University of California, San Diego, School of Medicine in La Jolla.

If you've swallowed something toxic, go immediately to a hospital emergency room, where your stomach can be drained and cleaned out using a tube, Dr. Goldberg says. Vomiting could cause the stomach to rupture, he warns.

▶SOLUTIONS

Absorb relief. Many times nausea may be relieved or eliminated with the use of an absorbent like activated charcoal, bentonite clay (available at health food stores), or even Pepto-Bismol, says Steven Bailey, a naturopathic doctor at the Northwest Naturopathic Clinic in Portland, Oregon, and a member of the American Association of Naturopathic Physicians. Living up to its hype, Pepto-Bismol is a great nausea remedy because it contains bismuth, an element now used to treat ulcers.

Sip a syrup. You also can take over-the-counter Emetrol, which is basically flat cola syrup (without the caffeine) with a little phosphoric acid added, says Cynthia M. Yoshida, M.D., assistant professor of gastroenterology and hepatology at the University of Virginia Digestive Health Center in Charlottesville. It promotes burping, which can help relieve gas.

Push away from the table. "Nausea is usually a sign that the stomach is not interested in more food, so I would avoid foods until hunger returns," says Edwin J. Zarling, M.D., associate professor of medicine at Loyola University Medical Center in Maywood, Illinois.

When you do eat, you can eat and drink whatever you like, but you might feel most comfortable starting with bland foods, like saltine crackers or toast, says Dr. Yoshida. But more important, drink liquids you can tolerate, she says. This is especially good if your distress is caused by a gastric irritant; the fluids will help dilute it.

Take up hurling. If your stomach is irritated by something you've eaten or drunk, then vomiting may provide relief, Dr. Goldberg says. "Once you get rid of it, the stomach will have a chance to heal. And the faster you get rid of it, the faster you get better," he says.

▶ALTERNATIVE APPROACHES

Do the peppermint twist. Suck on a couple of strong peppermints (such as Altoids), eat a few peppermint patties, or drink one cup of peppermint leaf tea, following package directions on how to prepare. Whatever your peppermint preference, they usually work equally well to settle your stomach, says Dr. Yoshida. Peppermint is an antispasmodic, so it can regulate stomach rhythms, she says. Be aware, however, that peppermint does promote gastroesophageal reflux, and that can result in heartburn or burping. So if you're susceptible to

History Lesson

The inevitable wish-I-hadn't-done-that post-gorge agony has consumed us all at some point. But even in our nauseated, unbuckled states, most of us wouldn't dare offend the host by vomiting up the evening's pot roast. Yet that's exactly what the ancient Romans did—and often.

When feasting in their "vomitorium," these early Romans would stuff themselves then have their slaves tickle their throats after each course to purge and make room for the next dish.

heartburn, you may decide that the side effect would be worse than your current problem.

In that case, one of your best bets is essential oil of peppermint (available at health food stores or through natural-products catalogs). You should not eat or drink this oil, though. Instead, you inhale it, says Dr. Bailey. This form of aromatherapy can soothe your stomach without putting you at risk for heartburn. Dr. Bailey recommends putting a couple drops of the oil in your bath water or steam bath or on a lightbulb before turning it on.

Let ginger soothe you. A digestive aid, ginger can soothe nausea, which often is triggered by digestion problems, Dr. Bailey says. To make ginger tea (found in health food stores), steep one tea bag for five minutes in warm, not boiling, water. Or combine half a ginger capsule with eight ounces of warm water, or with apple juice. Persons with gallstones should consult a doctor prior to use.

Down beet juice. "Beet juice has been used for at least 40 years for correcting liver and gallbladder congestion, which are common sources of nausea," Dr. Bailey says. Use fresh juice or bottled beet juice (available at health food stores). One popular preparation is Biotta beet root juice. One caution: Never drink it at full strength but, rather, dilute it with other vegetable juices like carrot juice or celery juice, according to Dr. Bailey. He suggests using about one part beet juice to two parts of another juice. The reason for this is that it is a very dramatic liver enzyme stimulant that can make you feel ill if you drink it straight. Otherwise, follow package directions.

▶PREVENTIVE MEASURES

Cut the fat. Fatty foods actually slow down the digestive process, trapping food in the stomach for longer periods of time and making you feel bloated, a condition known as distention, says Dr. Bailey. "That's why, for example, when you eat very fatty stuff, you often get nauseated."

Feed your needs. In some cases, nausea can be caused by a deficiency in certain vitamins or minerals, says Dr. Bailey. Vitamin B_6 plays a key role in the production of hydrochloric acid, so it's especially important in protecting against nausea. Inadequate amounts of hydrochloric acid can lead to incomplete protein digestion, which can trigger feelings of nausea. Dr. Yoshida recommends taking the Daily Value of 2 milligrams.

Magnesium is also frequently missing in diets and that, too, can cause nausea, says Dr. Bailey. For most people, eating well-balanced meals and taking a daily multivitamin supplement should be enough, he says.

Ward off the bug. Pepto-Bismol can work preventively for travelers, who are at risk of picking up all sorts of gastrointestinal illnesses. "Chew one tablet a day while you are traveling to fend off foreign bacteria," Dr. Bailey advises. Another option is to take one to three capsules of acidophilus to prevent nausea during travel, he says. Dosage as well as strains of acidophilus vary between manufacturers, so follow package directions for best results. You can find acidophilus at most health food stores.

Neck/Shoulder Pain

▶PROBLEM

The pain's not only in your neck but also down into your back and upper shoulders. It hurts to turn your head. You live in dread of sudden noises that might cause you to involuntarily jump and crane your neck.

▶CAUSE

It could be a strained tendon, sore muscle, or a compressed nerve from a car accident, sports injury, poor posture, or even sleeping in an odd position.

▶HOW SERIOUS

If you have dull, achy pain, you probably have nothing more than a muscle-tendon strain or spasm. Constant, sharp, burning pain is indicative of a pinched or inflamed nerve. Both conditions usually clear up after a few days, although nerve pain can last longer—until the inflammation eases, says Karlis Ullis, M.D., assistant clinical professor at the University of California, Los Angeles, UCLA School of Medicine. "But if you have pain day and night, or shooting pain down to the elbow or fingers, go see your doctor. That may involve a disk in the upper back," says Dr. Ullis. A constant burning pain that lasts for more than two to three weeks is also serious; have it checked by a doctor.

▶SOLUTIONS

Stretch where it's sore. When your neck is tight and sore, bend your head in the opposite direction of the soreness, suggests Jerome F. McAndrews, D.C.,

DO THIS NOW

When pain strikes, put your head into a "neck-neutral" position, says Karlis Ullis, M.D., assistant clinical professor at the University of California, Los Angeles, UCLA School of Medicine. Hold your chin parallel to the ground, and pull back with your chin. You'll look somewhat like a chicken, and you should have made a double chin.

If the pain is still sharp, put some ice in a rolled-up towel and drape it around your neck. Alternate, ice on for 15 minutes, ice off, as needed, suggests Dr. Ullis.

Did You Know?

"Burner" or stinger syndrome is a common neck injury in contact sports like wrestling and football. A burner is an overstretching or compression of a nerve at the base of the neck. It not only causes neck, shoulder, and arm pain, but weakness in the arm and hand on the injured side. About 65 percent of college football players have suffered burners, according to one study.

spokesman for the American Chiropractic Association. "Don't force it so that it's painful. Just establish a gentle 'pull' on the troubled area, and as it relaxes, let it bend more to the side," he advises. "Hold this for 20 seconds. Your neck will start to loosen up." Repeat this as needed, depending on how tight your neck feels. Generally, doing this four times a day is enough. Stretching not only restores mobility but also moves fresh blood into the area to flush out wastes and toxins coming from injured muscles, he adds.

Use your head. Your neck muscles usually don't get much of a workout except for holding up, bending, or turning your head, asserts Dr. McAndrews. To strengthen these muscles or loosen them up after long hours of driving or computer work, Dr. McAndrews suggests that you tilt your head to one side, hold for a few seconds, and then return your head to the starting position. If just one side is sore, repeat on that side. If not, stretch to the other side.

"You'll feel those muscles relax because they just aren't used to it," says Dr. McAndrews. "Do this a few times a day or as needed when your neck hurts."

Heat it up. You can get a stiff neck and pain that radiates down into the shoulder blades from a spastic muscle, one that is in a state of contraction and unable to relax and lengthen. This may happen after you've really exerted yourself, says Alison Lee, M.D., a pain-management specialist and acupuncturist with Barefoot Doctors, an acupuncture and natural-medicine resource center in Ann Arbor, Michigan. Try applying heat to the area with a heating pad or hot towels, 15 minutes on and 15 minutes off, suggests Dr. Lee. Repeat as needed. To make a hot towel, soak it in comfortably hot water. You can then put the towel in a plastic bag if you want to stay dry.

Roll up the towel. When you're hurting, sleeping is a pain in the neck. You need to support the space between the head and back created by the curve of the neck, says Mary Kintz, an orthopedic physical therapist at Raleigh Community Sports Medicine and Physical Therapy in Raleigh, North Carolina. Roll up a towel, four to six inches in diameter, and place it inside your pillowcase on top of your regular pillow. Then lay on your back or your side with the towel roll supporting your neck. "With a little support, those neck muscles can relax," Kintz says.

▶ALTERNATIVE APPROACHES

Massage it. The trapezius, the muscle that runs from the shoulder up to the neck, is a common site of neck and upper-shoulder pain. Its trigger point lies halfway between the neck and either shoulder, says Dr. Lee.

"I call it the Vulcan Death Grip point. It isn't hard to find because it hurts when you squeeze it," says Dr. Lee.

If you apply pressure to the trigger point for 30 seconds, the muscle will relax and lengthen, says Dr. Lee. If that seems a little brutal and heat isn't working, take a bag of frozen vegetables from the freezer, wrap it in a thin towel, and hold it over the trigger point for 15 minutes, she says.

Find magnetic north. You've probably heard of athletes wearing magnets to speed healing. Magnets are reported to increase blood flow to the sore area and may have some effect on bone, muscle, and tissue factors associated with healing. Dr. Lee uses magnetic therapy and lets her patients be the judge. "Some people swear by them, and I think they can help," she adds.

Dr. Lee suggests that you place the magnets on the trigger points of the affected neck and shoulder muscles. To find the trigger point, feel your way along the muscle until you come to a particularly tender area. Follow label directions. Don't use magnets if you have a pacemaker or other implanted device, she adds. If you can't find magnets at your health food store, you could write to the North American Academy of Magnetic Therapy for a list of manufacturers and product information. Their address is 28240 West Agoura Road, Suite 202, Agoura Hills, CA 91301.

▶PREVENTIVE MEASURES

Change positions. One of the greatest causes of stiff neck and shoulders is holding the same position—staring at the computer or a long stretch of highway—for hours on end. Stop it already. If you're at work, take a break or shift positions every 15 minutes. Shift positions on the road, too. But also make sure that you take advantage of those highway rest areas and rest your neck and shoulders at regular intervals, says Kintz.

Give your neck a break. Much neck and upper-shoulder pain comes from poor posture that rounds the shoulders and juts the head forward, says Kintz. "It puts a lot of pressure and stress on the ligaments, nerves and muscles of the neck," she says.

To give your neck a break, Kintz suggests that you put your hands behind your head, pull your shoulders back, bring your shoulder blades together, and lean your neck back slightly. You can do this standing or sitting.

"If you're having a lot of neck pain, I would do this for five minutes every hour," Kintz says.

Nicotine Addiction

▶PROBLEM

Considered one of the most addictive substances in the world, nicotine keeps more than 47 million Americans puffing away on cigarette after cigarette. Only about 23 percent of smokers are able to quit. If you have to smoke every day, if you smoke your first cigarette within 10 minutes of waking up, or if you experience withdrawal symptoms when you try to quit smoking, then you are addicted to nicotine.

▶CAUSE

When you inhale a cigarette, the drug travels to the brain and triggers a release of neurotransmitters—chemicals that transport messages from your brain to your body—that make you feel good. But after awhile, the brain becomes dependent on nicotine to release these feel-good substances. Eventually, you need more nicotine to get the same pleasurable effects. And if you go without the drug, the brain goes into withdrawal, causing you to feel irritable and downright ill.

▶HOW SERIOUS

Cigarette smoking has been associated with almost every serious disease in the human body. Lung cancer and heart disease are the biggest two, but smoking has also been linked with pancreatic cancer, dementia, colon cancer, and stroke. In a study at the Royal Free Hospital School of Medicine in London, researchers followed 7,735

DO THIS NOW

Set a quit date. Pick a special milestone like your birthday or an upcoming holiday to be the first day in the rest of your smoke-free life. That way, you're not always saying you'll quit someday—a day that might never come. By picking a date, you'll also give yourself time to prepare for the trying times ahead. "People actually do better when you give them time to prepare. Look one or two weeks down the road," says Douglas E. Jorenby, Ph.D., assistant professor of psychology and clinical services program leader of the Center for Tobacco Research and Intervention at the University of Wisconsin Medical School in Madison.

History Lesson

No question: John P. "Honus" Wagner earned his place as a member of the Baseball Hall of Fame. The Pittsburgh Pirates shortstop entered the majors in 1897 by hitting .344 and then batted over .300 for the next 17 years. He won the National League batting title eight times in his 21-year career, with a lifetime average of .329.

When his great career ended in 1917, he had accumulated 3,415 hits, 640 doubles, 252 triples, 101 home runs, and 722 stolen bases. Yet it was Wagner's aversion to smoking cigarettes, not his exceptional baseball prowess, that makes one of his baseball cards among the most valuable in existence.

In the late 1800s and early 1900s, cigarette companies routinely placed pictures of baseball players inside cigarette packs as a marketing ploy, thus inventing the million-dollar collectors' industry of baseball cards. But Wagner, a nonsmoker who thoroughly disliked cigarettes, objected to his likeness being used for cigarette promotions because he thought he was setting a bad example for children. In 1910, Wagner threatened to sue the Sweet Caporal cigarette brand if they continued to publish his baseball card. Production of the card ceased, leaving only 150 in existence. The "Wagner 1909 T206" is known throughout the baseball collectors' world as the king of baseball cards. The last card sold at auction for $451,000.

---

middle-aged men for 15 years. Only 42 percent of those who smoked could expect to live to age 73, compared to 78 percent of those who were nonsmokers. Smokers also report having more problems with sleeping disorders and impotence than nonsmokers.

If you try the following strategies to quit smoking but can't kick the habit, you should seek help, says Douglas E. Jorenby, Ph.D., assistant professor of psychology and clinical services program leader of the Center for Tobacco Research and Intervention at the University of Wisconsin Medical School in Madison. Many hospitals and clinics offer smoking-cessation programs, where you learn coping skills and get to hang out with other would-be ex-smokers who know exactly what you are going through.

Or you can make an appointment with your own doctor, who can offer you some prescriptions to help you fight your addiction. One option to ask about is an antidepressant called Zyban, Dr. Jorenby suggests. Although it contains no nicotine, it has been approved by the U.S. Food and Drug Administration to be used as a smoking-cessation medication after studies showed that it helps smokers kick the habit, he says.

▶SOLUTIONS

Go cold turkey. It's not the most effective way to quit: Only 5 out of every 100 who go cold turkey successfully kick the habit. But giving up cigarettes all at once, as opposed to gradually weaning yourself off them, is the *cheapest* way to quit. And it may just work for you, says Dr. Jorenby "If you have never tried to quit before, going cold turkey is a great way to start. If it works, it's cheap and doesn't need a lot of resources," he says.

Distract yourself. No matter what method you use to quit, you are going to be hit with an urge from time to time. The best way to beat these urges is to have a line of defense ready, Dr. Jorenby says. First, figure out when and where you are most likely to be hit by an urge to smoke. Classics include right after you wake up, while you're driving, and after a meal. Then, think about what you are going to do when you get that urge: drink a tall glass of water; take a few deep, relaxing breaths; chew a piece of gum; or whatever it takes to distract you from your desire for a cigarette.

"Urges can be pretty strong when they hit, but they don't last long. Within a few minutes, the urge is going to pass regardless of whether you smoked. Having a distraction ready allows you to step out of the way of the urge and let it pass," Dr. Jorenby says.

Clean house. The night before your quit date, throw out all your packs and clean out your ashtrays. "That butt that looks disgusting right now when you have a fresh pack is going to look a whole lot more attractive as soon as you try to quit," Dr. Jorenby says.

Search for forgotten stashes. Rummage through all your closets, desk drawers, or any other places where you may have inadvertently left a pack. Search high and low for all cigarettes.

"You may have put a coat away last fall with a pack in it and never thought about it. But if you stumble upon it in a couple months, it's going to be a big temptation for you. Check the house and the car; just don't leave any around," Dr. Jorenby says.

Stay out of bars. "If I had a dollar for every one of my patients who has relapsed in a bar, I'd be wealthy and retired by now," Dr. Jorenby says.

Cigarettes and a drink go hand in hand. And bars are filled with smoke and even more smokers, putting your willpower to a Herculean test. Do yourself a favor and avoid the temptation for at least a few weeks, if not longer, says Ken Leonard, Ph.D., senior research scientist and clinical psychologist at the Research Institute on Addictions in Buffalo. When you've kicked the habit and can cope with the sights, smells, and easy availability of cigarettes, then take your seat at the bar.

Patch it up. If going cold turkey fails, give one of the many over-the-counter nicotine patches (like Nicoderm) a try, Dr. Jorenby says. Or try nicotine gum, such as Nicorette, which does the same thing as the patch. Most drugstores carry these easy-to-use products, and you don't need a prescription.

▶ALTERNATIVE APPROACHES

Make a quit list. Think about why you want to quit. Maybe you want to see your grandchildren grow up, or you want to run a race, or you just want to breathe freer and feel healthier again. Then write it down on a piece of paper or an index card and stick it in your wallet. The next time you feel close to taking a puff, take the list out and remind yourself why you want to quit. "When you are in the middle of one of those big urges, it's not always obvious to you why you decided to quit. Remembering what you stand to gain by quitting is critical," Dr. Jorenby says.

Breathe deeply. Slowly breathe in, then breathe out. It may be what you do every second of the day to stay alive, but it can also calm you down and help fight the temptation to grab a cigarette. "It's a relaxation skill and can help you cope with urges caused by stress," Dr. Jorenby says. Instead of reaching for a cigarette the next time you are stressed out, sit back, relax, and breathe deeply until the urge passes.

▶PREVENTIVE MEASURES

Get juiced. Starting the day with orange juice may be a good way to deter the craving for a morning cigarette, Dr. Jorenby says. The combination of most citrus juices and tobacco makes for an awfully unpleasant taste in the mouth. Many patients have told Dr. Jorenby that even the thought of a cigarette after a glass of orange juice makes them sick. Carry some citrus juice around with you and take a swig when you feel a craving coming. But don't use orange juice as a deterrent if you use nicotine gum, Dr. Jorenby warns. The citrus changes the chemicals in the mouth and will inhibit the effectiveness of the gum. Wait to use the gum at least 20 minutes after a glass of citrus juice or any acidic beverage, such as coffee or cola drinks.

Go for a jog. Getting some exercise may help quell your urges before they start. A study at the University of Wisconsin Medical School found that ex-smokers who got regular aerobic exercise said that their cravings for cigarettes were less severe than those who didn't exercise, Dr. Jorenby says. For an even bigger plus, regular exercise reduces stress and may help keep off the pounds that many people gain when they try to quit, he adds.

Nosebleed

▶PROBLEM

For such a relatively small body part, the nose can spill a lot of blood. Just a small nick in the inside lining of your nostril can open up what seems like a never-ending river of red. Despite the appearance that you're bleeding to death, you'd lose at most about a half-cup of blood, but this is rare.

▶CAUSE

Your nose is filled with hundreds of blood vessels. This constant and quick blood flow helps the nose humidify and cleanse the air you breathe. "The blood flow to the nose is wonderful," says Sanford Archer, M.D., associate professor of otolaryngology at the University of Kentucky A. B. Chandler Medical Center in Lexington. But when one of those blood vessels opens up because it has been dried out, injured, or picked at, all that blood flows down onto your shirt.

▶HOW SERIOUS

Most nosebleeds can be treated within a few minutes right at home. "The majority of people have nosebleeds every once in awhile," Dr. Archer says. If you have been experiencing frequent nosebleeds for three weeks or more, you should get it checked out by a doctor. In extreme and rare cases, nosebleeds can be signs of a tumor or a blood disorder.

▶SOLUTIONS

Blow gently. A quick and gentle blow may remove the small blood clots that prevent the broken blood vessels from sealing, Dr. Archer says. But make sure that it's a mild honk or you may rupture other blood vessels, he warns.

Stuff it. Use a cotton ball moistened with phenylephrine to stop the blood flow, suggests Alan J. Sogg, M.D., an otolaryngologist in private practice in

History Lesson

Using something cold to stop a nosebleed has been held as a tried-and-true technique since ancient times. But other methods of halting blood flow have thankfully come and gone. During the Middle Ages, people inserted a nasal plug of "cranial moss," the fungus that grew on the skulls of hanged corpses exposed to the weather for a long time. Others used "mumia," a black oily substance made of Egyptian mummies. It didn't get much better in the early 1800s when some people used an inflated balloon made of animal intestines to stop nosebleeds.

Cleveland. Phenylephrine is the main ingredient in Neo-Synephrine, Duration, and Vicks Sinex brand nasal sprays, as well as others that you can purchase at your local drugstore. So just use one of those products to moisten the cotton. "Place the cotton ball in the side of the nose that's bleeding and then pinch the nostrils together firmly. You want a lot of pressure," Dr. Sogg says. As you do this, tilt your head forward and hold it for about five minutes. Leave the cotton in for about a half-hour, Dr. Sogg says. But don't blow your nose afterward. It will reopen the closed blood vessel and put you back at square one. (If you suspect that your nose is broken, see Broken Nose on page 589.)

Get cottonmouth. That's right, your mouth—not your nose. This old folk remedy actually works, Dr. Archer says. Roll a piece of tissue or a cotton ball and place it right under your nose between your gums and your upper lip for 5 to 10 minutes. The cotton applies pressure to the blood vessels located there that send blood to the nose.

▶ALTERNATIVE APPROACHES

Make a pork plug. Tired of doctors telling you to lay off the bacon? Here's a good excuse to always keep some around. Take a piece of uncooked bacon (any brand will do just fine) and fold it in half lengthwise, says Jean D. Miller, D.O., holistic medical director of BodyCentered in New York City. Fold it in half again lengthwise over a section of string, letting an inch or so of it hang out either side. Mold the bacon into a small pencil-like shape and put it in the freezer. When your next nosebleed strikes, place a slightly defrosted plug in your nose (allowing the string to hang out of your nose). Gently tug on the string to remove the plug when the bacon melts or gets soft. Compounds in the bacon called leukotrienes will stop the bleeding, Dr. Miller says.

Eat your C rations. Improve your nostril well-being by getting enough vitamin C through food or supplements. The Daily Value is 60 milligrams, but it's considered safe to take up to 1,200 milligrams a day. Vitamin C helps maintain capillary health, which gives the mucous membrane lining of the nose an advantage in fighting off infections by improving circulation, Dr. Miller says. Vitamin C also aids in the creation of collagen and mucus, which give your nostrils a moist, protective lining.

▶PREVENTIVE MEASURES

Pick your friends, not your nose. The most common cause of nosebleeds is what Dr. Archer euphemistically calls digital trauma. "Don't stick your finger in your nose. Nothing should go in your nose," Dr. Archer says. This also goes for bleeding that has already started. Many patients come into the hospital emergency room "with everything stuck up their nose to stop the bleeding. When you try to take it out, it doesn't always come out," Dr. Archer warns. The only exceptions are the bacon or the cotton soaked with phenylephrine that we mentioned earlier.

Keep the air moist. Nosebleeds usually increase during the winter months when the heater runs full blast. The hot, dry air consequently sucks all the moisture out of your nose. Use a humidifier during the winter to keep the air and your nostrils moist, Dr. Archer says. Warm-mist humidifiers do a better job than cold-mist humidifiers, he adds.

Drink up. "The nose is very sensitive to moisture," Dr. Archer says. To keep your airways moist from the inside, drink 8 to 10 eight-ounce glasses of water or noncaffeinated beverages during the day, he suggests.

Give your nostrils a lube job. Put a dab of petroleum jelly inside your nose to keep the nostrils from drying up, Dr. Archer says. Or you can use over-the-counter saline nasal sprays, such as Ocean or Pretz. Use the spray every one to two hours during the dry season, he says.

Oily Hair

▶PROBLEM

The Tin Man envies you. The oil that your head is producing could keep him limber all the way up the yellow brick road. Your hair is limp, slick, lifeless, and dirty looking from all that 10W-30 up top.

▶CAUSE

A big part is genetics, says Fredric S. Brandt, M.D., clinical associate professor of dermatology at the University of Miami School of Medicine. Perhaps your ancestors lived in a highly arid environment that needed all that extra oil. Stress and a poor diet can also be the culprits. Whichever is the case, the sebaceous glands in your scalp are working overtime, pumping out more oil than a Texas gusher.

▶HOW SERIOUS

Health-wise, it's not serious at all. But the social embarrassment can be significant. If, despite all your best efforts, you simply can't get a handle on the excess oil, Dr. Brandt suggests that you seek out a dermatologist.

▶SOLUTIONS

Water it down. If you have oily hair, you'd think that using a shampoo marked for oily hair would be a no-brainer. Think again. It may not help, and you could be trading one problem for another. That's because shampoos for oily hair often contain harsh detergents that could dry your hair, says

DO THIS NOW

If you want to cut back on excess oil in your hair, try mouthwash, says David H. Kingsley, a certified trichologist (a specialist in hair and scalp) and owner of British Science Corporation, which counsels and treats people with hair and scalp problems, on Staten Island, New York. But don't gargle with it. Instead, make a hair treatment by diluting 1 part unflavored mouthwash with 10 parts water. Wet your hair, work the mouthwash mixture into your scalp, and leave it on for 15 minutes. Rinse your hair thoroughly, then shampoo. Do this more frequently at first, once or twice a week, then once a month when your hair is less oily.

History Lesson

Your hair troubles may be minor compared to the legal woes that faced the original musical *Hair*. Simulated intercourse, nudity, and desecration of the flag as components of the show were all cited in the legal attempts to keep the antiwar show off stage.

The Broadway version had been raising eyebrows since 1968, but not until the show went on the road did it face court battles. Then-District Attorney Garrett Byrne tried to shut down the Boston production in 1970, saying the show was too "lewd and lascivious." The Massachusetts Supreme Court finally cleared the way for the show to perform several months later by a tied 4-4 vote.

In Chattanooga, Tennessee, a similar outcry blocked the opening of a production there in 1975. This case landed in the U.S. Supreme Court, which refused to rule on whether the show was obscene but did say that the city board that blocked the show did not follow the correct procedures.

Fortunately for the nation's crowded court system, Quentin Tarantino and Oliver Stone weren't making movies then.

David H. Kingsley, a certified trichologist (a specialist in hair and scalp) and owner of British Science Corporation, which counsels and treats people with hair and scalp problems, on Staten Island, New York. If you have oily hair shampoo, water it down by filling the bottle about a quarter-full of H_2O, he suggests. Otherwise, just use a shampoo for normal hair.

Shampoo daily. "I would really recommend washing at least every day," says Kingsley. Even twice a day if you're going out at night.

Find a means to the ends. Some people with longer hair have oily scalps but dry ends. Condition only the ends, says Kingsley, and then sparingly. Rinse it out well or it could add to the limpness of your hair.

Eschew fatty foods. Too much oily food doesn't mean more oil in your hair. But eating a healthy diet full of fruits and vegetables, says Kingsley, and cutting way back on the greasy, fatty foods not only is important for overall health but also may affect hair health. And make sure that you drink lots of water. Experts say that you need eight, eight-ounce glasses a day.

Go with the flow. Consider yourself lucky. Just think how much money NBA coach Pat Riley has to spend on hairstylists to look so slick. If you can't shut the oil pump off, consider going whole hog, suggests Stephen Moody, assistant general manager of the Vidal Sassoon Academy in Santa Monica, California. Get yourself some Brylcreem, or similar hair fixative, and make the shiny look your hallmark. "With the right haircut and the right look, it works. It looks good," says Moody. You'll look more like Bing than Sting, but, hey, who has made a greater contribution to music? Hair oils, gels, and mousses are available at drugstores, grocery stores, and wherever hair products are sold.

▶ALTERNATIVE APPROACHES

Bewitch your hair. Witch hazel is good for getting excess oil out of your hair. Mix 1 part witch hazel with 10 parts water and dab the mixture on your scalp with a cotton ball after shampooing, Kingsley suggests. It doesn't have to be rinsed out. Try this once or twice a week at first. When your hair feels less oily, switch to twice-a-month treatments. When your hair feels less greasy, do it only once a month.

▶PREVENTIVE MEASURES

Forget the hat trick. Some people with oily hair wear a hat continuously, says Kingsley. That's good on hot, sunny days, but if your bean is bearing a baseball cap all the time, your scalp sweats more, dumping water on your hair. The added water makes your hair look even more oily. Besides, it's good manners to remove your hat at the dinner table.

Can the Cajun food. "If you're going out on a hot date, stay away from spicy foods," says Kingsley. "They make you perspire, and the extra water on the bottom of your hair strands added to the oil that's already there can make your hair go limp."

Keep your hands off. If you run your hands through your hair often, you're trailing an oil slick in your wake. Excessive head-handling encourages your scalp to produce more oil, says Kingsley.

Comb, don't brush. Brushes can overly stimulate your scalp, Kingsley says. Get a good-quality wide-tooth comb. And check the teeth: You want a comb that has smooth edges, not one with sharp corners left from the mold. Kingsley prefers rubber combs.

Oily Skin

▶PROBLEM

Oily skin feels greasy and looks shiny. It isn't, however, the opposite of dry skin, which lacks moisture, not oil. "Oily skin is a result of excess sebum production," says Joseph W. Rucker Jr., M.D., a plastic and reconstructive surgeon in private practice in Eau Claire, Wisconsin. "Sebum is an oily substance that coats the outer layer of our skin."

Sebum provides a barrier for the skin. It slides across the body to create a thin layer of oil that prevents dirt from getting inside. But people with oily skin have overactive sebaceous glands (the place where sebum is produced).

"Your skin is a little more resilient and protected against harsh things when it's thicker and oilier," Dr. Rucker says. "On the other hand, it's more prone to breakouts because the oil is more likely to trap bacteria and become infected."

This excess oil creates a shiny look. Worse, though, is that when the excess bacteria mixes with the oil, the skin becomes inflamed with pimples or just clogged with blackheads and whiteheads.

▶CAUSE

Some people, such as brunettes and other dark-haired people, just naturally produce too much oil. Their skin type is thicker than blond-haired people, and they actually have more sebaceous glands throughout their bodies than thin-skinned blonds.

Some people think that people with oily skin have larger pores, but that isn't the case. "If you have oily skin and your skin becomes inflamed, it will swell up around the pore; and when the light hits the skin, it creates a shadow,"

DO THIS NOW

Twice a day wash your face with a made-for-oily-skin soap that contains salicylic acid, advises Patricia Farris, M.D., a dermatologist in private practice in New Orleans. "Salicylic acid helps loosen dirt and dead skin cells from the pores, which will allow the excess oil to be washed off," she says. "Also, it won't add extra oil to your face." Be sure to rinse well.

Did You Know?

True, oily skin may cause you some degree of social embarrassment. But isn't that a small price to pay for your immortal soul? Next time you're feeling self-conscious, recall the words of Falstaff, the garrulous buffoon in Shakespeare's comedy *The Merry Wives of Windsor:* "I think the devil will not have me damned, lest the oil that's in me should set hell on fire."

explains Dr. Rucker. "If you remove the swelling, the look of 'enlarged pores' will also go away."

▶HOW SERIOUS

Oily skin, like dry skin, is only serious if it's not cared for properly. "It's important to know what skin type you have in order to protect it," Dr. Rucker says. "If you have oily skin, you need to clean it well to prevent it from becoming infected." The most serious problem that oily skin can lead to is acne.

▶SOLUTIONS

Clean well. Your mission, should you choose to accept it, is to clean your face of dead skin cells, impurities, and excess oiliness but not to strip it so much as to upset the balance of moisture in the skin. Look for antibacterial soaps with benzoyl peroxide (triclosan is a good over-the-counter ingredient) and washes containing alpha hydroxy acids (citric acid, lactic acid, or glycolic acid) since the use of these together will cut down oil in the cells and reduce the chance of infection, says Patricia Farris, M.D., a dermatologist in private practice in New Orleans.

Numerous products are available in drugstores with these ingredients, but they can be priced very differently. The amount of money you spend doesn't determine how helpful a product will be. A less expensive product can be just as effective as a high-price item if it has the same ingredients as a name brand, Dr. Farris says.

Be Mr. Natural. Soaps with glycerine, cucumber, witch hazel, or citrus acids can help keep your skin healthy. "I like natural ingredients in skin-care products," Dr. Rucker says.

Soaps made with these ingredients can be found in drugstores (Clearly Natural is one brand) as well as the "natural" beauty products stores, such as The Body Shop and Bath and Body Works that have sprung up in many shopping malls.

Tone your face. After you wash your face, try using a toner—an alcohol-based product that you apply with a cotton ball. "It's very important to use a toner or astringent after you cleanse because that will reduce the amount of soap left on your skin and further reduce the chance of infection," Dr. Rucker says. Once again, he recommends toners with natural ingredients, particularly cucumber, witch hazel, or citrus acids. You can find these products in most stores that sell cosmetics.

▶ALTERNATIVE APPROACHES

Fight oil with oil. Essential oil, that is. John Steele, an aromatic consultant for Lifetree Aromatix in Los Angeles, recommends adding two drops of lemongrass essential oil to a half-ounce of carrier oil such as apricot kernel, flaxseed, witch hazel, or hazelnut oil (available in most health food stores). Apply the mixture to your face after every cleansing, but be certain not to use more than two drops of lemongrass essential oil, Steele cautions. It can irritate sensitive skin. The lemongrass helps degrease the skin and regulates overactive sebaceous glands, he says. Keep the mixture away from your eyes. You may use it on a daily basis, if necessary.

▶PREVENTIVE MEASURES

Keep your balance. Some guys think that if they scrub hard enough, they can actually wash every drop of oil off their face, reducing the occurrence of pimples. Not true, says Dr. Farris. "Men can create a new problem of dry skin if they overbathe and overcleanse in their attempt to get rid of oil," she says. "Then the skin is constantly fighting to rebalance itself."

One of the best ways to tell if you're getting your skin to a proper balance is to wash it as you normally do, and then see how it feels a few hours later, Dr. Farris suggests. Are you greasy? Then you need to find a different, more effective cleanser. Does your skin feel tight? Then ease up on the grease-cutting products. Your skin's not as oily as you thought.

Overweight

▶PROBLEM

Since 1960, the number of U.S. adults who are overweight and obese has risen. According to government guidelines, based on body mass index (a simple ratio of height to weight), the percentage of overweight and obese adults had reached 55 percent of the population by 1998. And in the 13 years that *Prevention* magazine published its annual health survey (using the standard height/weight tables produced by Metropolitan Life Insurance Company), the results were even more alarming. According to *Prevention*, the share of adults who are overweight (10 to 20 percent above ideal body weight) jumped from 58 percent in 1983 to a whopping 68 percent in 1995.

▶CAUSE

It's one of those irrefutable laws of nature: Consume more calories than you expend in physical activity, and you're going to gain weight; consume *lots* more calories than you expend, and you're going to get fat.

▶HOW SERIOUS

It has reached epidemic proportions in the United States, says Albert Craig, M.D., emeritus professor of physiology and pharmacology at the University of Rochester School of Medicine and Dentistry in New York. "Heart disease, high blood pressure, high cholesterol, diabetes, cancer—all are at least indirectly related to carrying excess weight," he says. No less an authority than former U.S.

Surgeon General C. Everett Koop has stated that if he had stayed in the office longer, he would have launched the same attack on obesity that he did on smoking.

▶SOLUTIONS

Audit your lifestyle . . . honestly. A man who's serious about slimming down should start by writing it down, says Felicia Busch, R.D., spokesperson for the American Dietetic Association and a dietitian in St. Paul, Minnesota. "Keep a log of what you eat and drink every day for a week, and emphasize the portion sizes since men often underestimate the amount of food they eat," she says. "They also tend to gloss over the details. For example, you had a sandwich. Fine, but what was on it? Cheese? Mayonnaise? It all adds up, so write it all down."

Log in any physical activity as well. If you're thorough, Busch says, you'll end up with a clear picture of what you need to change. Maybe you're a habitual snacker who eats too much in the evenings; maybe you're getting less exercise than you think. Whatever your story, a log will spell it all out for you.

Build a pyramid. Forget all those exotic diets; the simplest and best eating strategy is to follow the Food Guide Pyramid, says Connie Crawley, R.D., nutrition and health specialist at the University of Georgia Cooperative Extension Service in Athens. In a nutshell, that means generous helpings of fruits, vegetables, and whole-grain breads; choosing lean meats and fish; low-fat dairy products; and going easy on the fats, oils, and sweets.

"Learning to eat right takes an attitude adjustment for most men, especially with regard to low-fat," Crawley says. "The key is the first four to six weeks. Make it that far and your body will learn to prefer low-fat foods."

Stay home. "If you're really serious about weight loss, don't eat out more than once or twice a week," advises Crawley. "By frequenting restaurants, you're setting yourself up for failure because you're much more likely to choose high-fat items." When you do dine out, have a piece of fruit on the way to the restaurant. "This will take the edge off your appetite. When you're ravenous, you tend to eat until you're overfull, which is trouble," Crawley says.

Go halfsies. "When you sit down to dinner, right off the bat fill half your plate with nutritious, low-calorie vegetables," Crawley says. "Broccoli, cauliflower, green beans, peas—but no butter." You'll still be able to enjoy your meat and potatoes (it's *not* about denial), but just not as much of them.

Get walking. Majid Ali, a certified personal trainer, licensed acupuncturist, and sports nutritionist in Reseda, California, likes to tell his clients that when you're in your twenties, you can just look at your running shoes and lose weight; but by the time you hit 40, you actually have to use them.

You say that you couldn't possibly run? That's easy—walk. "Even the classic couch potato can do that," says Ali. "Start with 30 minutes every other

History Lesson

Germany, 1956: Dr. H. A. Nemec invents the ultimate weapon in the war against obesity. The Nemectron is an electrical apparatus that converts household current into "stimulating voltages" that are applied to the body via applicator pads. The result is "precision slimming and toning (of anything from spare tires to double chins and thick ankles) unattainable by the usual methods of exercise or diet." Before you rush out to your nearest Nemectron dealer, here's the bad news: The device was seized by federal agents in the United States in 1961 and labeled fraudulent. If you're curious, however, you can check out the Nemectron and other assorted pieces of quackery at the Museum of Questionable Medical Devices in Minneapolis.

day, and gradually increase your distance and pace. It's the perfect way to start toning your muscles in a gentle way." Once you've built up a little stamina, mix in some running. You may soon discover that there's a full-time runner inside you. Remember that you should check with your doctor before beginning a new exercise plan.

Start small. Making relatively minor changes to your eating habits can make a major difference in weight loss. "You can exercise eight hours a day, but if you don't eat right, it's a losing battle," says Kevin Maselka, certified conditioning specialist and president of both Elite Physique and Planet Fitness in Rockville, Maryland. Pay particular attention to fats. Get yourself in the habit of doing the little things: Remove the skin from chicken, pass on the butter and cream sauces, avoid deep-fried or breaded foods, skip the pepperoni on your pizza. Over the long haul, you'll greatly reduce the amount of fat in your diet.

Wage a two-front war of sweat. To shed pounds and keep them off, you need a combination of aerobic and strength training. "You should have two exercise objectives. First, burn as many calories as you possibly can. Second, build muscle to increase your body's metabolic rate," says Annette Lang, a certified personal trainer at Equinox, a fitness club in New York City. "Any aerobic activity—like running, biking, or stairclimbing—satisfies the first objective by getting your blood pumping," she says. Aim for 30 to 45 minutes of aerobic exercise four or five days a week.

Lang stresses, however, that the goal is to work out as hard as you can for as long as you can. Strength training takes care of the second by helping your body be stronger. Lang recommends that you train your major muscle groups two or three times a week. Go for about 12 repetitions of each exercise with a challenging resistance, taking a day off in between to rest the various muscles. Always get medical clearance first, Lang adds.

▶ALTERNATIVE APPROACHES

Fill up with psyllium. Can a natural fiber normally used for constipation keep you from overeating? Yes, according to Ray Sahelian, M.D., a family physician in Los Angeles and author of *Creatine*. "Just mix a teaspoon of psyllium with an eight-ounce glass of water and take it with a meal," he advises. "It makes you feel satiated, fuller in the stomach—and, thus, less likely to overindulge." Psyllium is safe for everyone except those who have a severe gastroenterological disorder (check with your doctor if you are not sure), says Dr. Sahelian. He suggests using it once or twice daily with a meal.

Stay motivated with creatine. If sticking with an exercise program has always been a sticking point for you, the supplement creatine may be the answer. Dr. Sahelian recommends it to anyone starting a program. "Within a couple days of using it in conjunction with working out, there's a marked increase in muscle size. The benefit is twofold: The results spur you to continue on, and the increased muscle mass burns more fat," he says. Creatine is available in powder form and can be taken with juice; three to five grams mixed into an eight-ounce glass daily will do the trick. Dr. Sahelian recommends going off the creatine one week a month and then taking one month off every three months. Creatine is not recommended for those who have chronic kidney disease or liver problems. People with diabetes should also be careful, since creatine is often taken with a sweet drink like fruit juice.

▶PREVENTIVE MEASURES

Make a commitment. An excellent way to keep your weight under control is by resolving to make a small, steady commitment at the start of every day. "A quick 10-minute walk when you wake up, followed by 10 pushups and 10 crunches, will burn a modest 35 calories. But over the course of a year, that's three pounds you've lost," Maselka says.

Performance Anxiety—Sex

▶PROBLEM

A guy is so concerned about how he will perform sexually that it affects his lovemaking. Some sex therapists call this spectatoring because a man is essentially watching himself perform rather than becoming fully involved in the lovemaking. If he worries that he won't get an erection or be able to sustain one, it may become a self-fulfilling prophecy. Other sexual concerns, such as fear of ejaculating too quickly or being up to performing on exactly the right days when trying to conceive a child, also can keep a good man down. "It's common because the physiology of sex requires a man to perform in one sense: He needs to have an erection," says Martin Goldberg, M.D., clinical professor of psychiatry at the University of Pennsylvania School of Medicine in Philadelphia. "A woman can be a passive participant and still be fairly successful sexually."

▶CAUSE

There is a lot of pressure on men to perform well in the sack. Whether it's a James Bond flick or a cologne advertisement, the relentless message is that a

Did You Know?

Bill Margold has never had performance anxiety, and it's a good thing. His career depended on getting erect and ejaculating readily. Margold, you see, has appeared in perhaps 500 sex scenes in roughly 300 adult films with names like *Cunning Coeds*.

"I never had much anxiety about performing. I was more concerned with forgetting my lines," says Margold, whose career began in 1972 and has petered out to just an occasional role. "I could have sex with somebody in the Coliseum—the Roman one or Los Angeles Memorial. I've had enough sex in my life for 10 lifetimes."

How has Margold done it? By not taking sex too seriously and by taking care of himself. "The trick is one five-letter word: relax. Let nature take over," he says.

"You shouldn't be ashamed of your nudity but, instead, try to recapture the innocence you had as a child," he says. So what really turns him on? Kissing. "That's the guaranteed way to get me up," he says. "I like kissing."

---

man ought to be bedding babes and doing so with aplomb. That's tough enough, but with the advent of the women's movement, our partners rightfully started demanding that we please them in addition to ourselves. It's no wonder that when Junior lets us down—as inevitably he will, on occasion—some of us lose confidence and worry that he won't rise to the occasion in our next romp between the sheets. And the more we fret about this, the more limp he remains. The more limp he is, the more we worry about it. It's a vicious cycle.

▶HOW SERIOUS

Performance anxiety can bring your sex life to a complete halt, says Robert Hawkins Jr., Ph.D., professor emeritus of health sciences in the School of Health Technology and Management at the State University of New York at Stony Brook. "There is no question that the way some people deal with performance anxiety is that they don't even attempt to perform," he says. "It's just easier for them not to deal with it or to deal with it by not doing it."

▶SOLUTIONS

Hit bottom. The next time you and your partner have intercourse, let her be on top. It is perhaps the most relaxing sexual position there is for a man and may help him achieve and sustain an erection, says Dr. Hawkins.

Block out other thoughts. You're in over your head at work, and the debts are piling up at home. Don't bring these or other worries into the bedroom with you, Dr. Goldberg says. Think instead about the pleasurable business at hand—and other parts of the anatomy.

Create the right ambiance. One way to keep your mind on your woman and not your worries is to create the right setting for lovemaking, says Dr. Goldberg. Candlelight, music, or whatever works for you and her.

Get away. Soft lights and Barry White crooning on the stereo won't help a bit if the two of you are interrupted by your young children barging in or the telephone incessantly ringing. A quiet, peaceful setting free of distractions is essential, says Dr. Goldberg. One solution that is fun and not too expensive is to hire a babysitter and spend a weekend at a local hotel being pampered and pampering each other, he says.

Lower your expectations. Don't make it more difficult for yourself by trying to live up to unrealistic expectations, Dr. Goldberg says. "You have to give up the image of the great lover. You have to say, 'I'm not a great lover; I'm just a student of the art,'" he says.

▶Alternative Approaches

Rub out the anxiety. Sensate massage can take the pressure off a guy to perform sexually, says Dr. Hawkins. Here's how it works: Each of you takes turns massaging the other. Both of you are nude, and the massage is done with oils, powders, or whatever the recipient prefers. No sex may occur during the massage, even if the man gets an erection.

"What you're after here is some kind of setting where you can interact with each other in sensuous ways but where there is no pressure to perform," Dr. Hawkins says. "When you do that, very often the anxiety is gone and things happen." He suggests that a couple do this massage-only regimen on three or four separate occasions with the man getting erect before attempting a resumption of intercourse. If the man has a relapse of anxiety, repeat the procedure again. If massage isn't your thing, you can substitute caressing and kissing, again refraining initially from intercourse, Dr. Hawkins says.

▶Preventive Measures

Don't dare compare. Comparing your sexual prowess to other guys—whether it's the boasting of buddies or the torrid sessions you see on the silver screen—is "one sure way to increase performance anxiety," warns Dr. Hawkins. Besides, it's hard to really know how other men fare. "Not many people are going to tell you the truth about how they're performing sexually. Even friends are not going to tell you the truth," he says.

Performance Anxiety—Sports

▶PROBLEM

Performance anxiety is a chronic fear of doing anything—making a speech, eating, playing music—in front of other people. Sports performance anxiety is pretty much the same thing. Before or during the event, you might sweat buckets, your mouth may go dry, your heart may pound, or you may even panic. And you're not the only one. "Even professional athletes get nervous," says Shane Murphy, Ph.D., owner of Gold Medal Psychological Consultants in Monroe, Connecticut; head of sport psychology for the U.S. Olympic Committee between 1987 and 1994; and author of *The Achievement Zone.* "When I work with a team and they're in the locker room before an event, everybody is nervous. There are guys in the bathroom throwing up, other guys pacing, and others nervously telling jokes to get their minds off what's ahead."

▶CAUSE

Most often, performance anxiety is brought on by the fear of failure, says Robert N. Singer,

History Lesson

April 14, 1996: Professional golfer Greg Norman blows a six-stroke lead and loses the Masters golf tournament in Augusta, Georgia, the worst collapse in the history of golf. At the 18th green, his opponent, Nick Faldo, holes a 15-footer for a birdie, then gives the shaken Norman a sympathetic hug. Later, a comedian performing at a Pro-Am dinner puts Norman's debacle this way: "You remember Faldo hugging Norman on the 18th at the Masters? That wasn't a hug. That was the Heimlich Maneuver."

Ph.D., chairman of the department of exercise and sport sciences at the University of Florida in Gainesville. Other reasons include letting down your team or coach, being intimidated, or looking stupid in front of others.

▶HOW SERIOUS

You need some anxiety to perform well. It gets your adrenaline pumping and sharpens your mental focus. But if you can't tame your anxiety, it can keep you from performing at your peak. Even worse, it can make you choke.

▶SOLUTIONS

Use a card trick. Athletes with performance anxiety often forget that they're supposed to be having fun. To remind yourself, list on an index card the reasons you like to play your particular sport, Dr. Murphy suggests. (Any reason is a good reason, he says. Maybe you just like hanging out with friends on the golf course on a sunny afternoon.) A few minutes before you play, look at the card (or just "read" it in your mind). "It will help remind you what you're doing out there, especially during those times when you're calling yourself an idiot," Dr. Murphy says.

Stick to your routine. A routine is a two- or three-step plan that focuses you, mentally, before every stroke, swing, serve, or shot. Devising a routine will keep your attention on the game rather than on your performance, thereby reducing your anxiety, says Dr. Murphy. If you play tennis, for example, you might take a deep breath, decide on your goal (Should you hit a swinging serve wide at the forehand or draw it down the backhand line?), and give yourself a verbal cue (such as "Go for it" or "Relax, let it happen"). "Using a process like this helps you to be ready to do your best at all times," Dr. Murphy says.

Talk to yourself. Weeks, days, or even minutes before the event, use a technique called positive self-talk, suggests Dr. Singer. Basically, you're giving yourself a silent, mini pep rally designed to ignite your self-confidence. "Tell yourself, 'I can't wait to get there. It's going to be exciting. I've prepared well, and I expect to do well,'" Dr. Singer says. But make sure that your inner dialogue is truly positive, he adds. It should focus on your performance and expectations rather than on crushing your opponent.

Know the territory. A more tangible way to reduce your anxiety is to study the layout and physical conditions of the court, track, or field the day before an event. "Go to the tennis court to see what the courts look like," suggests Dr. Singer. "If it's a clay court, what kind of clay? Is it in good or poor condition? If you're a golfer, visit the course and get the lay of the land. Familiarity reduces anxiety."

▶ALTERNATIVE APPROACHES

Imagine your personal best. If the root of your anxiety is a fear of performing badly, a technique called visualization can help you "play" your best in your head—before you ever set foot on court, green, or track, Dr. Singer says. No fancy stuff: Just set aside 10 to 15 minutes every other day in the late afternoon or early evening for a week before the event to imagine yourself in action and performing well. If you're a golfer, for example, "visualize your fairway shots, your tee shots, your putting," says Dr. Singer. "The idea is to relax and see yourself playing to the best of your ability."

Tai one on. Often described as "moving meditation," tai chi has been practiced in China for thousands of years. Because it combines relaxation with rhythm and physical movement, tai chi can be a great help to anxious athletes, says Jerry May, Ph.D., professor of psychiatry and behavioral sciences at the University of Nevada School of Medicine in Reno, who served as the sports psychologist for all the U.S. athletes at the 1992 Olympics in Barcelona, Spain. "It's a wonderful way to practice mental states and get into the rhythm and sensation of movement, which can help your sport," he says. You'll find books on tai chi in the health or fitness section of any large bookstore. One to try, suggests Dr. May, is *Step-by-Step Tai Chi* by Master Lam Kam Chuen.

▶PREVENTIVE MEASURES

Enjoy the game. Don't focus on winning and fearing losing. Learning to let go of the outcome and trusting yourself can go a long way toward reducing anxiety. "Go for the exhilaration of the challenge and let the winning or losing take care of itself," says Dr. Singer.

Be your own best critic. If you're a serious athlete with a confidence problem, do what top-level performers do, suggests Dr. Murphy: Relentlessly critique your game and work to improve any flaws in your technique. Performance anxiety can stem from a weakness in performance, he notes. "A golfer may have a bad swing; a tennis player may have a weak backhand that's being exploited by opponents," he says. "Trying to raise your confidence level without fixing the underlying problem is really shortchanging yourself."

Personality Conflicts

▶PROBLEM

For whatever reason, a certain person in your life rubs you the wrong way. It might be a backstabbing co-worker, an arrogant boss, a nosy next-door neighbor, or a critical mother-in-law. Ignoring their existence isn't an option, and it takes every ounce of your self-control not to punch them out when you're in their presence.

▶CAUSE

Personality conflicts often stem from the relationships we had with our families, says Fred P. Piercy, Ph.D., director of the marriage and family therapy program at Purdue University in Indianapolis. For example, a strong, overbearing mother might raise a kid who grows up to dislike "pushy" women, while people whose fathers were emotionally reserved might grow up to be uncomfortable with gregarious, "emotional" folks. Another hypothesis is that the characteristics you loathe in others represent a part of you that you have suppressed or can't accept. Or you might unconsciously wish that you possessed those very characteristics.

▶HOW SERIOUS

Most of the time, dealing with someone who pushes your buttons is merely unpleasant. But a true feud might cost you a promotion at work or cause a rift in your family. The mental strain of dealing with this person can even lead to stress-related symptoms, such as headaches.

DO THIS NOW

Ask someone who gets along with your foe for pointers on how to work with him successfully, suggests Michael H. Smith, Ph.D., founder of Michael H. Smith, Ph.D., and Associates, a consulting firm in Oakland, California, that specializes in conflict management. "I worked with a vice president of engineering who was having a terrible time with the president of his company," recalls Dr. Smith. Acting on Dr. Smith's advice, this man sought advice from a colleague who got along just fine with the president. Once the vice president understood what "worked" with his boss and what didn't, the problem disappeared.

Did You Know?

If you think office politics is brutal, imagine feuding with professional wrestlers. "Our business is conflict," says "Hacksaw" Jim Duggan, the 6'3", 297-pound carrier of the World Championship Wrestling banner. Here's his advice on managing on-the-job disputes.

Put up or shut up. "Get out there and tell him what you're gonna do to him and when." The bigger the threat, the better.

Deliver the low blow. "If a guy has a weak point—a bald spot, being short, being heavy—jump right on it."

Make the collar. If you really want to end that office feud, chain yourself to your antagonist, suggests Duggan. In a "dog-collar match," the opponents buckle dog collars around their necks and connect the collars to a chain. "Sometimes I wish I could handle my normal life the way I do in the ring," Duggan says. "Life in the ring is so clear-cut."

We know what you mean, big guy.

▶SOLUTIONS

Be agreeable. The next time your foe attacks you, agree with whatever he says, Dr. Piercy suggests. This technique is called fogging. Say that, visiting your family over the holidays, your brother-in-law starts in on how you should run your life—a lecture you've heard every Thanksgiving for years. This year, when he starts in about your dead-end job and asks when you're going to make a change, tell him he has a point and that you're considering doing just that. Remember: If you don't take the bait, he can't reel you in.

Beat it. When a kid has a tantrum or otherwise can't behave, he often gets a time-out—a few minutes alone to cool off. Similarly, grown-ups with flaring tempers should take a break, says Robert Bolton, Ph.D., chief executive officer emeritus of Ridge Associates, a national training and consulting firm based in Cazenovia, New York, and author of *People Skills*. "If you're really out of control, leave the situation," he says. "You might tell the other person, 'I'm so angry I can't see straight, and I don't want to say something I'll regret. So let's talk tomorrow.'"

Be a great communicator. Being involved in a dispute with someone who pushes your buttons can be aggravating. These tips from Dr. Bolton can make it less frustrating and may even lead to a truce.

• Hear him out. This doesn't mean waiting until he has stopped speaking so that you can attack what he has just said. To listen effectively, you have to understand what he's saying, understand how he feels about what he's saying, and repeat what you've heard back to him to show him that you've understood.

Often, what you think he said isn't what he meant, says Dr. Bolton. "When you really try to understand where the other guy is coming from, he calms down," he says. Listening can also help you keep your cool. You can't be enraged if you're concentrating on what he's saying.

• Keep it short and sweet. Now it's your turn to talk. Keep your rebuttal brief and present your points in bite-size chunks. "If you have five points that you want to make, make the most important one first, let him respond, then go on to the next one," says Dr. Bolton.

• Find common ground. Before you give your side of the story, mention a few points on which you both agree. "When people are in conflict, they usually don't think about how they agree with each other," says Dr. Bolton. "It's important to say, 'We have some things in common.'"

▶ALTERNATIVE APPROACHES

Return to center. When your least-favorite person is working your nerves, discover your center, advises Thomas F. Crum, in his book *Journey to Center: Lessons in Unifying Body, Mind, and Spirit.* "To be centered is to feel emotions, to suspend your knee-jerk reaction to fight back or shrink," writes Crum. "When you are centered, you feel a heightened sense of balance, relaxation, and calmness. You are able to recognize that we've all had bad days that push us over the edge into rage." There's no real technique involved, explains Crum. Just focus on where your deepest natural breathing originates. As you concentrate on your breathing, you'll automatically recover your center without trying to figure it out.

▶PREVENTIVE MEASURES

Devise an early-warning system. If you and your antagonist can agree that some topics (say, politics or religion) are too hot to get into, you can devise a code word (*red*, for example) that either of you can say to remind the other to change the subject, Dr. Piercy says. That way, you can continue your conversation without missing a beat.

Phobias

▶PROBLEM

You have an excessive, unreasonable fear connected to a specific object or situation.

▶CAUSE

There's probably no single, underlying cause. You may carry a phobia from childhood, instilled by a parent who feared water or snakes, or whatever you're fearful of, says S. Lloyd Williams, Ph.D., professor of psychology at Lehigh University in Bethlehem, Pennsylvania. Phobias sometimes appear in adulthood with little warning. And they can be linked to an unpleasant event. You may become afraid to driving on expressways after being in a traffic accident.

▶HOW SERIOUS

When confronted with your phobia—such as talking in front of a large group—your heart may race and you may break out in a sweat, feel afraid, and try to avoid the situation. The physical symptoms are a bit like a panic attack, but with specific phobias, you know that the fear is irrational, that it really doesn't make sense, says Katherine Shear, M.D., professor of psychiatry at the University of Pittsburgh Medical Center.

"Still, many people can only cope with their phobias by avoiding situations, and eventually, that begins to interfere with your life," says Dr. Shear. Phobias become a problem when, for example, you turn down a promotion because your new office is on the fifth floor and you can't stand heights. Or your fear of insects keeps you from walking across grassy areas. Or, from a single

DO THIS NOW
Expose yourself. The single, most effective method for overcoming phobias is exposure or desensitization therapy—in other words, "facing what you fear" so that eventually you are no longer afraid of it, says S. Lloyd Williams, Ph.D., professor of psychology at Lehigh University in Bethlehem, Pennsylvania. "The bottom line is that you have to face it. Phobias don't go away on their own. You have to do it to get over it. And the sooner you get started the better."

History Lesson

G. Gordon Liddy, the unrepentant Watergate conspirator and right-wing talk-show host, recounts in his autobiography how he was so phobic of rats as a child that when he once saw one he "felt an extreme urge to urinate." The G-Man couldn't tolerate this weakness in himself. One day, he roasted a dead rat that the cat had dragged home, ate the rodent's haunches, and thought, "From now on, rats could fear me."

phobia—fear of crowds—you develop multiphobias. People who experience agoraphobia (fear of public places) may not be able to shop, use public transportation, or even leave their homes, says Dr. Shear. In that case, you may need the help of a trained therapist.

If you find that, despite your best effort, you are simply unable to face your fear on your own, you should seek professional help. A psychiatrist, psychologist, or social worker who utilizes a behavioral approach to tackling the phobia is an excellent choice, suggests Dr. Williams.

▶SOLUTIONS

Rationalize with facts. Because your fear is out of proportion to the situation, you can use facts and rationality as ways to overcome the phobia, says Richard M. Glass, M.D., clinical professor of psychiatry at the University of Chicago Division of the Biological Sciences Pritzker School of Medicine and deputy editor of the *Journal of the American Medical Association.*

Calm yourself with positive self-talk, Dr. Glass says. Quote yourself the very low risk of being in an airplane crash. Go to an airport and watch dozens of planes and their passengers arriving and departing safely. Stand beneath a bridge you're afraid to cross and tell yourself it has stood for decades and will stand for decades more.

"There's the old adage that familiarity breeds contempt. It also decreases anxiety. Learn all about what you're afraid of, and use as much rationality as you can when you're in a phobic situation," suggests Dr. Glass.

Learn technique. If fear of public speaking is your problem—as it is for a lot of men—then join a group, like Toastmasters International or Dale Carnegie, to learn the technical aspects of giving a speech and to practice talking in front of a supportive group, says Dr. Glass.

"A lot of social phobias are rooted in a fear of looking foolish. These groups work at getting you to relax and be comfortable with yourself," says Dr. Glass.

Look at pictures. If you can't face your fear in the flesh, you can begin by looking at pictures of what you're afraid of. Let's say that you want to go camping, but you're afraid of being bitten by insects. You can get an insect guide at the library, look at pictures of the bugs you abhor, and begin to think about being exposed to these rather harmless creatures, says Dr. Glass.

"At first, even the pictures may cause you revulsion and fear. But the more you look at them, the less that happens," says Dr. Glass. "It makes you ready to take the next step—to actually see and touch insects."

Bring a friend. When you're facing your fears, it can be comforting to have a friend along to provide reassuring words and encouragement, says Dr. Williams.

"Sometimes you can do much more with a friend or spouse than you can do alone," Dr. Williams says. If you fear driving on expressways, your friend can sit in the passenger seat, keep an eye on the road and talk you through the traffic. That person isn't there just to reassure you but also to push you a little to take the next step, says Dr. Williams. "And eventually the friend has to withdraw from the situation entirely," he says. In the case of agoraphobia, the friend may take you grocery shopping a few times and then, one day, wait outside the door of the store while you shop on your own, suggests Dr. Williams.

▶ALTERNATIVE APPROACHES

Relax on cue. When you get the anxiety symptoms of a phobia, sometimes you need to back off and take a few seconds to relax, says Andrew A. Sappington, Ph.D., a clinical psychologist at the University of Alabama at Birmingham.

Try this technique: Breathe deeply through your nose, hold for a few seconds, and then exhale slowly. Let your shoulders sag, unclench your fists, and let gravity tug at your limbs. Repeat this until you feel relaxed. You can also mentally repeat a cue word during each exhalation, a word or phrase such as *relax* or *calm down*, suggests Dr. Sappington.

▶PREVENTIVE MEASURES

Push yourself. Throughout the exposure therapy (doing what you fear until it becomes easy), you're probably going to have some uncomfortable moments of anxiety and fear, says Dr. Williams. "If you're getting really terrified, you may need to back off and catch your breath," he says. "But you don't want to back off as soon as you start feeling afraid. The old saying 'no pain, no gain' applies here."

Push yourself when you can, and realize that most people find that whatever they fear is not as frightening as they once expected, says Dr. Williams.

Pneumonia

▶ PROBLEM

Basically, your lungs are drowning in a sea of pus, phlegm, and other junk. This debris congesting your lungs makes it hard for them to do their job, which is to remove carbon dioxide from the blood and replace it with oxygen.

▶ CAUSE

Pneumonia is caused by a variety of organisms, including bacteria, viruses, and mycoplasma (neither bacteria nor virus, but somewhere in between). Some types of pneumonia are classified as atypical. These include Legionnaires' disease (a bacterial pneumonia), *Pneumocystis carinii* (a fungal pneumonia that commonly strikes people with AIDS), and some more unusual strains of viruses or mycoplasma. Other diseases, such as tuberculosis, can also cause pneumonia.

▶ HOW SERIOUS

It depends on your age and overall health, says Ronald Greeno, M.D., co-director of respiratory therapy pulmonary function at Good Samaritan Hospital in Los Angeles. Guys over 65 or who have underlying health problems, including lung or heart disease, diabetes, or kidney problems, have a higher risk of pneumonia. (If you're in this group, ask your doctor about getting pneumonia and flu shots, advises Dr. Greeno.) In generally healthy people, bed

DO THIS NOW

Drink, drink, drink. "Staying well-hydrated is extremely important," says Ronald Greeno, M.D., co-director of respiratory therapy pulmonary function at Good Samaritan Hospital in Los Angeles. Drinking lots of water or juice will help thin the secretions in your lungs, making it easier to cough them up and out. The old eight-glasses-a-day rule doesn't apply when you have pneumonia. If you're big or have a very high fever, you probably need to drink more.

Not sure? Scrutinize your urine. If it's dark and concentrated (or you haven't had to go in the last two hours), you need to drink more, says Dr. Greeno. But avoid soda, beer, or coffee.

History Lesson

Martha Jane Canary Burke, also known as Calamity Jane—American folk heroine, girlfriend to "Wild Bill" Hickok, sharpshooter, and all-around hell-raiser—died of pneumonia following a bout of heavy drinking in 1903. She was 51. Her last words: "It's the 27th anniversary of Bill's death. Bury me next to Bill." (Bill, by the way, had a less painful and arguably more pleasant death. He was shot through the head while playing poker in 1876.)

rest, "productive coughing" (a polite term for hawking up phlegm and other fluid from your lungs), and antibiotics (if necessary) can clear up the condition in a few weeks. But you still need to see a doctor since pneumonia can be serious even when its symptoms aren't. Symptoms of viral pneumonia include fever, a dry cough, muscle aches, fatigue, and breathlessness. The more serious bacterial pneumonia debuts with high fever; chills; a cough that produces thick, rust-colored or greenish phlegm; and occasionally, chest pain.

▶SOLUTIONS

Reach for relief. "It's usually the muscle aches and fever that make you feel the worst, and you can control these symptoms with aspirin or a nonprescription nonsteroidal anti-inflammatory drug like ibuprofen," says Dr. Greeno. Follow the label directions.

Unplug the heating pad. It won't help the chest pain associated with pneumonia, which is caused by inflammation of the lining of the lung (the pleura). "If you have chest pain, and not everybody does, treat it with aspirin or ibuprofen, which will reduce the inflammation and relieve the pain," says Dr. Greeno. Follow the label directions.

Try a new position. Sometimes a change of position helps reduce chest pain, Dr. Greeno says. "If it hurts when you're lying down, try sitting up. If it hurts when you lie on your left side, try rolling over onto your right," he says. There's no "right" position for relief; "it depends on where the inflammation in your lung is," says Dr. Greeno. So roll around until you find your sweet spot.

Get it up. Your phlegm, that is. Make yourself cough strongly several times an hour, Dr. Greeno says. This should be helpful in clearing the secretions from your lungs.

Move it. Get out of bed a few times a day to sit in a chair, recommends Dr. Greeno. "People with pneumonia who move around improve faster than people who don't because the secretions don't pool in the lungs and get infected," he says. Walking around for short periods, or following a normal daily routine as much as possible, will help clear the secretions in your lungs, he says.

▶ALTERNATIVE APPROACHES

De-mucus with mullein. In herb lingo, mullein is a demulcent—a substance that relieves irritated tissue, especially mucous membranes, says Amy Rothenberg, a doctor of naturopathy in Amherst, Massachusetts, and editor of the *New England Journal of Homeopathy.* Besides soothing the mucous membranes lining the lungs, mullein also acts as an expectorant, "so when you cough, the mucus slides out a little bit more easily," Dr. Rothenberg says. Tinctures—liquid herbal preparations typically sold in health food stores—are often the simplest and most effective way to take herbs, says Dr. Rothenberg. She recommends taking 7 to 10 drops of mullein tincture mixed in a quarter-cup of water every two to three hours during the infection. This remedy, along with other alternative treatments, should be a complement to, not a substitute for, a doctor's care, Dr. Rothenberg says.

Protect your plumbing. Women on antibiotics often develop yeast infections; men get urinary tract infections, says Dr. Rothenberg. So if you're taking antibiotics, take supplements of *Lactobacillus acidophilus* (available at drugstores and health food stores). Dr. Rothenberg recommends taking one capsule two or three times a day while taking antibiotics and for two weeks afterward. This "friendly" bacteria, which is found in your gut and added to brands of yogurt, helps replenish the helpful bacteria in your intestines that's killed off by antibiotics. However, don't use yogurt instead of the supplements, Dr. Rothenberg says, because it isn't strong enough for this purpose and can actually contribute to your mucous problems.

Maximize your immune system. The herb echinacea has long been used to boost the immune system, says Dr. Rothenberg. Another herb, goldenseal, helps fight viruses and bacteria. Both of these herbs come in tincture form. Dr. Rothenberg recommends taking 15 to 20 drops of each herb in tincture form in a glass of water every two to three hours while the infection persists. Do not use echinacea for more than eight weeks or goldenseal for more than three weeks in a row.

▶PREVENTIVE MEASURES

Swallow supplements. Antioxidants such as vitamin C, beta-carotene, vitamin E, and zinc have been shown to stimulate the immune system, which can help you avoid infection, says Dr. Rothenberg. She advises taking 1,000 milligrams of vitamin C per day, along with 25,000 international units of beta-carotene, 200 international units of vitamin E, and 25 milligrams of zinc. Doses of zinc above 20 milligrams per day should be taken only under medical supervision.

Poison Ivy/Oak/Sumac

▶PROBLEM

You never heard the old adage, "leaflets three, leave it be," and pitched your tent atop a soft carpet of shiny vines. By the time you got out of the woods, you were ready to scratch off your arms and face. Unfortunately, you're part of the 67 percent of Americans allergic to poison ivy and its cousins, poison sumac and poison oak.

▶CAUSE

Some plants of the genus *Rhus* contain urushiol—an oily, toxic irritant. Once your skin cells absorb urushiol, a process that takes just 5 to 10 minutes, the body mounts an immune inflammatory response. This response, called delayed hypersensitivity, takes between four and six hours, with the end result being a blistering rash.

Typically, you get poison ivy when you brush up against the plant. Sometimes, you can pick up the resin from a contaminated pet, clothing, or garden tool.

▶HOW SERIOUS

Within 24 hours and sometimes even a few minutes, redness and blistering show up as thin lines on the skin, peculiar to the way you brushed against the plant or infected yourself by scratching with resinous hands. The blisters itch severely and weep a yellowish fluid for a few days until they begin to dry out and crust over.

This allergic reaction can be uncomfortable and even maddening, but there's no long-term damage, says Abraham R. Freilich, M.D., a dermatologist and assistant clinical professor of dermatology at Downstate Medical Center in

DO THIS NOW

Once the resin that causes poison ivy, oak, or sumac rash is on your skin, you have to get it off quickly or try to counteract the allergic effect, says David Winston, professional and founding member of the American Herbalists Guild and a clinical herbalist in Washington, New Jersey. He recommends scrubbing down with an old-fashioned brown soap such as Fels Naphtha, which you can get at some drugstores. Be careful to keep it out of your eyes since it can be irritating.

Did You Know?

Of all the villains Batman has battled over the years, few have been as personally toxic as Poison Ivy.

Along with a vine whip, this human-plant hybrid wields extraordinary powers. She has all plant life at her bidding (what a garden she must have) and is immune to poisons, fungi, and bacteria (no worry about athlete's foot). Unfortunately, her touch and kisses are deadly to all human beings. (No wonder she never gets a second date.)

In the fourth Batman movie, Poison Ivy, portrayed by Uma Thurman, attempted to create an all-plant world. But Batgirl dispatched her with the remark, "I kicked her botanical butt."

Brooklyn, New York. If discomfort, swelling, redness, blistering, or crusting is severe, you should see your doctor. He can prescribe oral cortisone and strong antihistamines, if necessary.

If you inhale the smoke of burned poison plants, you can get poison in your respiratory system, which can also be quite serious, adds David Winston, professional and founding member of the American Herbalists Guild and a clinical herbalist in Washington, New Jersey.

▶SOLUTIONS

Get naked. The resin can remain on clothes for some time, and re-expose you if not washed off, says David D. Madjar Jr., M.D., a dermatologist in private practice in Holiday, Florida. If you've possibly been exposed to poison ivy or its related cousins, remove and wash all your clothes and take a shower. Wash your dog, too, if he was out walking with you, especially if he has been off the leash.

Don't scratch. It's natural to want to scratch any allergic reaction, but breaking open blisters could lead to infection, says Dr. Freilich.

What's more, since the resin can get under your nails, it is possible to spread the poison ivy to other parts of your body by scratching, adds Dr. Madjar.

Pretend it's an allergy. To relieve poison ivy itch, take a recommended dosage of an over-the-counter antihistamine or allergy medication such as Benadryl, suggests Dr. Freilich.

Caution: Antihistamines can cause drowsiness, so avoid any activity where alertness is imperative (such as driving) when taking this drug.

Dry out. Once the rash is full-blown, you'll develop blisters that leak a watery fluid. The fluid isn't contagious, but you can speed healing and dry out the blisters by applying a compress using Domeboro (acetic acid). To use, dissolve a powder packet of it in two cups of water. Then saturate a clean white cloth in the solution, squeeze it out, and apply it loosely to the affected area, repeating every 15 to 20 minutes as necessary. You can also use an over-the-counter hydrocortisone cream, calamine lotion, or both, says Dr. Madjar. If the rash is severe or widespread, or becomes infected, see a dermatologist.

▶ALTERNATIVE APPROACHES

Bathe in your breakfast. Grandma knew what to do. Mix one to two tablespoons of plain oatmeal into a bath or basin of water and immerse the affected area, suggests Dr. Freilich. Alternate your oatmeal bath with cold compresses of plain water. "The oatmeal gives you some relief from the itching and helps dry out the lesions when they are blistered and crusted," Dr. Freilich says.

▶PREVENTIVE MEASURES

Clean up. To keep from reinfecting yourself, clean whatever gear you had with you when you were exposed, says Dr. Madjar. Besides clothes, that means cleaning shoes, glasses, or any garden tools or camping equipment.

Shelter your skin. When you're going into the woods and fields, always wear long pants and a long-sleeve shirt, says Dr. Freilich. That will help keep you from brushing exposed skin against an offending plant.

Bone up on botany. Don't like walking around pink-faced with dried calamine lotion on your mug? Then learn to recognize the three poisonous plants of the *Rhus* genus, says Dr. Freilich. "Knowing these plants and staying away from them is really the best strategy," he says.

Poison ivy can take on many different forms. It can be an erect shrub up to six feet tall; it also can creep along the ground and even climb up trees. As a vine, it tends to have hairy aerial roots. Other than its telltale trifoliate leaf arrangement, these plants can have differing leaf shapes and textures, ranging anywhere from glossy to hairy and toothed, lobed, or untoothed.

Poison oak is the bushy West Coast cousin of poison ivy and is nearly identical in appearance. Both have small red leaves in spring, which turn green in summer and yellow in fall.

Poison sumac (also known as poison elder and poison dogwood) is easier to recognize but far less widespread. This narrow shrub or small tree with greenish flowers grows mainly in eastern North American swamps. The 7 to 13 leaves are arranged on a branch like the quills of a feather, alternating and opposite of one another.

One of the common distinguishing characteristics of all three of these plants is their whitish berries. Keep a watchful eye out for these whenever you are outside, says Dr. Madjar.

Block the resin. Before you go into the woods, protect your exposed skin. You can rub on a lotion containing the active ingredient bentoquatam, such as the over-the-counter product called IvyBlock, says Dr. Freilich. "You put it on like suntan lotion before you go into the woods. It blocks the absorption of urushiol by the skin."

Premature Ejaculation

▶PROBLEM

You are ejaculating during intercourse more quickly than you and your partner would like. How long this is varies from couple to couple, says Robert Birch, Ph.D., a sex therapist in Columbus, Ohio, and author of *Male Sexual Endurance*. The average man ejaculates perhaps as soon as 2 minutes after penetration. "I see guys who go 12 minutes and think they ought to be able to go an hour. It all depends on expectations," Dr. Birch says. He prefers the term *rapid ejaculation* rather than *premature ejaculation*, which has a more negative connotation.

▶CAUSE

Some men are just really excitable. "They're in an altered state of consciousness" during sex, says Dr. Birch. Others are overly anxious. And some men may just have unusually sensitive penises, he says. Premature or rapid ejaculation isn't limited to young guys either. "I'm seeing a 72-year-old man who is a rapid ejaculator even on the second episode in the same evening," says Dr. Birch.

▶HOW SERIOUS

It can be pretty devastating if a guy's partner believes that the only way she can have an orgasm is via vaginal stimulation. If he ejaculates quickly, she may feel he is depriving her of an orgasm. Hard feelings may ensue.

DO THIS NOW

Switch positions, advises Robert Birch, Ph.D., a sex therapist in Columbus, Ohio, and author of *Male Sexual Endurance*. By stopping and switching positions every so often, you're helping to moderate the amount of stimulation you're getting, which will help you prolong intercourse. Ultimately, though, the idea is to find positions that better enable you to postpone ejaculation. For many men, lying passively on their back with their partner on top does the trick, says Dr. Birch. Relax and let her do the thrusting. Not only will you be less apt to pull the trigger too quickly but also she can move in ways that provide the most stimulation of her clitoris, says Dr. Birch.

Did You Know?

If you're feeling a little sensitive about your sexual staying power, here's something that may console you: Pioneering sex researcher Alfred Kinsey, among others, concluded that a man, on average, ejaculates two minutes after penetration. Here's something that may make you feel even better. Some of our fellow primates finish the sex act faster than you can peel a banana. Here are some average times.

Chimpanzee: 7 seconds
Lemur: Less than 10 seconds
Gibbon: 15 seconds
Gorilla: 1.1 minutes

And of course, there are show-offs in any group. Among us primates, it's these guys.

Orangutan: Nearly 11 minutes
Baboon: Multiple mountings lasting more than 10 minutes
Rhesus monkey: Multiple mountings lasting 10 to 20 minutes

▶SOLUTIONS

Take a hands-on approach. If a guy who ejaculates quickly isn't having sex as often as he would prefer, then he should masturbate, says Dr. Birch. "One of the things that will lead to superexcitability is deprivation," he says. "A man needs to be keeping track of frequency and filling in any gaps."

Start and stop. If you feel yourself reaching the point of ejaculation too quickly, pull out and relax for as long as it takes to regain control, says Dr. Birch. This may be a good time to slow the pace and change positions.

Get squeezed. When you are nearing ejaculation, withdraw and have your partner gently but firmly squeeze the tip of your penis, where it meets the glans or head of the organ, between her thumb and first finger, advises Neil Baum, M.D., associate clinical professor of urology at Tulane University Medical School and Louisiana State University School of Medicine, and director of the Impotence Foundation, all in New Orleans. When you've regained control, resume intercourse. If you are about to climax too quickly again, have your partner repeat the squeeze. "It requires a very cooperative partner to help do it," says Dr. Baum. Of course, you can always do the squeezing yourself, too.

Sheath the shaft. Many men find that they last longer if they wear a condom, says Dr. Birch. If this is why you are going to wear a condom, make it one that is not lubricated, he says. Those that are lubricated are warm and slippery, and you know how that sensation affects you.

Call the squeeze play. Doing Kegel exercises can help pump more blood to the penis and provide more ejaculatory control, says Dr. Baum. Contract the muscles you use to hold in urine or to stop the flow—that's a Kegel—for three to five seconds and then relax. Dr. Baum recommends doing a set of 10, four or five times a day.

Tighten up. Some guys wear a constriction band, commonly called a cock ring, at the base of their penis, says Dr. Birch. It doesn't delay ejaculation, but it keeps you from going soft after you do climax by trapping all that blood in the penis that made you erect in the first place. Never wear one for longer than 30 minutes, Dr. Birch warns. He also advises that you avoid using a constriction band when you are drinking because you might fall asleep with it on. Depriving your penis of blood and oxygen for any length of time can prove disastrous, he adds. He suggests using adjustable rings that are easily removable.

▶ALTERNATIVE APPROACHES

Take a breather. Breathing exercises may help you maintain some measure of control, says Marty Klein, Ph.D., a sex therapist in private practice in Palo Alto, California. He suggests deliberately slowing down your breathing during sex so that it's deep and relaxing (it'll take some effort, we know). This breathing technique will reduce anxiety and help delay ejaculation.

Be sensitive to potential problems. Some men apply desensitizing creams to the penis in order to delay ejaculation. Dr. Birch doesn't recommend them because they are simply not very effective. You can never be sure how much to use, he adds, and there is a good chance that the cream will rub off on your partner, desensitizing her as well (definitely not the goal you are shooting for). But if you do go this route, he adds, look for a penis desensitization cream—preferably with Novocain—that has specific instructions for penile application and be sure to follow the directions carefully.

▶PREVENTIVE MEASURES

Don't look. Men are notoriously visual in matters sexual, so keep your eyes closed during at least part of intercourse, advises Dr. Birch. Let's say you're in the woman-on-top position that he recommends. The sight of your partner's breasts bobbing like buoys may quickly bring on a tidal wave of lustful feelings and—uh-oh!—you're to the point of no return again. When you feel that you're under control, then you can try opening your eyes again, says Dr. Birch.

Psoriasis

▶ PROBLEM

You have red, scaly patches of skin. They can be almost any size, depending on the variety of psoriasis you have. Sometimes it looks like a splatter pattern of red drops, and sometimes it's big splotches. Although psoriasis can occur on almost any part of the body, you're most likely to find it on your scalp, elbows, and knees, says Giulio Leone, M.D., a dermatologist in private practice in Arlington Heights, Illinois.

"Psoriasis can be relentless," Dr. Leone adds. "You can distinguish it from other skin problems, such as dandruff, because while those come and go, psoriasis continues to produce thicker skin with a heavier feel."

▶ CAUSE

"We used to think psoriasis was simply a disease of the skin," Dr. Leone says. "Now we realize that it's a very complex disease of the skin, immune system, and joints in some patients."

For some reason, people with psoriasis have immune systems that are overactive, in terms of the growth of their skin. While normal skin cell division and growth takes 28 days, that growth and attempt at shedding happens much more rapidly in people with psoriasis. In fact, psoriasis causes the skin cells to replicate 10 times faster than average skin cells. Because they duplicate so rapidly, they don't have enough time

Did You Know?

The acclaimed author John Updike suffers from psoriasis. He devotes a chapter of his memoirs, *Self-Consciousness*, to the problem and calls it "At War with My Skin."

Updike recounts how ashamed of his skin he was as a child and how it inspired his move, as an adult, to a Massachusetts town with a beach, where the sun could heal his skin. In fact, the sun was really the only thing that helped him. He planned his days and years around psoriasis, going to the Caribbean in the winter and sunning himself in the Northeast during the summer.

As Updike grew older, new and better treatments became available for psoriasis, and it was no longer something to be ashamed of. He writes: "Fifty years have demythologized the disease, to an extent; it is mentioned on television commercials and its 'heartbreak' is publicly joked about. . . . For the first time in my life I own a house within walking distance of a beach, and I walk there scarcely three times a summer. Life suddenly seems too short to waste time lying in the sun."

---

to shed properly. That's why psoriasis is, and looks like, an accumulation of dead skin cells—silvery and clumpy.

Psoriasis also seems to appear in places where there has been an injury to the skin, says Dr. Leone.

▶HOW SERIOUS

Psoriasis will not lead to another illness or problem, but it can greatly affect a person's quality of life. Psoriasis outbreaks can determine which clothes you'll wear and how comfortable you are shaking hands or meeting strangers. If you have it on your genitals, psoriasis can interfere with your sex life.

"In this day and age, no one has to live with debilitating psoriasis," says Alan Menter, M.D., chief of dermatology and director of the psoriasis center at Baylor University Medical Center in Dallas. "We can't cure psoriasis, but there are four or five systemic therapies that can certainly keep the problem under control."

The remedies here can soothe a psoriasis breakout, but anyone with psoriasis should be under a doctor's care, Dr. Menter says.

▶SOLUTIONS

Don't pick, scrub, or scratch. These are three of the most important facts about psoriasis, says Dr. Menter. "Be gentle," he says. "You can use a number of things to relieve the flaking and discomfort, but touching the patches with your hands incessantly will only make the problem worse."

Use cream, not lotion. "You should put a moisturizing cream on just after your bath or shower," says Dr. Menter. He recommends Cetaphil or Eucerin. Creams are thicker and more emollient (soothing) than lotions. Only use a lotion if you need relief on hairier parts of your body, such as the legs or chest. Psoriasis patches should receive liberal applications of cream once, and maybe twice, a day, depending on your level of discomfort.

Use special shampoo. Medicated shampoos will help you if you have psoriasis on the scalp, says Gary White, M.D., chief of the department of dermatology at Kaiser Permanente Hospital in San Diego. T/Gel tar shampoo by Neutrogena or T/Sal, which has salicylic acid, can help, he says. Use the shampoo daily initially, then reduce its use as you are able. Continue using it at least twice a week, leaving it on for five minutes at a time, Dr. White says. Use your regular shampoo the other days.

▶ALTERNATIVE APPROACHES

Get sun cautiously. The oldest and most traditional treatment for psoriasis is the sun. So why is it listed under "alternative"? Because skin cancer cases are reaching epidemic proportions. We now know that we can't sit in the sun for endless hours baking psoriasis away without suffering far more serious side effects.

"You have to be careful and put sunscreen on your face, on the top of the hands, and on uncovered skin, at the very least," says Dr. Menter. "You should have a dermatologist determine how much sun you should get and what SPF [sun protection factor] to use and check any moles before you start sunning. This way, he can watch for changes in the skin."

By the way, tanning booths don't provide the right wavelength to fight psoriasis.

▶PREVENTIVE MEASURES

Send stress packing. "I tell all my patients to exercise and meditate," Dr. Leone says. "Stress clearly aggravates psoriasis, and it's something that we have a great deal of control over."

The doctor's recommendation? If you don't yet have a regular exercise routine, get to a gym, hire a personal trainer, or just start walking 20 to 30 minutes every day. For meditation, read *How to Meditate* by Lawrence LeShan, says Dr. Leone. "So many people hesitate to do this, but I do it and it feels great," Dr. Leone adds.

Avoid alcohol. Alcohol flushes the skin and turns it redder, Dr. Leone says. "I really think it aggravates psoriasis outbreaks," he adds.

Public Speaking

▶PROBLEM

Men fear public speaking more than anything else—more than marriage, more than divorce, even more than death. About half the people who fear public speaking feel their first butterflies by age 13, with the rest getting their first dose of stage fright by age 20.

▶CAUSE

Public-speaking jitters start the minute you think about something going wrong. Examples include: I'll sound stupid. My hands will shake. No one will laugh at my jokes. I'll forget what to say. Such fear forms a vicious cycle. Once you notice your squeaky voice, sweaty pits, or trembling hands, you start to focus more on your anxiety and less on your actual speech. So you wind up forgetting important main points, confusing your audience, and eventually bringing about the result you initially feared—a poor presentation.

▶HOW SERIOUS

About 5 percent of those who fear public speaking get the jitters so badly that they lose important jobs and pass up fun social activities. In fact, the speech communication department at Pennsylvania State University designed a special course for such people when professors realized that some students would rather drop out of school than take the required Speech 100. You can easily overcome mild jitters with the mental and behavioral strategies listed in this chapter. If you're so fearful of public speaking, however, that you avoid even small conversations such as telling a joke to a couple buddies, you ought to con-

DO THIS NOW

Practice, practice, practice. And practice again. Performing your speech over and over again—yes, out loud—gets your mouth and voice used to saying the words, trains your body to say them in a somewhat relaxed manner, and helps you feel confident that you'll make a coherent presentation, says Lawrence Welkowitz, Ph.D., assistant professor of psychology at Keene State College in Keene, New Hampshire, and co-author of *The Hidden Face of Shyness*.

History Lesson

Talking longer doesn't necessarily mean that you have more to say—especially in Washington, D.C. Just consider U.S. Senator Strom Thurmond, a South Carolina Democrat at the time (now a Republican) who, starting on August 28, 1957, filibustered his way to the record for the longest speech ever made in the upper chamber. Thurmond jabbered on for 24 hours, 18 minutes in an effort to block a vote on what later became the Civil Rights Act. Thurmond read the voting laws of 48 states, large portions of the U.S. Criminal Code, and various long-winded federal statutes.

---

sider seeking professional help from a psychologist or public speaking expert, advises Tony M. Lentz, Ph.D., assistant professor of speech communication and director of the Reader's Theatre at Pennsylvania State University in University Park.

▶SOLUTIONS

Know the lay of the land. If possible, check out your speaking location. Know what the microphone sounds like. Figure out how far you'll have to walk to get to the podium. Find out who will introduce you and what he'll say. "The more things you can control beforehand by knowing what's expected, the lower the threat of the situation," Dr. Lentz says.

Hit the pause button. To keep nagging fears under control just before a presentation, take a deep breath and look over the audience for a couple of seconds before actually launching into your speech, says oral communication course director Melissa Beall, Ph.D., professor of communication studies at University of Northern Iowa in Cedar Falls.

See what the audience sees. If during your speech you notice your hands shaking, hear your voice quivering, or feel your mouth drying, remind yourself that your audience isn't paying attention to your hands, voice, or mouth. They are listening to your words. "Usually, the audience will only notice such things if you call attention to them," Dr. Beall says. If you don't believe her, try practicing in front of a video camera. Be sure to have a friend or two present to make you sufficiently nervous. Then watch the tape. You won't look as bad as you think, Dr. Beall says.

Use visuals. Slide shows, pie charts, and handouts give the audience something else to look at so you won't feel them staring at you, Dr. Beall says. Also, you'll have to physically move around to hand out paper, point to charts, or run a slide projector—all of which help burn off muscle tension.

Master your technology. If you're planning on a multimedia show beamed onto a screen by a laptop computer loaded with PowerPoint software, bring two of everything, says Robert Stephens, chief inspector of the "Geek Squad," a computer task force in Minneapolis that repairs computers, offers online technical support, and helps ensure that technical presentations go smoothly. "Assume that your equipment will fail because it probably will," Stephens says.

If you don't own two laptops, rent or borrow a second one for the day, he says. Also, back up your presentation on more than just a plain old floppy disk. For instance, putting it on a removable storage drive, such as Iomega Jaz or Zip, provides another layer of backup.

Repeat yourself. As you deliver your speech, the last thing you want to see is a sea of scrunched up, confused faces. So forget everything you learned in your college basic composition class. Redundancy makes good speeches. Repeating yourself is good. "During a speech, an audience only has a couple of seconds to hear a word and then it's gone," Dr. Lentz says. "So repetitions and catch phrases help key the audience in." Say important points more than once. And outline your main points in the beginning and summarize them at the end, Dr. Lentz says.

▶ALTERNATIVE APPROACHES

See yourself through their eyes. Visualizing your speech while you're relaxed trains your body to stay relaxed when doing the real thing, Dr. Lentz says. To do so, sit down and relax. Then, imagine yourself giving a speech. See the attentive faces of the audience. Hear them laugh at your jokes. Watch them applaud after your conclusion. Take yourself through the visualization a few times before attempting the real thing.

Exercise your butt. And your abs. And your legs. To relieve muscle tension, squeeze your muscles tight, and then release. Do it over and over just before and even during your speech. No one will be able to tell, says Dr. Beall.

▶PREVENTIVE MEASURES

Sweat the small stuff. Instead of starting out with a big presentation in front of a huge auditorium full of nameless people, break yourself in slowly, Dr. Lentz says. For instance, if you severely fear public speaking, you might start out with a short speech to just one person—say, convincing your landlord to fix your leaky roof. Then you might move up to a more-prepared speech to a very small group, like explaining to your son and his friends why they shouldn't throw rocks at passing trains. Eventually, you might read Bible verses in church or present a proposal at work. "You need to establish realistic, achievable goals," Dr. Lentz says. "Put yourself in a situation where you can succeed. The more goals you accomplish, the more confident you feel and the more comfortable you are tackling a threatening situation."

Rashes

▶PROBLEM

In 1995 alone, about 12.3 million people visited a dermatologist because of skin rashes, making them the second biggest reason that people see skin specialists, according to a study from the U.S. Department of Human Services.

▶CAUSE

Getting a rash indicates that your body is having a problem, says J. Greg Brady, D.O., a dermatologist and partner at Advanced Dermatology in Allentown, Pennsylvania. The redness, caused by the dilation of blood vessels in your skin, is a warning or a stop sign. If you are working with a substance that makes your skin turn red, stop and wash the substance from your skin as soon as possible. But skin redness can also indicate an allergy to a food or a medication—or may be a sign of illness, Dr. Brady says. To help find the cause of the rash, you have to be a detective and figure when, where, and what you were doing for the 24 hours prior to the rash's appearance.

▶HOW SERIOUS

If you have no symptoms other than an isolated rash, you can treat yourself at home. But if after a day or two the rash gets worse, you should see a doctor, says Karl Kramer, M.D., clinical professor of dermatology at the University of Miami School of Medicine. If your body is covered by a rash and you also have a fever, a headache, joint pain, or trouble breathing, get to a doctor right away. You may be having a severe allergic reaction, he warns.

History Lesson

The next time you get the urge to mud wrestle, you might want to check out what actually is in the mud first. Twenty-four men and women jumped at the chance to mud wrestle at the University of Washington. Within 36 hours, seven of the wrestlers were covered with patches of pus-filled red bumps. The rest of the crew fell victim soon after. The rash developed where the wrestlers did not wear clothing. Unfortunately, one unlucky victim rolled around naked. The diagnosis was dermatitis palastraie limosae, or "muddy wrestling rash," believed to be caused by manure-tainted mud.

▶SOLUTIONS

Cover it with cortisone. A 1 percent hydrocortisone cream should calm the itch of a rash, says Vail Reese, M.D., a dermatologist with the Dermatology Medical Group of San Francisco.

Stick with it. Combining different anti-itch products can further irritate the skin, so once you've started using a particular cream, don't switch to another to see if you can get better results, says Dr. Kramer. It may take several days for cortisone creams to work, he says.

Soak in oatmeal. Use a colloidal oatmeal bath product in water as cold as you can tolerate to help calm your itchy skin, says Don W. Printz, M.D., president of the American Society of Dermatology and a dermatologist in Atlanta. Soak for 5 to 10 minutes, he recommends.

Cool with cornstarch. Powdering the rash with ordinary household cornstarch can also be soothing, Dr. Printz says. Just sprinkle some on the affected areas of the skin.

Take your Bs. B vitamins can revitalize flaky, itchy skin beset by a rash. B_{12} nourishes the skin and helps new skin cells form, says Kenneth Singleton, M.D., a physician in private practice in Bethesda, Maryland. Take 1,000 micrograms of a vitamin B_{12} supplement every day for two weeks, he says. Then cut back to 1,000 micrograms twice a week. You can continue taking this dosage indefinitely; even huge dosages are harmlessly excreted in your urine.

Tie your hands together. Although it may take all your willpower, don't scratch the living daylights out of your itch. "If you scratch a rash, you make it worse," Dr. Reese says.

▶ALTERNATIVE APPROACHES

Oil up from the inside. A skin problem may signal an omega-3 fatty acid deficiency, says Dr. Singleton. Omega-3 fatty acids are healthy fats found in fish (like salmon, sardines, and tuna) and flaxseed. Ideally, you should get your omega-3's from eating fish three times a week. But if that's not appealing, Dr. Singleton recommends taking 3 to 6 grams of fish oil in a capsule every day. When the rash clears, cut back to 2 to 3 grams a day. You can safely continue taking this lower dose indefinitely, says Dr. Singleton. Or take a teaspoon of refrigerated flaxseed oil three times a day to replenish your omega-3 count and calm the rash. Both products can be found in health food stores.

Scratch the itch internally. The homeopathic remedy sulfur provides relief for people with eczema and can also aid people who have the itch of a basic rash, says Michael Carlston, M.D., assistant clinical professor in the department of family and community medicine at the University of California, San Francisco, School of Medicine. Take one dose (usually two or three pellets) of a 30C potency sulfur product four times a day initially. Reduce the frequency of the dosage as the itching goes away, and stop when the rash is gone, Dr. Carlston suggests. You can buy sulfur in many health food stores.

▶PREVENTIVE MEASURES

Pamper your skin. Dry, irritated skin falls prey to rashes, Dr. Reese says. Keep your skin smooth and moist by using a moisturizing lotion every day. Apply the lotion after a shower but before you dry off. The water seals the lotion into the skin, keeping it moist for hours.

Become Columbo. Rashes pop out a few days after your exposure to the irritating substance or to a substance to which you are allergic. To find out what triggered your reaction, go back over what you have done differently in the last few days, Dr. Kramer says. Rashes form after exposure to an external irritation, such as soaps (especially laundry detergent), creams, or plants. Allergic rashes from external sources, such as cream medications or plants, may not develop until several days after the exposure and may last three to four weeks—even after you've stopped using the offending agent. Once you pinpoint what caused the rash, stay away from it. When the rash has disappeared, you solved the case and now know to stay clear of it forever.

Shampoo your chest. Hairy men frequently develop rashes in the center of their chests, Dr. Printz says. Out-of-place dandruff, just like the stuff on the top of your head, causes these rashes. Wash your chest with any dandruff shampoo to prevent this irritation, he recommends.

Razor Burn and Cuts

▶PROBLEM

Each morning, many barely coherent men take a sharp razor to their face to shear off layers of skin and hair. And you wonder what the problem is?

▶CAUSE

Each time you run that blade across your face to take off the hair, you also scrape off some of the skin cells that protect your skin. "You are removing the cells that form the outermost layer of the skin," says J. Greg Brady, D.O., a dermatologist and partner at Advanced Dermatology in Allentown, Pennsylvania. These are the cells that help your skin retain moisture and form a barrier against irritating substances. Without this protective layer, the underlying skin becomes dry, feels tight, and is easily irritated. This sensation is called razor burn. Cuts are caused by moments of inattention, haste, increased blade pressure, or slight protrusions on the skin's surface, says Dr. Brady.

▶HOW SERIOUS

Other than redness and discomfort, you can live with razor burn and cuts without ever having to set foot in a doctor's office. Men with curly beard hair and African-Americans—who tend to suffer the most from razor bumps—may want to see a dermatologist if the pain becomes severe and they can't find relief at home.

▶SOLUTIONS

Wake up first. If you're stumbling around nearly comatose, dreaming of that first cup of coffee, don't pick up your razor. Give yourself a few minutes to wake up before you shave, advises Dr. Brady.

History Lesson

Hans N. Langseth of Norway didn't have to worry about razor burn and cuts. That's because he didn't shave. His beard measured 17½ feet at the time of his burial in 1927.

Be sharp. When using a safety razor, make sure that your blade is sharp, Dr. Brady says. The increased pressure you must apply when using a dull blade is one cause of razor cuts. Change blades every three to four days, he advises.

Jump in the shower. If you cut yourself shaving, hop right into the shower, says Vail Reese, M.D., a dermatologist with the Dermatology Medical Group of San Francisco. The hot water hitting your face constricts the blood vessels, stopping the bleeding. Shaving before you shower also makes it easier to wash off the blood.

Vary your shaving methods. Switching back and forth between an electric and a wet razor cuts down on razor burn, says Don W. Printz, M.D., president of the American Society of Dermatology and a dermatologist in Atlanta. "Using either an electric or a regular razor doesn't seem to make a difference. But periodically varying the two for some reason does," he says. Use each method four to six weeks and then switch, Dr. Printz suggests.

Apply hydrocortisone. Cover your bearded area right after shaving with a 1 percent hydrocortisone cream every four or five days, Dr. Reese says. The cream decreases the pain and inflammation from razor burn.

Don't dab. If you do cut yourself, don't dab at it. "When people cut themselves, they dab the wound for a few seconds. All they are doing is perpetuating the bleeding," says Karl Kramer, M.D., clinical professor of dermatology at the University of Miami School of Medicine. Remember that pressure is the key.

▶ALTERNATIVE APPROACHES

Cure trauma with Traumeel. A homeopathic cream remedy named Traumeel, available in health food stores, soothes the pain of razor burn and razor bumps, says Kenneth Singleton, M.D., a physician in private practice in Bethesda, Maryland. Apply a pea-size dab of Traumeel to your face each day after shaving, he suggests.

Mind your own beeswax. "For shaving, the best product I have ever used is a mixture of olive oil and beeswax," says Steven Bailey, a naturopathic doctor at the Northwest Naturopathic Clinic in Portland, Oregon, and a member of the American Association of Naturopathic Physicians. The combination of the two contains healing agents that soothe your irritated skin, he says. It also makes for a good moisturizer.

You can buy ready-made olive oil and beeswax mixtures that contain a variety of herbs in health food stores. Dr. Bailey offers the following recipe to make it yourself. Over low heat, warm eight ounces of olive oil with one tablespoon each of the following dried herbs: calendula, comfrey, lavender flowers, and thyme. The calendula and comfrey are soothing herbs, and the lavender and thyme are antiseptic. When the herbs become a little crisp and the olive oil takes on some color from the herbs, strain the mixture and add two ounces of beeswax, stirring until the beeswax melts. Let cool. Store in a jar at room temperature away from sunlight. Apply this healing salve to cuts or abrasions after you shave.

Cream it with calendula. The calendula flower has been used through the years to treat various skin problems, and razor burn is no exception. Apply a calendula cream, which can be found in health food stores, to your face when suffering from razor burn, says Michael Carlston, M.D., assistant clinical professor in the department of family and community medicine at the University of California, San Francisco, School of Medicine.

▶PREVENTIVE MEASURES

Wash your face. Cleaning your face with soap and water before you shave removes a superficial skin layer and softens the beard, Dr. Reese says. Both protect the skin from razor burn and razor bumps.

Washing your face exclusively with an antibacterial soap helps prevent secondary infection, says Dr. Printz.

Get ready for the razor. You'll need to ready your beard for harvesting, but how you prepare depends on which type of razor you're using. If you're shaving with a blade, hold warm water on your face (either with or without a washcloth) for a few moments. This makes the hair swell and stand up stiffer, making it easier to razor them off. If razor burn plagues you, try a shaving cream made for sensitive skin, says Dr. Reese.

An electric shaver needs a dry, stiff surface to work on. So make sure that your face is completely dry. Otherwise, it'll irritate the skin, cautions Dr. Reese.

Stay moist. After you shave, splash your face with water. Before the water dries, apply a layer of moisturizing lotion, Dr. Reese says. The lotion and water combination keeps the skin smooth and protects it from razor burn.

Avoid products with high alcohol content, though. They'll burn and irritate your skin, Dr. Brady warns.

Go with the grain. It may not give you as close a shave, but it will save you from the irritation of razor burn. Shave with the flow of your hair, usually with downward strokes, Dr. Printz says. Shaving with the grain takes off less skin, giving it more protection against infection, he adds.

Skip a day. If you can get away with it, shave every other day, Dr. Reese says. The free day allows the skin to be replenished between shaves and lessens the inflammation. If you can't do it every other day, take a day off every few days. Taking an occasional break also relieves razor bumps.

Rectal Itch

▶PROBLEM

The name says it all: You have an itch in a place where it ain't polite to scratch. Its formal name is *pruritus ani*, but even doctors often just call it itchy butt. "If you look at it, it looks like a really terrible case of diaper rash," says David Beck, M.D., chairman of the department of colorectal surgery at the Ochsner Clinic in New Orleans. "The skin just looks painful." We'll take your word on that, Dr. Beck.

DO THIS NOW

Sprinkle cornstarch or baby powder on a cotton ball and dust around your anus to keep it dry and alleviate itching, advises David Beck, M.D., chairman of the department of colorectal surgery at the Ochsner Clinic in New Orleans.

▶CAUSE

There are three primary reasons that you have an itch you can't ditch: excessive anal hygiene, not enough anal hygiene, or diet. Each can cause your anus to be chronically moist. "It's akin to having your hand in dishwater for a period of time, or soldiers walking in a swamp and getting trench foot," Dr. Beck says. The skin thickens, develops folds, itches, and becomes more easily injured. Occasionally, itchy butt may be caused by a skin disease such as eczema or psoriasis and may require a visit to the dermatologist. Prolapsed hemorrhoids and scar tissue from an earlier surgery also can cause moistness.

▶HOW SERIOUS

Rectal itch is not serious. Perhaps no malady lends itself so well to home remedies. Most of the time these home treatments will alleviate your itching, so a trip to the doctor is not necessary. "However, if after trying these home remedies your itching doesn't stop, consult your primary care physician, a colorectal surgeon, or a dermatologist," advises Dr. Beck.

▶SOLUTIONS

Blow-dry your buttocks. After a bath, a sweaty workout, or any other time your anus may be moist, set your blow-dryer on the cool setting, spread

History Lesson

It wasn't so long ago that our forefathers were putting newspapers, department store catalogs, pamphlets, and advertisements to double duty in outhouses and bathrooms, where they served as both reading material and toilet paper.

The first commercially packaged toilet paper in America was introduced in 1857 but was available only in packages of individual sheets and sold poorly. Toilet tissue on a perforated roll was marketed in England in 1879, but it also fared poorly, perhaps because advertising such an unmentionable product during the Victorian era was so difficult.

In the 1880s, brothers Edward and Clarence Scott began selling rolls of toilet paper in the United States in unmarked, plain brown wrappers. With many homes, restaurants, and hotels beginning to convert to indoor plumbing at about the same time, their toilet paper—later called ScotTissue—was a success. It claimed to be "soft as old linen." Competitors followed, and so did advertising wars. Stated one ScotTissue ad: "They have a pretty house, Mother, but their bathroom paper hurts."

those cheeks, and gently dry the area, advises Steven Wexner, M.D., director of the anorectal physiology laboratory at Cleveland Clinic Florida in Fort Lauderdale.

At *Men's Health*, we would add a caveat: Don't do this in the locker room in front of the guys at your gym.

Wear boxers, not briefs. Briefs tend to hold in sweat, while boxers let more air circulate, Dr. Beck says. For the same reason, he also advises against exercising in tight clothes and wearing bicycle shorts if you have rectal itching.

Change undershorts often. If you're engaged in a sweaty activity in which you are still wearing your undershorts, put on a fresh, dry pair when you are finished exerting yourself, Dr. Beck advises.

Wipe sufficiently. If you don't wipe thoroughly, "the stool is sitting on the skin and irritates it," says Dr. Wexner.

Don't wipe excessively. Some guys, however, "try polishing their bottoms, rub it and scrape it, and denude the skin," says Dr. Wexner. For some men, eliminating itchy butt can be as simple as "calming down a bit and not being so anally compulsive about trying to sterilize their anus after a bowel movement," Dr. Wexner says.

Dr. Beck recommends wiping with dampened toilet paper to help loosen and remove the stool and then patting dry. "Then if you wipe too hard, it kind of falls apart. It's self-limiting."

Don't reach for Vaseline. Vaseline and certain other balms and lotions may make your itchy bum feel better, but they are waterproof and hold moisture in—exactly what you should be trying to avoid, says Dr. Beck. Instead, look for one of the over-the-counter mild steroid creams, he suggests. One on the market that Dr. Beck recommends is ProctoCream, a 1 percent hydrocortisone cream, available over the counter at drugstores nationwide. Follow the package directions carefully, but don't use it every day. Chronic use of steroid creams may weaken the rectal skin permanently, he cautions.

▶ALTERNATIVE SOLUTIONS

Be a foot soldier. Foot powder is designed to keep your feet dry. But here's a little secret: It also works on your butt, says Dr. Beck. Just sprinkle a bit down there once or twice a day.

Try aloe. Aloe gel or lotion is water-soluble, allowing your skin to breathe, and some people find that it soothes rectal itch, says Dr. Beck. But he cautions that other folks have an adverse skin reaction to it. Test a small patch of skin first, and if there is no adverse reaction, you can use it once or twice a day until your symptoms have resolved, he advises.

▶PREVENTIVE MEASURES

Give your food some thought. Certain foods and beverages can cause you to have a stool that burns or itches. Some of the culprits are spicy foods, caffeine and cola products, foods that contain tomatoes, and alcoholic drinks, Dr. Wexner says. "There is even some evidence that beer may lower the sphincter pressure and allow for more leakage," he says.

Dr. Wexner suggests eliminating these foods from your diet one at a time, then add them back in moderation until you find those that cause you problems. He and Dr. Beck both recommend a diet that includes plenty of fiber—fruits, vegetables, bran cereal, and nuts—for healthier, less troublesome bowel movements.

Red Nose

▶PROBLEM

Rosacea, in its different stages, can look like a lot of things: a sunburn, blushing, pimples, even a swollen nose. In fact, the problem is most commonly associated with W. C. Fields, whose bulbous nose was considered a sign of alcoholism, says Patricia Farris, M.D., a dermatologist in private practice in New Orleans. But the acerbic comedian's nose was really the final-stage symptom of a long-running disorder, and not a funny one at that.

"The first changes a man will notice with rosacea is a diffuse reddening that almost looks like a sunburn across his nose and cheeks," says Dr. Farris. "Most men miss the early stages, and that's when we can do the most to treat it." Rosacea also appears as broken blood vessels, or sometimes little pimples or red bumps, across the nose and cheeks and less commonly on the forehead.

Rhinophyma, or nose growth, is one of the last-stage symptoms of rosacea, and it can be accompanied by pustules and bloodshot eyes. At first, the symptoms of rosacea come and go. But eventually, they become more difficult to suppress and last for longer periods of time.

▶CAUSE

"If I knew what caused rosacea, I'd be a rich man," says Vail Reese, M.D., a dermatologist with the Dermatology Medical Group of San Francisco. "We know very little about it. It's chronic, doctors can prescribe antibiotic treatments

DO THIS NOW

"Protecting yourself from the sun is the number one thing you can do to prevent a flare-up of rosacea, which causes a red nose and blotchy skin," says Vail Reese, M.D., a dermatologist with the Dermatology Medical Group of San Francisco. "If you're going to be outside, make sure that you wear sunscreen and a hat."

Sunscreen should be applied at least a half-hour before you go outside. Look for an SPF (sun protection factor) of at least 15, although 30 is preferred. Re-apply the sunscreen whenever you get wet or sweat a lot, or if you've been outside for more than a couple of hours, Dr. Reese says.

History Lesson

In 1996, President Bill Clinton was diagnosed with rosacea. Of course, anyone used to seeing the bulbous-nosed caricatures of Clinton drawn by those paragons of sensitivity, editorial cartoonists, could have figured that out for themselves.

that suppress it, and there are things you can do to help control it. But as to why it happens to some people and not others, no one really knows."

All that's really known about rosacea is that it begins to occur when fair-skinned, blond adults are in their thirties and forties. Although its proper full name is acne rosacea, the disease is less of a skin problem and more of a vascular (vein) disorder. The redness doesn't occur because of clogged pores but from enlarged blood vessels.

Unfortunately, because rosacea can very much resemble pimples, guys will try to treat the rosacea the same way they used to treat their teenage acne, but that tends to make the problem worse. And, although women are more likely to get rosacea, men are more likely to suffer from rhinophyma.

▶ HOW SERIOUS

Other than the symptoms it presents, rosacea doesn't lead to more serious problems. However, having a nose like W. C. Fields is a pretty big problem. Basically, some people who aren't in the know will assume that a person with rosacea drinks too much, which doesn't help anyone's career or social life.

Although these home remedies will help you prevent flare-ups of rosacea, you need a doctor's care and, possibly, prescriptions to truly keep the problem at bay, Dr. Reese says. If you're in your thirties or forties and suddenly find yourself breaking out, see a dermatologist. Only he can determine if you have rosacea or if it's another disorder. Then, too, only he will be able to give you the proper antibiotics to fully fight it, Dr. Reese says.

▶ SOLUTIONS

Go easy on the alcohol. Rosacea may not be a sign that W. C. Fields drank too much, but there's no question that if he did drink, the alcohol made his problem worse. "Alcohol causes outbreaks of rosacea because it engorges the blood vessels," Dr. Farris says. "That makes your face look redder."

Watch your diet. Avoid hot and spicy foods as well as caffeine and you'll avoid the two leading causes of rosacea outbreaks, Dr. Reese says. But because there are so many foods that are reputed to cause rosacea flare-ups, Dr. Reese advises his patients to keep a record of what they eat.

"If your rosacea begins to act up, you can look back a day or two at your record to try to figure out what caused it," he says. "Patients are usually willing to cut out certain foods if they can be sure about what causes the problem."

Keep cool. Heat is a cause of flare-ups. So dress in layers of light clothing that you can remove to keep your body cool, says Mary Lupo, M.D., associate clinical professor of dermatology at Tulane University School of Medicine in New Orleans. Also, don't head for the sauna or hot tub.

▶ALTERNATIVE APPROACHES

Get bitter. "I believe that most of my patients with rosacea don't produce enough hydrochloric acid," says Eugene Zampieron, a doctor of naturopathy in Middlebury, Connecticut, and a professional member of the American Herbalists Guild. Drinking or eating bitters helps wake up their digestive systems, he adds.

Look for bitter herb combinations sold at health food stores. They will most likely include gentian, dandelion root, barberry or Oregon grape root, prickly ash, and centaury. These are often found in tincture form. Put about a quarter-teaspoon in about two ounces of warm water and sip it about a half-hour prior to eating heavy meals, like lunch and supper, Dr. Zampieron says.

Caution: People with stomach irritation, inflammation, or ulcers should not use gentian. People with gallbladder problems should not use dandelion root.

Hit the salad bar. Try a salad with bitter greens, including escarole, dandelion leaves, broccoli rabe, chicory, radicchio, and arugala, Dr. Zampieron says.

▶PREVENTIVE MEASURES

Stay cool. Just as hot and spicy foods bring on rosacea, so does being too overheated from exercise or hot weather. "Don't get overheated from exercise or lifting something that's too heavy," Dr. Farris says. "Any situation that has ever caused you to get red in the face is likely to bring on a flare-up, so try to adjust your habits accordingly."

Stay calm and collected. Stress also will bring on rosacea flare-ups. Think about it: Lots of angry or frustrated people describe themselves as "steamed" or "hot under the collar." If you have acne rosacea, look for ways to relax, such as meditation or long walks, Dr. Zampieron recommends.

Restless Legs

▶PROBLEM

When you have restless legs, you just gotta move. It's the only way to relieve the creepy-crawly sensation in your legs that happens when you lay down in bed or have to sit still at a movie or business meeting. In its mildest form, sensations occur around bedtime (as they may be tied to your circadian rhythm) or when you are sitting still for any prolonged period of time, says Peter Fotinakes, M.D., director of the University of California—Irvine Sleep Disorders Center. In severe cases, the sensation is ever-present, he adds.

▶CAUSE

Doctors don't know the causes of restless legs. It sometimes runs in families or may be associated with iron deficiency, rheumatoid arthritis, kidney disease, diabetes, and neurological malfunctions in the brain or spinal cord.

▶HOW SERIOUS

Not necessarily painful, but certainly extremely unpleasant, restless legs is an annoyance, usually relieved without medications. In the early stages, you only get the "crawlies" around bedtime because the problem occurs when you're at rest. In its severe stages, the symptoms will appear during the day whenever you are sitting still for a time. The key point is that symptoms can range from extremely mild to extremely severe, says William Ondo, M.D., assistant professor of neurology at Baylor College of Medicine in Houston. At its worst, people with restless legs are driven to distraction, by the sensation of swarms of ants running under their skin. And in extreme cases, it can cause disruption in daily functioning.

It can really drive you crazy, adds Mark Buchfuhrer, M.D., a physician and medical advisor to the Southern California Restless Leg Syndrome Support Group in Los Angeles. He explains that restless legs usually will get worse as you get older, although many people remain at the milder stage of the syndrome.

When you find yourself pacing the lobby while your wife watches a movie alone, or you no longer fly because you can't stay put in your seat, it's time to see a doctor—probably a neurologist or sleep specialist, says Dr. Ondo. The doctor may treat you with L-dopa (Sinemet) or other drugs developed for Parkinson's disease. Other prescription drugs have proven helpful: opiates like codeine and methadone, and antiseizure medications and sleeping pills like clonazepam. "In some combination, the drugs usually do the trick. Probably 90 percent of people can be satisfactorily treated," says Dr. Ondo. "But it's no cure. Drugs only relieve the symptoms."

▶SOLUTIONS

Work out the bugs. Exercise and physical activity seem to relieve restless leg symptoms by stimulating the nerves in the legs or simply taking your mind off the sensations, says Dr. Fotinakes. "I have patients with exercise bikes right by their beds," he says. "They ride for 30 minutes before lying down. If they wake up, they ride again until the sensations go away."

Caution: Exercise right at bedtime can pump up your metabolism and may make you less sleepy, warns Dr. Fotinakes. What you may want to do is exercise in the late afternoon so that you're more fatigued at bedtime. Then your tiredness may be more powerful than the sensations. "Experiment to see what works for you," he suggests.

Iron out the problem. A shortage of iron, folate, and vitamin B_{12} may trigger restless legs. You can increase folate and iron levels by eating green vegetables, liver, kidney beans, lentils, and wheat germ, says Dr. Buchfuhrer.

"We usually associate iron deficiency with women of menstruating age; men usually are not anemic. So if I have a male patient with low iron levels, I always check into other possible conditions," says Dr. Buchfuhrer. "Restless legs caused by an iron shortage may actually be a sign of another disease like a bleeding ulcer."

Before considering supplements, have your doctor test your blood and eliminate other causes of iron deficiency, suggests Dr. Buchfuhrer.

▶ALTERNATIVE APPROACHES

Have a kava. Some people with restless legs syndrome find relief with kava (*Piper methysticum*), an herbal remedy known for its for antispasmodic properties, says David Winston, professional and founding member of the American Herbalists Guild and a clinical herbalist in Washington, New Jersey. Kava is available at most health food stores in two forms: as a standardized extract in capsule form, or as a tincture. If you use the tincture, take two to three milliliters (about 40 to 60 drops) three times a day. Tincture is an acquired taste, says Winston. He recommends mixing the tincture into a little juice or tea (about two to three ounces). If using the capsule form, take one or two capsules (about 1,500 milligrams total) a day.

"Kava acts as an anti-anxiety medicine," says Winston. He does not recommend using kava for preventive reasons but to treat restless legs syndrome as needed. Kava, if taken at these recommended doses, for short periods of time is perfectly safe, Winston adds. But when taken in extremely high amounts, kava can cause a chronic skin problem. Do not take kava if you are currently taking benzodiazepines (such as Valium). And if you are a regular drinker (more than two drinks a day), you should know that kava intensifies the effects of alcohol.

Stop spasms with skullcap. Skullcap (*Scutellaria lateriflora*) is another effective herb used for treatment of restless legs as well as spasms, palsies, and twitches, explains Winston. Buy it as a fresh tincture (available at most herbal stores) and take five milliliters (one teaspoon) two or three times a day as needed, he says.

▶ PREVENTIVE MEASURES

Engage your brain. Help your kid with her algebra, dispatch an angry letter to the gas company, or defend your end of a political debate at dinner and you probably won't be aware of your restless legs, says Dr. Buchfuhrer.

"When the brain's really engaged, it's able to inhibit the sensations. But the activity has to be mentally challenging. Watching TV and reading are too passive," says Dr. Buchfuhrer. Video and computer games work. Some people can tolerate long car trips and airplane flights by playing games on laptop computers, says Dr. Buchfuhrer.

Road Rage

▶PROBLEM

About 96 percent of road-ragers are men. Road rage is expressed anger on the highway: horn blowing, hostile stares, retaliation through tailgating, flicking headlights, and screaming and throwing things at other drivers. You're not just driving fast; you're driving recklessly and lashing out at anyone who gets in your way, says Arnold P. Nerenberg, Ph.D., a clinical psychologist and road-rage expert in private practice in Whittier, California. "In a road-rage episode, you're actively expressing and communicating your hostility directly at another driver," he says.

▶CAUSE

What set you off could have been that jerk furiously blinking his lights and riding within a hair's breadth of your rear bumper. Or maybe you were late for an appointment or mad at your boss or just bummed that the Cold War is over, and this traffic jam was just the last straw.

What triggers road rage is a combination of stress and frustration. It may have very little to do with traffic conditions, says E. Scott Geller, Ph.D., professor of psychology at the Virginia Polytechnic Institute and State University in Blacksburg. "Frustration leads to aggression, and when some people are in their cars, they just let their aggressions go," Dr. Geller says. "You can feel anonymous dealing with anonymous folks you'll never see again. Under those circumstances, you may do things you would never do face-to-face."

DO THIS NOW

Imagine that jerk is a pothole. Most events that set off road rage are accidental or careless but rarely personal, says Andrew A. Sappington, Ph.D., a clinical psychologist who facilitates the Anger Management Group at the University of Alabama at Birmingham. The other driver is not out to get you. Treat a bad driver as a road hazard, akin to a pothole or truck tire tread lying on the highway, Dr. Sappington says. "You deal with it, go around it, and then forget it," he says. "You don't get mad at a pothole and try to do it harm. The same should be true of other drivers."

▶How Serious

If you're flipping the bird to old ladies, spewing spittle on the dashboard, and exhibiting other road rage–type behaviors more than twice a year, then you have a mild case of road rage. Doing these things 20 to 30 times a year puts you in the moderate category. And if you're expressing your hostility toward other drivers more than 40 times a year, you have a severe case of road rage, Dr. Nerenberg warns.

And that anger probably results in behavior that is dangerous to other drivers, your passengers, and yourself, Dr. Nerenberg says. It might seem harmless to toss off a few obscene gestures or drop-dead glares at other drivers, but someday that object of your scorn may pull out a gun or a crowbar or follow you home.

"Often one retaliation leads to another, and people end up getting killed over the most trivial of incidents," says Dr. Nerenberg. Most men are able to stop their road rage–type behavior once they recognize that they have a problem, he says. But if you realize that you're a road-rager and you can't seem to change your behavior even though you've tried, you may want to seek the help of a psychologist, Dr. Nerenberg advises.

▶Solutions

Turn the other cheek. In the first *Rambo* movie, Sylvester Stallone told the small-town sheriff, played by Brian Dennehy, "Let it go." The sheriff, of course, didn't listen and Rambo blew up the town in revenge, justifying his mayhem with the excuse "but they drew first blood."

Retaliation and revenge are at the heart of a road-rage incident, Dr. Nerenberg says. One reckless or deliberate act leads to another. You may feel like playing Rambo on the roads some days, but you'd be better off taking his advice to just let it go. If you're in a tangle with a road-rager, don't do anything to escalate or aggravate the situation.

"Don't make obscene gestures at angry drivers. Avoid making eye contact, and just get out of their way," Dr. Nerenberg adds. "Give them a wide berth."

Use your blinker. Maybe you don't flip out on the highway, but the way you drive makes others do so. You change lanes suddenly, don't maintain a good speed, and eat breakfast and yak on the phone during your commutes.

Be a more attentive driver, says Dr. Geller. Think the bigger picture: You're not alone out there but are part of a fast-moving, bumper-to-bumper system. "A lot of drivers are unconsciously discourteous. They cruise along in their own little world not thinking or caring about how their behavior affects anyone other than themselves," he explains. "When you're dialing a cellular phone and slow down or weave into another lane, you're affecting, maybe scaring, a lot of other people."

Act civil to avoid war. We're quick with an obscene gesture, but when someone does you a good turn out on the highway, signal that you appreciate

Did You Know?

The most popular weapons used during road-rage incidents are guns and motor vehicles, according to a study on aggressive driving conducted by the American Automobile Association Foundation for Traffic Safety. Between 1990 and 1996, ramming with a motor vehicle led to the deaths of 48 police officers and 38 drivers and passengers in the United States. About 96 percent of the incidents reported in the study involved men. In more than half of the incidents involving women, a vehicle was used as a weapon. "Men are more likely to be shooters; women are more likely to use passive-aggressive tactics, like tapping their brakes to scare off a tailgater," says E. Scott Geller, Ph.D., professor of psychology at the Virginia Polytechnic Institute and State University in Blacksburg.

it, says Dr. Nerenberg. And if you screw up, show the offended party that you're sorry you goofed.

Dr. Nerenberg advises that you do not slap your forehead or make any kind of gesture because it could be misinterpreted by another driver as an obscene gesture. Instead, he suggests that you have a sign that says "sorry" in your car to hold up when you've made a mistake.

In 1997, Dr. Nerenberg surveyed close to 600 road-ragers, and 64 percent of them said that seeing such a sign would calm them down. "Just like when you bump into someone in a crowd, an apology or acknowledgment that you made a mistake quickly defuses a situation," he says.

▶ALTERNATIVE APPROACHES

Relax on cue. Don't take your anger from home or work out on the highway. Take a few seconds to relax before turning the key, suggests Andrew A. Sappington, Ph.D., a clinical psychologist who facilitates the Anger Management Group at the University of Alabama at Birmingham.

Breathe deeply through your nose, hold for a few seconds, and then exhale slowly. Let your shoulders sag, unclench your fists, and let gravity tug at your limbs. You can also mentally repeat a cue word or phrase during each exhalation, such as *relax* or *calm down*, Dr. Sappington suggests. "You may have to practice using the cue word at home, but when it becomes part of your routine, it can help you relax more quickly before you put the car in gear," he adds.

Control your environment. The car really is a cocoon, a microenvironment. Make it a relaxing place to be with pleasant scents and sound. Put on some relaxing music—country ballads, Gregorian chants, whatever—and spray the car with a vanilla scent, suggests Avery Gilbert, Ph.D., scientific affairs director of the Olfactory Research Fund in New York City. Heliotropin, an active ingredient in vanilla, reduces anxiety and stress, Dr. Gilbert says. "It seems to calm because it is a familiar, safe smell, sort of ingestible, and inviting," he adds.

Other aromas that might work include cocoa, chocolate, caramel, maple syrup, or berry scents.

▶PREVENTIVE MEASURES

Leave early. Did you ever notice that when you're cruising the speed limit, and a guy blows by you, you think, "What a jerk"? But when you're in a hurry and someone's poking along at 55 miles per hour, they're a "menace on the highway."

Aggressive driving and road rage frequently happen when you're in a hurry, running late, and traffic is bad, Dr. Geller says. "So leave early, and give yourself the time you need to get to your destination," he recommends. "Expect some hassles along the way, and when they happen, it won't be a catastrophe."

Remember your screwups. Before leaving the driveway, remind yourself of the time you ran a red light while singing along with "Annie's Song" or the day you smashed your rental car into the back of your brother's van while following him home from the airport.

"No one is a perfect driver. We've all made mistakes on the highway, and remembering those mistakes makes us more tolerant of other people's lapses," Dr. Geller says.

Saddle Sores

▶PROBLEM

Saddle sores didn't die out with the cowboys in the Old West. A new breed of men inherited this malady: bicyclists. Part pimple, part nodule, and part boil, saddle sores creep up where the leg meets the crotch area, explains Karl Kramer, M.D., clinical professor of dermatology at the University of Miami School of Medicine. Although less prevalent with the advent of specialty bicycling clothing and gear, these mounds can keep a rider in pain for weeks. You may not feel it sitting in an office chair, but as soon as you jump onto the saddle, it'll send a quick reminder of its presence.

DO THIS NOW

Doughnut your butt. Take a moleskin patch with a hole in the middle—the kind used to cover up blisters—and place it on the saddle sore. "That will relieve some of the pressure," says Ed Burke, Ph.D., professor of exercise science at the University of Colorado at Colorado Springs and author of *Serious Cycling*.

▶CAUSE

A good deal of your weight rests upon that little saddle. Combine that pressure with the constant rubbing created by pedaling and you have an abrasion. Bacteria find an opening into the layers of your skin through the abrasion, and manifest themselves as a painful infection.

▶HOW SERIOUS

To take care of saddle sores properly, take time off the bike. And if you develop fever, increasing redness around the sore, or increased pain, see a doctor. If ignored, the sores grow deeper into the skin. Eventually, they may have to be removed by a surgeon. "They can get to 1½ inches deep. When you take them out, you basically have a cavity left," says Dr. Kramer.

▶SOLUTIONS

Take a bike break. "If you have a saddle sore, you have to get off the bike," says Len Pettyjohn, Ph.D., former coach and trainer of the Coors

History Lesson

A nice, thin, juicy steak may seem the perfect way to cap off a long bike ride. But for members of the 1928 Olympic bicycling team, that juicy steak was better appreciated when it was in their pants. According to the diary of Emile Fraysse, the 1928 U.S. bicycling team coach and manager, the cyclists developed saddle sores from riding cobblestone surfaces in Amsterdam. Fraysse ran out to a local butcher for thin-sliced steaks. He told the riders to place the raw pieces of meat in their shorts to heal the sores. "A French trick that works very well," he wrote.

Light Cycling Team. If you keep pedaling, you'll make them bigger and deeper.

How long you need to take a riding vacation varies from person to person. If you hop on the saddle and still feel pain, you need more time to heal, Dr. Kramer says.

Climb the hills. If for some reason you can't or won't resist the road, take to the hills, says Ed Burke, Ph.D., professor of exercise science at the University of Colorado at Colorado Springs and author of *Serious Cycling*. When hill-climbing on a bike, you spend most of your time pedaling out of your saddle. You take pressure off your saddle sore and improve your hill-climbing technique at the same time, Dr. Burke says.

Bathe bumps away. Because saddle sores are similar to boils, you can try to bring them to the surface. Soak in a comfortably hot bath for 10 minutes three times a day. This may help the sores drain faster, says Dr. Kramer.

Don't play with them. It seems to be human nature to want to squeeze out whatever infectious goo the body produces. "I've seen people try to stick needles in them," Dr. Pettyjohn says.

But popping a saddle sore only pushes the infection further down into the skin. Let the sore heal by itself, advises Dr. Kramer.

▶ALTERNATIVE APPROACHES

Rub in relief. Professional riders usually rub an antibacterial ointment or cream like Noxzema or petroleum jelly into their chamois (padding in bicycle shorts) before each ride to reduce friction, Dr. Pettyjohn says.

Treat with tea tree. Oil from the Australian tea tree costs a bundle, but a small bottle will last for years, says Eve Campanelli, Ph.D., a holistic family practitioner in private practice in Beverly Hills, California. The oil soothes the saddle sore and has antibacterial properties to fight the infection. Soak a cotton ball in water and then put a few drops of oil on it. Apply the solution to the saddle sore, Dr. Campanelli says. Use it every day until the sore heals.

▶PREVENTIVE MEASURES

Pad your padding. Bicycling shorts contain extra padding called a chamois that prevents chafing. When buying shorts, make sure that they fit, Dr. Pettyjohn says. They should be tight yet smooth, and they should not bunch anywhere, he says.

Go natural. "The biggest problem with novice riders is that they wear underwear," Dr. Pettyjohn says. Bike companies design shorts so that you don't need underwear. The padding near the crotch on bicycle shorts has no seams. But underwear has seams right on the crotch where your weight bears down on the saddle. These seams cause more friction when you pedal, enhancing the conditions for a saddle sore.

Give your shorts a bath. Unwashed bike shorts provide a wonderful breeding ground for bacteria. "It amazes me that people will change their underwear every day but wear the same bike shorts two or three days in a row," Dr. Pettyjohn says. After every ride, give them a good wash.

Mix alcohol and water. Immediately after a sweaty ride, wipe your bike's seat area with alcohol. Some riders carry alcohol moist towelettes (like Handi Wipes) for this purpose. The alcohol kills bacteria looking for a place to enter the skin, Dr. Kramer says. Then jump right in the shower and wash with antibacterial soap, like Dial or Lever 2000.

Size up your saddle. Proper saddle fit prevents saddle sores. First, test a number of saddles and choose one you feel comfortable with. Once you pick out your saddle, position it correctly. To determine height, get on and push one pedal down toward the ground. When the pedal is at the bottom, you should have a slight bend in your knee. No bend means that the saddle is too high; a major bend means it's too low, Dr. Pettyjohn says.

Or ride and have someone watch you from behind, Dr. Burke says. If your hips rock back and forth or you bounce out of the saddle when you peddle, then your seat needs adjustment.

You can always ask your professional bike shop personnel for help in fitting your saddle, Dr. Pettyjohn adds.

Sciatica

▶PROBLEM

You have pain that radiates down the leg, usually below the knee, and sometimes clear to the foot and toes. In severe cases, some leg muscles may become partly or completely paralyzed.

▶CAUSE

Usually, sciatic pain is caused by a herniated disk. Disks are pads of cartilage filled with a thick mucus that help absorb shock and act as a cushion between the vertebrae. Sometimes this inner portion of the disk breaks through the outer ring and presses on the sciatic nerve, the widest and longest nerve in the body, running from the lower spine through the buttocks and into the knee. Pressure in the lower back can inflame the entire course of the nerve.

Sciatica may also occur from irritation and contraction of the piriformis, a muscle deep within the buttocks. After a lot of bending, stooping, lifting, or sitting, the muscle may freeze up and trap the sciatic nerve, says Richard M. Bachrach, D.O., medical director at the Center for Sports and Osteopathic Medicine in New York City.

A spasm in your psoas major, another muscle in the lower back, may also cause your pain, says Jerome F. McAndrews, D.C., spokesman for the American Chiropractic Association.

DO THIS NOW

Lie down on your back on a firm bed and rest the foot of the painful leg off the side of the bed on the floor, says Jerome F. McAndrews, D.C., spokesman for the American Chiropractic Association. Make sure that the buttock on the side of the spasm is half off the bed. Then let your leg and pelvis relax completely so that your leg's weight begins to pull on the muscles in the lower abdomen. At the same time, reach above your head with the hand on the same side as the leg on the floor, hold onto the headboard, and pull. Use only your arm and shoulder muscles on that side. Do the stretch for 5 minutes, and then rest 30 minutes before doing it again, suggests Dr. McAndrews.

Did You Know?

If you have any two of the following symptoms, you may have a recurring problem with sciatica-type nerve pain, says Jerome F. McAndrews, D.C., spokesman for the American Chiropractic Association.

- You've had a "weak back" for years with recurring pain.
- When you bend, take a misstep, or lift a grocery bag, you feel pain in one of your legs.
- When you sneeze or cough, a sharp pain travels into your leg.
- You have to frequently change positions to get rest and feel comfortable.
- One or both legs ache painfully at the end of the day.
- After driving for any length of time, you feel a pain in your leg.

▶HOW SERIOUS

Sciatica can be very painful, and debilitating if some leg muscles become paralyzed. You'll walk with a limp or drag along a bum leg. The inflammation can take weeks or months to dissipate, and in the meantime, you may be unable to find a position where you can get complete relief, says Dr. Bachrach. "If you have this kind of pain, I wouldn't wait too long. If it doesn't clear up on its own within two or three days, see a doctor," he says.

▶SOLUTIONS

Identify the problem. First, take this test to find out if a spasm in your psoas major muscle might be causing the pain running down your leg, Dr. McAndrews says. Lie on your back on the floor and reach your arms above your head (so you look like you're about to sing The Village People's "YMCA." Have another person stand behind your head and pull equally on both arms as though you are being stretched in a straight line from toes to fingertips.

If you have a spastic psoas major muscle, one arm will not pull as far as the other because the muscle restricts the ability of the body on one side to extend, Dr. McAndrews says. The spastic muscle will be on the side of the "shorter" arm.

Break the spasm. If a spastic psoas major muscle is your problem, you can try stimulating the muscle to relax, says Dr. McAndrews. If the muscle is in a spastic state, it may ultimately result in the pinching of a nerve, he says.

"The muscle may stay in permanent contraction unless some outside force is applied," Dr. McAndrews says. "If you can get to the center of the muscle and apply pressure, you can restore its normal function."

To relieve the spasm, bend the leg opposite the "short" arm so that the heel of the foot is flat on the bed or floor. Keep the other leg straight. Your helper should stand or kneel on the side opposite the bent leg and then pull the knee of your bent leg across your body toward him while at the same time pressing in the spot midway between your hipbone and navel (on the side of the bent leg). The muscle is deep in the back portion of the abdomen, so the person will need to use a good deal of pressure. Initially, the skin and underlying abdominal muscles will be sensitive; this will pass in a moment or two, Dr. McAndrews says. Pressure can be applied either with the tips of the fingers of the hand not holding the knee, or with the knuckles of that hand.

Occasionally, the helper can actually feel the psoas muscle let go, or relax. If the arms appear to be equal in length when the helper pulls them again, you've hit the spot. And once the muscle relaxes, it will not ordinarily re-spasm unless it is challenged in an abnormal or stressful manner, Dr. McAndrews says.

Get out of that chair. If you have leg pain, the worst thing you can do is sit all day because of the pressure that sitting places on the buttocks and sciatic nerve, says Dr. McAndrews. Also, when you sit for long periods, your hamstring muscles contract and shorten. When you stand up, the hamstrings pull, perhaps unevenly, on the pelvis and apply pressure to the sacroiliac joint, which, in turn, can result in pelvic muscular imbalance, he explains.

"You should get out of your chair for at least five minutes every hour—longer if you can," says Dr. McAndrews. "Take a walk to relieve the pressure on the nerve and to allow those hamstrings to stretch. You should make it a habit to do this regardless of whether you have any problems."

▶ALTERNATIVE APPROACHES

Ease pain with potassium. For reasons that aren't completely understood, some people with sciatica have relieved the pain by eating large amounts of potassium, according to Julian Whitaker, M.D., founder and president of the Whitaker Wellness Institute in Newport Beach, California. Dr. Whitaker suggests making bananas, oranges, and potatoes—all potassium-rich foods—a regular part of your diet.

Let ginger make it better. According to James A. Duke, Ph.D., the world's foremost authority on healing herbs and author of *The Green Pharmacy*, the Egyptians used this remedy for sciatic pain: Mix two tablespoons of grated fresh ginger with three tablespoons of sesame oil and one teaspoon of lemon juice. Rub it where it hurts.

▶PREVENTIVE MEASURES

Throw away your credit cards. Whether your wallet is stuffed with cash or overdue bills from creditors, a bulging billfold can be a big pain in the butt—literally.

"It's the wallet-in-the-back-pocket syndrome. We see it with men," explains Dr. Bachrach. "When you sit down, your wallet presses right on the sciatic nerve. A thick wallet can bruise it so badly that it takes months to heal."

Seasonal Affective Disorder (SAD)

▶PROBLEM

For some people, the overcast days and fewer hours of daylight in fall and winter are depressing. We're not talking about the kind of grousing most of us do when we set our clocks back an hour in late October but, rather, a listless, irritable mood characterized by poor concentration, excessive sleeping, and a craving for carbohydrates and sweets. How appropriate then that seasonal affective disorder is often known by its acronym SAD, says Anthony Levitt, M.D., associate professor in the department of psychiatry and nutritional science at the University of Toronto and head of the mood disorders program at Sunnybrook Hospital in Toronto.

▶CAUSE

It's not known why some people get SAD. Theories about biological and social catalysts abound. One says that society is geared toward summer activities, so when summer ends, some people have a letdown. Another is that people with SAD have a special sensitivity to light.

DO THIS NOW

Go outside every morning for a half-hour, advises David Avery, M.D., associate professor of psychiatry and behavioral sciences at the University of Washington School of Medicine in Seattle—even if it's so dreary that you don't want to leave the house. People with seasonal affective disorder respond well to light, which is measured in lux. A cloudy day radiates from 1,000 to 10,000 lux, says Dr. Avery. Most homes have a light intensity of 100 to 200 lux, while a brightly lit office may have 400 to 600 lux.

456

Others say that their melatonin is out of sequence. Melatonin is a hormone produced in the pituitary gland in response to light, which acts as a timekeeper for the internal clock, explains Dr. Levitt.

▶HOW SERIOUS

People with SAD tend not to be as severely depressed as folks with non-seasonal depression, says Dr. Levitt. Some can be so depressed, however, that they become suicidal, he warns. "It still can and does occur with alarming frequency," Dr. Levitt says. If your symptoms are severe enough to make you think about taking your life, see a doctor or therapist.

▶SOLUTIONS

Make yourself exercise. Some studies show that exercise helps lift depression. Running, walking, and aerobics are particularly good forms of exercise, says Joanne Brown, Ph.D., a psychologist in private practice in Salt Lake City.

Outdoor activity is especially good because it exposes you to potentially therapeutic light, too, says David Avery, M.D., associate professor of psychiatry and behavioral sciences at the University of Washington School of Medicine in Seattle.

The problem, of course, is that the primary symptom of SAD is lethargy. How, then, are you going to manage to get yourself moving? Dr. Brown suggests starting an exercise regimen in the spring, with the hope that you can carry it over into the fall and winter. Remember that before beginning any exercise program, it's always best to check with your doctor.

Be a snowbird. If gloomy days have you feeling gloomy, take a vacation where it's sunny. "Getting closer to the equator appears to be helpful," says Dr. Levitt.

Get ripe. "Discipline yourself to avoid going overboard on carbohydrates, and make a weekly visit to a produce market instead," suggests Dr. Levitt. Since you're craving the sun, your spirits might be lifted by produce grown under that ball o' fire. The fruits' sweet smell and golden colors may remind you of the brighter-lit seasons, and they will give you loads of healthy vitamins to keep up your endurance. Be sure to eat two to four fruit servings a day, and also take hearty portions of vegetables so that you're getting (at the very least) three to five servings daily, Dr. Levitt advises.

Enlist family and friends. Tell people close to you about your winter blues. Ask them to come over on your darkest days. Perhaps they can cook for you or encourage you to go for a walk. "Sometimes it helps to have a roster of friends because it can be quite a heavy burden for one or two people," says Dr. Levitt.

Moderate your life. Don't take on extra projects and responsibilities during the months that you have SAD symptoms, advises Dr. Brown. "If you learn to moderate your life according to the season, your self-esteem may be less damaged."

Did You Know?

No symptom of seasonal affective disorder is so overwhelming as that of lethargy and a lack of energy to do anything. For one of our fellow mammals, every day is like that, no matter what season of the year. The three-toed sloth, found in South America, rarely even comes down from its tree.

It is little wonder. This homely little flat-faced creature is the slowest mammal in the world. The poor devil has an average ground speed of six to eight feet per *minute*, making him easy pickings for jaguars and other predators. So he's content to cling to tree trunks and branches or hang upside down for hours on end, occasionally rotating his head up to 270 degrees to survey the world he doesn't dare explore.

▶ALTERNATIVE APPROACHES

Work with the wort. Conventional researchers say that there is insufficient information on whether herbs such as Saint-John's-wort may help people with SAD, but herbalists swear by the powers of this natural antidepressant. One of the best mood-lifters for those with SAD is Saint-John's-wort combined with equal parts lemon balm, according to David Winston, professional and founding member of the American Herbalists Guild and a clinical herbalist in Washington, New Jersey. He recommends taking about 40 to 60 drops of the liquid tincture form of each herb (mix in a glass of water or juice), three times a day, until your mood improves. You can find both tinctures in most health food stores. And give it some time: You need to take Saint-John's-wort for a few weeks before you may notice any effect, Winston adds. Don't take Saint-John's-wort if you are on any monoamine oxidase (MAO) inhibitor drugs. Saint-John's-wort also can make you more sensitive to the sun, particularly if you're fair-skinned.

Mimic the dawn. A device that helps a lot of people with SAD is a dawn simulator, says Dr. Avery. You program a dawn simulator like a digital alarm clock, and it releases light gradually and at increasing wattage during the last hour of your sleep. It works through the eyes—closed eyelids are translucent to light—which have a direct connection to one's internal body clock, says Dr. Avery.

Dawn stimulators can be purchased by mail order from several companies throughout the United States specializing in lighting or light therapy and cost between $100 and $200. You can receive information on purchasing light therapy devices by writing to the National Institute for Mental Health (NIMH). Send your request for an "SAD information pack" to NIMH, Public Information, 5600 Fisher's Lane, Room 7C02 MSC8030, Bethesda, MD 20892-8030.

Light up your life. Researchers say that there is no doubt that sitting in front of an intensely bright light helps most people with SAD "It works in about two-thirds of people," says Dr. Levitt. Special units called light boxes, at costs of $250 to $600, can be purchased that emit sufficient light to be beneficial. A person sits near the box for at least 30 minutes, preferably in the morning. You can also buy head-mounted portable light units to accomplish the same purpose, which cost $75 to $400.

A light box or visor can be purchased through several companies specializing in light therapy. Ask your doctor for a list of sources, or write to the Society for Light Treatment and Biological Rhythms to purchase their information pack for a small fee: 10200 West 44th Avenue, Suite 304, Wheat Ridge, CO 80033-2840. If you plan on using either device, consult a doctor or therapist knowledgeable about SAD. Using either one without proper guidance could result in physical problems like eyestrain or damage to a preexisting eye condition.

▶PREVENTIVE MEASURES

Don't drink the blues away. Some guys resort to alcohol to melt away the winter doldrums. "Not a good idea," says Dr. Avery. "Alcohol is a very subtle drug in that it may lift the depression and the anxiety, but there is a crash after that. People obviously can become dependent upon it." And remember that alcohol isn't a stimulant. It's a depressant.

Sex Addiction

▶PROBLEM

Ask yourself this question: Do you constantly pursue sex, even when it might cause you or your family harm? If you answer yes to this question, you may have a sexual addiction. Real sex addiction rivals the ugliness of all the chemical addictions: Your highs are followed by cavernous lows, and your entire being is consumed with getting more. It can ruin your love life, your family, your career, your reputation, and even your bank account. A true sex addict will neglect his job, his family, and even his own physical health to pursue his desires. Whether it's masturbation, pornography, 1-900 numbers, or picking up prostitutes, the actual sex act doesn't matter. It's an addiction when it is not reliably controlled and when it continues despite significant harmful consequences, says Aviel Goodman, M.D., director of the Minnesota Institute of Psychiatry in St. Paul.

▶CAUSE

Sex addicts share the same condition as those who have other addictions such as alcoholism and drug abuse: Something is out of kilter with the part of the brain that regulates emotional states, Dr. Goodman says. And there is some evidence that certain people seem to be more prone to addictions—sexual and otherwise—than others. In a survey of sex addicts in the early 1990s, 42 percent said that they also had a chemical dependency; 38 percent had an eating disorder; and 26 percent reported that they were compulsive spenders.

DO THIS NOW

If you feel an overwhelming sexual urge sweeping over you, reach out for help. Call someone. Just make sure that the number doesn't start with 1-900. This should be someone you trust, someone who knows that you're struggling with this extremely sensitive problem, says Suki Hanfling, a licensed social worker, certified sex therapist, and founder and director of the McLean Hospital Human Sexuality Program in Belmont, Massachusetts. In other words, it should be a close friend who will help talk you through the urge, she says.

Sexual abuse or a person's home environment can also factor in to a person becoming a sex addict, Dr. Goodman says. "They learned somewhere early in life that sexual stimulation can regulate emotions," he says.

▶HOW SERIOUS

Sex addiction can destroy every facet of a person's life. Frequent sex with multiple partners puts addicts at an increased risk of sexually transmitted diseases, including AIDS, that can also be passed on to unsuspecting wives or partners. Some sex addicts use their family's very last dime on prostitutes and telephone sex, incurring thousands of dollars of debt. They spend so much time focusing on their addiction that they lose jobs or find themselves in the middle of a sexual harassment lawsuit. In the survey of sex addicts, 40 percent said that they lost a partner or spouse; 58 percent have had severe financial consequences; and 79 percent said that their job productivity suffered. Many sex addicts get themselves in trouble with the law for frequenting prostitutes, for exposing themselves, or for sexually abusing others.

If you have a sexual addiction, you should seek help from a therapist who is experienced in psychiatry and psychology as well as in addictions, Dr. Goodman says. Ask your primary care physician, your clergyperson, or a trusted friend for a specialist in your area, he says. You may also find specialists listed in your local phone book.

▶SOLUTIONS

Ask yourself some questions. There's a difference between being sexually compulsive and having a large sexual appetite, says Suki Hanfling, a licensed social worker, certified sex therapist, and founder and director of the McLean Hospital Human Sexuality Program in Belmont, Massachusetts. Knowing what you're dealing with is the first step toward solving your problem. You have already answered one question about sexual addiction in the beginning of this chapter. Answer a few more to confirm if you are addicted to sex.

- Do you have trouble resisting the behavior?
- Do you feel bad about it afterward?
- Does a lot of tension build up before you do it?
- Do you spend an inordinate amount of time planning for sex, having sex or thinking about it?
- Have you ever wanted to stop the behavior but haven't been able to?

If you answer yes to three or more questions, chances are that you have a problem and it is important for you to seek professional assistance.

Write it down. Perhaps you don't even know why you indulge in your addiction. To get a handle on what triggers an episode, keep a journal. When you get hit by an urge or you engage in the addictive behavior, write down everything you feel and what happened to you before and after. You can use the

History Lesson

Today we have therapy and the self-help school of thought to help the sexually addicted deal with their problems. But back in the nineteenth and even early twentieth centuries, torturous devices were invented to "help" control those who engaged in "self-abuse." Daniel P. Cook invented one such product called the Self-Protector in 1870. Cook described it as "a device for so covering up the sexual organs of a person addicted to the vice of masturbation . . . that he or she must refrain from the commission of the vicious self-degrading act." Similar to a jockstrap, the invention consisted of a series of cloth, rubber, or leather bands, plus a padded metal cup to shield the genitals. Cook said, "The edges of the cup fit close against the person so that it will be impossible for the wearer to touch the confined organ." The cup was then padlocked, and the "person who has charge of the masturbator" held the key. Cook was kind enough to install a small hole so that wearers could relieve themselves.

---

journal to spot patterns or to help you avoid triggers. "You need to get a sense of what your risky situations are. Keep a journal of when you engage in the behavior or you feel a strong urge. Then study what might have triggered that situation," Dr. Goodman says.

Stay out of temptation's way. It may not be as simple as "out of sight, out of mind," but limiting your exposure to temptation can greatly help control your addiction. If pornography is your downfall, throw out all your magazines and stay away from places that sell it. Get a phone block on 1-900 numbers. "If a person uses prostitutes, he may need to avoid certain parts of town," Dr. Goodman says. You can also quell urges by avoiding your triggers, he adds. For instance, if you feel sex urges after you've been drinking, don't drink or hang out in bars.

Give yourself your just desserts. Fighting your addiction may seem more like self-denial than self-improvement. But it doesn't have to. "It's important to build in rewards so that the recovery process is enjoyable," Dr. Goodman says. Give yourself prizes and rewards along the way, he suggests. It could be as simple a buying a CD at the end of each week that you did not engage in addictive behavior.

▶ALTERNATIVE APPROACHES

Picture yourself on a beach. Get away from all the stresses and urges without leaving your chair. Visualization and imagery make for a quick getaway from life's troubles, says Larry Anthony, Ed.D., academic coordinator of the addiction studies program at the University of Cincinnati. Take a deep breath and picture yourself on a sandy beach, or in the deep woods near a stream. Imagine not just the sights but also the sounds and smells. Once the stressful feeling passes, you'll come back to reality a little more relaxed and refreshed.

Plan your day. Lack of sleep, lack of time, lack of good food—all lead to a hectic out-of-balance life and leave you in a weakened state. "If we are strung out, if we are tired, if we are hungry, if we are under stress, those are the times that we are most likely to lapse into addictive behavior because our lives are out of balance," Dr. Goodman says.

Scheduling your day will help maintain your balance, says Jay L. Glaser, M.D., medical director of the Maharishi Ayur-Veda Medical Center in Lancaster, Massachusetts. Set a time to go to bed and get up so that you develop a healthy sleep pattern, he says. Then set aside blocks of time each day for nutritious meals and stick to the schedule like you would an important meeting. Plan for exercise, leisure activities, reading, even watching TV. Schedule your work day the same way. Getting your day organized will help you fit in everything while staying relaxed and healthy, Dr. Glaser says.

▶PREVENTIVE MEASURES

Plan your fire drill. If you find yourself in the throes of an uncontrollable urge, you may not be prepared to fight back. That's why you should rehearse your plan of action ahead of time, Dr. Goodman says. "In the midst of the urge, there's such a rush of adrenaline that if the fire drill isn't well-rehearsed, then it's hard to come up with a plan in the heat of the moment," Dr. Goodman says. Think of what you will do: call a friend, take a walk, recite a positive phrase—whatever takes you away from the urge. Practice it enough that it becomes an automatic response in times of temptation, Dr. Goodman suggests.

Balance work and play. When sex addicts load their plate with too much work and not enough leisure time, they tend to stress out and grow resentful—perfect fuel for a sexual outburst. "A backlog of resentment and entitlement can build up to the point where we do something compulsive to 'reward' ourselves with the addictive behavior," Dr. Goodman says. Schedule fun and relaxing activities into your week, such as going to a ballgame or a movie. Needless to say, stay away from those rated XXX.

Sexual Monotony

▶PROBLEM

When you first met her, you were like a rutting deer. You had sex in the car. In the woods. In the basement. In the kitchen. Even in the bedroom, on those occasions when you summoned the Herculean willpower to wait that long. But these days, the only thing in a rut is your sex life.

▶CAUSE

You've grown comfortable with one another. That's perfectly natural and, in many ways, even healthy. We like to be comfortable. But you can become so used to being around one another, so much a part of each other's routine, that you stop really noticing each other. "It's like the brain sort of goes to sleep," says marriage and family therapist Patricia Love, Ed.D., author of *Hot Monogamy*.

When sex becomes familiar and routine, you get bored. "In general, human beings have incredibly short attention spans," says Doreen Virtue, Ph.D., a relationship expert and psychotherapist in Newport Beach, California, and author of *In the Mood*. "We need variety in all aspects of our lives—in our jobs, in the foods we eat, and even in our sex lives."

▶HOW SERIOUS

"Sometimes what's needed is to simply recognize that you're in a rut. A lot of people are afraid to admit it. They think that there's something wrong with them or that they're being hurtful to the other

Did You Know?

Wondering why it's so tough to remain true to one sexual partner over the long haul? Blame it on biology. "You're fighting a genuine restlessness born from millennia of having sexual variety being part of basic human reproductive strategy," says Helen Fisher, Ph.D., research associate in the department of anthropology at Rutgers University in New Brunswick, New Jersey. "I don't think the human animal was built to be with one person for the rest of his life. So the sexual boredom that can set in with monogamy is real."

Dr. Fisher says that promiscuity delivered a Darwinian payoff for our primitive relatives by rewarding those who "spread their seed" with survival. And some of that genetic programming is still swimming in our DNA soup today. But that doesn't mean that you are a prisoner of your genes. Human beings naturally tend to pair off, even in cultures where multiple partners are permitted.

"There's a very deep need in the human psyche to build an intimate, sexy, happy relationship," Dr. Fisher says. "And, to my amazement, many of us succeed."

person to admit it," says Steve Manley, Ph.D., staff psychologist for the Male Health Institute in Irving, Texas.

▶SOLUTIONS

Make your move. Don't assume that your partner will be unwilling to consider ways to break the monotony. Remember, if you're bored, odds are that she is, too. "People don't get bored by themselves; relationships get boring," says Helen Fisher, Ph.D., research associate in the department of anthropology at Rutgers University in New Brunswick, New Jersey, and author of *Anatomy of Love*. "If you come up with a good idea, she'll probably go for it."

Lay down the law. Setting fun rules is a great way to spice up your sex life, says Dr. Virtue. Declare tonight Three Positions or Bust Night. Or maybe Sex Standing Up Night. Whatever turns you—and your partner—on.

Make boredom illegal. While you're setting rules, go ahead and outlaw those comfortable old positions you've been relying on, Dr. Virtue suggests. Impose a three-month ban on the missionary position, for example. Or go a week without making love in your bed. The idea isn't to restrict your love lives but to open your minds to new and exciting possibilities.

Pick her up. If you want to experience the thrill of seducing a sexy woman you've just met, go ahead and do it. Just make sure that it's your partner, suggests Lonnie Barbach, Ph.D., assistant clinical professor of medical psychology at the University of California, San Francisco, School of Medicine and author of *The Erotic Edge: Erotica for Couples*. Arrive separately at a bar or hotel and strike up a conversation. Flirt. Turn on the charm full wattage, just like you did the first time you saw her. Then take her to a hotel room and ravish her. Just make sure that your partner is as open to the idea of role-playing as you are.

▶ALTERNATIVE APPROACHES

Go to the videotape. Erotic films—also known as blue movies or just plain old porn—can spark your imaginations and fire up your lovemaking. But only if you both are open to it. So talk to her about it before you head down to the video store to rent *Debbie Does Dallas*. "You have to communicate with her on this," says Robert Birch, Ph.D., a sex therapist in Columbus, Ohio, and author of *Male Sexual Endurance*. "Every woman is unique, with different appetites and desires."

For many women, finding an X-rated flick with a plot—yes, there actually *is* such a thing—is the key. "Seeing 90 minutes of mindless screwing isn't going to do much for her. On the other hand, movies with some story line, some erotic language, are going to arouse her," says Anne Semans, one of the owners of the adult store Good Vibrations in San Francisco, and co-author of *The Good Vibrations Guide to Sex*. Among the favorites at *Men's Health* are *Behind the Green Door* and the "Emmanuelle" series available on video.

Play with toys. You may be all grown up, but there are still toys for girls and boys. For her: a vibrator. For you: a constrictor ring. Vibrators range from battery-powered "self-massage" units to big, electric, phallic-shaped, pulsating objects with multiple attachments for different sensations. This is one shopping trip where you'll definitely want to go along with her. Constrictor rings, also known as cock rings, are placed on the base of the penis, trapping blood in the erectile chamber. The result: You stay harder longer. "It's sort of the male equivalent of lingerie," Semans says. "It adds kind of a visual element to sex play."

Just make sure that you never wear a constrictor ring for longer than 30 minutes at a time because they cut off blood flow to the penis. If fresh blood doesn't get pumped in there, you risk tissue damage.

▶PREVENTIVE MEASURES

Make sex a priority. One of the saddest things about the frenetic schedules that many of us keep is that sex can be relegated to an afterthought. You work, she works, and you have kids. So if your regular time for sex is midnight after yet another exhausting day, those twin demons of boredom and routine are lurking just outside the bedroom door. "How can you enjoy sex when you're in no condition to enjoy anything?" asks sex therapist Theresa Crenshaw, M.D., author of *The Alchemy of Love and Lust*. "You can't operate on burnout and expect sex to function."

The answer is to make time to make love, says Timothy Perper, Ph.D., a Philadelphia biologist and independent sex researcher who wrote *Sex Signals: The Biology of Love*. "It's a ghastly cliché, but you have to set aside quality time for your sex life together," Dr. Perper says.

Shingles

▶PROBLEM

Shingles (herpes zoster)—the second coming of the chickenpox virus (varicella zoster)—inflames nerves, causes severe localized pain, and produces skin blisters, usually along one side of your chest, stomach, or head. The sores eventually erupt and leak a contagious fluid.

▶CAUSE

"Shingles is not chickenpox, but it's caused by the same virus," says Stephen Straus, M.D., chief of the Laboratory of Clinical Investigation in the National Institutes of Health Allergy and Infectious Diseases in Bethesda, Maryland. After your childhood bout with chickenpox, the virus goes dormant and takes up residence in nerve cells near the spinal cord. For reasons not well understood, but probably relating to the strength of your immune system, the virus may reactivate decades later, says Dr. Straus. About 20 percent of the people who once had chickenpox will someday get shingles. Other serious illnesses, a tumor, a medical operation, or the use of immune-suppressing drugs, seem to be factors in shingle outbreaks, but the most common link is age. The majority of the more than 500,000 Americans who get shingles each year are age 50 and older, says Dr. Straus.

▶HOW SERIOUS

See a physician promptly if you suspect shingles, recommends Dr. Straus. The doctor can prescribe an antiviral medication that limits the duration and severity of the outbreak. But this medication only helps if it is begun during the

DO THIS NOW

Wash gently. You should clean the blisters and any sores that may have opened by lightly sponging them with a mild soap and water one or two times a day, says Stephen Straus, M.D., chief of the Laboratory of Clinical Investigation in the National Institutes of Health Allergy and Infectious Diseases in Bethesda, Maryland. **Wear clean, loose, cotton clothing** so that you don't pinch or chafe the rash. Breathable clothing and airflow also keep the lesions dry, adds Dr. Straus.

Did You Know?

About 9 out of 10 Americans have had chickenpox—usually in childhood—but this disease may not be so common in the future. In 1995, doctors began inoculating children with a new chickenpox vaccine. The vaccine is expected to be 70 to 90 percent effective, but there's no proof yet that it will prevent shingles. That question will only be answered when today's toddlers are aging adults.

first three or so days of the outbreak, so don't hesitate to take action. "You also want an accurate diagnosis because the pain can feel like something else, and the doctor can rule out a more serious, underlying condition," Dr. Straus adds.

Shingles usually last three to five weeks before the sores heal completely and the pain subsides. Most people never have a recurrence. The biggest complication is postherpetic neuralgia, or pain that may last for months while the inflamed nerves heal. Elderly people are the most likely to have lingering pain.

After you've seen your doctor, the following tips might help make the duration of the disease a bit more comfortable.

▶SOLUTIONS

Take a bath. The itching associated with the blisters can be as maddening as the pain. You can relieve some of the itching and dry skin symptoms with an occasional colloidal oatmeal bath, such as Aveeno, an over-the-counter product, recommends Jessica Severson, M.D., a clinical researcher in dermatology at the University of Texas Medical Branch at Galveston. For the consistency of the bath, follow the directions on the product. Just don't bathe any more than you normally would, Dr. Severson cautions. The skin needs to be kept clean, but excess bathing could be irritating. "An oatmeal bath probably works best in the beginning and end stages of shingles. But if you have open sores, you may not want to put anything on them and risk irritation," Dr. Severson says.

Seek out Sarna. After the bath, you can rub on Sarna, a topical lotion that prevents itching. Sarna is sold over-the-counter, so you don't need a prescription. Use it as needed, says Dr. Severson.

Motion for the lotion. If dry skin is your problem, be certain to use a moisturizing lotion frequently (especially after a bath), says Dr. Severson. Again, only apply the lotion when the sores aren't weeping. Most moisturizers are good, but keep away from any containing alpha hydroxy acids, which will sting any break in the skin, she adds.

Chill out. Cool compresses can give temporary relief to the pain and itching, says Norman Levine, M.D., chief of dermatology at the University of Arizona College of Medicine in Tucson and author of *Skin Healthy*. Soak clean towels in ice water, wring out, and apply to the blisters for 30 minutes, three or four times per day, suggests Dr. Levine.

Push back the pain. The pain from inflamed nerves can last for weeks and be so severe that it can feel like you've been slammed against a wall. To get some immediate pain relief as well as to bring down inflammation, you can take anti-inflammatory medications like aspirin or ibuprofen as well as analgesics like acetaminophen, says Dr. Levine. He recommends two aspirin (325 milligrams each) every four to six hours, two acetaminophen (325 milligrams each) every four hours, or two ibuprofen (400 milligrams each) every six hours.

▶ALTERNATIVE APPROACHES

Take tea topically. A strong tea made out of licorice, lemon balm, or both can be applied topically to the sore areas as an antiherpetic agent (shingles is a form of herpes), says David Winston, professional and founding member of the American Herbalists Guild and a clinical herbalist in Washington, New Jersey. To make the licorice application, add one teaspoon of dried licorice to eight ounces water, and simmer on the stove until the liquid reduces to half (four ounces). To make the lemon balm application, add eight ounces of boiling water to two teaspoons of the dried herb and steep, covered, for 20 minutes.

These teas can be refrigerated and used the next day. Apply the herb teas with cotton balls, and let them dry on the skin. Try to remember to apply them two to four times a day, Winston advises.

Seek Saint John's help. Another approach is to take Saint-John's-wort tincture, Winston says. Three times a day add 30 to 60 drops of the tincture to water or juice, and drink it as an antiviral agent. Look for the high-quality tincture, which should be burgundy-red with a strong, fragrant smell. Saint-John's-wort oil (hypericum oil) applied topically, directly to the inflamed skin, can help with pain, too, Winston says. The oil is available by mail order through herb companies, and the teas and tincture should be available at health food stores.

Burn out the pain. If your blisters have dissipated but the pain has not, you can try Zostrix, an over-the-counter cream containing capsaicin, the ingredient that makes hot peppers hot. There is one uncomfortable side effect, however. It burns going on, says Dr. Levine. Many drugstores have house brands similar to Zostrix. Look for a cream with 0.075 percent capsaicin concentration, and apply four or five times daily, says Dr. Levine.

▶PREVENTIVE MEASURES

Treat yourself well. There's no guarantee that you won't get shingles, but you're less likely if you maintain a strong, healthy immune system, says Dr. Straus. Get plenty of rest, eat a healthy diet, take a multivitamin, and avoid unnecessary stress, he suggests. And if you still get shingles, this advice is still sound. "Shingles can change your mood, disrupt sleep, and make you feel terrible," he says. "Lighten up on your schedule and you may get over it quicker."

Shinsplints

▶PROBLEM

Shinsplints is a catchall phrase for a muscle or tendon strain along the tibia, the bone on the inside of the lower leg. It usually involves the soleus muscle (on the back of your lower leg) or an inflamed posterior tibialis tendon, where it attaches to the bone midway down the inside of your lower leg, says Rick Hammesfahr, M.D., a physician at the Center for Orthopaedics and Sports Medicine in Marietta, Georgia.

▶CAUSE

Shinsplints are an athletic injury caused by repeated running on a hard surface, switching to a different running surface, or wearing worn-out shoes that have lost their shock absorption. You're also more likely to get shinsplints if you have a gait or stride that causes your feet to pronate or turn outward, which forces your tendons to compensate, says Richard M. Bachrach, D.O., medical director at the Center for Sports and Osteopathic Medicine in New York City.

DO THIS NOW

Take an ice cube or a small bag of ice chunks and massage the painful area for a few minutes, suggests Duane Iverson, a physical therapist, certified athletic trainer, and director of the sports medicine department at the University of Oregon Student Health Center in Eugene. "Ice massage or cold packs can be great for decreasing the swelling and pain associated with this inflammation," he says.

▶HOW SERIOUS

You'll first notice some pain in your shins while you're exercising, but it usually goes away when you stop. It may return the very next time you work out, however. And if you've really irritated the muscle and tendon—perhaps by running an unusual number of miles or playing tennis all day—you may find yourself limping about for several days afterward, says Dr. Bachrach.

Shinsplint pain is usually diffuse over a three- to four-inch-wide area, says Dr. Hammesfahr. If it's sharp and localized, you may have a stress fracture of the bone. In that case, you'll want to see a doctor.

History Lesson

He won the silver medal in the 5000-meter race at the Montreal Olympics, but for seven years, New Zealand runner Dick Quax had been plagued by an Olympic-size case of shinsplints. It was so bad, it appears, that he finally had to undergo surgery to get rid of them. It turned out that he had run so much that the muscles in his legs had grown too large for the very membranes in which they were encased. So Quax reportedly had a surgeon cut the membranes, alleviating the terrible pressure, and curing that particular case of shinsplints for good.

▶SOLUTIONS

Support your foot. While overuse is typically the cause of shinsplints, some people seem to be more prone to getting them, says Duane Iverson, a physical therapist, certified athletic trainer, and director of the sports medicine department at the University of Oregon Student Health Center in Eugene. Men who pronate their feet (collapse their arches) excessively seem to be in a higher-risk category, he says. While pronation is a normal part of the gait, when it occurs too much or for too long, it can cause problems. "A really easy solution is to place an insert made of foam, cork, or plastic into your shoe," he says. "These inserts give support to your arch and limit the extent of the pronation." The inserts are available at most drugstores or sporting goods stores.

If you have excessive pronation, you can also try wearing motion-control sneakers, Iverson suggests. Most shoe manufacturers make at least one model of motion-control shoe, he says, and you should go to a sports store to get an experienced salesperson to help you. For motion-control running shoes, check out *Runner's World* magazine's semiannual shoe reviews, which usually appear in the March and October issues. Or go to the magazine's Web site (www.runnersworld.com) to see an extensive list of training shoe reviews.

Switch sports. Shinsplints take time to go away, but in the meantime, you may still want to get in your exercise. If pounding the pavement while jogging caused the problem, try swimming and riding a stationary bike, says Dr. Hammesfahr. "Rest will make it heal faster, but you don't have to give up exercise," he says. "It's a good idea to change activities and to avoid the sport that caused the shinsplints."

▶ALTERNATIVE APPROACHES

Move the blood. You can bring down the inflammation of chronic shinsplints and speed healing by taking ginkgo biloba, a common herbal treatment available at drugstores and health food stores, says Alison Lee, M.D., a pain-management specialist and acupuncturist with Barefoot Doctors, an acupuncture and natural-medicine resource center in Ann Arbor, Michigan. Ginkgo biloba dilates blood vessels and increases blood flow to soft-tissue injuries. Fresh blood brings in nutrients needed for healing and also carries away waste products (oxidants) manufactured by injured cells, explains Dr. Lee, who recommends a product with standardized extract of 24 percent. Take 40 milligrams three times a day, she recommends. Ginkgo is safe to take every day, and you may have to take it for a few weeks to notice a difference, Dr. Lee says. One caution, however: Ginkgo may increase the effect of monoamine oxidase (MAO) inhibitor drugs, so talk to your doctor about using ginkgo if you are taking these.

Squeeze out the pain. To combat shinsplint pain, try blending a pineapple with a half-inch-thick piece of fresh ginger and drinking a little of the mixture three times a day, Dr. Lee says. One blenderful should last about two days.

▶PREVENTIVE MEASURES

Stretch deep. The posterior tibialis muscle is the most frequent culprit in shinsplints, but it's a very difficult muscle to stretch, says James Waslaski, sports massage therapist at the Center for Pain Management and Clinical Sports Massage in Tampa, Florida, and author of *International Advancements in Event and Clinical Sports Massage*. "Most athletes never stretch this muscle because you have to do it with the leg in a 90-degree position," he says. To stretch the posterior tibialis and treat shinsplints on the inside of the lower leg, sit on the floor and bend one knee to a 90-degree angle, keeping your other leg straight. Grab the foot of the bent leg with both hands and turn the foot outward slightly so that your toes are pointing outward instead of straight ahead. At the same time contract the muscles in the outside of your lower leg to release the muscles on the inside of your lower leg. Hold the stretch for 5 to 10 seconds and repeat a few times.

Shyness

▶PROBLEM

The French philosopher Jean-Paul Sartre said, "Hell is other people." Shy people can relate. Nearly half (48.7 percent) of all Americans report being shy, a form of extreme self-consciousness that interferes with quality of life. Some shy people are shy only in certain situations—say, being at a party or giving a talk (situational shyness). Others feel shy in virtually any social situation (chronic shyness).

▶CAUSE

The root cause of shyness is low self-esteem, says Frank J. Bruno, Ph.D., professor of psychology at San Bernadino Valley College in California and author of *Conquer Shyness*. "If you don't have a good opinion of yourself, it's hard to feel self-confident in social situations," he says. Often, shy men try to hide their shyness by acting the "strong, silent type" or by being loud and aggressive. "This acting out is actually a defense against shyness," says Dr. Bruno.

▶HOW SERIOUS

An estimated 30 million Americans are so severely shy that it affects their quality of life. They're said to have social phobia, reported as the third most common mental health problem, behind depression and alcoholism. Men make up 60 percent of those treated for social phobia, says Lawrence Welkowitz, Ph.D., assistant professor of psychology at Keene State College in Keene, New Hampshire, and co-author of *The Hidden Face of Shyness*.

"Society expects men to be self-confident and aggressive, and men who

DO THIS NOW

Take the elevator at every opportunity—at the office, at the mall—and chat with whomever you find there, says Lynne Henderson, Ph.D., director of the Palo Alto Shyness Clinic in Portola Valley, California. You might start by making eye contact and smiling at someone on every ride. Gradually, work up to commenting on your immediate surroundings, the weather, or a headline (if a fellow rider is reading the paper). It's always good to talk about a situation you might commonly share at the moment.

Did You Know?

Shyness originates in the brain. The amygdala and the hippocampus—two clusters of nerve cells located in the limbic system, the part of the brain responsible for emotions—are responsible for the social anxiety part of shyness.

aren't tend to have a lot of problems," Dr. Welkowitz says. "The consequences of shyness for men are particularly severe." Studies show, for example, that men with social phobia achieve less in their careers, marry later in life, have less stable marriages when they do couple up, and are more prone to depression than less self-conscious men. If your shyness is keeping you from doing the things you want to in life, make an appointment with a therapist specializing in cognitive-behavioral treatment of social phobia, says Dr. Welkowitz.

▶SOLUTIONS

Give shyness the slip. If you find yourself thinking, "I'm going to make an ass of myself at the meeting" or "I have no friends," you're giving in to automatic thoughts—ideas that you accept as true without question. And they tend to paralyze shy people, says Dr. Bruno.

"An automatic thought is like a flying fish that jumps out of the water of your subconscious, hangs briefly in the air, and plops back into the water again," Dr. Bruno says. Learning to "net" these thoughts, he says, will rob them of their power. Every time you catch yourself in a distorted thought, write it on a slip of paper, Dr. Bruno says. Keep the slips in one place. "Then, at your leisure, actively reflect on whether these thoughts have a basis in reality," Dr. Bruno suggests. "Most of the time, you'll find that they don't."

Be a host with the most. In the movie *Only the Lonely*, shy John Candy woos a *very* shy Ally Sheedy by focusing on her feelings instead of his own. If you're shy around women, follow Candy's lead: Try to make the woman on your arm as emotionally comfortable as you can. Research shows that women like a man who acts like a "host" while on a date, says Lynne Henderson, Ph.D., director of the Palo Alto Shyness Clinic in Portola Valley, California. "When you behave like a host, you're thinking about helping others feel more comfortable, which takes your mind off yourself," she says.

Be like Mike . . . or Joe . . . or Bob. When you're in a situation that makes your heart pound and your stomach churn, think of a person you know who isn't shy and who is quite effective in similar situations. Just imagine what he would do in your place, Dr. Welkowitz suggests, "then act like you think he would."

▶ALTERNATIVE APPROACHES

Use the power of the pen. Dr. Bruno once had an acquaintance who studied graphology, the scientific system of assessing a person's character by studying his handwriting. "He believed that not only does handwriting reveal character but also it can be used to build character," Dr. Bruno says. One of his recommendations: When you write the pronoun *I*, consciously use a bold handwriting—one strong vertical line with two firm crossbars.

"My acquaintance said, 'If you will make a big, bold, block letter *I*, it is like saying, 'Here I am, world.' The printed *I* is ego-enhancing. It brings the self forward in a confident way," adds Dr. Bruno.

Build up buttercup. It sounds strange, but the flower essence buttercup can help treat shyness that's rooted in low self-esteem, says Patricia Kaminski, co-director of the Flower Essence Society in Nevada City, California, and author of *Healing with Flower Essences* and co-author of *Flower Essence Repertory*. Flower essences—liquid preparations distilled from plants—are used for emotional healing, Kaminski says. You can buy flower essences in health food stores or directly through mail order. To find a store in your area, contact the Flower Essence Society, P. O. Box 459, Nevada City, CA 95959. The recommended dose is four drops (placed under the tongue) four times a day. Flower essences can be used on a short-term basis for acute situations, but if you want to effect a long-term change, you should generally use them for about one month. The amount of time an individual may need to stick with it can vary from person to person. You don't need to worry about overdosing on a flower essence because they only contain traces of actual physical substances—much like homeopathic remedies. Of course, if you drank it in huge quantities, the alcohol in it which is used as a preservative may have some effect.

▶PREVENTIVE MEASURES

Talk to strangers. Although talking to people you don't know can feel like you're buffing your ego with coarse-grade sandpaper, do it as often as you can, Dr. Bruno advises. "Learning to take the initiative—to break the ice—has a desensitizing effect on shyness," he says. Don't worry about being witty. (In fact, *don't* be witty, advises Dr. Bruno, because that puts pressure on the other person to make a clever comeback.) It's enough to ask for a mini review of a movie you're in line to see or to comment on the selection at the buffet table.

Side Stitch

▶PROBLEM

It's that pain in the gut you got in gym class when the teacher made you run the cross-country course. And that's who usually gets side stitches—distance runners.

▶CAUSE

No one really knows why we get side stitches, but it may have something to do with gravity; the jostling of your internal organs; a spasm of the diaphragm, the domed-shape muscular partition that separates the chest from the abdominal cavity; or any combination of these.

The diaphragm inflates and deflates your lungs. When you exercise, it has to work harder. And like any muscle, it can cramp, says Owen Anderson, Ph.D., exercise physiologist and editor of *Running Research News* in Lansing, Michigan. "One clue is that elite athletes don't tend to get stitches, possibly because they have stronger, better-conditioned diaphragm muscles," he says.

The other culprits may be your stomach and liver, both attached to the diaphragm by some fibrous tissues. When you run, your organs may bounce, pull on the diaphragm, and cause a stitch, Dr. Anderson says. "The liver is a really heavy organ, and most stitches do tend to be on the right side," he notes.

If you get a stitch on the left or middle of your abdomen, you may have eaten too soon before running. The weight of the undigested food may simply make the stomach a heavier organ, causing the same effect as the bouncing liver.

"There seem to be a lot of causes. You may be really tense or your muscles aren't properly stretched or you could be dehydrated," says Karlis Ullis, M.D., assistant clinical professor at the University of California, Los Angeles, UCLA School of Medicine.

DO THIS NOW

Putting your legs up is an almost foolproof solution, but you must stop running to do it, says Owen Anderson, Ph.D., exercise physiologist and editor of *Running Research News* in Lansing, Michigan. "Lie down on your back and pull your knees up to your chest," Dr. Anderson suggests. "It takes the pressure right off the diaphragm, and the stitch goes away within a minute or so."

Did You Know?

What do camel jockeys and joggers have in common? Side stitches. Camel racing, a popular sport in wealthy Persian Gulf countries, uses young boys as jockeys because of their light weight and a belief that their high-pitched, juvenile voices make the animals run faster. Apparently, the jostling effect of riding a seven-foot tall camel galloping at 12 miles per hour shakes the internal organs of the young riders so much that they get the jogger's familiar gut ache.

▶HOW SERIOUS

In nearly all cases, a side stitch is just a temporary inconvenience. If you stop what you're doing, it goes away after a minute or so. But don't be too casual about stitches if you're up in years or have a heart condition. Side stitch pain may mimic the early symptoms of a heart attack, so it is important to recognize the symptoms of both, Dr. Ullis says. A side stitch does not radiate to the neck, back, or arms. It does not produce nausea or chest pressure. It will go away within a short period of time, and you can continue to exercise, Dr. Ullis explains. If the pain does not go away almost immediately after you stop exercising, seek immediate medical attention, he adds.

▶SOLUTIONS

Change your breathing pattern. Most people are right-footed breathers, inhaling and exhaling when their right foot strikes the ground. The shock of the impact travels up the right side of the body, and puts downward pressure on the liver, Dr. Anderson says.

"The impact accentuates the pull the organ has on the diaphragm. When you're exhaling, the diaphragm is going up while the liver is going down," Dr. Anderson says. "By switching to left-footed breathing, the jostling effect is less significant. It may be enough to make a stitch disappear."

Switching to left-footed breathing isn't hard, he says. "Most people aren't aware how they breathe anyway, so it's easy to make the change," he says.

Breathe easy. Panting, gasping, and mouth breathing can bring on a side stitch and hasten dehydration, which may also lead to cramping, Dr. Ullis says. "Try to breathe through your nose for a time. You'll conserve fluids and warm the air going into your lungs, and it may give you a more rhythmic, controlled breathing pattern," he says.

Massage your gut. Stitches can occur when the diaphragm becomes restricted by fascia, the fibrous tissue that surrounds muscles and organs. Fascia can be rather stiff and ungiving until warmed and made pliable by exercise or massage, says James Waslaski, sports massage therapist at the Center for Pain Management and Clinical Sports Massage in Tampa, Florida, and author of *International Advancements in Event and Clinical Sports Massage.*

Take a deep breath while you're running and reach up, under your rib cage where the pain seems to be coming from, and rub the region, he suggests. "You're not just rubbing on the stitch, but actually reaching up under the ribs to get to the fascia," Waslaski says. "Sometimes, all you have to do is release that fascia to get rid of the stitch, then focus on deep breathing to keep the stitch from recurring."

▶ALTERNATIVE APPROACHES

Grunt like a pig. Making a loud noise on an exhale seems to break a cramp by forcing the diaphragm to loosen up, Dr. Anderson says. Grunting may allow you to keep running. And who knows? Maybe it will scare the daylights out of that runner you're trying to pass.

▶PREVENTIVE MEASURES

Build those abs. If you build up your abdominal muscles and thus stabilize your internal organs, you're less likely to get side stitches, Dr. Anderson says. Any exercise that makes abs stronger seems to work, but Dr. Anderson recommends the old standby of crunches. Lie flat on your back with your hands cupped behind your ears, elbows out. (Avoid pulling your head up with your hands; it may cause injury to the neck or upper back.) Bend your knees at about a 45-degree angle. Place your feet flat on the floor, shoulder-width apart and about six inches from your buttocks. Keeping your lower body stable, curl your upper torso in toward your knees to the count of two, raising your shoulder blades no more than four to six inches off the floor. And don't arch your lower back since that takes the strain off your midsection. Concentrate on the contraction of the abdominal muscles. Then count to two again as you return to the starting position. Finish your set without resting between repetitions.

"I'd say start with two sets of 10 crunches per day and eventually and comfortably work your way up to three sets of 45 per day," Dr. Anderson says.

Eat light, digest fast. If you tend to get stitches on your left side or in the middle of your abdomen, they're probably related to your stomach and what you ate before exercise, Dr. Ullis says. Eat easily digestible foods and eat at least one to two hours before you work out, suggests Dr. Ullis. That way, your stomach is mostly empty.

"Have simple carbohydrates like crackers, toast, a jelly sandwich, or rice, and maybe some complex carbohydrates such as fruit, fruit juice, or a sports drink," Dr. Ullis says. "What you don't want is much protein or fat because that stays in your stomach a lot longer."

Silent Treatment

▶ PROBLEM

Whoever coined the old saying, "The silent dog is the first to bite," must have experienced the silent treatment firsthand. In a way, enduring your partner's icy politeness and refusal to make eye contact can be as brutal as going 12 rounds with Evander Holyfield. Maybe worse, because you don't have to crawl into bed at night with Holyfield.

▶ CAUSE

So why isn't your partner talking? You have probably made her mad or hurt her feelings. You may have decided to go golfing when your partner's third cousin's wedding was on your calendar. Golf may have been a great escape from a boring wedding, but at your partner's expense. Shutting you out is your partner's way of giving up on the relationship, at least for an hour or two, because of your insensitivity. But whatever the cause, you need to find out what's bothering your partner and how you can fix it in a way that's acceptable to both of you, says Willard Harley Jr., Ph.D., a clinical psychologist and expert on marital therapy in Whitebear Lake, Minnesota, and author of several books on marriage, including *Give and Take*.

▶ HOW SERIOUS

In a healthy relationship—that is, one in which both partners can resolve their conflicts in a mutually acceptable way—an occasional episode of the silent

---

DO THIS NOW

As soon as you realize that your partner is talking in monosyllables (or not at all), ask her what's wrong, says William F. Fitzgerald, Ph.D., a psychotherapist who specializes in marital and sexual psychotherapy at the Silicon Valley Relationship and Sexuality Center in Santa Clara, California. Approach her in a calm, nonjudgmental way. "You might say to her, 'I obviously hurt you in some way or did something to make you angry, but I don't know what. Please help me understand how you feel; I really want to get a better perspective,'" Dr. Fitzgerald suggests. "What woman wouldn't respond to that?"

History Lesson

Chicago, 1905: Joe Tinker, the shortstop for the Chicago Cubs, and Johnny Evers, the Cubs' second baseman, get into a pregame argument that culminates in a fistfight at second base. They give each other the silent treatment for the next 12 years.

Tinker, Evers, and Frank Chance, the Cubs' first baseman, are credited with inventing baseball's double-play combination while they played with the Cubs in the club's glory years (1906–1910). A New York City sports columnist immortalized the deed—and the phrase "Tinker to Evers to Chance"—in the poem "Baseball's Sad Lexicon" in 1910, the year the Cubs won their fourth National League pennant.

But while Tinker, Evers, and Chance were a well-oiled machine on the diamond, off it they couldn't stand each other. Ironically, all three were inducted into the Baseball Hall of Fame in 1946 ... together.

treatment is nothing to worry about, says Dr. Harley. But beware, he says, if you find your partner regularly distant and cold. That scenario spells trouble because it means that your spouse is learning how to live without you.

▶SOLUTIONS

Stand your ground. "The silent treatment is a power play designed to coerce someone into submission," says William F. Fitzgerald, Ph.D., a psychotherapist who specializes in marital and sexual psychotherapy at the Silicon Valley Relationship and Sexuality Center in Santa Clara, California. If your partner frequently uses the silent treatment to get her way, inform her that you're not playing that game anymore. Dr. Fitzgerald suggests saying something along the lines of, "You seem to be giving me the silent treatment. But I won't reward your behavior by changing mine. When you're ready to tell me what's wrong, so that we can work together to fix it, you'll have my undivided attention."

Go back in time. One of the best ways to solve a problem is to think back to the time when it didn't exist. So ask yourself: When was the last time she was talking to you and things seemed fine? Once you have that clear in your mind, pinpoint precisely when she stopped talking to you. Then, think about what happened in the time in between. You may identify something you did or didn't do that is directly linked to your being cast in the starring role of her silent movie.

Wait it out. If your initial apology and expression of willingness to resolve the problem doesn't break the ice, wait it out. While some spouses may be willing to break out of withdrawal immediately and are willing to start discussing the problem, others are not able to lower their defenses that quickly. If your partner wants to continue to be left alone, keep a respectful distance until she is ready to talk to you again, says Dr. Harley. But before you leave her alone, let her know that you will be ready to solve the problem whenever she feels ready.

▶ALTERNATIVE APPROACHES

Do something nice. While waiting for your partner to warm to the idea of talking again, give her evidence that you are serious about taking her feelings into account. Be willing to help with something she needs help with. Run an errand, fold the laundry, brew some coffee. Your thoughtful gesture may demonstrate your willingness to be more thoughtful in the future, and that will go a long way toward thawing your partner out, Dr. Harley says.

▶PREVENTIVE MEASURES

Shut off the silencer. Overcome behavior that pushes your partner's buttons, says Dr. Harley. Does she go mute when you snap at her? Next time, think before you speak. Does she zip her lip without fail the day after your regular all-night poker game? Don't go to the poker game if it makes her unhappy. Learn to fill your leisure time with activities that you can enjoy together. Avoiding "hot buttons" not only prevents a chilly silence but also lets her know that you care about her.

Sinus Problems

▶PROBLEM

Sinusitis is an inflammation or infection of the sinuses that affects an estimated 35 million people in the United States, 14 million of them men. The symptoms include nasal stuffiness, facial pain, throbbing headaches, and postnasal drip, an annoying leakage of mucus from the back of the nose into the throat. Sinusitis can also cause some nasty drainage from the nose—thick, yellowish-white stuff that looks like custard. Sinusitis comes in two flavors: acute and chronic. Acute sinusitis commonly follows a cold and can last up to three weeks. After continuing for three months, and after an x-ray shows evidence of inflammation of sinuses, it's officially chronic sinusitis.

▶CAUSE

The sinuses—eight hollow, air-filled pockets above, below, and behind the eyes—lighten the weight of our skulls and give our voices resonance. They also make mucus, and here's where the problem starts. The sinuses are lined with cilia, tiny hairlike projections that beat like waves. Normally, the cilia move the mucus into the nasal cavity and you blow it out. But viruses, bacteria, allergens, and cigarette smoke can cause the membranes that line the nose to swell, trapping the mucus in the sinuses. This backup of mucus then becomes infected, and the torture begins.

DO THIS NOW

Boil a gallon of water to sterilize it, let it cool, and stir in one tablespoon of salt. Then, pour some into your hand and sniff it into your nostrils. You may do it to both nostrils at once or one at a time, says Sanford Archer, M.D., associate professor of otolaryngology at the University of Kentucky A. B. Chandler Medical Center in Lexington. You can do this as often as necessary. This saltwater mixture will help reduce stuffiness, soothe irritated membranes in the nose, and moisten the sinuses. Keep the extra solution in the refrigerator, although it's probably best to make it fresh every day.

Did You Know?

Normal sinuses produce about a quart of mucus every day. Inflamed or infected sinuses, on the other hand, can produce a half-gallon or more.

▶HOW SERIOUS

Most of the time, acute sinusitis clears up on its own. But if you're not better in 10 to 14 days, you need to see a doctor, who will prescribe antibiotics and perhaps some other medications, says Wellington S. Tichenor, M.D., an allergist in private practice in New York City who specializes in allergies, asthma, and sinusitis. Rarely, acute sinusitis can lead to meningitis or clots in the blood vessels of the brain. Chronic sinusitis can be serious for people with chronic lung conditions. Because these folks can't cough the infected mucus up and out, it may settle in the lungs and lead to pneumonia.

▶SOLUTIONS

Hit the showers. Take a hot shower, advises Sanford Archer, M.D., associate professor of otolaryngology at the University of Kentucky A. B. Chandler Medical Center in Lexington. "The steam will help open up your nose and sinuses and help them drain," he says. Stay in the shower for 10 to 15 minutes.

Go ahead—inhale. If you'd rather keep your clothes on, boil a pot of water and inhale the steam, Dr. Archer suggests. Before inhaling, take the pot off the stove and let it cool so that no active boiling is taking place. (If the water is actively boiling, it can scald your face.) Hold your face about a foot away from the pot and cover your head and shoulders with a towel to trap the steam.

Be a man of the cloth. Lay a hot, wet washcloth over your eyes and cheekbones for fast relief, Dr. Archer says. Wet the washcloth with hot tap water and wring it out, but make sure that the cloth isn't too hot because it could burn your skin. Rewet it every few minutes to keep it warm, says Dr. Archer.

Buy a humidifier. Run a humidifier at your bedside every night, Dr. Tichenor says. It will keep your nasal and sinus passages from drying out, which can aggravate your symptoms. While most people with sinusitis prefer hot-mist humidifiers, he says, opt for a cold-mist model if there are children in your household to prevent scalding accidents. Cool-mist humidifiers are magnets for fungus, so clean yours out daily with soap, water, and about one teaspoon of bleach. Be sure to rinse the humidifier thoroughly until the bleach smell is gone. Hot-mist humidifiers also need to be cleaned, but not as often—about once every two or three days.

Fill your glass. Drink as much water as you can—at least eight, eight-ounce glasses every day, says Dr. Tichenor. "Water helps thin out mucus, so the more you drink, the better off you'll be," he says.

Soothe with a spray. Nasal sprays such as Afrin can relieve congestion and pain, says Dr. Archer. But don't use them longer than two or three days at a time, and follow the label directions. While these products initially shrink nasal passages and relieve stuffiness, overuse can cause nasal passages to swell even more than before, a condition called rebound congestion.

Stage a counter attack. The cold-remedy aisle of virtually every drugstore in America is bulging with over-the-counter medications for sinus problems. You might start with a decongestant that contains pseudoephedrine hydrochloride, such as Sudafed. If you have high blood pressure, check with your doctor before taking decongestants, says Dr. Archer. And don't take antihistamines to treat a sinus infection. " Antihistamines dry up mucus, and you don't want that," he says.

▶ALTERNATIVE APPROACHES

Root out sinus pain. "My favorite home remedy for sinusitis is to sniff horseradish," Dr. Archer says. He recommends one or two quick sniffs of prepared hot horseradish two or three times a day. Stay four to six inches from the jar because the strong smell can be very powerful, and avoid breathing into the jar, which could contaminate it for other family members, says Dr. Archer. This spicy root contains allyl isothiocyanate, a chemical similar to one used in decongestants. Freshly grated horseradish will knock the socks off anyone, "but the stuff in the jar is just as good," says Dr. Archer. It doesn't matter whether you use white or purple horseradish, but the white variety tends to be hotter.

Slurp some herbs. Drink a cup of goldenseal tea twice a day for 14 to 21 days, suggests Scott Gerson, M.D., an expert in Ayurvedic medicine in private practice in Brewster, New York, and New York City. This herb is classified as an antimicrobial, meaning that it helps kill viruses and bacteria that can lead to infection. To make goldenseal tea, put one teaspoon of the loose herb in a tea ball and put the ball in an eight-ounce cup. Pour boiling water over the ball, let the tea steep for five to seven minutes, and drink. Buying a box of prepackaged goldenseal tea bags is okay, too, says Dr. Gerson. They're available at many health food stores. But make sure to use the tea within four months because herbs' healing properties weaken with age. Goldenseal should not be used for longer than three weeks at a time, especially if you suffer from a chronic kidney disease. Otherwise, it is quite safe, says Dr. Gerson.

▶PREVENTIVE MEASURES

Allergy-proof your turf. Many people with sinusitis also have allergies, says Dr. Tichenor. If you're one of them, avoid as many allergens as you can. If you're allergic to dust, use mattress and pillow covers and remove carpeting in the bedroom. If pollen is the problem, close the windows and turn on the air conditioner. If you're allergic to animal dander, keep pets out of the bedroom.

Sloppiness

▶ PROBLEM

Your house or office lies somewhere beneath junk mail, dirty clothes, unused exercise machines, recyclables, the remains of last night's dinner, and lots of other stuff.

▶ CAUSE

Odds are that you have a clutter problem because you lack systems for organizing all this stuff and you don't have much time to get it done, says Susan Sussman, a professional organizer in Lafayette Hill, Pennsylvania. "People just don't have a lot of time today because both men and women are out working," she says. "When there isn't as much time, you simply have to be more organized. Otherwise, clutter will just take over."

DO THIS NOW

Put your stuff in containers: shoe boxes, plastic bins, drawers, files, and baskets. "Containing things is a trick of the trade," says Ann Saunders, a professional organizer who is president of S.O.S.—Simple Organizing Solutions in Baltimore. "It gives organization to the clutter and enables you to keep like items together."

▶ HOW SERIOUS

Being a disorganized pack rat may be just a personal preference. Your desktop is strewn with unfiled reports, banana peels, and newspapers, but you can plunge your hand into the mess and come up with exactly what you need. And that's okay, says Ann Saunders, a professional organizer who is president of S.O.S.—Simple Organizing Solutions in Baltimore. But sometimes clutter compromises your life. You don't pay bills on time because you can't find them. You pay extra interest on credit cards because your payments are always late. And you don't bring home guests because your home is a disaster.

In its worst case, disorganization and sloppiness may be a symptom of depression, attention deficit disorder (ADD), or some type of neuropsychiatric problem, says Charles Gant, M.D., medical director at the Holistic Center of Central New York in Syracuse. If you think that your sloppiness problem might

be caused by one of these more serious conditions, see your doctor.

▶SOLUTIONS

Schedule yourself. You may
get to business meetings or doctor
appointments on time, but when it

comes to scheduling personal tasks, you're a slacker. Get an appointment
book and block out time during the week to pay your bills, do your laundry, or
sweep out the garage, says Sussman. This is not a to-do list but a real schedule,
she adds.

"A schedule forces you to prioritize and make time estimates," Sussman
says. "It makes you much more realistic about what can get done."

Relocate home. Clear everything out of a given space. Pretend that you've
just moved to your house and it's time to plan how you'd like the area to look
and function, advises Saunders. Then fill and organize the space accordingly.
Dispose of everything else.

Reinvent the system. "You may need to rethink your systems. Just because
you've always done something one way, doesn't mean that it works," Saunders
explains.

You may decide to hang your ties on one rack, put your shirts on another,
and keep your sports jackets together. Or, maybe you'll find it easier to coordinate a tie, clean shirt and jacket on one hanger, suggests Saunders. "It doesn't
matter what system you choose, as long as you're consistent in following
through," she says. "You may have a good system, but it doesn't work if you
keep throwing your clothes on the floor."

Take a small bite. When faced with a huge pile, your natural tendency is
to try to do it all at once. Break down your organizing into manageable tasks,
starting with the most immediate, says Sussman.

"If you don't, it will get overwhelming, and you'll leave it half done,"
Sussman predicts. "It's better to chip away at it."

If your mail has piled up for weeks, just sort out all the bills, says Sussman.
Deal with those, and then start on the book club responses or credit card solic-
itations.

▶ALTERNATIVE APPROACHES

Toss away that old life. *Feng shui*, the Chinese art of placement, advocates
that you throw away nine objects per day for nine days or, even better, for 27
days, says Steven Post, chief executive officer of the Geomancy/Feng Shui Education Organization in San Francisco and author of *The Modern Book of Feng
Shui*. The numbers of days—all multiples of three—are important because to
the Chinese they represent completeness, Post explains.

As you toss out the items, think about ways to open your life to new opportunities, to clear out any obstructions that are impeding the benefits that could be flowing to you from the surrounding world, says Post.

"You link the physical act with your intention of getting more control of your life," Post says. "By organizing space, you are also clearing the mind."

▶PREVENTIVE MEASURES

Make time to save time. Maybe you don't think you have the time to be neat and ordered, but a few minutes spent organizing saves much more time later on, says Sussman. Take 5 minutes every hour or 30 minutes at the end of the working day to clean up and prepare for upcoming tasks," she suggests.

Snoring

▶PROBLEM

The problem is a hoarse, rasping sound produced during sleep by drawing air through the mouth. Most snorers are men, middle-aged or older, and overweight. Smoking and drinking makes the problem even worse.

▶CAUSE

During sleep, the muscles in the throat relax, the tongue slips back a bit, and your airway narrows. Usually, that's not a problem. But if the opening is so constricted that you have to draw hard to breathe, the airflow vibrates the soft tissues of your palate. This giant sucking sound is akin to wind howling down a narrow canyon, says Neil Kavey, M.D., director of the Sleep Disorders Center at Columbia-Presbyterian Medical Center in New York City.

▶HOW SERIOUS

We all snore sometimes: when we're extremely tired, lying on our backs, or after an evening of beer drinking with the boys. But if you snore every night, loudly enough that your bedmate complains or a business associate refuses to share a motel room with you on the road, you may have a problem, says Dr. Kavey.

"When you or your wife has to sleep in another room, that's a problem right there," says Dr. Kavey. "But loud, chronic snoring also may mean that all is not right with your sleep."

The warning signals to watch for are restless sleep (tossing and turning) and

DO THIS NOW

If you snore in bed but not on the recliner, it could be your attitude—meaning the tilt of your body. When you're sprawled out flat on a bed, gravity is more likely to pull your tongue down into the airway, says Neil Kavey, M.D., director of the Sleep Disorders Center at Columbia-Presbyterian Medical Center in New York City.

Try tilting your bed by placing bricks or phone book–size blocks under the headboard. Or put an extra pillow under your head. "That angle may make your airway fall just a little differently and smooth out the airflow," says Dr. Kavey.

History Lesson

When your wife and kids complain that your snoring sets the house to vibrating, you can mention Kåre Walkert of Sweden, the world-record holder for the loudest snore. At 93 decibels, Walkert's snore is almost as loud as standing about 11 yards away from an iron worker who's riveting together steel beams. That's louder than the din of city street traffic (68 decibels) and just below the percussion of a hammer striking a steel plate (114 decibels).

When Walkert recorded his snore at a hospital in 1993, he suffered from sleep apnea.

---

extreme daytime sleepiness, says William Finley, Ph.D., director of the Sleep Disorders Center at St. Mary's Medical Center in Knoxville, Tennessee. Heavy snorers often experience apneas (Greek for "without breath"), complete blockages of the airway that literally choke off your wind. You may struggle for breath and wake up frequently at night, although you may not be aware of these nocturnal arousals, says Dr. Finley.

"Apneas are a real health risk, associated with heart problems, high blood pressure, stroke, and automobile accidents caused by falling asleep while driving," says Dr. Finley. "And many heavy snorers, who now only have partial blockage of their airways, will eventually progress to full-blown apneas." If you suspect that you have sleep apnea, see a doctor right away, he advises.

Even if you don't have sleep apnea, loud snoring may damage the muscles in your throat, according to a study by Swedish researchers.

▶SOLUTIONS

Cut the smokes and suds. A night on the town makes for noisy sleep. Smoking swells throat tissues and narrows the airway, while alcohol so relaxes the neck muscles that it makes a partial collapse more likely at night, says John Galgon, M.D., medical director of the Sleep Disorders Clinic at Lehigh Valley Hospital in Allentown, Pennsylvania.

"You shouldn't drink in the evening before bed, and, of course, for a lot of health reasons, you should quit smoking," Dr. Galgon says. "Smokers almost always have inflamed, swollen throat tissues."

Put the squeeze on. Sleep doctors call them external nasal dilators, but you know them as those fancy pieces of tape that football players wear on their noses. "Dilators open a normally narrow portion of the nose," explains Dr. Finley. "They increase airflow, and for some folks, that's all that's needed." Nasal dilators such as Breathe Right are available at drugstores.

Hose your nose. If you wake up in the morning with dry mouth, the problem may be in your nose, not your throat, Dr. Galgon says. Many snorers have deviated septums, chronic congestion, postnasal drip, or nasal polyps that force them to breathe through their mouths. Try to clear a path through your plugged proboscis with an over-the-counter nasal spray or allergy medication. These sprays can be effective but may be addicting, so be sure not to use them more than three times a day or for more than three days, advises Dr. Galgon.

Go for a run. When the muscles of the upper airway lose their tone and strength from aging or inactivity, they may be more likely to sag during sleep, says Dr. Finley.

Vigorous aerobic exercise and physical fitness may put the tone and tautness back in your upper airway muscles. Aerobic exercise activates muscles that dilate the upper airway so that you can take in more air and, in so doing, may also strengthen upper airway muscles.

For those who are overweight, weight reduction often leads to marked improvement of snoring by removal of fat from the walls of the upper airway, says Dr. Finley. "Physically fit people, like runners, rarely appear at the sleep center complaining of loud snoring or breathing pauses while they sleep," he says.

For most of us, aerobic exercise such as brisk walking, jogging, or playing basketball 30 to 40 minutes a day three or four times a week will lead to improved physical fitness. Choose a form of exercise you really enjoy doing because if you don't, you're unlikely to stay with it long enough to tone up sagging muscles and to lose weight, says Dr. Finley. As an added bonus, being physically fit is associated with better, more restful sleep, he adds.

▶ALTERNATIVE APPROACHES

Back off. You're most likely to snore on your back. Stay off your back by stuffing Styrofoam peanuts (packing material) into a sock and then sewing the sock onto the back of a tight-fitting night shirt, Dr. Kavey says. "Each time you lay on your back, you'll be prodded by the Styrofoam and forced to turn onto your side," says Dr. Kavey. "Some people recommend several tennis balls, but those get heavy."

▶PREVENTIVE MEASURES

Taper the neck. Most snorers are overweight guys with big necks. If you're carrying extra pounds around the middle, then you probably have fat deposits in the back of your throat, which narrows the space behind your tongue. When you're asleep, your throat muscles relax and narrow that space even more, causing you to snore, says Dr. Galgon. "If you want to stop snoring, try losing some weight," he says. "Sometimes just 25 to 30 pounds can make a difference in some patients."

Sore Throat

▶PROBLEM

Your throat is reacting to an intruding germ by swelling and getting red, hot, and sore, says David Rooney, M.D., a family physician with Southern Chester County Family Practice Associates in Oxford, Pennsylvania. "The mucous membranes that produce saliva make your throat a very sensitive spot on your body," explains Dr. Rooney. "There are a lot of nerve endings there, which is why you feel even a minor infection so promptly."

▶CAUSE

Your throat could be responding to a strep or cold virus as well as simply some postnasal drip, Dr. Rooney says. If your voice is hoarse, it could be due to "gastroesophageal reflux," or heartburn, he adds. Other possible causes of sore throats and hoarseness are smoking, yelling too much, or using your voice improperly.

Finally, a worst-case scenario for a sore throat is a growth or problem in the neck that's causing pain in the throat. This is very rare, though, Dr. Rooney says.

▶HOW SERIOUS

You should see a doctor if there are changes in your voice that last longer than two weeks, or if your sore throat is accompanied by symptoms, such as coughing up blood, a lump in the neck, or difficulty swallowing, Dr. Rooney says.

DO THIS NOW

Soak a small towel in very warm water, wring it out well, and wrap it around your neck. Cover the cloth with a piece of wool (such as a scarf) and leave both on until your neck is quite warm. Then, take the cloth and put it in cold water. Wring it out very well and wrap it around your neck, again covering it with wool. This time, leave both on until the cloth dries.

"This will promote circulation in your neck and throat," says Devra Krassner, a doctor of naturopathic medicine and homeopathy in private practice in Portland, Maine. "Increased circulation naturally promotes healing." Repeat one or two times a day for the duration of the sore throat.

Did You Know?

Legend has it that Saint Blaise once saved the life of a boy who had a fish bone stuck in his throat. To commemorate this event, Catholics to this day celebrate the blessing of the throat on Saint Blaise's Feast Day each February 3.

In U.S. churches that observe this feast day, the blessing is given while two unlit candles are held under the throat in the formation of the cross. In Germany, where the throat blessing ceremony is more widespread, the candles are lit.

You also should see a doctor if you think you have strep throat. Here are the signs: severe pain, pus in your throat, swollen glands (tender spots on the sides of your neck, just below your jaw and ears). And you should see a doctor if you have a high fever (over 101°F) or pain behind your eyes and ears, adds Dr. Rooney.

▶SOLUTIONS

Gargle salt water. It's one of the oldest and most common home remedies; and the good news is, it really works. Mix a half-teaspoon of salt in four ounces of warm water for best results. Gargle it four times a day. "The bacteria germs can't survive in salt water," says Leif Christiansen, D.O., a physician with the Perkiomen Internal Medicine Group in Mount Penn, Pennsylvania. "But more than that, the salt water acts as a disinfectant to any open sores in your mouth. Finally, it also breaks apart the thickened mucus and helps you breathe better and feel better."

Find relief the hard way. When it comes to sore throats, candy *is* dandy. There's no medicinal effect here, but sucking on hard candy such as lemon drops will produce saliva, which will soothe your sore throat, Dr. Rooney says.

Follow your nose. Breathe through your nose whenever possible. It acts as a natural air humidifier. Your throat is healthiest when it's moist, and breathing through your mouth dries out your throat, says Jerome C. Goldstein, M.D., visiting professor of otolaryngology/head and neck surgery at Johns Hopkins University School of Medicine in Baltimore and Georgetown University School of Medicine in Washington, D.C.

Spray it. Those over-the-counter spray remedies, such as Cepacol Spray or Sucrets, do work to numb the throat and temporarily relieve pain, Dr. Rooney says. "The problem is that it's difficult to get it in the right place," he adds. So, if you have good aim or the pain doesn't seem localized in the far reaches of your throat, by all means, spray away.

If you do want to give the medications a try, look for sprays with dyclonine hydrochloride, which is also found in many throat lozenges.

▶ALTERNATIVE APPROACHES

Knock back a mixed drink. Of honey, lemon juice, and ground red pepper, that is. "Pour about a teaspoon of honey into a tablespoon, top off the spoon with fresh lemon juice and then add a pinch of ground red pepper," says Elson Haas, M.D., director of the Preventive Medical Center of Marin in San Rafael, California.

Take this mixture, straight up and without water, every few hours until your throat feels better. Each ingredient helps a different symptom. Honey coats the throat, lemon cleanses by its astringent action and may reduce inflammation, and the ground red pepper promotes blood circulation in the area, Dr. Haas says.

Slip in some slippery elm. You can buy this herb as a lozenge in most health food stores and some drugstores, says Devra Krassner, a doctor of naturopathic medicine and homeopathy in private practice in Portland, Maine. Officially, it's considered a demulcent, which means that it soothes your throat because it's, well, slippery, and relieves that dry, scratchy feeling. Use the lozenges as needed.

▶PREVENTIVE MEASURES

Stop shouting already. It's easy to get carried away while cheering on the home team. But going home without a voice simply means that you've been yelling enough to annoy everyone around you, and now it's time to pay. "There's no warning sign to tell you that you're using your voice too much or incorrectly," Dr. Rooney says. "Being hoarse is the sign, and by then, it's too late." So, keep it down.

Sperm Problems

▶PROBLEM

Female and male problems can be equally to blame when there is infertility, but in this case, it's your sperm that are in a slump.

▶CAUSE

A man may have too few sperm. His little guys could be poor swimmers who poop out before they reach the finish line. They may have deformities or other abnormalities. Or the man could have too little seminal fluid with which to guide his sperm on their difficult journey. Lots of things can adversely affect your sperm, from contracting the mumps to getting a hard kick to the testicles. A common culprit is a varicocele—veins near the testicle that may drive up the temperature of your testicles, damaging sperm production and their motility or movement.

There also is some evidence that men everywhere may be producing less sperm than they once did. A 10-year study of middle-aged men in Finland, for example, found that the percentage of men with normal sperm production dropped from 56 percent to 27 percent from 1981 to 1991. Some researchers suspect that pollutants and chemical pesticides in the water and food supply increase environmental estrogens—compounds that act like the female hormone. Others, however, say that it simply hasn't been established yet if sperm production is really disappearing as fast as the rain forest. These researchers say that more studies are needed.

▶HOW SERIOUS

For many men, learning that they are infertile is a huge blow to their self-esteem. The truth is that, even if a guy's sperm are sputtering, it has no bearing on his masculinity, says Neil Baum, M.D., associate clinical professor of urology at Tulane University Medical School and Louisiana State University School of Medicine, and director of the Impotence Foundation, all in New Orleans. "Men can be very virile and very sexually active but can be infertile," he says A couple is considered infertile when they have been trying to conceive a child and had unprotected intercourse for one year without success. You may want to get a semen analysis even sooner, however, if your partner is in her mid-thirties or older, since the ticking of her biological clock is growing ever louder by now. About five million American couples have trouble conceiving—about one out of seven will have problems doing so sometime during their reproductive years.

> ### MEN'S HEALTH INDEX
>
> **Sperm are amazing little devils. Here are a few things you might not know about them.**
>
> 1. **A man's testicles produce 50,000 sperm per minute around the clock from puberty on into old age.**
> 2. **During each ejaculation, a man typically releases between 80 million and 300 million sperm.**
> 3. **All 300 million or so of those sperm can fit on a pinhead.**
> 4. **Sperm and fluid from the testicles make up only 3 to 5 percent of a man's semen. The rest is fluid produced in the seminal vesicles and the prostate.**
> 5. **A single sperm needs four to five days to learn to swim and swims only one to two inches an hour. Very few will make it to a woman's Fallopian tube, home to a woman's egg.**

▶SOLUTIONS

Get loose. Men who have a borderline sperm count or low motility of their sperm can also benefit from wearing loose-fitting underwear, suggests Dr. Baum.

Drink in moderation. One glass of wine or two beers per day is considered moderate. Any more than that may harm sperm production, says Larry Lipshultz, M.D., professor of urology at Baylor College of Medicine in Houston.

Use a condom. Not if you're trying to make a baby, of course. But protecting yourself against a sexually transmitted disease when you're younger could protect your sperm when you're older, says Dr. Lipshultz. That's because some diseases, such as gonorrhea and chlamydia, can occasionally impair fertility, he says.

Forgo the high life. The use of recreational drugs such as marijuana can be a downer for sperm production, says Dr. Lipshultz.

Lose the lube. Avoid using lubricants if you're trying to father a child, says Dr. Baum. "The sperm get caught in the jelly. Any of the lubricants can affect sperm motility," he says.

De-stress for success. Learning a relaxation technique to deal with stress could help your sperm. One study suggests a relationship between stressful events and changes in sperm production, says Dr. Lipshultz. "It's hard to isolate stress as a single variable," he says. "But people who are under stress do things that aren't healthy. They won't sleep enough, they won't eat correctly, they won't exercise." In other words, things that could impair their sperm.

▶ALTERNATIVE APPROACHES

Add some C. Vitamin C is an antioxidant that stabilizes cell membranes and may promote healthy sperm, says Dr. Lipshultz. He recommends getting at least 500 milligrams a day.

Put the E in sperm. Similarly, vitamin E is an antioxidant that may be helpful to sperm. Dr. Lipshultz recommends 400 international units a day.

▶PREVENTIVE MEASURES

Stay off Tobacco Road. Tobacco can produce oxidants that adversely affect the shape of your sperm, and possibly its DNA, says Dr. Lipshultz. Here's yet one more reason to quit smoking or refrain from starting.

Protect yourself. If injury to the testicles can impair sperm production, it pays to wear a protective cup when you're engaging in contact sports or any sport where you might get hit in the groin, experts say.

Splinters

▶PROBLEM

You have a foreign object lodged in your skin.

▶CAUSE

Everything from stacking split wood to sliding your bottom across an old park bench to breaking a glass while washing the dishes can give you a splinter.

▶HOW SERIOUS

Splinters hurt because they're usually in your fingertips—not your posterior—where there are lots of nerve endings. It's best to remove splinters sooner than later, says Howard Backer, M.D., a physician who practices emergency sports and wilderness medicine for Kaiser Permanente Medical Centers in the San Francisco Bay area and teaches wilderness medicine through the Wilderness Medical Society. Metal and glass splinters are less of a problem than wood slivers because wood is reactive and nearly always causes an infection, says Dr. Backer.

"If it's wood, you should remove it right away. If you don't, it will become infected; and then you'll need a doctor to drain the abscess and remove the sliver. And that's painful," explains Dr. Backer.

▶SOLUTIONS

Use the right tool. Your mother probably wielded a sewing needle or straight pin to dig for a sliver, while you did your best to squirm away. Needles work, but they tear at the tissue to get to the sliver. There are better products available: tweezers with serrations to grasp the splinter or short-handled

> ### DO THIS NOW
>
> **Scrub up. Before you operate on yourself or someone else to get a splinter out, wash your hands and the area around the imbedded splinter with soap and water, says Warren Bowman, M.D., medical director for the National Ski Patrol who lives in Cooke City, Montana, just outside Yellowstone National Park. That'll help prevent an infection that could be even worse than the pain of a splinter.**

Did You Know?

Your skin has a built-in splinter-removal system. It's in a constant state of re-generation and deterioration. The outer layer—the epidermal—consists of cells born 35 to 45 days earlier in the dermis, the deeper skin layer, that binds the body together like a body stocking. If you get a small splinter in this outer layer of your skin, the constant sloughing of skin cells will eventually force the splinter up to the surface. Of course, you shouldn't wait a month for that to happen, no matter how small or superficial the splinter.

tweezers with pointed tips, such as the Splinter Grabber, that give you excellent control, says Carl Weil, an emergency medical technician and director of Wilderness Medicine Outfitters in Elizabeth, Colorado. Tweezers with serrations are available at most drugstores. You can get the Splinter Grabber at some outdoor stores or through B&A Products, Route 1, Box 100, Bunch, OK 74931-9705. There's also a tool called a lance—basically a three-cornered, tapered needle—which you can slide into the skin parallel to the splinter and use to lift out the splinter, Weil says. CFM Technologies sells a Splinter-Removal Kit that comes with tweezers and a lance. The company's address is 192 Worcester Road, Wellesley, MA 02181.

Whatever you use, be sure to sterilize the item before probing. To do that, you can scrub it with soap and water, put it in rubbing alcohol for 30 seconds, or hold it over a clean flame, such as from a gas stove, says Weil. Just be sure to let tweezers you put in a flame cool for a minute or so before using, he adds.

Don't slice and dice. Most slivers—at least one end anyway—lodge in the epidermis or outer layer of dead skin cells where it doesn't really hurt much to probe around. But don't get too carried away if you have a lance, says Weil. "You don't want to be slicing and dicing yourself. That will just make things worse," says Weil.

The best strategy is to get at one end of the sliver, lift up, and pull with tweezers. If the splinter goes under the fingernail, you may have to cut a small V notch into the nail to get at the splinter. Then grasp one end of the splinter with tweezers and pull, Weil says.

Patch the hole. When you get the sliver out, clean the wound and the surrounding skin with hydrogen peroxide, a povidone-iodine solution such as Betadine, or just plain soap and water, says Warren Bowman, M.D., medical director for the National Ski Patrol who lives in Cooke City, Montana, just outside Yellowstone National Park. Or you can use Hibiclens—a germicidal soap like the ones used in hospitals to prepare the skin for surgery, he says. All these products are available at drugstores. After cleaning the area, flush it with clean water. "Then apply a small bead of antibiotic ointment and cover with a bandage," Dr. Bowman adds.

▶ALTERNATIVE APPROACHES

Soak it. If you have trouble getting at the sliver (if it is deep in the skin), try soaking the affected area in a solution of Epsom salts and warm water, which will soften the skin and draw the sliver closer to the surface, says Weil. "Then you may be able to get at it with tweezers," he says.

Sacrifice a plant. You can also make effective drawing poultices from the common houseplant aloe, says Weil. "Simply cut off part of a leaf of the plant, lay the cut edge over the splinter, tape it in place with an adhesive bandage and leave it there for several hours, says Weil. The aloe will help to draw the splinter out of the skin so that you can more easily remove it with a tweezers, he says. Some people are allergic to aloe, so before using it as a poultice, put some of the gel from the leaf on a small area of your skin and make sure that the area doesn't become red or irritated, says Weil.

▶PREVENTIVE MEASURES

Protect yourself. One of the best, simplest ways to prevent most splinters is to simply wear leather gloves when you're hauling wood or nailing up a two-by-four, says Weil.

Don't let things slide. Whether it's your buttocks on a bench or a hand along a split-rail fence, let common sense guide you: Try not to slide your skin along a rough, splintery surface. That's just asking for trouble.

Sports Addiction

▶PROBLEM

You know the names and vital statistics of the entire Dallas Cowboys offensive line (not to mention their cheerleaders) but can't remember your own kid's name or birthday. If sports dominate your life to the point where they're virtually all that you watch and think about—negatively affecting your family, job, and social life—you may be a sports addict.

▶CAUSE

Put a guy in a roomful of other guys he has never met and all someone has to say is "How about those Bulls?" The next thing you know, they're talking like they have known each other for years. "It's tremendous bonding. When men get together, they have an immediate conversation. Men are more comfortable talking about those things," says Leonard Jason, Ph.D., professor of clinical and community psychology at DePaul University in Chicago and co-author of *Remote Control.* But in order to keep up with the other guys, you also have to be right on top of the latest stats, scores, and deals, leading some men to become compulsive. And, like other addictions, sports can be a way to avoid dealing with other problems.

▶HOW SERIOUS

At the least, you can become a bore. At its worst, sports addiction has brought many a couple to the marriage therapist's office. "I have had women threaten divorce," says Robert Pasick, Ph.D., a clinical psychologist at the Ann Arbor Center for the Family in Michigan and author of *Men in Therapy*.

In extreme cases, men can become so obsessed with sports that it can cause them to avoid problems in their own lives, says Merrill J. Melnick, Ph.D., sport sociologist and professor of physical education and sport at the State University of New York at Brockport. "It's like a sweaty Land of Oz for them," he says. If sports obsession interferes with your daily routine or takes precedence over your family or work responsibilities, you may need professional help, says Dr. Melnick.

▶SOLUTIONS

Go cold turkey. Take a week off from sports. That's right—no baseball, no ESPN SportsCenter, no *USA Today* sports page—for at least a week. And no fair picking the week after the Super Bowl, when nothing happens anyway. Keep breathing; this isn't going to kill you. But it will force you to find something else to do with your life, Dr. Pasick says. "A lot of times, people just fall back on watching sports because they don't have anything else to do and they get stuck there," he says. Spend your sports time reading a good book, going to the movies, catching a show, or just getting out of the house. Or maybe something really wacky, like talking to your wife and kids.

Play in your own old-timer's game. You may know all of Joe DiMaggio's stats, but wouldn't it be fun to talk with someone who has actually seen "The Yankee Clipper" in action? Call your local nursing home or community center and ask if you can volunteer time with residents similarly interested in sports, Dr. Melnick says. Perhaps you could start a sports group to watch a game each week or just find a single fan who wants to share his sports knowledge as much as you do.

Go from couch to coach. Maybe your days of running the base paths are over. That doesn't mean that you shouldn't be out there in the middle of the action. Put your extensive sports knowledge to good use by coaching the local Little League team or a school sports team, says Dr. Jason.

"Serve in a voluntary capacity with youth sports. They need informed coaches," Dr. Melnick adds.

Suit up. If you enjoy the thrill of victory and agony of defeat from your couch, imagine how intense it feels when you actually play. Okay, so the company softball tournament may not be as exciting as the NBA playoffs, but it's a great way to enjoy sports, socialize, and get fit at the same time, says Joel H. Fish, Ph.D., a sport psychologist and director of the Center for Sport Psychology in Philadelphia. Bring the wife and kids along and make sports a fun activity for everyone to enjoy.

Read the other sections of the paper. Unless you want your grave inscription to read, "He knew all the winners of every major PGA tournament from 1985 to 1995 as well as the batting averages of the 1980 Philadelphia

History Lesson

To hear most women tell it, sports addiction is strictly a male thing. How, then, do you explain 65-year-old Katherine Eldridge, who chose to go into heart failure rather than miss her beloved University of Kentucky Wildcats' basketball game?

During the Kentucky-Tulane game on March 18, 1995, the *Lexington Herald-Leader* reported, Eldridge felt short of breath. But it wasn't the fast-paced nature of the game that had her gasping for air. She knew what it meant. Three years earlier, a leaky valve in her heart caused fluid to build up in her lungs. It led to heart failure and open-heart surgery.

But when she experienced the same signs during the game, she didn't call the hospital. "I wanted to see my Cats play," she told the *Lexington Herald-Leader* at the time. Even after the Wildcats romped Tulane's Green Wave 82 to 60, she waited until the next morning to go to the hospital.

Phillies starting lineup," you need to become a bit more well-versed in other areas. Start your re-education with the rest of the daily paper you may throw away after you grab the sports section, suggests Philip Levendusky, Ph.D., clinical psychologist at McLean Hospital in Belmont, Massachusetts. Catching up on politics, world events and local goings-on will expand your personality and your mind, making you more interesting to those who aren't interested in sports. (Yes, such people do exist.) The entertainment and local sections will also help you find other things to do with your new free time.

As Dr. Melnick says, it's not a crime that you know a lot about sports; but it is a shame if it's the only thing you know.

Educate your partner. Teach your wife the finer points of your favorite sports, Dr. Melnick says. "Tell her, 'I could teach you some of the basics. You might even come to enjoy this activity that I enjoy,'" Dr. Melnick says. She may actually have a better eye for it than you.

▶ALTERNATIVE APPROACHES

Figure out what's missing. According to the Indian practice of Ayurveda, sports addiction is similar to an affliction called vigil, or staying up late. If a person practices vigil, he doesn't want to retire at bedtime because he feels that he hasn't gotten satisfaction out of his day. In men with sports addiction, perhaps their work life, home life, or even spiritual life isn't what they want it to be, says Jay L. Glaser, M.D., medical director of the Maharishi Ayur-Veda Medical Center in Lancaster, Massachusetts. So they turn to sports to live vicariously through others, he suggests. Think about what may be bothering you. Is your work not satisfying? Are you not happy about your body? Your spirituality? Then, instead of watching sports, focus all your attention on making that part of your life better, Dr. Glaser says. "One of the most important teachings in Ayurvedic medicine is that whatever we put our attention on is what grows in our lives," Dr. Glaser says.

▶PREVENTIVE MEASURES

Revisit your youth. For many men, sports evoke happy childhood memories: playing stickball with the neighborhood kids, tossing a football with your old man, going to your first big-league game. But dig deeper back into your mind and remember the other things you enjoyed when you were a kid. Maybe you built model airplanes, worked in a wood shop, or rode your bike all the time. "As men fade into sports addiction, they often drop hobbies they used to like," Dr. Pasick says. Pick up some of your old hobbies and rekindle some other fond memories of your youth.

Sprains

▶PROBLEM

Ligaments connect your bones and cartilage with each other, like a hinge on a gate, allowing you to enjoy a wide range of motion in your knees, ankles, elbows, shoulders, and wrists. But the flexible connective tissue can only bend and move so much. When those ligaments give way, you have a sprain.

▶CAUSE

If you take a thin rope and pull on it hard enough, the fibers in the rope start to tear. Keep pulling on the rope and, eventually, the fibers may break completely. That's what happens during a sprain: Pressure pulls on the ligaments, causing them to tear or rip apart. The ligament rupture brings about the swelling, pain, and instability of the joint.

▶HOW SERIOUS

Orthopedic surgeons grade sprains in three categories: Grade one is a small tear; grade two, a larger partial tear; and grade three, a complete tear. No matter what the degree, the treatment remains the same—just wait. "Even a complete tear will heal on its own," says Quinter Burnett, M.D., orthopedic surgeon and team physician with the Western Michigan University athletic department in Kalamazoo. Scar tissue eventually reconnects the torn ligaments. If the swelling is severe, see a doctor and get an x-ray to rule out a fracture, says Dr. Burnett.

▶SOLUTIONS

Put the freeze on. Place an ice pack wrapped in a thin towel on the sprain for 15 to 20 minutes, Dr. Burnett says. The ice reduces the swelling by contracting the blood vessels.

> ## DO THIS NOW
>
> Get off it. Using a sprained ligament can turn a partial tear into a full one. Rest the sprained area immediately and do not move or use the joint for a few days, says Quinter Burnett, M.D., orthopedic surgeon and team physician with the Western Michigan University athletic department in Kalamazoo.

Did You Know?

Only when the knee's anterior cruciate ligament (ACL), the ligament that runs through the center of your knee, tears does a sprain need serious surgery. Any swelling of the knee, especially if it's immediate, should be checked by a doctor because that may indicate an ACL tear, says Quinter Burnett, M.D., orthopedic surgeon and team physician with the Western Michigan University athletic department in Kalamazoo. Doctors can replace the ligament with some of your own tissue.

Reapply the ice pack every few hours for 36 hours, says Kevin Pugh, M.D., assistant professor of orthopedics at the University of Kentucky College of Medicine in Lexington.

Go with your Ace. Wrap up the sprain with an Ace bandage or any piece of material that applies moderate pressure, Dr. Pugh says. After the initial 36 hours, use the bandage to keep the swelling down while you're up and about. The pressure shuts down the blood flow from the damaged blood vessels and decreases the swelling.

Lie down and lift up. When you tear ligaments, blood can pool in the broken vessels, causing swelling and bruising. By elevating the injured area above your heart, you slow down the blood flow to the injured area. Lie down on the ground and prop up the injured part, Dr. Burnett adds. It makes it more effective to elevate an injured body part above heart level.

Take it easy . . . for awhile. Keep the injured joint immobile for a few days after the sprain. But sprains actually heal faster when you use the joint, Dr. Burnett says. So after a few days, get up and get moving—slowly. Let pain be your guide. If it hurts too much and you can't use it, lay off it for another few days. But if you can withstand some pressure with minimal pain, use it carefully, Dr. Burnett says.

▶ALTERNATIVE APPROACHES

Find comfort in comfrey. Although hard to find, leaves of the comfrey plant, also known as knitbone or *Symphytum officinale*, can soothe a bruised, swollen sprain, says Eve Campanelli, Ph.D., a holistic family practitioner in private practice in Beverly Hills, California. Look in homeopathic stores for the leaves, or try and grow them in your garden. Crush a fist full of them, then place the crushed leaves around the sprain and keep them in place with a bandage overnight, Dr. Campanelli says. If tinctures are more your speed, take one dose of homeopathic comfrey tincture or the pellet form, as the label recommends, every 15 minutes during the first hour after a sprain, she advises. After the first hour, continue with the dose recommended on the bottle three times a day until the sprain heals. You can find the remedy in health or homeopathic stores. Comfrey shouldn't be used on broken skin. Also, avoid using it for prolonged periods or if your skin is sensitive; it may trigger an allergic reaction.

Aid with arnica. South American Indians used the herb arnica to combat injuries from climbing. Arnica reduces swelling, bruising, and pain, says Andrea D. Sullivan, Ph.D., a doctor of naturopathy; president of Sullivan and Associates Center for Natural Healing in Washington, D.C.; and author of *A Path to Healing*. You can buy arnica cream at most health and homeopathic stores. Apply the cream to the sprain area as soon as possible. It should be applied three or four times a day for five days, says Dr. Sullivan. Do not use arnica on open wounds or broken skin. Also, it can cause allergic dermatitis if you have sensitive skin or use it for a prolonged period.

▶Preventive Measures

Band together. This quick and simple exercise won't completely prevent you from suffering another sprained ankle, but it may decrease your chances. Find a six-inch rubber loop or piece of tubing or purchase flex bands at a sporting goods store. While sitting with your feet together, wrap the tubing around the balls of both feet, Dr. Burnett says. Bend your knees slightly. Keeping your heels together, slowly rotate your feet apart and then bring them back together. Repeat this 10 to 20 times. This exercise can be done daily, or at least three days a week. It strengthens the muscles around the ankle joint, giving the ligaments better protection the next time they take a hit, Dr. Burnett says.

Wear protection. For one to two weeks after the sprain, wear a protective bandage such as an Ace bandage around the sprain. Wrap it snugly, but not so tightly that it causes swelling. Other products such as air and lace braces also protect the sprained body part. After a few weeks, only wear the bandage when you play sports or put extra force on the injured joint. Keep that up for two to three months, Dr. Burnett says.

Stretch before you sweat. When you jump right into an athletic activity without warming up, your ligaments may just snap, says Michael Bemben, Ph.D., associate professor of exercise science in the department of health and sport sciences at the University of Oklahoma in Norman. Begin with a slow five-minute jog, or ride your bike to the company softball game. Then, once you have increased your body temperature, take a few minutes to stretch your muscles. The increased body temperature warms up the muscles and ligaments, allowing them to stretch more easily and making them less likely to get injured.

Stomachache

▶PROBLEM

"Where's the pain?" and "What does it feel like?" are the two questions a doctor will ask if you complain of a stomachache. So, in order to treat yourself, you'll need to learn how to decipher your pain. Doctors divide the "stomach" (or what most people think of as their stomach, meaning their abdominal area) into four quadrants:

Middle of your chest, under the breastbone: You probably feel burning and are most likely burping. This usually signifies acid indigestion or heartburn. (For tips on dealing with heartburn, turn to page 277.) You could also possibly have an ulcer, if the pain happens when your stomach is empty or in the middle of the night. (For tips on dealing with ulcers, turn to page 551.)

Upper right side of the abdomen: There's probably pain but no other symptoms. You might need to have your gallbladder checked out. See a doctor, advises David Peura, M.D., a gastroenterologist and professor of medicine in the division of gastroenterology and hepatology at the University of Virginia Health Sciences Center in Charlottesville.

Under your belly button: Discomfort in this area is usually accompanied by bloating, cramping, and diarrhea. Your lower intestine is probably irritated.

Lower right quadrant: If there's gas, bloating, and diarrhea, it's still your lower intestine. But if it is severe and persistent or associated with a fever or it hurts to walk, it could be your appendix, says Dr. Peura. See a doctor.

DO THIS NOW

Take a walk. Since there's a good chance your stomachache is due to overeating, you'll want to help gravity get whatever is bothering your stomach to move out of your system.

"Don't lie flat," says David Peura, M.D., a gastroenterologist and professor of medicine in the division of gastroenterology and hepatology at the University of Virginia Health Sciences Center in Charlottesville. "The food wants to go south, but if it can't, it's going to go north. If you lie down or bend over, there's more of a chance that the food contents will come up."

▶CAUSE

Two things tend to cause stomach problems: putting something in your mouth (food, cigarettes, alcohol, coffee, and the like) or *not* putting something in your mouth, namely, food, says Malcolm Robinson, M.D., a gastroenterologist at the University of Oklahoma Health Sciences Center and director of the Oklahoma Foundation for Digestive Research, both in Oklahoma City. Determining if it's food or the lack of food that caused your stomachache is the first step toward treating yourself. It's good to know, for example, that heartburn is worsened with certain foods, while most ulcers hurt when you don't eat, Dr. Robinson says.

"A lot of stomachaches are due to misbehavior," Dr. Robinson says. "Overeating, eating too fast, swallowing air, drinking a lot of hot and cold beverages, and smoking all give people stomachaches," he says.

On the other hand, not eating also can cause a stomachache, but that usually feels more like a gnawing or burning sensation. If the burning is in the upper abdomen, suspect an ulcer, Dr. Robinson says. If it's heartburn, the burning is behind the breastbone, higher than where an ulcer hurts.

▶HOW SERIOUS

Some warning signs scream, "See a doctor!" These include severe and unrelenting abdominal pain, a high fever, blood in your stool (which will look very dark), vomiting blood, and pain moving around your abdominal area, says Dr. Peura.

On the other hand, most of us get stomachaches once in awhile, and it doesn't usually mean anything serious is wrong. You either ate too much, didn't eat enough, or ate, drank, or smoked the wrong thing.

▶SOLUTIONS

Spit out the gum. If your stomach problem is gas, bloating, and diarrhea, it could be caused by sorbitol (a sugarless, artificial sweetener used in gum and even some medicines), Dr. Peura says. Our stomachs can't absorb sorbitol, but the bacteria in our stomachs thrive on it. The bacteria break it down, which releases a lot of gas.

Three sticks of gum a day can have 6 grams of sorbitol, which is about the amount that can cause problems. Other sources of sorbitol include some milk of magnesia, cough syrups such as Sudafed and Dimetapp, asthma medications, antibiotics, and even some vitamins. So read your labels if you haven't found an obvious cause for your stomachache.

Think pink. "One medicine very likely to help people quickly is Pepto-Bismol," Dr. Robinson says. "It was developed to help fight cholera in the eighteenth century, but we're learning more and more about all the positive benefits that it has. It blocks inflammation, affects motility (fights cramping), and protects against noxious chemicals. Pepto-Bismol may also be helpful for var-

Did You Know?

Which is more acidic: stomach acid or battery acid? Believe it or not, stomach acid is just about as acidic as the corrosive battery "juice." In fact, gastric juice—which is what stomach acid is—is more acidic than lemon juice, vinegar, tomato juice, cola, or black coffee.

Your stomach secretes gastric juice to digest the food you've eaten. This colorless fluid consists, for the most part, of hydrochloric acid, rennin, pepsin, and mucin. Adding acidic liquids or eating so much food that your stomach begins to overproduce gastric acid to deal with it really creates a bubbling mess.

On the other hand, if you add a base liquid to your stomach, you can neutralize the acid. If you remember your high school chemistry, liquids exist on a continuum from base to acid, with neutral in the middle. Maalox, Mylanta, and baking soda are bases, which is why they soothe a stomachache.

ious forms of indigestion, nausea, or diarrhea. Just follow the instructions on the bottle, whether you use the liquid or the tablets."

Use antacids and acid-blockers sparingly. They work, there's no question about that, but medicines such as Tagamet, Zantac, Axid, and Pepcid AC, sometimes "cause tolerance," Dr. Robinson says. In other words, if you take them regularly over long periods of time, you might have to keep using them, and using more of them, to get relief.

You have two options when it comes to antacids. You can block the production of the acid by using Tagamet, Zantac, Pepcid AC, or Axid. Or you can neutralize the acid with Mylanta, Maalox, or Tums. Either way, you should consider these short-term solutions, Dr. Robinson says.

There are two potential problems with using antacids long-term. First, they can mask a more serious problem. "It's okay to reach for these medicines for fast relief, but if you find yourself using them more and more often, go see a doctor," says David Rooney, M.D., a family physician with Southern Chester County Family Practice Associates in Oxford, Pennsylvania.

Second, some antacids don't interact well with other medications. "If you take other medicines regularly, ask your doctor which antacid would be safest for you," suggests Dr. Rooney.

Reach for the baking soda. Dissolve a teaspoon of baking soda in warm water, toast to a calmer belly, and drink up, Dr. Peura says. Baking soda has been used to relieve upset stomachs for generations, and with good reason: It works. Just don't use it every day, he says.

▶ALTERNATIVE APPROACHES

Sip soothing teas. For stomach upset, try brewing up some licorice root, marshmallow root, and meadowsweet flowers, says Priscilla Skerry, a naturopathic and homeopathic doctor in private practice in Portland, Maine. "This tea is a demulcent, which means that it can heal and soothe irritated and inflamed mucous membranes," she explains. Mix equal parts of the herbs so that you have a heaping teaspoon, and steep the mixture in a cup of boiling water. This tea should be used after or in between meals, three times a day, for several days. But if your stomach continues to bother you, see your doctor, Dr. Skerry advises. Licorice may interact with some drugs and is not recommended for long-term use, nor should it be used by people who have diabetes, hypertension, liver disorders, severe kidney insufficiency, or hypokalemia (consult with your doctor before using if you have any of these conditions).

If cramping and diarrhea accompany your stomachache, drink a tea made from chamomile or valerian, Dr. Skerry recommends. A cup or two at the onset of your discomfort or until your stomach settles will help your stomach recover from the stress of spasms. People who are allergic to closely related plants like ragweed, asters, and chrysanthemums could be allergic to chamomile, too. If so, drink the tea with caution.

▶PREVENTIVE MEASURES

Don't stuff yourself. Overeating is the major cause of acid reflux, which causes heartburn, Dr. Robinson warns.

"The stomach is a very adaptable organ and will relax and expand to accommodate what's in it," says Dr. Robinson. "If you eat a lot more than you usually do, however, it will have difficulty expanding that quickly."

Line up vitamins. Foods high in the antioxidant vitamins A, C, and E are very important to maintain the integrity of the intestinal lining, Dr. Skerry says. Fruit is vitamin-rich, but since you don't want to irritate your stomach with sugar (or pesticides), focus mainly on organic vegetables, she adds. To load up on vitamin A, eat orange vegetables such as carrots, sweet potatoes, and squash. Cold-pressed salad or cooking oils are one of the top sources of vitamin E (it is important they are labeled "cold-pressed" to assure that the vitamin is preserved). Almonds and sunflower seeds are also vitamin E–rich. Broccoli, cauliflower, potatoes, cabbage, and green and sweet red peppers are high in vitamin C. Try to eat four to six servings of vegetables daily and some fruit in season to keep your stomach running smoothly.

Think zinc. This antioxidant mineral does wonders for the stomach, Dr. Skerry adds. "The most absorbable form is zinc picolinate. If you take it as a supplement, make sure that the tablet has some copper in it. A good ratio is seven to one. Your daily dose of zinc can be up to 15 milligrams, which means that you also need to take approximately 2 milligrams of copper."

Stress

▶PROBLEM

At precisely the moment you need a clear head, steady hands, or deep voice, stress makes you feel jittery, sweaty, and confused. More than half of us admit to feeling stressed, though only 9 percent of men seek professional help. Stress is more common among the highly educated and well-paid and among Whites than among ethnic groups.

▶CAUSE

Stress is a biological response designed to sharpen the senses and heighten alertness during life-threatening situations. When your brain perceives imminent danger, it signals the body to secrete stress hormones, which speed up your heart rate, breathing, and sweating, later leaving you feeling exhausted. When man's worries were primal, like avoiding being eaten by a shark, this was a very good thing, indeed. But in these more civilized times, when the most dangerous sharks wear three-piece suits and carry cellular phones, it can be destructive.

The brain misinterprets benign events—an angry boss or wife, a looming deadline—as life-threatening and triggers the stress response. And it usually can be traced back to a thought: My wife is going to kill me. I'm gonna lose my job.

"Stress is all in your mind," says Peggy Kileff, a wellness consultant at the Institute for Preventive Medicine in Houston. "You always have a thought before you have a feeling."

▶HOW SERIOUS

Stress is more than a nuisance. Stress can be deadly. Chronic stress raises levels of hormones in the body that can damage blood vessels, raise cholesterol,

> ### DO THIS NOW
>
> "Sensations of heaviness are relaxing for people," says Peggy Kileff, a wellness consultant at the Institute for Preventive Medicine in Houston. So take a short break and sit or lie down for five minutes. Imagine that your body weighs 600 pounds. Feel that weight press into the floor. The more you allow your body to plaster itself to the floor, the more stress will sink away.

spike blood pressure, impair immunity, and generally make you feel wiped out, says Michael Babyak, Ph.D., assistant clinical professor of medical psychology at Duke University Medical Center in Durham, North Carolina. Also, we usually don't take good care of our health when stressed. We eat lots of junk, don't get enough sleep, and blow off our workouts. If you are constantly experiencing headaches, bowel or bladder problems, tension and pain in your neck or lower back, heart palpitations, irritability, or depression, you should talk with your doctor, says Dr. Babyak. Everyone gets these symptoms occasionally, but if they become chronic, that's when it is time to take action.

▶SOLUTIONS

Take a cue. Stop everything. First, quickly evaluate the situation. Will your stress help you achieve anything useful, like sprinting to rescue a loved one from an oncoming car? If not, then try to slow down your breathing and be aware of your heart rate and level of muscle tension, says Dr. Babyak.

Then, take 10 to 15 minutes to pace your breathing and let your mind and body relax. "You are soothing and slowing yourself down by repeating a cue word or visualizing a pleasant place," says Dr. Babyak You need to practice this before you get stressed for it to be most effective. While visualizing yourself in a quiet, restful place, relax your muscles and slow your breathing. Use a cue word such as peace when you do. That way, when stress hits, you can repeat your cue word and your body will already know how to relax, he explains.

Look at the big picture. Usually, we stress out over trivial matters—arriving late for an important date, making a good impression, getting a work assignment in by deadline. To put things in perspective, Kileff suggests, ask yourself: "In five years, what difference will it make if (fill in the blank)?"

Breathe slowly. To slow your breathing, you must pay attention to your breath, which means that you can't pay attention to all the other things that made you feel stressed out to begin with. Slow breathing also helps you physically feel relaxed. Inhale deep into your belly for a count of four. Slowly exhale for another count of four. "You breathe in and out thousands of times a day, so you have lots of chances to practice slow breathing," Kileff says. "Whenever you're stuck at a traffic light, on hold, or waiting for the elevator, practice."

Turn on your radio. Music—any music—will relax you as long as you like it. John Tesh might work for some (although, frankly, that's hard to imagine), the Red Hot Chili Peppers for others. "We don't believe that there is any magical type of music that is going to be relaxing for everyone," says Valerie N. Stratton, Ph.D., professor of psychology at Pennsylvania State University in Altoona. "If someone really likes hard rock or rap, that's what would relax them."

▶ALTERNATIVE APPROACHES

Cheer up with oats. For a remedy that is mild enough for everyday use but plenty strong to help you deal with intense stress, try a tea made from oat straw,

Did You Know?

The average Fortune 1,000 worker sends and receives 178 messages a day. Instead of saving time, new communications tools such as e-mail, voice mail, and faxes have further stressed workers, according to a joint study by Pitney Bowes, the Institute for the Future, the Gallup Organization, and San Jose State University in California. Because sending and receiving messages takes up so much of the workday, many employees must take real work home at night and on the weekends, the study found.

says Susun S. Weed, an herbalist and herbal educator from Woodstock, New York, and author of the *Wise Woman* series of herbal health books. To make the tea, put one ounce (by weight) of dry oat straw in a quart jar and fill it with boiling water. Screw on the lid and let it steep overnight or for at least four hours before straining off the liquid. "I drink one to four cups a day to strengthen my nerves and relieve stress The only side effect," says Weed," is increased libido." Oat straw is available in health food stores.

Accept some mothering. "When I am acutely stressed, I use tincture of flowering motherwort," says Weed. It's important to use a tincture of motherwort prepared from fresh (not dry) plants. A dose of 15 to 20 drops in about a half-cup of liquid promptly relieves symptoms of stress. "If I don't feel better in five minutes, I take another dose," says Weed. "Motherwort brings the calm of sitting in your mother's lap. No matter how hard life gets, it helps me cope," she says. You can find motherwort tincture at health food stores, or they can order it for you.

Reduce stressful effects. Ginseng is noted for helping those under stress. It won't necessarily make you feel calmer, but it does help with the physical effects that accompany stress, says Weed. She prefers American ginseng, the root, at least five years old, dried or a tincture. When under stress, chew a chunk of dried root, "the size of the last joint (closest to the tip) of your little finger" or take a dropper of the tincture as the bottle directs, says Weed. Ginseng is available at health food stores and drugstores.

Slack off. Set aside time each day to do absolutely nothing. Just kick back and let your mind wander nowhere in particular. Usually, your mind will eventually take you to various worries. "You have to put yourself in a situation where you are relaxed so that you can view these things with a clear head. Usually, you'll realize that the problem isn't as big as you thought," says Andrew Yiannakis, Ph.D., professor and director of the laboratory of leisure, tourism, and sport at the University of Connecticut in Storrs.

Morning is the best time of day to do nothing. Get up earlier than usual, make a cup of tea or coffee, and sit in a comfortable chair while you leisurely drink, Dr. Yiannakis suggests. Though not as beneficial, you can also try doing nothing every once in awhile at work, providing you turn off your e-mail and phone and mentally give yourself permission. Or, use part of your lunch break to walk to a park, sit on a bench, and relax.

Train for action. When you work out, your heart rate quickens, your blood pressure jumps, your breathing speeds up, and your pores sweat. When you feel stressed out, your heart rate quickens, your blood pressure jumps, your breathing speeds up, and your pores sweat. Sound familiar? "Exercise is like a fire drill," Kileff says. "People who exercise seem to handle stress better." Any exercise is better than no exercise. So if you can only motivate yourself to take a walk now and then, you'll still do yourself some good. The more strenuously you exercise, however, the more relaxed you'll feel, says Kileff. Aim for a 30- to 45-minute workout three times a week.

Remember to play. Yes, exercise is an effective stress-buster, but only if you enjoy it. If you're overly competitive, one of those winning-is-everything guys, then even your playtime will be stressful. "The goal of playing should be to enjoy the process," says Dr. Yiannakis. "People who are outcome-oriented want to win. People who are interested in doing the activity because it is fun are less concerned with competition and winning."

Changing your mindset won't be easy. You'll have to consistently remember to go easy on yourself when you make a mistake. Also, give your teammates a break as well. Allow a month to adjust to this new way of playing. If at the end of the month you still play to win, try switching to a less competitive activity such as hiking, dancing, or stationary cycling.

▶PREVENTIVE MEASURES

Read good books. On a regular basis, reading helps you dissociate yourself from the troubles of the world, providing a healthy escape from reality, says Dr. Yiannakis.

Make a list. The simple habit of keeping a daily to-do list can help organize your life as well as make you feel competent. You can keep one for your personal life (get groceries, mail birthday card, pick up kid from soccer) as well as one for your career (ask for a raise, complete report, schmooze with the new guy). As you complete tasks, cross them off, says Kileff. Just make sure that you're realistic. Stack your to-do list too high and it, too, will become a source of stress when you can't get everything done.

See your way through. If you have a stressful event looming—an important presentation, a confrontation with your boss, a divorce settlement—imagine how smoothly things will go. For instance, see yourself presenting your idea to the chief executive officer. Take note of your confident posture, your authoritative voice, and your intelligent sounding ideas. The more you mentally rehearse, the less stressed you'll feel when the real-life event occurs, says Kileff.

Sunburn

▶PROBLEM

In the early part of the twentieth century, tanning (and consequently sunburn) weren't much of a concern for men. Bathing suits barely exposed skin, and (among Caucasians anyway) white, sunless skin was a sign of high station. Only common laborers and field hands wore tans. The change came after World War II with bikinis, beach blanket movies, the Beach Boys, and the accompanying strange notion that tanning was healthy. Exposure to the sun, products to soothe such exposure, and, eventually, cases of skin cancer boomed.

▶CAUSE

Sunburn is an inflammation of the skin from overexposure to the sun. The body protects itself against foreign invaders—in this case, the sun's ultraviolet rays—by flooding the skin with white blood cells. This inflammatory response makes your skin red and sore.

Anyone can get sunburn, but the lighter your skin color, the quicker you'll fry. Some guys get red-faced after eating a lunch in the park; others need to lounge on a beach all afternoon.

You're most likely to burn on a clear, summer day between the hours of 11:00 A.M. and 3:00 P.M., when sunshine is most intense, says David D. Madjar Jr., M.D., a dermatologist in private practice in Holiday, Florida. This is especially true of fair-skinned people, he adds.

"That doesn't mean that you can't burn on a cloudy day. A lot of ultraviolet light gets through the clouds," Dr. Madjar explains.

Water, sand, concrete, and snow can intensify the ultraviolet rays. Latitude makes a difference, too. The sun rays are much stronger the further south you go toward the equator, says Dr. Madjar. "You get the same intensifying effect when you go up in altitude. Backpackers, climbers, and skiers have to protect themselves when they're in the mountains," he adds.

▶How Serious

Usually, you just get some redness and stinging/itching sensations that recede after a few days. A more severe case of sunburn causes blistering. And like any second-degree burn, the wound will be quite painful, require weeks to heal, and probably give you permanent scars, says Abraham R. Freilich, M.D., a dermatologist and assistant clinical professor of dermatology at Downstate Medical Center in Brooklyn, New York. He advises that you see a dermatologist if you experience blistering, severe pain, or excess swelling. Your doctor may want to start you on a short course of oral cortisone, if necessary, he adds.

Repeated sunburns or years of tanning prematurely ages the skin and can lead to increased risk of melanoma and other skin cancers.

▶Solutions

Reach for relief. Six to 12 hours afterward, you'll realize that you spent too much time in the sun, Dr. Freilich says. That's when your skin will turn red, burn, and itch. You can take away some of the sting and pain with over-the-counter anti-inflammatories such as aspirin or ibuprofen, he says.

Taking them as soon as possible after a sunburn will actually minimize burn tissue damage, says Vail Reese, M.D., a dermatologist with the Dermatology Medical Group of San Francisco. "Symptoms of a burn can really be minimized by shutting down the inflammation process. By taking anti-inflammatories as soon as you can, you fool the inflammatory process into thinking that nothing's wrong," Dr. Reese says.

Follow the package label and start taking the anti-inflammatory as soon as possible after the burn. Continue taking it for the first two days after a burn, suggests Dr. Freilich.

Ease it with vitamin E. If you know that you've been burned, take 400 international units of vitamin E every four hours (while awake), starting immediately, and continue for one day, says Karen Burke, M.D., Ph.D., a dermatologist in private practice in New York City. "The d-alpha-tocopherol form is best," she adds. Check with your doctor first before taking large amounts of vitamin E, especially if you are on some blood-thinning medications or on aspirin therapy.

Soak in oatmeal. Pick up some colloidal oatmeal, such as Aveeno, at your local drugstore. Follow the manufacturer's directions, and add it to a tubful of cool or tepid water to relieve the itchiness of dried, sunburned skin, says John E. Wolf Jr., M.D., chairman of the department of dermatology at Baylor Col-

Did You Know?

During World War II in the Pacific, sailors and soldiers working on flight decks while fighting on coral atolls needed protection from the equatorial sun. Red petrolatum, an inert refining residue from gas and home heating oil, blocked ultraviolet rays quite effectively but stained the soldiers' skin reddish-bronze. Dr. Benjamin Green, a scientist who helped develop the petroleum sunscreen for the military, believed that there was a postwar market for tanning products. Since it was unlikely that bathers would slather themselves with red petroleum, Dr. Green came up with a more pleasing snow-white lotion scented with jasmine. He gave it a more marketable name as well: Coppertone.

---

lege of Medicine in Houston. You can do this as often as needed for sunburn relief with no adverse effects, he adds.

Salve the skin. Only time cures sunburn, but you can relieve some of the itching and burning with over-the-counter skin lotions such as calamine or Caladryl Clear Lotion, says Dr. Freilich. Follow label directions carefully, and apply the lotion where it itches, when it itches, he adds. Moisturizing creams will also help get rid of dead skin when you start to peel, says Dr. Freilich. Apply two or three times a day or as directed on the label.

If your burn is severe enough to blister, apply some lubricant such as petroleum jelly or bacitracin two or three times a day and keep the area clean, says Dr. Freilich. Test a small area of your skin first to make sure that you are not allergic to bacitracin. You should see a doctor if there is excessive discomfort, redness, swelling, or blistering.

▶ALTERNATIVE APPROACHES

Apply aloe. If houseplants are your thing, you should always have some aloe growing as a balm for most types of burns, says David Winston, professional and founding member of the American Herbalists Guild and a clinical herbalist in Washington, New Jersey. "It's really easy to grow. It takes neglect very well," he says.

The gel is most soothing when it comes from a fresh plant, rather than the bottled gels sold in many drugstores and health food stores. Cut the end of an aloe leaf, squeeze or express the gelatin, and apply it lightly to the sunburn, suggests Winston. "Do this two or three times a day for the first couple of days after the sunburn until the pain is gone," Winston says.

And if you add a drop or two of essential oil of lavender to the aloe, you'll create a powerful antiseptic and antibacterial formula, Winston says. "That will help speed up the healing process," he says.

Shrink the skin. White vinegar applied directly on the skin with a cloth two or three times a day or a weak tea made from plantain, a common backyard plant, may take away the sting of sunburn, as will any of the many herbs that acts as astringents, says John Crellin, M.D., Ph.D., John Clinch professor of the history of medicine at Memorial University of Newfoundland Faculty of Medicine in St. John's.

To make the tea, simply grind a few leaves of plantain (*Plantago major*), place the mulch in a cup of boiling water, and steep for a few minutes. When the mixture cools, use it as a soothing wash for your skin, Dr. Crellin says. You can do this once or twice a day while your symptoms persist, he adds. Plantain leaves are available at some health food stores and through mail order. Do not confuse the plant plantain with the banana-like fruit also called plantain.

Plantain, like most astringents, contains tannins, substances that pucker the skin, Dr. Crellin says.

▶PREVENTIVE MEASURES

Take cover. When outdoors, wear a long-sleeve shirt and a hat with a wide brim. Make sure that the shirt has a tight weave. If you can hold it up to the sun and see daylight, then ultraviolet rays will have no problem getting through, says Dr. Madjar.

Smear on the sunscreen. If you do expose your skin to the sun, liberally apply a sunscreen with an SPF (sun protection factor) of 15 or better, says Dr. Madjar. Apply sunscreen 60 minutes before you go outside, to let it soak in, and reapply every hour or two, especially when you are swimming. Don't forget to apply the sunscreen to the tips of your ears and your lips, he adds.

Swimmer's Ear

▶PROBLEM

Soldiers fighting in the South Pacific during World War II called it jungle ear. But whatever you call it, this infection of the outer ear, caused by fungus or bacteria, is mighty painful. At first, the affected ear may feel blocked and itchy. Soon, however, it becomes swollen and tender to the touch and may drain a thin, milky fluid.

▶CAUSE

In most cases, trapped water from swimming or showering causes swimmer's ear. When you get water in your ears, you also get a dose of bacteria or fungus. If the water runs right back out, your ear dries out and these microorganisms don't cause problems. But if water gets trapped in the ear canal, the skin gets soggy, creating a moist environment that allows bacteria and fungus to multiply. That said, you don't have to be anywhere near water to get swimmer's ear. "Some people are prone to it because they don't make enough earwax, which protects the ear canal," says Mark K. Mandell-Brown, M.D., an otolaryngologist in private practice in Cincinnati.

▶HOW SERIOUS

Swimmer's ear isn't generally dangerous, but it can make you exceedingly grumpy. "Swimmer's ear begins with an itch that progresses to great pain, so that pulling on the ear will hurt," says Evany Zirul, D.O., professor of clinical medicine at the University of Health Sciences in Kansas City, Missouri, and assistant professor of clinical medicine at the University of Kansas in Kansas City. Once you have an acute infection—if your ear is excruciatingly painful or if the

> **DO THIS NOW**
>
> Set a heating pad on low, and place it over the painful ear as long as needed until you feel relief. The dry heat can help ease the pain of swimmer's ear, says Mark K. Mandell-Brown, M.D., an otolaryngologist in private practice in Cincinnati. Heat promotes blood flow, bringing infection-fighting white blood cells to the area. You can do this as often as you want, he says.

History Lesson

On August 24, 1875, Captain Matthew Webb became the first man to swim the English Channel, covering the distance in 21 hours, 45 minutes. But his time in the water wasn't confined to the breaststroke. From the time he entered the water in Dover, England, to the time he touched land at Cape Gris-Nez, France, Captain Webb sang, sipped coffee and beer, ate steaks, was stung by a jellyfish, and fought his way through a storm.

Almost 51 years later, on August 6, 1926, Gertrude Ederle became the first woman to swim the English Channel. She whipped Webb's time, covering the distance in 14 hours, 31 minutes. But her trip wasn't nearly so pleasant: She went deaf as a result of damage to her eardrums during the swim.

---

glands in your neck are swollen—you'll need to go to the doctor, who will likely prescribe antibiotic eardrops, she says.

▶SOLUTIONS

Reach for the vinegar. Make your own antiseptic eardrops by mixing equal parts of rubbing alcohol and white vinegar. Then insert three or four drops into the infected ear using an eyedropper or a small-bulb syringe (either of which you can buy at a drugstore).

"The alcohol dries out the dampness in the ear, and the vinegar changes the pH of the ear environment so that it's inhospitable to the bacteria that cause the infection," says Dr. Zirul. "It's this dampness in a long, dark tunnel and all that delicious ear goo to feed on that starts the infection." To ward off future bouts, use this solution immediately after you swim or shower. You can use this solution every day if you want to, she says. If you're just beginning to feel pain or tenderness, use the drops four times a day.

Keep 'em dry. Avoid getting your ears wet for 7 to 10 days, Dr. Mandell-Brown says. Don't worry; you won't need to wear a shower cap. "Stick a cotton ball covered with a little petroleum jelly in your ear," he says. "Petroleum jelly repels water." Don't use just the cotton ball, though. "You'll just end up with a soggy cotton ball in your ear," he says.

Hit the drugstore. Pick up a bottle of antiseptic eardrops, such as Swim Ear, says Dr. Zirul. These over-the-counter drops can help kill the fungus or bacteria causing the infection. Follow the directions on the label.

▶ALTERNATIVE APPROACHES

Oil your ear. Oils made from herbs can help relieve the pain of swimmer's ear, says Amy Rothenberg, a doctor of naturopathy in Amherst, Massachusetts, and editor of the *New England Journal of Homeopathy*. "Using an eyedropper, insert one or two drops of mullein oil or garlic oil into the painful ear," suggests Dr. Rothenberg. According to herbalists, mullein (available in health food stores) is used as an anodyne, a substance that reduces pain.

Arm your immune system. Antioxidant vitamins, which help boost the immune system, can help speed the infection out of your system, Dr. Rothenberg says. She advises taking 500 to 1,000 milligrams of vitamin C three times a day. She also recommends 50,000 to 100,000 international units of beta-carotene, 200 international units of vitamin E, and 50 milligrams of zinc a day until the infection clears up. If the infection has not cleared in a week, seek medical help, Dr. Rothenberg says. Excess vitamin C (more than 1,200 milligrams) may be enough to cause diarrhea in some people. Doses of zinc above 20 milligrams a day should be taken only under medical supervision.

▶PREVENTIVE MEASURES

Blow-dry soggy ears. The key to avoiding swimmer's ear is to deprive bacteria and fungus of the moisture they need to thrive. So, after your next swim or shower, aim a blow-dryer into your ears, Dr. Zirul suggests. "But use a low setting so that you don't burn your ears, and keep the dryer 12 to 18 inches away from your ear," she says. Thirty seconds or so should be long enough to dry them.

Leave your wax be. No matter how desperate you are, do not use cotton swabs to remove earwax, advises Dr. Zirul. "Using cotton swabs can contribute to swimmer's ear by scratching the ear canal, giving the infection a place to start," she says.

Technophobia

▶PROBLEM

"About 85 percent of the population has moderate to severe discomfort with technology," says Larry D. Rosen, Ph.D., an expert on the psychology of technology and co-author of *Technostress*. Some technophobes experience actual physical symptoms when they think of or use electronic gadgets, including a queasy stomach, headaches, and heart palpitations. Others experience emotional symptoms of anxiety or dread. "They think, 'I'm never going to figure this out,' or 'I'm going to hit the wrong key and blow up the computer,'" says Dr. Rosen.

▶CAUSE

Highly anxious people, or people who tend to resist change, may be more prone to technophobia than relaxed types, says Timothy Jay, Ph.D., professor of psychology at Massachusetts College of Liberal Arts in North Adams, who has conducted studies on computerphobia. Generally speaking, "technophobes have a negative view of the impact of technology on society," Dr. Jay says. "They believe that technology dehumanizes people. Feeling uncomfortable about using a computer, or cyberphobia, is part of a bigger skepticism—or, in some cases, paranoia—about using technology."

▶HOW SERIOUS

Technophobia isn't serious at all, if you're Amish. But for most other folks, preferring "While You Were Out" slips to voice mail, or a legal pad to a

DO THIS NOW

Kids learn about the world through their play. So do adults. So, this very second, turn on your computer and try to make it do something cool. Look for a computer game in your directory. Type a fake ransom note and try to print it out. In short, fool around. "Think of a computer as a toy," suggests Timothy Jay, Ph.D., professor of psychology at Massachusetts College of Liberal Arts in North Adams, who has conducted studies on computerphobia. "You just can't make mistakes when you're playing with a toy."

History Lesson

January 12, 1997: HAL, the soft-voiced ubercomputer who turns murderous in Arthur C. Clarke's classic sci-fi novel *2001: A Space Odyssey*, is born. In the 1968 movie, directed by Stanley Kubrick, HAL is born on January 12, *1992*. According to Clarke, this discrepancy may have been caused by one of the actors bungling his lines. Leave it to humans.

ThinkPad, can be hazardous to your professional health. "You can no longer escape technology at work," says Dr. Rosen. It's getting harder to avoid at home, too. "I used to say that technophobia couldn't affect your private life because you could just avoid technology—and many people did," Dr. Rosen says. "But it's getting harder to ignore. As soon as any household item breaks, you're confronted by new technology. You can hardly even buy a coffeepot that doesn't have an embedded computer in it."

▶SOLUTIONS

Find a hook. "People accept computers and technology when they see that they will enhance their lives," says Dr. Jay.

And Scott Adams, creator of the comic strip *Dilbert*, says the biggest boon of technology is "that it will allow you to work at home while you're naked."

Write up your own short list of benefits. Learn to navigate the World Wide Web, for example, and you'll be able to file your taxes electronically and get your refund quicker. Decipher the office voice-mail system, and you can ignore people you don't want to talk to (or don't have answers for).

Ask the right people for help. If you're less than comfortable with technology, it's important to trust your teacher, Dr. Rosen says. The best teacher is often a calm, relaxed, noncritical friend who teaches you a specific task, then backs off so that you can try it yourself. The worst teachers are technoweenies and kids. "Technophiles tend to use their knowledge to make you feel like an outsider," Dr. Jay says. And kids, who were practically born with joysticks in their hands, "tend to get frustrated with your incompetence, so they do it for you, which keeps you from learning on your own," he says.

Confront your destiny. Anxious people often feel powerless. But try to push past that helpless feeling. "Tell yourself, 'I can master this. And the more I know about technology, the more power I'll have,'" Dr. Jay says.

▶ALTERNATIVE APPROACHES

Get used to it. If you're intimidated by your computer, take a few days to get to know it, suggests Dennis Gersten, M.D., a San Diego psychiatrist, author of *Are You Getting Enlightened or Losing Your Mind?* and publisher of *Atlantis: The Imagery Newsletter.* Try this six-day exercise.

- Days 1 to 3: Sit down at your computer, but don't turn it on. Just put your hands on the keyboard for several minutes. Do this twice a day.
- Days 4 to 6: Turn on the computer, sit in front of it for several minutes, then turn it off. Do this twice a day.

Visualize success. After your six days of courting, it's time to run off with your computer. But relax; it's only in your mind. A technique called mental imagery can help you master your discomfort with using a computer, Dr. Gersten says. "When you realize that a computer is merely a vehicle to help you communicate or gather information, your fear will change to anticipation," he says. Here's how.

1. Turn on your computer and sit down in front of it. Close your eyes. Notice any anxiety that you feel.
2. Take long, deep breaths to release tension. Use "4-4-8 breathing"—inhale to the count of four, hold to the count of four, exhale to the count of eight. Using this technique, inhale and exhale four times.
3. Imagine any remaining tension turning to liquid. Watch it ooze out of your feet.
4. Open your eyes and look at the computer screen for a minute. Then close your eyes again. Imagine the computer connecting you to people and places all over the world. Visualize those positive connections. You might think of them as golden threads that emanate from your computer, connecting you with faraway places or loved ones. Repeat this visualization as often as you need to.

▶Preventive Measures

Get some class. The best way to master your distrust of computers is to enroll in a computer class. But not just *any* computer class, says Dr. Rosen. You want a class that's very hands-on so that you're learning not from a lecture but from using the keyboard. "The instructor should be calm and relaxed and avoid using computer jargon," Dr. Rosen says. "There should be a lot of opportunity for you to play around and make mistakes. And the class shouldn't be too long—maybe an hour or two at the most." If you're nervous about taking a class, don't be. The others won't know any more about computers than you do.

Teeth Grinding

▶PROBLEM

Also called bruxism, the grinding or clenching of teeth often occurs during sleep. You may be unaware that you're doing it unless a bedmate tells you. It has been estimated that the average person with bruxism has five eight-second episodes of teeth grinding per night. Some people also gnash their teeth during waking hours. Clenching teeth, it should be noted, is not as serious as grinding, though. "Clenching is putting the teeth together forcefully but not actually letting them slide over each other and making that noise," says William Howard, D.D.S., assistant professor of dental hygiene at Western Kentucky University in Bowling Green. "Clenching is not usually detrimental; grinding is."

▶CAUSE

People who grind their teeth in their sleep suffer from a disorder that occurs as they pass from deep sleep into lighter phases of slumber, says Sheldon Gross, D.D.S., past president of the American Academy of Orofacial Pain and a dentist in Bloomfield, Connecticut.

People who are under stress, who are chronic worriers, or who have hard-driving, impatient personalities seem to be prone. So, too, are people whose teeth or jaws are out of alignment. Just before their mouths are fully closed, one or more upper teeth make contact with lower teeth. It can be a maddening feeling, which prompts sufferers

> ### DO THIS NOW
>
> Slowly stretch out your sore jaw muscle, advises Sheldon Gross, D.D.S., past president of the American Academy of Orofacial Pain and a dentist in Bloomfield, Connecticut. Do this in a hot shower. Start by loosening up your neck muscles, which also can become stiff from teeth clenching or teeth grinding. Move your head around, looking first over your left shoulder, then the right shoulder. Open your mouth. You should be able to place two, and preferably three, fingers stacked vertically inside. If not, try using your fingers to gradually open your mouth wider. If this only makes the pain worse, then seek professional help.

525

History Lesson

Centuries ago, false teeth were hand-carved and tied in place with silk threads. They were so unstable that people who wore full sets of dentures had to remove them before eating. Upper and lower plates were held together with steel springs and could spring suddenly out of a wearer's mouth.

Early dentures were usually made of animal bone or ivory, especially from elephants or hippopotamuses. But some people bought teeth from the mouths of the poor for a negotiated fee. The transplanted molars soon rotted, turning brown and rancid.

Thousands of teeth were yanked from the mouths of dead and even wounded soldiers during the French Revolution and the American Civil War for use as dentures. The advent of porcelain teeth ended that practice. Today, dentures are either plastic or ceramic.

---

to try and grind down the offending teeth, altering their jaw movements, says John C. Brown, D.D.S., past president of the Academy of General Dentistry and a dentist who practiced for 35 years in Claremont, California.

▶HOW SERIOUS

Teeth grinding can cause headaches, pain when chewing, limited jaw opening, temporomandibular disorder, and tooth sensitivity. (For more information, see separate chapters on Temporomandibular Disorder on page 528 and Tooth Sensitivity on page 548.) A teeth-grinder on average exerts 162 pounds per square inch of biting force. Guys who grind at night often do themselves more harm than their daytime counterparts, says Dr. Gross. "The grinding is so loud that you cannot voluntarily make that noise," he says. "Grinders are able to exert such excessive force at night that they can even break or loosen teeth. During the day, the pain or discomfort would make you stop. When he's awake, even under stress, a person still has some conscious control over it." In short, teeth grinding can cause permanent, irreversible damage to your choppers. So if you routinely have tooth or face pain when you wake up, see a dentist, Dr. Gross says.

▶SOLUTIONS

Apply moist heat. This helps alleviate general soreness, says Dr. Gross. You can do this for 15 to 20 minutes at a time, two or three times a day. Wet towels with warm water and wring them out or wrap a wet, wrung-out towel around a hot-water bottle and apply to your face, Dr. Gross advises. Be sure to check your skin often to make sure that it's not getting burned.

Watch what you drink. Reduce or eliminate stimulants in your diet, such as caffeine beverages like colas, coffee, and tea, says Dr. Brown. A guy on edge is more apt to have disturbed sleep at night and grind his teeth. Nor should you drink alcoholic beverages before bed, says Dr. Gross. "It makes you sleepy, but actually, alcohol has been shown to disturb your sleep rhythms," he says.

Work out. "Probably any kind of exercise is a stress-reducing mechanism," says Dr. Brown. "The important thing is to exercise enough so that you go to sleep tired."

Sleep around. Try sleeping in different positions, advises Dr. Brown. You may find one in which you don't grind your teeth or you do less of it. If your bed partner sees or hears you gnashing your teeth, have her tell you what position you were sleeping in when you did so, and try to avoid that position. Waking up to tired, aching jaws is another clue that you were probably grinding your teeth in your sleep, Dr. Brown says.

Get a wake-up shake. This one can be difficult, but have your bedmate awaken you every time you start grinding your teeth in your sleep. It's called aversive conditioning and can reduce the amount of nighttime grinding you do. "It definitely has proved beneficial in a lot of ways," says Dr. Brown. Of course, the woman you sleep with must be a light enough sleeper to hear your nocturnal gnashing or stay awake all night in order to wake you.

Clench until it hurts. In a technique called massed negative biofeedback, you voluntarily clench your teeth for five seconds, then relax the jaws for five seconds. Repeat the exercise five times in succession, several times a day, for two weeks. It helps some people, says Dr. Brown. "They condition themselves by clenching until it's almost painful, to the point where the brain says, 'I don't want to do that.'"

▶ALTERNATIVE APPROACHES

Play that tune. Listen to a relaxing tape or CD before you turn in. Doing this in the evening before going to bed can help produce restful sleep, says Dr. Gross.

Practice breathing exercises. "Good deep breaths with abdominal breathing is much more relaxing," says Dr. Gross. "Take a slow, easy breath letting the air puff out your abdomen (not your chest). Then count to 10 and exhale. Do this up to 10 times. And don't worry about taking really deep breaths; it's the slowing of your breath that matters."

▶PREVENTIVE MEASURES

Veto instant replay. Don't rerun the day's activities in your head as you try to fall asleep, which may cause disturbed sleep later, says Dr. Gross. Instead, jot down your thoughts, then allow yourself to drift off to dreamland.

Temporomandibular Disorder (TMD)

▶PROBLEM

You have a popping or clicking sensation in your jaw. Perhaps your jaw locks in the open or shut position. Or you feel pain radiating forward from an ear or have excruciating headaches behind the eyes, in the temples or the back of the head. Maybe you have difficulty or pain when chewing or using your jaws, or your jaws regularly feel stiff and tired. You may have temporomandibular disorder, a broad term for problems with the temporomandibular joint, located just in front of your ear, and with muscles used in chewing. It is such a pain to pronounce that it's simply called TMD.

▶CAUSE

A single event that caused trauma to the jaw, such as a punch or a sharp elbow in a basketball game can cause TMD. So can repetitive behavior such as grinding your teeth, chewing on a pencil, or biting your nails. Emotional stress seems to make the pain worse for some people. Most ominous is that "over-rambunctious sexual activity using the mouth can strain the jaw," says Greg Goddard, D.D.S., a dentist; assistant clinical professor of restorative dentistry at the University of California, San Francisco, in the Center for Orofacial Pain; and author of *TMJ—The Jaw Connection, the Overlooked*

> ### DO THIS NOW
> **Rest your jaw. Don't clench your teeth. "You want to have your teeth apart, lips relaxed," says Greg Goddard, D.D.S., a dentist; assistant clinical professor of restorative dentistry at the University of California, San Francisco, in the Center for Orofacial Pain; and author of *TMJ—The Jaw Connection, the Overlooked Diagnosis*.**

Diagnosis. We can hear you now: "Uh, sorry, babe. My TMD is flaring up, and I can't do that tonight."

▶ HOW SERIOUS

TMD can be quite painful, making it difficult to yawn or chew. It also can be embarrassing. A woman we know says that the romantic mood was ruined when her date's jaw began clicking like a telegraph during a passionate embrace. It's time to see a dentist if you have pain, can't chew, or have difficulty opening your mouth, Dr. Goddard says.

▶ SOLUTIONS

Eat a soft diet. Until the pain subsides, stick to foods like scrambled eggs and pasta and avoid crunchy and chewy foods such as hard nuts, chips, and carrots, says Sheldon Gross, D.D.S., past president of the American Academy of Orofacial Pain and a dentist in Bloomfield, Connecticut, who specializes in jaw-related problems. "It's the same as if your ankle hurts. Doctors say to sit down and put your foot up, but certainly don't go jogging uphill."

Exercise regularly. How can working out help your sore jaw feel better, you ask? TMD, like lower-back pain, is a chronic condition, says Dr. Goddard. "When you get chronic pain and you become sedentary, you deplete your own endorphins, your own painkiller in your body," he says. "By exercising and producing your own natural opiates, you reduce the pain that you feel." He recommends low-impact exercises to minimize pressure on the joints, three or four times a week for 20- to 30-minute intervals.

Hold the phone. Do not cradle the phone between your neck and shoulder; it irritates jaw and neck muscles, Dr. Goddard says.

Apply cold. For severe episodes of chronic pain, injuries of less than three days, and reinjured areas, apply cold. Ice serves as a "counterirritant"; that is, the cold overwhelms nerve endings carrying pain messages to the brain, says Dr. Goddard. Use ice wrapped in a towel for 10 minutes at a time three or four times a day, he recommends.

Try heat for chronic pain. To promote healing, apply moist heat (hot towels or a hot shower) for 20 minutes for mild to moderate pain to increase circulation and muscle relaxation, says Dr. Goddard. This doesn't conflict with the last tip.

"You can put hot on it, then cold on it, and just keep alternating that," says Dr. Goddard. Ice is especially effective for initial TMD symptoms, such as if you hit your jaw on something in an accident, while heat works well on chronic TMD pain. Alternating hot and cold therapy is appropriate for chronic pain but not new injuries, he says.

MEN'S HEALTH INDEX

Number of times women are more likely than men to seek medical treatment for temporomandibular disorder symptoms: Three to nine times

Avoid opening too wide. Limit how far your mouth opens during yawns. And eat small bites, advises Dr. Goddard.

Massage the jaw and temple muscles. This stimulates circulation, relaxes muscles, and decreases soreness, says Dr. Goddard.

▶Alternative Approaches

Give your face some slack. If the key to minimizing TMD pain is to reduce stress, few things fit the bill like meditation. Try to set aside time every day (as little as five minutes will work) where you can sit quietly, let your thoughts and worries go, and turn your mind inward. Become aware of your body, particularly of the muscles in your face. Allow them to relax. Such techniques open up the body to energy flow, says Dr. Goddard. "When people are under stress, they hold tension." Making time to relax every day can help you let go some of that tension.

▶Preventive Measures

Beware of the chair. Of course, you should visit a professional for any serious tooth or jaw problems you have. But if it looks like you're going to spend more time in a dentist's chair than in your easy chair, take frequent rests. Leaving your mouth wide open for prolonged periods can be a real jaw-breaker, says Dr. Goddard.

Maintain good posture. Avoid leaning your head forward when you sit or stand. That forward head posture may increase jaw and neck muscle activity and soreness, says Dr. Goddard.

Sleep on your side. "Find a pillow that fits you, one that will keep your neck and shoulders in a straight line," Dr. Goddard says. Or sleep on your back with the neck curve supported, he says.

Testicular Trauma

▶PROBLEM

You take a hit to the groin and the pain is so all-consuming that you feel like curling up in the fetal position and dying.

▶CAUSE

Blows to the scrotum during sports such as basketball and football are probably the most common, along with the occasional kick there during a fight, says James Nolan, M.D., a urologist in private practice in Fayetteville, North Carolina. Straddle-type injuries involving bicycles and falls also are common.

▶HOW SERIOUS

A shot to the scrotum and testicles usually feels awful, but "how much it hurts doesn't mean much," Dr. Nolan says. An injury to the testicles (one or both) can be serious. There can be bleeding on the inside, and rarely, one testicle can be ruptured, he says. Fortunately, this seldom happens. "I look at that as a pretty significant injury that needs to be evaluated by a urologist." Dr. Nolan says. If it isn't attended to, the ruptured testicle may eventually wither and die. If there is evidence of bruising, bleeding, or severe pain, especially associated with nausea, then seek medical attention right away, Dr. Nolan adds. A severe blow to the family jewels also can cause a man to lose (or lessen) the ability to father a child, he says. If you have a major discoloration of the scrotum and nausea and discomfort that don't subside within 15 minutes, you should see a doctor immediately, says Thomas Douglas, M.D., staff urologist at DeWitt Army Community Hospital in Fort Belvoir, Virginia.

> ## DO THIS NOW
>
> Apply an ice bag to your scrotum to ease the pain and swelling, says James Nolan, M.D., a urologist in private practice in Fayetteville, North Carolina. Place the ice in a resealable plastic storage bag and wrap a hand towel around the bag as a buffer to deaden the shock of the cold. Do this for 10 to 20 minutes at a time, for two or three times immediately following the injury. If pain persists or is severe, you should see a doctor.

History Lesson

Here's a testicular problem you don't see every day. The story was related by William A. Morton Jr., M.D., a retired urologist writing in the July 1991 issue of a medical journal.

A patient came to Dr. Morton with his left testicle missing and eight rusty staples in his scrotum, which was "swollen to twice the size of a grapefruit and extremely tender." The man explained he had injured himself in the machine shop where he worked and closed the laceration himself with a heavy-duty stapling gun.

The man later disclosed that he regularly stayed alone at the shop during the lunch hour, at which time he masturbated by holding his penis against the canvas drive-belt of a large piece of running machinery. One day, as he approached orgasm, he leaned too close to the belt. His scrotum became caught between the pulley wheel and the drive belt, throwing him in the air and ripping off his testicle. He then stapled the wound and resumed work.

Concluded Dr. Morton, "I can only assume he abandoned this method of self-gratification."

▶SOLUTIONS

Get them up. Elevate your scrotum by lying down and putting a rolled-up towel between your thighs, says Dr. Nolan.

Go rest, young man. If you get hurt during an athletic event, don't be a hero. Take yourself out of the game and get some rest right away, advises Dr. Douglas. By all means, avoid heavy lifting or straining until you are symptom-free, and then gradually resume your usual activities, adds Dr. Nolan.

Try a pain-reliever. An over-the-counter pain-reliever can help, says Dr. Nolan. "I usually tell patients to take Tylenol or a nonsteroidal anti-inflammatory such as Motrin if there is only mild to moderate pain as a result of the injury," Dr. Nolan says.

Keep 'em snug. For the next few days after a testicular injury, wear snug-fitting, supportive underwear, if you don't already, says Dr. Douglas. This takes weight off the tender cord of the testicle, he says.

▶ALTERNATIVE APPROACHES

Do a self-exam. Guys should inspect and feel their testicles every one to two months, says Dr. Nolan. Learn their shape and size. Then, if you do get injured or, worse, develop a tumor there, you will be able to recognize any changes that would prompt consultation with a doctor.

▶PREVENTIVE MEASURES

Place your jewels in a cup. Baseball catchers normally wear a protective cup to spare them the agony of a foul ball to the testicles, and other athletes should do the same, when possible, says Dr. Douglas. "You don't have to be a catcher. A ball can take a funny hop on the infield," he says. He advises wearing a cup if you play any sport where you might get hit in the groin.

Wear an athletic supporter. Okay, maybe you don't wear a protective cup because you can't run as well with one. You should at least wear a jockstrap, says Dr. Douglas. You already know that it keeps the boys secure, but it may offer some protection, too. "I think that you see more injuries in guys who are not wearing them," says Dr. Douglas. "It does make a difference. I think testicles are more likely to get injured hanging down in the heat of battle."

Tick Bites and Lyme Disease

▶PROBLEM

You can get Lyme disease (a bacterial infection) anywhere in the United States, but more likely in the Northeast, northern California, and the North Central states, especially Wisconsin and Minnesota—places where there are high deer populations, growing forests, and suburban development in formerly rural areas. This includes areas like Lyme, Connecticut, where the disease was first identified in 1975 after large numbers of children were being diagnosed with juvenile rheumatoid arthritis. The common link was that each child had been bitten by a tick.

▶CAUSE

The tick itself doesn't make you sick; rather, it is the bacteria (*Borrelia burgdorferi*) living within the tick. The tick picks up the bacteria from another host, usually a white-footed mouse or a white-tailed deer, and then passes it on to you, says Bruce Paton, M.D., past president of the Wilderness Medical Society based in Indianapolis. "Not all ticks are

DO THIS NOW

If you've been bitten by a tick, watch for a red, circular patch that appears near the bite three days to one month after infection. That's the mark of Lyme disease. As the rash gets larger, the central portion usually clears, while the outer edges redden. After a few days, it resembles a bull's-eye, says John Stein, D.V.M., an epidemiologist for the Centers for Disease Control and Prevention, division of vector-borne illnesses, in Fort Collins, Colorado. "If you get anything like this in the first month of a bite, go see your doctor," he says.

infected with disease, but worldwide ticks are known to be disease-carriers," he says.

A tick doesn't just bite. It buries its head in your skin and, if you don't remove it, feeds on your blood for up to 72 hours. If the tick carries Lyme disease, the bacteria invade the host's body through the tick's saliva. The longer the tick is attached to you, the more opportunity it has to make you sick, says John Stein, D.V.M., an epidemiologist for the Centers for Disease Control and Prevention, division of vector-borne illnesses, in Fort Collins, Colorado.

▶How Serious

A tick bite is no guarantee of Lyme disease. Unless the disease is common in your part of the country, the tick probably isn't infected, says Dr. Stein. If you think you have Lyme disease, go see a doctor, he says. If you recognize the early signs—fatigue, joint pain, flulike symptoms, and a peculiar-looking rash—Lyme disease is easily cured with antibiotics like doxycycline and amoxicillin. Doctors can misdiagnose Lyme disease, however. And if the disease progresses, you may experience severe fatigue, Bell's palsy (a numbness on one side of the face), and other neurological problems. Even then, Lyme disease is almost always curable, says Dr. Stein.

▶Solutions

Get ticked off. Research shows that a tick must be attached for at least 24 hours before it can pass on the bacteria, but since you may not know how long a tick has been hanging on you, you'll want to remove that sucker as soon as possible.

If a tick is burrowed into your skin, take a pair of tweezers, grasp the tick right where it is attached, and pull gently, instructs Howard Backer, M.D., a physician who practices emergency sports and wilderness medicine for Kaiser Permanente Medical Centers in the San Francisco Bay area and teaches wilderness medicine through the Wilderness Medical Society. "But don't get in a hurry and break off the head in the skin. If that happens, use a needle or splinter forceps to dig it out." Splinter forceps are tweezers specifically designed to pull out ticks and splinters; you can find them at some outdoors stores. After removal, wash the bitten area with soap and water or wipe with an antiseptic.

Stay centered. Tick nymphs tend to reside in leaf litter on the forest floor, while adult ticks hang out on tall grass and brush waiting until a mammal (a big one like you) brushes by, says Dr. Stein. "Ticks can't jump, so you should stay to the center of the trail away from overhanging vegetation," he says.

Go long. Always wear long pants, and tuck your cuffs inside your socks, says Dr. Stein. The less exposed your legs are, the less chance a tick will have of getting onto your skin.

Make them easy to spot. When you're out in the woods, wear light colored clothing—that will make it easier to see a tick if you do pick one up. Usu-

Did You Know?

The tick's odd lifestyle extends to its sexual habits as well. The male, lacking the normally essential appendage of a penis, relies instead on his nose to accomplish copulation.

First, he pushes his snout into the female's vagina to enlarge her opening, and then turns about to deposit a packet of sperm into the entrance. Using his nose once again, he pushes the sperm deep inside the female's body. All of this must occur while the female is actively taking a blood meal from a host.

ally, you can see an adult tick. But in the nymph stage, the tick may be no bigger than the period at the end of this sentence, says Dr. Stein. So before you go out in the woods, give yourself every advantage to improve your visibility.

Do a tick check. When you come out of a wooded area or overgrown field, check your body for ticks and, if you're with a partner, check each other, suggests Dr. Backer. Ticks often climb on your ankles or lower legs and then dig in wherever they can attach. They're really not particular about where. "You'll need to look hard. Don't miss hairy areas. I'd strip off my clothes and do a thorough check," advises Dr. Backer.

▶ALTERNATIVE APPROACHES

Fight back with herbs. When he was bitten by a tick and developed the telltale bull's-eye, James A. Duke, Ph.D., the world's foremost authority on healing herbs and author of *The Green Pharmacy*, took six capsules of 450 milligrams of the immune-boosting herb echinacea, and garlic capsules equivalent to 1,200 milligrams of fresh garlic every day for three weeks to fight the infection while it was in its early stages. He did this in conjunction with the doxycycline that his physician had prescribed. By the end of three weeks, his bull's-eye had disappeared.

Mince the mint. Dr. Duke swears by the mountain mint plant as a natural tick repellent. He crushes the leaves and rubs his skin with the juice. This perennial herb is commonly found in dry thickets in the eastern and southern United States. It can be identified by its lance-shaped leaves that appear in pairs opposite of one another and small whitish or purplish flowers that form in small, dense clusters. The plant itself has the aroma of pennyroyal and is often used as a substitute for pennyroyal oil.

▶PREVENTIVE MEASURES

Repel the invaders. Before you go into the woods, says Dr. Backer, spray bug repellent on both your clothes and your skin. It'll keep more than mosquitoes away. When spraying clothing, make sure that you have the kind that's meant for use on clothing; otherwise, you could end up with stains. Permanone and Duranon are two repellent products safe for clothing. They contain the chemical permethrin and are available at some sporting goods stores. (For more information on repellents, see Insect Bites and Stings on page 323.)

Create a tick-free zone. The clearer you keep your property of leaf litter and brush, the less chance ticks will find a home in your yard. Ticks like to winter under leaf piles, says Dr. Stein. So keep your property clean. Rake up leaves where you or your children frequent. Prune low-lying bushes to let in more sunlight, and remove any brush piles near your house.

Toenail Injuries

▶PROBLEM

Pain, swelling, and discoloration have settled into your toenail, or at least that's how it appears. "It's not actually the nail that hurts," explains Edward Beckett, D.P.M., a podiatrist in private practice in Lehighton, Pennsylvania. "It's the skin around and underneath the nail. Toenails are dead tissue, which is why it doesn't hurt to clip them."

It's not uncommon for a guy to first spot a toenail injury by finding blood on his sock rather than on his foot. "A lot of us look at our socks more than we look at our feet," Dr. Beckett says.

Another symptom to watch for is thickening of the nail. If a toe is continually bumping against the inside of a shoe, the nail may respond by growing thicker in order to better protect itself against injury.

▶CAUSE

There are at least three things that can cause a toenail injury, says Dr. Beckett: sudden impact, such as dropping a two-by-four on your foot; repetitive injuries, such as constant pressure from running with shoes that are too small for your feet; and, finally, genetic predisposition. Perhaps you were born with Morton's foot, so your second toe is longer than your big toe, which causes your shoes to press on some toes more than others.

To help determine the type of care you might need to give your toes, ask

DO THIS NOW

If your toenail is black and elevated, it's probably because blood has pooled underneath the nail. To fix this (and take away the pain), thoroughly heat one end of an unfolded paper clip with a match or lighter, says Edward Beckett, D.P.M., a podiatrist in private practice in Lehighton, Pennsylvania. "While the tip of the paper clip is still hot, put it through the nail plate," Dr. Beckett explains. "This will melt the nail so that the fluid will escape." Keep the drainage hole in the nail clog-free (that means no ointment or bandages) in case more liquid wants to ooze out. And don't burn your fingers with the heated paper clip.

yourself if the problem was caused suddenly or over time. "You can have either acute or chronic trauma," Dr. Beckett says. "Even picking your toenails or cuticles can be considered a trauma if it ultimately causes pain or an infection."

Knowing the cause of the pain will allow you to determine how to fix the problem and how to keep it from happening again.

▶How Serious

Usually, a guy stubs his toe or drops something on his foot and can connect that injury to the pain or redness in his foot. Not a big deal. Sometimes, however, there's pain or a change in the color of the nail, but the person can't remember dropping that brick on his foot. "That's when you need to see a doctor," Dr. Beckett says. "Changes in a toenail could actually be showing the signs of another problem, such as heart disease, melanoma, or skin cancer. It's not common, but it happens."

It's also time to see a doctor if the pain doesn't feel as if it's coming from the skin of the toe but from inside the toe. "You can fracture the bones in your toe but not realize it and only treat the toenail injury," Dr. Beckett says. "This is especially important because if the skin is broken and there's a broken bone, you're particularly susceptible to a dangerous bone infection, which could require intravenous antibiotics, amputation of the toe, or both."

Also, it's worth noting that nail injuries could initiate or lead to gout attacks if the person has a history of gout. And anyone who has diabetes should always see his doctor for foot problems.

▶Solutions

Cut it loose. It's all right to clip the nail if it's detached from the skin, provided you don't see any blood, Dr. Beckett says. "If it's very far down on the nail, though, you might be getting into a part of the nail that's very close to the nail bed, which is skin," Dr. Beckett warns. "Don't cause yourself more pain." If the toe is too painful to cut the nail immediately, soak the toe in table salt and water (one teaspoon of salt added to one quart of warm water) two or three times a day and cover with a bandage between soaks. After a few days, the pain, redness, and swelling (if any) should go down. You can attempt to trim the nail, but if it is still too painful, get professional help.

In some cases it's better to use antibiotic ointment (follow label directions), let the nail grow a bit, and then cut it when it's past the point of pain. The whole idea is to figure out what course of action is least likely to cause infection, Dr. Beckett says.

Take it off. This is pretty serious business, but if your toenail is about to fall off, the best thing to do is take charge and care for it yourself rather than wait for your sock or something to catch on it and painfully tear the nail from its attachments, says Richard Braver, D.P.M., a sports podiatrist and head of the Active Foot and Ankle Care Centers in Englewood and Fair Lawn, New Jersey.

Did You Know?

Your toenail grows at a rate of about 1 millimeter per month. "If you lose your nail, it will take anywhere from 12 to 18 months to grow from underneath the skin to the free edge, depending on age and general health," says Edward Beckett, D.P.M., a podiatrist in private practice in Lehighton, Pennsylvania.

You'll want to clean the nail with soap and water, then clip it as close as possible to the underlying skin, says Dr. Braver.

"Don't do this unless the toenail is very loose and about to come off anyway," Dr. Braver says. "Put some antibiotic cream on the skin and nail and bandage it fairly snugly." Keep a close eye on it, too. If the toe becomes red and swollen, exudes pus, or remains painful after a few days, see your podiatrist for treatment of a probable infection.

If you notice an off-yellow or red watery drainage from the nail bed (not yellowish-green pus), then you should soak your foot in warm water with a few capfuls of Betadine antibiotic solution. Add a few tablespoons of Epsom salts to promote drainage. Soak for 10 minutes twice a day. Regardless of whether you soak, apply a small amount of antibiotic cream to the toe and change the bandages twice daily for three weeks. If, after this time, the nail is still loose or you notice fluid under the nail, see your podiatrist.

Soak with salt. To cleanse the area and prevent an infection, soak your foot in a saltwater solution, made with one teaspoon of table salt added to a quart of warm water, says Dr. Beckett. Do this a couple times a day for three or four days. This is a general approach to promote drainage of an infected toe. It also adds a soothing effect on the irritated area.

▶ALTERNATIVE APPROACHES

Believe the hypericum. If you drop something on your toe, try hypericum, a homeopathic remedy specifically recommended for nerve-rich areas of the body, such as fingers and toes. "Take a low potency of 30C every few hours as needed for the pain," says Nancy Dunne-Boggs, a doctor of naturopathy at Bitterroot Natural Medicine in Missoula, Montana. "It should be apparent within six doses or so that the hypericum is working. You probably won't need to take this for more than two or three days." Follow label directions for dosage information.

Take your quercetin. Quercetin is a bioflavonoid, or plant compound, that is sold as a dietary supplement in tablet form. "Quercetin controls the body's response of excessive inflammation," Dr. Dunne-Boggs explains. "I usually tell people to take 300 milligrams three times a day after they sustain an injury." You can find quercetin supplements in drugstores and health food stores. You'll only need this for a few days or up to two weeks.

▶PREVENTIVE MEASURES

Wear protective shoes. They're called work boots for a reason. If you're doing work, wear the right boots. "You need to protect your feet the same way you protect your skin and eyes," Dr. Beckett says. "If you're carrying something heavy, then put on a good pair of boots. Sandals aren't going to protect your toes if you drop something."

While we're on the subject of sandals, it's a good idea to wear them if you're going to be anywhere close to rocks in water. "Waterproof sandals can really protect a guy who's trying to walk through a stream," Dr. Beckett says.

The point is that you not go barefoot if there's a chance you'll be walking across anything hot (pavement), sharp (rocks and glass), slippery (rocks in water), or uneven.

Wear shoes that fit. It's not enough to wear a strong shoe. You have to wear one that fits correctly. "Runners develop runner's nails (black nails) because of the constant irritation of their nails against the toe box of their shoes," Dr. Braver says. "Sometimes the shoe is too big, which allows the foot to slide forward. Other times, the shoe may be too stiff, which causes the heel to slide upward and the toes grip downward while running. You shouldn't feel the shoe around your toes, no matter what kind of step you're taking.

"If you're a dedicated runner or athlete, go to an athletic shoe store with trained salespeople to help pick out your shoes," Dr. Braver says. "Once you've found a brand that fits, you can shop for a better price or convenience through a catalog or at a discount store. But by picking out the brand, size, and style at a quality store, there are less headaches and hopefully less footaches down the road."

Toothache

▶PROBLEM

You have a sharp pain sometimes accompanied by swollen gums. It can be triggered when eating hard foods, such as carrots.

▶CAUSE

You could have an abscess or an infection in a tooth that is dying internally. It could be a cavity. Or it might be from an injury to your mouth that occurred years earlier but that is just now starting to cause the decay of the tooth. Whatever the cause, the damage starts to irritate the delicate nerves in the tooth, and those nerves let you know about it.

▶HOW SERIOUS

A toothache can signal a significant problem that requires a visit to the dentist. In the case of an acute infection, "you're talking about bring-me-to-my-knees type of pain," says Charles Perle, D.M.D., spokesman for the Academy of General Dentistry, a member of the Council on Communications for the American Dental Association, and a dentist in Jersey City, New Jersey. You don't want to mess with that, but you can't overlook prolonged discomfort either. "Sensitivity can be caused by something as simple as irritating your gums and exposing a portion of the tooth that has never been exposed before. If the sensitivity continues more than a day or two, see a dentist," Dr. Perle says. "Bleeding gums are generally also a sign of problems."

▶SOLUTIONS

Keep your mouth at rest. "Lips together, teeth apart," advises Dr. Perle. That'll keep pressure off the injured tooth.

DO THIS NOW

Take aspirin or ibuprofen (follow the dosage directions on the label) for some immediate relief, says William Howard, D.D.S., assistant professor of dental hygiene at Western Kentucky University in Bowling Green. Do not, however, stick an aspirin or other oral medication directly against the sore tooth. "It burns the gum and makes the condition worse," says Dr. Howard of this old home remedy.

History Lesson

Here's something to think about the next time you're ruining a perfectly good shirt as you sweat in the dentist's chair. If you lived in third-century Egypt, you might have had all your pearly whites removed from your mouth, and we don't mean gently. That's what is said to have happened to Saint Apollonia.

Described by one admirer as a "marvelous aged virgin," she was attacked by a mob in Alexandria and hit repeatedly in the face until all her teeth were broken. The attackers then lit a bonfire and threatened to burn her if she did not renounce her Christianity. Instead, she said a quick prayer and walked into the fire.

Later legend made Apollonia a beautiful girl whose teeth were extracted with pincers. She traditionally is painted as a young woman and often holds a tooth in a forceps. It is little wonder, then, that Apollonia is the patron saint of dentists.

Rinse it. If the area around the tooth is swelling, rinse your mouth with warm water and get to a dentist, Dr. Perle says. Posttreatment swelling can be controlled with ice. Apply an ice pack wrapped in a thin towel (so that the pack won't hurt your skin) to the side of your face for intervals of 10 minutes for an hour or so, Dr. Perle recommends.

Warm it. For some people, applying ice can make the pain worse, says William Howard, D.D.S., assistant professor of dental hygiene at Western Kentucky University in Bowling Green. If that's you, a warm compress might help. Or it may only work for a while, and then you'll want to try the ice. "It's a trial-and-error sort of thing," says Dr. Howard.

Floss it. That pain may be emanating from your gum, not the tooth. Sometimes a tough little food particle like a popcorn kernel may be lodged in your gum, says Dr. Howard. Flossing can dislodge it and make you feel better.

▶ALTERNATIVE APPROACHES

Chew out a bud. Chew on a few cloves—dried flower buds from a tropical tree used as a spice—and let the oil in it penetrate your teeth, says Richard D. Fischer, D.D.S., past president of the International Academy of Oral Medicine and Toxicology and a dentist in Annandale, Virginia. Tuck three to five cloves (you can buy them in the spice section of a grocery store) between your sore tooth and your cheek when not chewing. You can leave the cloves in your mouth for an hour or two and replace them as the pain recurs, Dr. Fischer says. "Oil of cloves is very soothing," he says.

Use bark for your bite. In a pinch, you can chew a wad of willow bark, then tamp it onto the tormenting tooth for temporary pain relief, says James A. Duke, Ph.D., the world's foremost authority on healing herbs, in his book, *The Green Pharmacy*. The bark contains salicin, a chemical relative of aspirin; so if you are allergic to aspirin, you need to avoid willow bark. You can find willow bark at some health food stores.

Spice the pain. A compress made with the spices ginger or red pepper, or with both, can also help relieve tooth pain, Dr. Duke says. To make a compress for your tooth, mix the powdered spice or spices in enough water to create a gooey paste. Then dip a small cotton ball into the paste and squeeze any excess out, advises Dr. Duke. Apply the cotton directly to the tooth without letting it touch your gums. If it feels too hot, rinse your mouth and try another remedy.

Do the hand jive. Here's an acupressure technique that may stem the ache. If you can feel a pea-size nodule or a granular texture in the area between your thumb and index finger, apply pressure or ice to it, says Dr. Fischer. This can relieve various head pains, including toothaches, he says. "You often have to do both hands," he advises. "It usually takes about three minutes per hand."

Lend an ear. Another place you can apply pressure to lessen tooth pain is the earlobe, says Dr. Fischer, but it's not as efficient. Still, squeezing each earlobe for a few minutes can help, he says. "I've had people in the dental chair put a clothespin on the ear instead of using anesthesia," he says.

▶Preventive Measures

Stop sucking. Hard candies and sugar-coated lozenges are among the most pervasive promoters of tooth decay; hence, if untreated, toothaches may develop, says Dr. Perle. "In my experience, sucking candies are more devastating than a chocolate bar. The solution gets in between the teeth and all over the place."

Stick a straw in your maw. If you must drink sugary sodas, do so only with a straw and take small sips. Don't swish the soda around your teeth, and you won't cause further decay to the tooth. "Your throat is thirsty, not your teeth," says Dr. Perle.

Tooth Discoloration

▶PROBLEM

Your teeth look as yellowed as an old newspaper clipping.

▶CAUSE

A lot of things can stain teeth: smoking or chewing tobacco, coffee or tea, the acidic juice of certain berries (especially blueberries). Getting older does it, too. As we age, our teeth lose some of their outermost layer, the enamel. The material below the enamel is darker, so teeth lose some of their whiteness.

▶HOW SERIOUS

If a single tooth is becoming discolored, it may mean that the tooth is dying within—perhaps from an old injury—and you need to see a dentist, says Richard D. Fischer, D.D.S., past president of the International Academy of Oral Medicine and Toxicology and a dentist in Annandale, Virginia. If, however, your teeth are generally discolored from coffee or tobacco stains, it's only serious to the extent that your appearance concerns you. But teeth that look grayish or translucent may be the result of a loss of calcium, says Dr. Fischer. Calcium can leech out of the teeth and into the bloodstream. In healthy teeth, it works the other way around. You may need more calcium if you have more muscle cramps than usual (facial tics, charley horses) or if your teeth seem very sensitive to cold. If you're concerned about this, you should see a doctor or nutritionist, Dr. Fischer says.

▶SOLUTIONS

Chew gum. Chew a stick of sugarless gum after you drink coffee or tea. Doing so will produce more saliva to help wash away the beverage's residue be-

> ### DO THIS NOW
>
> Use a toothbrush with soft bristles and brush thoroughly. It's important not only to brush often but also to brush effectively, says William Howard, D.D.S., assistant professor of dental hygiene at Western Kentucky University in Bowling Green. A good rule of thumb is to replace your toothbrush every three months, or whenever the bristles are looking frayed.

History Lesson

Ancient peoples might be forgiven if they didn't brush after every meal. Toothbrushes found in Egyptian tombs dating to 3000 B.C. were little more than pencil-size twigs with one end frayed into a soft and fibrous material. These "chew sticks" were rubbed against the teeth. It would be another 1,000 years before the first known toothpaste appeared, also in Egypt. It was made from powdered pumice stone and wine vinegar.

As bad as that sounds, it had to taste better than what the early Romans were using—human urine in their toothpaste and as a mouthwash.

---

fore it stains your teeth, says Carole Palmer, R.D., Ed.D., professor and co-head of the division of nutrition and preventive dentistry at Tufts University School of Dental Medicine in Boston.

Brush after lunch. Sure, you may feel a little foolish brushing your teeth in the men's room at work after lunch, but it can help, says Charles Perle, D.M.D., spokesman for the Academy of General Dentistry, a member of the Council on Communications for the American Dental Association, and a dentist in Jersey City, New Jersey. A certain amount of tooth staining can be thwarted by diligent dental care. He advises using toothpastes that carry the American Dental Association Seal of Acceptance.

Switch toothpastes. Try a whitening toothpaste, like Colgate Platinum, says William Howard, D.D.S., assistant professor of dental hygiene at Western Kentucky University in Bowling Green.

Floss. Regular flossing—like brushing—wipes out plaque, the filmy crud that collects on our teeth and causes not only decay but also discoloration, says Dr. Howard. Floss every tooth at least once a day, he advises. "A toothbrush will not remove the plaque that is between the teeth," Dr. Howard says. "So effective plaque removal with brushes and floss will definitely cut down on the amount of tooth discoloration."

Hit the bleach. If all your teeth have a general discoloration, you might want to think about bleaching, says Dr. Perle. You can buy over-the-counter bleaching remedies to whiten your teeth. They require wearing a device in your mouth at night that contains a chemical gel. But often people do not follow the instructions when using bleaching products, and in doing so, they may damage their teeth, he warns. He says that the American Dental Association and the Academy of General Dentistry recommend that you only bleach your teeth under the care of a dentist.

"I've heard mixed things about the bleaches," says Dr. Fischer.

"They are potentially harmful if used without supervision," says Dr. Howard.

▶ALTERNATIVE APPROACHES

Peel away discoloration. If you scour the shelves of health food stores, you might find Peelu, a tree root extract. "It's a natural whitener," says Dr. Fischer. It can be purchased as a toothpaste or powder. You can use Peelu every day as a regular toothpaste, or in addition to regular toothpaste, he says. Use the powder the same way as the paste.

▶PREVENTIVE MEASURES

Be a water boy. As soon as you finish that blueberry muffin or cup of coffee, swish some water around your mouth. Rinsing your mouth will help cleanse your teeth and prevent stains from building up, says Dr. Palmer.

Drink less. If you're a heavy drinker of alcohol or coffee, reduce your consumption. We already know that coffee can stain your teeth. But both it and alcohol are diuretics, and they make you lose water-soluble vitamins and minerals that are essential to healthy-looking teeth, says Dr. Fischer. In fact, cutting back on anything that you eat or drink that is staining your teeth will go a long way toward lessening how much they get stained.

Tooth Sensitivity

▶PROBLEM

Certain hot or cold foods or beverages send a piercing shot of pain through one of your teeth. "More often, the reaction is going to be to cold," says William Howard, D.D.S., assistant professor of dental hygiene at Western Kentucky University in Bowling Green.

▶CAUSE

A filling may have come loose. Or your gums may have receded some, exposing a sensitive nerve. Grinding or clenching teeth can also cause sensitivity, as can a "high spot" on a filling or a regular tooth, in which one tooth hits a little harder than the others when you bite down. Sometimes a tooth becomes sensitive when you chew a hard food such as a pizza crust or pretzels, and your gum gets pushed down, exposing parts of your tooth that aren't accustomed to feeling air.

▶HOW SERIOUS

Mostly, tooth sensitivity is a major annoyance. In extreme cases, it can indicate nerve damage. It can also be painful enough that some people get root canals unnecessarily, says Richard D. Fischer, D.D.S., past president of the International Academy of Oral Medicine and Toxicology and a dentist in Annandale, Virginia. See a dentist if your teeth are very sensitive for more than a few days, he says, especially if the sensitivity comes from heat rather than cold.

▶SOLUTIONS

Change your diet. Tooth sensitivity often is a sign that you are not getting enough calcium and magnesium, says Dr. Fischer. Increase your consumption

---

DO THIS NOW

Apply petroleum jelly to the tooth for short-term relief. "It doesn't feel really good in your mouth, but it beats the alternative," says Charles Perle, D.M.D., spokesman for the Academy of General Dentistry, a member of the Council on Communications for the American Dental Association, and a dentist in Jersey City, New Jersey.

History Lesson

1790: George Washington's personal dentist, John Greenwood, invents the first known "dental foot engine" by adapting his mother's spinning wheel to rotate a drill bit by rapid, foot-pedaled action. Greenwood's drill rotated 500 times a minute, and was revolutionary, when you consider that earlier drills were tortuously slow. The dentist, holding a metal spike between his thumb and index finger, manually worked it back and forth while forcefully pressing downward. Today, turbine-powered drills rotate at speeds of 300,000 to 400,000 revolutions per minute.

And remember this the next time you hear yourself whimpering about an upcoming dentist appointment: Nitrous oxide, or the "laughing gas" that makes so many dental procedures painless, has only been in use for little more than a century. Novocain wasn't introduced until 1905.

---

of dairy products to get more calcium and legumes (tofu, beans) to get more magnesium.

Take supplements. Dr. Fischer recommends taking 600 to 1,000 milligrams per day of calcium, depending upon one's diet, and half that amount of magnesium. Men with heart or kidney problems should check with their doctor before taking supplemental magnesium. Supplemental magnesium may also cause diarrhea in some people. Ingesting fatty acids by eating a handful of seeds or nuts or about a teaspoon of vegetable or olive oil may also help one better absorb the calcium if they are taken at the same time, says Dr. Fischer.

Brush away the pain. Try a toothpaste designed for sensitive teeth. They actually are effective, says Charles Perle, D.M.D., spokesman for the Academy of General Dentistry, a member of the Council on Communications for the American Dental Association, and a dentist in Jersey City, New Jersey. Look for one with the American Dental Association Seal of Acceptance.

"The key is to use it for several weeks," adds Dr. Howard. "It doesn't work right away."

Drop the pain. Liquid toothache preparations like Anbesol or Orajel contain a topical anesthetic that can deaden tooth or gum pain, says Dr. Howard. But if the pain persists for more than a few days, see your dentist, he adds.

Do the obvious. Stop doing whatever is causing pain in your tooth, says Dr. Perle. If a cold beer makes you wince, don't drink them at such a chilly temperature. If hot tea torments your tooth, let it cool down a bit before you sip.

▶Alternative Approaches

Extend an olive branch. If the sensitivity is from an abrasion or erosion along the gum line, dry the tooth with air or cotton, then dab warm olive oil on it, advises Dr. Fischer. He suggests pouring a small amount in a saucepan and heating it until it starts to smoke. Dampen a cotton swab in the oil and wave it in the air briefly to cool it off. Then dab the warm oil on your gum line a couple of times. "Most of the time, that sensitivity will go away," says Dr. Fischer. "One treatment with the oil usually lasts for months, sometimes years. The key is that the tooth must be dry. You can repeat this remedy when the effect of the oil wears off."

▶Preventive Measures

Use a softer brush. Teeth also can become sensitive by overly aggressive brushing, especially with a brush that has hard bristles, says Dr. Howard. This combination can push back the gum and expose the root surface, which is highly sensitive when first exposed. He suggests using a toothbrush with softer bristles and a gentler technique.

Take a hard look at soft drinks. If you're drinking enough colas and root beers to float an armada, cut back. "The darker sodas have much higher levels of phosphoric acid, which pulls calcium out of your body (and teeth) like crazy," says Dr. Fischer.

Ulcers

▶ PROBLEM

There's a lowly, but strong, bacteria. *Helicobacter pylori*, more informally known as *H. pylori*, has begun to create an open wound in the lining of your stomach or duodenum. (The duodenum is the first part of the small intestine. It's connected to the lower end of the stomach.) A duodenal ulcer is four times more common than a stomach ulcer, and they both are referred to as peptic ulcers.

Your ulcer has begun to make its presence known with pain and burning in the upper part of your abdomen.

▶ CAUSE

The *H. pylori* bacterium accounts for almost 80 percent of all ulcers. People seem to pick up the bacterium (and it is contagious) as kids.

In fact, *H. pylori* is present in almost 50 percent of adult American stomachs, but that doesn't mean that everyone will develop a full-fledged ulcer. No one knows why ulcers develop from the bacteria in some people and not others, although stress, smoking, and some foods may be a factor.

"A minority of ulcers are caused by a consistent use of aspirin and other painkillers," says David Peura, M.D., a gastroenterologist and professor of medicine in the division of gastroenterology and hepatology at the University of Virginia Health Sciences Center in Charlottesville.

DO THIS NOW

For quick relief from stomach pain that you think may be an ulcer, take antacids, says David Rooney, M.D., a family physician with Southern Chester County Family Practice Associates in Oxford, Pennsylvania. (Follow directions on the label.)

"Antacids can help you wait out the 'telling time.' If the pain melts away in two weeks and doesn't return, then you probably didn't have an ulcer. If you find that you have to keep taking the medicine after two weeks, suspect an ulcer and see your doctor," Dr. Rooney advises.

There's no major difference among the antacids you'll see on your drugstore shelf, says Dr. Rooney. "Buy whatever is on sale," he says.

History Lesson

Satchel Paige, the great Negro League star who became the first African-American pitcher in the American League in 1948, wasn't a doctor. But he intuitively understood the connection between stress, bad habits, and stomach woes. Here are his keys to the good life.

- Avoid fried meats, which angry up the blood.
- If your stomach disputes you, lie down and pacify it with cool thoughts.
- Keep the juices flowing by jangling around gently as you move.
- Go very light on the vices, such as carrying on in society.
- The social rumble ain't restful.
- Avoid running at all times.
- Don't look back. Something might be gaining on you.

▶HOW SERIOUS

Although ulcers aren't necessarily serious, the pain of an ulcer is famous for waking its sufferers up in the middle of the night. The discomfort is episodic, however. It lasts for a couple of days or weeks and then goes away, but it always returns. Ulcers sometimes grow so large or do so much damage that they produce bleeding as well as lots of scarring. If you see blood in your stool (it looks black) or have severe stomach pain and a high fever, then you should see a doctor, says Dr. Peura.

"Most ulcers will heal on their own," Dr. Peura says. "But only antibiotics can get rid of the underlying problem, which is the presence of *H. pylori*. If you don't take care of that, there's a good chance that you'll have another ulcer again." So if you have an ulcer, see your doctor and request to be tested for *H. pylori*.

Getting rid of the *H. pylori* bacteria involves a two-week series of three medications. However, there are many other ways to combat the actual pain and discomfort of an ulcer attack.

▶SOLUTIONS

Watch what you eat. Certain foods may incite your ulcers. In fact, one of the leading candidates—milk—was for a long time widely considered a home remedy. "Milk isn't good for ulcers because the proteins in it stimulate the secretion of stomach acid," Dr. Peura says. "We generally tell people to simply see which foods bother them and then to avoid those foods."

In fact, food allergies can exacerbate ulcer symptoms, and milk is a leading allergen. Other allergens include corn and wheat. "Try to eat whole grains lower in gluten, such as brown rice, millet, or buckwheat," says Priscilla Skerry, a naturopathic and homeopathic doctor in private practice in Portland, Maine.

Snack. Food can either be part of the problem or part of the solution. It's your choice. If you have late-night discomfort, a snack of bread or crackers can serve as a good sponge for stomach acid and bring temporary relief, says Thomas Gossel, Ph.D., registered pharmacist, professor of pharmacology and toxicology, and dean of the College of Pharmacy at Ohio Northern University in Ada.

Relax. Although studies relating ulcers to stress are inconclusive, it is certain that stress can aggravate ulcers, says Dr. Skerry. (It's not the stress so much as your reaction to it that causes the problem.)

Whether through exercise, relaxation techniques, or meditation, take time each day to de-stress your life. Your stomach will thank you. And so will everyone else in your life, adds Dr. Peura.

▶ALTERNATIVE APPROACHES

Guzzle glutamine. Drinking one liter a day of fresh, raw cabbage juice throughout the day may help, Dr. Skerry says. Cabbage is high in glutamine, a nonessential amino acid. "Glutamine helps the healthy stomach cells regenerate and stimulates the production of mucin, which protects the stomach lining," Dr. Skerry says.

To make your own, slice then juice or blend an ordinary green cabbage, says Dr. Skerry. "It's not bad tasting," she says.

Play an album. Arsenicum album is one homeopathic remedy available in health food stores that can help burning pain and the anxiety that often accompanies an ulcer. "Take three 30X or 30C pellets when the symptoms are acute," says Dr. Skerry. "You can repeat that in a half-hour if you need to, but if the symptoms don't ease within an hour, then discontinue its use because this isn't the right remedy."

▶PREVENTIVE MEASURES

Quit puffing. Here's another reason to give up smoking, but this one has nothing to do with the health of your lungs. "Smoking depletes your saliva, which is your own internal antacid," Dr. Peura explains. Without healthy saliva, your stomach acid can't neutralize the foods that irritate it. Smoking also stimulates acid, which can aggravate ulcer pain and slow healing, adds Dr. Peura.

Rethink your aspirin strategy. Numerous men take one aspirin a day to fight heart disease, and that's good. But about 1 percent of all regular aspirin users end up with problem ulcers.

"You should only take a daily dose of aspirin and other painkillers under the care of a physician, and he should be checking for signs of an ulcer," Dr. Peura says. "The worry isn't so much that the medication will cause an ulcer but that it will cause an ulcer to bleed, which can be very serious."

If you need to take a painkiller, use acetaminophen instead, suggests Dr. Peura. It provides relief without irritating your stomach.

Unruly Hair

▶PROBLEM

That cowlick suddenly heads off for greener pastures. Your bicycle helmet has left you looking like Bill Murray is your stylist. Or your hair is just generally contrary and resists staying in place more than a dog in a tub. Don't pull your hair out by the roots; there's help.

▶CAUSE

Most things about your hair—how much you have, its color, thickness, and character—are hereditary. If you have a shock of coarse blond thatch, chances are that one of your parents gave it to you. But some of the things men do to their hair make it even more unmanageable, says David H. Kingsley, a certified trichologist (a specialist in hair and scalp) and owner of British Science Corporation, which counsels and treats people with hair and scalp problems, on Staten Island, New York. Hair dyes, chlorine-laden pools, harsh sunlight, poor nutrition, and even improper shampooing can add to a litany of hair woes.

▶HOW SERIOUS

It's not very serious, medically speaking. Aside from mussing up your pride, unruly hair is rarely a sign of a deep-rooted medical problem when it begins in adulthood and involves the whole scalp, says Susan P. Detwiler, M.D., a dermatologist in private practice in San Diego. One exception: "If there has been an acute change in the character of the hair, I would suggest getting a thyroid test," she says. So if your hair suddenly becomes excessively coarse or dry, especially if it's coupled with hot or cold spells, lethargy, or irritability, Dr. Detwiler recommends that you see a doctor.

DO THIS NOW

Find a misting bottle like the ones used to spray plants. Fill it with clean water. "Then spray your hair with a little water, put some gel on it, and run a comb through it," says Fredric S. Brandt, M.D., clinical associate professor of dermatology at the University of Miami School of Medicine.

Did You Know?

Beautiful bouffants beat back big busts. Amazing, but true.

In 1995, *Allure*, magazine made a "boob-boo" when it ran a full-page Wonderbra ad right next to a Neutrogena ad. The problem was that the Neutrogena ad proclaimed "Having a Bad Hair Day?" over a hair-treatment product, while the Wonderbra ad showed a buxom woman in her skivvies with the headline "Who Cares If It's a Bad Hair Day."

Allure sheepishly apologized, but the mix-up got the folks at Neutrogena to thinking. The company commissioned a study to determine whether women would prefer having good hair over good cleavage.

Of the 500 women surveyed, a whopping 80 percent said they would choose having drop-dead gorgeous locks over an ample, upright set of sisters. Only 6 percent opted for better breasts. The rest said neither, both, or were undecided.

And, dispelling the myth that men's eyes never make it above shoulder level, a paltry 20 percent of men said that they would prefer their wives or girlfriends to have bustier profiles. Fifty-one percent chose a mate with a well-coiffed mane. Most of the remaining 29 percent couldn't decide—or had enough sense to know that either answer would get them in trouble.

▶SOLUTIONS

Go wrong. Going the opposite way with your hair can help get it going back in the right direction. Dr. Detwiler suggests the following technique: Wet a comb. Run it through your hair in the opposite direction of the way you typically style it. Do that a few times and then retrain the hair back in the normal direction.

Try a gel. While most gels will help keep your hair in place, finding the one that gives you the look you want may require trial and error, says Kingsley. Read the label for a clue, he suggests. If it promises that the wet, slicked-back look that works for you, give it a try. No matter which type of gel you choose, Kingsley recommends starting with less than the package instructs.

Cut it short. Unlike Nero, some men don't want to fiddle around too much. Stephen Moody, assistant general manager of the Vidal Sassoon Academy in Santa Monica, California, says that if that's the case, a short haircut is often easier to style and care for.

Undo the damage. Damaged hair makes for unruly hair. You can avoid that damage, adds Dr. Detwiler, by taking a few precautions. Wear a wide-brimmed hat in the sun. Use hair dyes judiciously or not at all. Ditto for hair straighteners and perms.

▶ALTERNATIVE APPROACHES

Spray away. A little hairspray may help tame that mane. Don't overdo it, though. Kingsley recommends that you start with just a touch and work up from there.

▶PREVENTIVE MEASURES

Become a beachcomber. Heck, you can even try this one at home. Brush your hair. Later, when your hair is messy again, comb it. You'll find the comb catching and snagging more than the brush. For this reason, says Kingsley, people comb much more carefully than they brush. The daily rigors of rough brushing can lead to hair breakage and damage, making your hair even more unmanageable. So brush gently when you want to style your hair but always comb first. Kingsley suggests only using a wide-tooth, good-quality comb, making sure that the teeth don't have sharp edges from the mold used to make it. He prefers a rubber comb. Metal combs can add static to your hair, making it fly off all over the place. Keep a small comb in your wallet for quick touch-ups in the men's room, recommends Kingsley.

Air it out. Dr. Detwiler was part of a group that studied the damage that can be caused by blow-dryers. She found that home dryers can generate heats of up to 300°F. The problem arises when you allow hair and other bathroom crud to build up on the air intake of your dryer.

Insufficient air flow jacks the internal temperature of the dryer through the roof. The resulting superhot air can damage your hair by forming bubbles in the individual shafts. Not only are those hairs going to be impervious to styling, they often break off at the level of the bubble. The solution is to keep your dryer clean and watch for signs of overheating, such as red coils or a burning smell.

Urinary Incontinence

▶PROBLEM

There are about two million men—perhaps many more since the condition often is not reported—who have a loss of bladder control. There are several types of incontinence with just as many causes, but all are usually a result of an underlying medical condition. About 85 percent of those with incontinence are women.

▶CAUSE

The most common cause of male urinary incontinence is from prostate gland surgery, which can weaken the sphincter muscle that goes around the urethra that helps to hold urine in, says James Cummings, M.D., chief of the department of urology at the University of South Alabama College of Medicine in Mobile.

An injury such as a pelvic fracture; an aging, unstable bladder; and an enlarged prostate can also be at fault. Diuretics that are prescribed for hypertension and congestive heart problems can worsen incontinence in some men who already have a tendency toward it. These are the most common causes of incontinence; there are many others, says A. Scott Klein, M.D., a urologist at the Gundersen Clinic in La Crosse, Wisconsin.

▶HOW SERIOUS

"It's a problem that directly impacts on a man's quality of life because he has to wear protection as well as limit his activities," says Raul Parra, M.D.,

DO THIS NOW

Pace yourself. Urinate at regularly scheduled, short intervals, even if you don't feel the urge. Then slowly increase the intervals between trips to the bathroom until you reach the maximum time frame that you can hold out, says James Cummings, M.D., chief of the department of urology at the University of South Alabama College of Medicine in Mobile. He recommends starting out with 2-hour intervals, and if that works, try going 2½ to 3 hours between bathroom breaks, and so on. "Doing this empties your bladder before it gets so full that it contracts on its own," explains Dr. Cummings.

History Lesson

Even guys who don't have urinary incontinence know that it can be tough making it through the night without making at least one pit stop in the bathroom. Imagine, then, what it would be like to go 30 years without relief. The makers of the 1997 comedy, *Austin Powers—International Man of Mystery*, did.

In the movie, the hairy-chested runt of a secret agent, portrayed by Mike Myers, is defrosted after being cryogenically frozen for three decades. In what must be one of the longest such scenes in cinema history, Myers proceeds to noisily pee for 51 seconds—starting and stopping his stream a half-dozen times—before there is a segue to another scene.

professor and chairman of urology at St. Louis University School of Medicine. It can cause him to develop skin problems such as fungal infections and, yes, diaper rash. "It also hampers his sexual activity," says Dr. Parra. Understandably, incontinence can be a big blow to a man's self-esteem. "Any man with urinary incontinence should be evaluated by a urologist in order to determine the cause of the incontinence as well as possible remedies," says Dr. Parra. "Ultimately, urinary incontinence in a male can oftentimes be corrected. But patients need to be individually assessed since the cause is often a combination of problems."

▶SOLUTIONS

Squeeze it. For men whose incontinence is due to prostate surgery, Kegel exercises can help strengthen the urinary sphincter muscle, says Dr. Parra. And they can be done anywhere. Squeeze the muscles that you use to stop the flow of urine for 5 to 10 seconds, then relax a few seconds and repeat. Do 10 of these contractions four or five times a day, gradually working up to 25 or 30 contractions each time, Dr. Parra advises.

Once a man develops his urinary sphincter muscle to the point where he no longer leaks urine, he must continue to do the Kegels, says Dr. Klein. Otherwise, like a weight lifter who stops working out, his muscle will atrophy.

Skip the nightcap. Naturally, you can't practice timed urinating when you're asleep, so it's wise to avoid drinking beverages of any kind during the hour before going to bed, says Dr. Parra.

Swathe yourself. Admittedly, this is no long-term solution, and the idea can make a guy cringe. But if your incontinence is more than a bit of dribbling, buy adult diapers until your condition improves, Dr. Parra says. At least they enable you to leave your house without telltale wet spots on your pants.

Watch your diet. If you are urinating into special undergarments, you might be able to mask any telltale odor by modifying your diet, says Dr. Parra.

Garlic, spices, and certain herbs are among the things that may produce a strong smell, he says.

Coffee, cabbage, broccoli, and brussels spouts may also have the same effect, while drinking cranberry juice may have a positive effect on urine smell, Dr. Klein says. "But the more you drink, perhaps the bigger the problem," he adds.

Claims of good and bad effects of various foods have not been scientifically proven, so you have to discover for yourself what works through trial and error, says Dr. Parra.

▶ALTERNATIVE APPROACHES

Make your own spread. Saw palmetto, pumpkin seeds, and Brazil nuts all are effective in preventing and relieving benign prostate hyperplasia, an enlarged prostate gland (also known as BPH), says James A. Duke, Ph.D., the world's foremost authority on healing herbs, in his book, *The Green Pharmacy*. For some men, BPH is a cause of excessive urination, especially at night. Dr. Duke touts a spread that you can smear on crackers and bread, prosnut butter, for treating an enlarged prostate. He says to place about a half-cup of fresh pumpkin seeds in a blender or food processor. Open one saw palmetto capsule (160 milligrams), pour in the contents, and blend until smooth. To make the mixture a little more spreadable, add a few drops of Brazil nut oil made by grinding about 10 Brazil nuts. Brazil nuts contain selenium and sitosterol, both proven useful in combating prostate problems, says Dr. Duke. He suggests eating a couple of tablespoons every day and advises not to make it in big batches so that it will always be fresh. Pumpkin seeds and Brazil nuts are available at supermarkets, and saw palmetto capsules can be found in most health food stores.

It must be stressed, however, that Dr. Duke recommends this treatment for men with an enlarged prostate, not those who have undergone prostate surgery. You should consult with your doctor regularly when using saw palmetto for treatment of enlarged prostate. In rare cases, people taking this herb have experienced stomach problems.

Be nettlesome. Take two to three teaspoons a day of stinging nettle extract. A group of 67 men with BPH who were given the extract reported a significant decrease in their need to get up at night and urinate, reports Dr. Duke.

▶PREVENTIVE MEASURES

Avoid alcohol and coffee. Both make you produce more urine, says Dr. Klein. And alcohol has the double whammy of dulling your senses so that you may be unaware that your bladder is becoming full until it overflows and begins leaking, he says.

Varicose Veins

Bluish veins make your legs look like a road map. In some cases, the veins aren't visible but your legs can ache or feel exceptionally heavy, especially after standing or sitting for an extended period of time. In advanced cases, the veins bulge and are very painful.

▶**CAUSE**

There are several theories on what the root cause of varicose veins is, but nobody is certain. Genetics play a big role. If your mother and grandmother have them, chances are good that you have some brewing. And, for some reason, Western societies have a much greater incidence of varicose veins. The mechanism at work, however, is painfully clear. The veins in your legs have nifty little one-way valves that prevent blood from backflowing when you stand. For some reason, these stop working in certain veins, allowing blood to pool and even flow the wrong way. The vein wall then starts breaking down, and before you know it, blue bulges are popping out of the side of your leg.

▶**HOW SERIOUS**

It depends. "If you have some small veins and you have no problems, leave them alone," says Howard C. Baron, M.D., associate professor of surgery at the New York University School of Medicine in New York City, attending

DO THIS NOW

Stop, drop, and elevate your legs. Leg elevation is a quick and effective way to counteract the throbbing ache that can come with varicose veins. Lie down, get yourself at least a couple of pillows, and put your feet on them. "You have to get them above the level of the heart," says Tamara D. Fishman, D.P.M., president and chief executive officer of the Woundcare Institute, a not-for-profit educational organization in Miami that disseminates medical information pertaining to wound management and diabetic foot care. Keep your feet elevated for at least a half-hour. If you're at work and have a chair that tilts back, use that and plop your feet on your desk.

Did You Know?

Perhaps it will offer a semblance of reassurance to know that your ancestors were bothered by varicose veins as well. Although varicose veins are widely considered to be a modern ailment—a product of Western society—they actually predate the Industrial Age by thousands of years.

An ancient Egyptian medical text written on papyrus paper around 3000 B.C. describes the problem. The ancient Greeks were also impressed enough with varicose veins to render them in a votive relief. This memorial is still on display in the National Museum of Athens.

---

vascular surgeon at the Cabrini Medical Center in New York City, and author of *Varicose Veins*. Home remedies should suit you fine to help keep them from getting worse. But if the veins bulge or you feel pain or heaviness, especially after sitting or standing for a long time, get yourself checked by a doctor. Untreated, varicose veins can turn into leg ulcers and even be life-threatening, Dr. Baron warns.

▶SOLUTIONS

Turn on the hose. Get some good therapeutic support stockings. "And I don't mean the cheap ones. You need proper stockings," says Alexander H. Murray, M.D., head of the division of dermatology at Dalhousie University Faculty of Medicine in Halifax, Nova Scotia. These stockings should be custom-fitted by a medical supply store (they will measure the circumference of your leg), or your doctor may prescribe them for you. The tight, supportive fit of these specialized socks helps your heart pump blood back out of the legs. Generic ones are available at many drugstores, but Dr. Murray says that if they don't fit properly, they can actually constrict the flow of blood rather than aid it.

Fight back with fiber. "We're a constipated society," says Dr. Baron. Because of that, the pressure of a permanently full colon on the upper leg veins can be a distinct aggravator of varicose veins, he says. He strongly recommends a high-fiber, low-fat diet. Keep in mind that the Daily Value for fiber is 25 grams and that a high-fiber food is one that has 5 grams of fiber or more per serving. To get this much fiber in your diet, Dr. Baron suggests eating foods like bran breads and cereals, sweet potatoes, asparagus, or leafy vegetables daily. A low-fat food has 3 grams or less of fat per serving. So you should be getting no more than 80 grams of total fat a day on a 2,500-calorie-a-day diet. Not only will your heart love you but also your varicose veins will sing your praises.

Take a seat. If your job requires you to spend a lot of time on your feet, you're making your leg veins work doubly hard. Take regular sitting spells, Dr.

Murray says. And avoid crossing your legs. Crossing your legs jacks up the pressure in your leg veins, making it harder for blood to circulate. If sitting down on the job is not an option, or if you're a Beefeater guarding Buckingham Palace, flex your calf muscles often and shift your weight from one foot to the other.

Make a stand. Conversely, if you're a full-time desk jockey like so many of us today, you're sitting right on your leg veins, constricting blood flow. Get up, move around, even lie down, at least every half-hour, says Dr. Baron.

Slim down. Carrying around excess weight increases the pressure on your legs, says Tamara D. Fishman, D.P.M., president and chief executive officer of the Woundcare Institute, a not-for-profit educational organization in Miami that disseminates medical information pertaining to wound management and diabetic foot care. This increases your chances of developing varicose veins and worsens them if you already have them.

▶ALTERNATIVE APPROACHES

Land a powerful combination. Taken together, vitamin C and bioflavonoids (natural antioxidants) may be a big help to your veins, says David Edelberg, M.D., assistant professor of medicine at Rush Medical College; section chief of holistic medicine at Illinois Masonic Medical Center and Grant Hospital, all in Chicago; and founder of the American Whole Health Centers in Chicago, Denver, and Bethesda, Maryland. Vitamin C aids circulation by reducing blood-clotting tendencies, while bioflavonoids may reduce venous fragility. He recommends 3,000 milligrams per day of vitamin C and 500 milligrams of bioflavonoids. Both are sold in drugstores and often sold in combination. A word of caution: Excess vitamin C may cause diarrhea in some people.

Supplement with vitamin E. Here's yet another good reason to take extra vitamin E: It improves circulation and may help prevent the "heavy" feeling that can come with varicose veins, says Dr. Edelberg. He recommends starting at 400 international units of vitamin E a day and slowly increasing that to 1,200 international units over three to six weeks.

Learn to like lecithin. Lecithin is available at health food stores and some drugstores. Dr. Edelberg recommends 1,200 milligrams three times a day to help emulsify fat and lower cholesterol.

Caution: At high dosages, lecithin may cause a reduced appetite, nausea, abdominal bloating, gastrointestinal pain, and diarrhea.

▶PREVENTIVE MEASURES

Walk away. You need exercise, says Dr. Baron. It gets the calf muscle pump in gear and forces blood back to the heart. "Walking is great," Dr. Baron says. "I think walking is the best exercise in the world. After that, swimming." Be sure to consult with your doctor before starting any exercise program.

Wandering Eye

▶ PROBLEM

Let's define our terms: We're not talking about strabismus, a condition that makes your eyes point in different directions. Then again, maybe we are. This chapter's about looking at women—on the street, at the mall, at the grocery store—and all those soft-skinned, pert-bosomed females in your field of vision can turn any red-blooded American male walleyed.

▶ CAUSE

Most men with a wandering eye aren't on the make. They simply admire a fine-looking woman, much the way they might appreciate a mint-condition 1968 Camaro. "There's nothing wrong with looking. We all look," says Frank Pittman III, M.D., a psychiatrist in Atlanta and author of *Man Enough* and *Private Lies: Infidelity and the Betrayal of Intimacy*. "Looking is only a problem if you start stumbling over the furniture or drooling on your tie. But even then, one would hope that your wife or girlfriend would be amused rather than threatened."

▶ HOW SERIOUS

Men in an otherwise happy, fulfilling relationship shouldn't sweat their desire to admire, and neither should their partners, Dr. Pittman says. Men in unhappy marriages who find their eyes wandering, however, may eventually find that other body parts follow suit. Yet what such men yearn for isn't a sexual connection but an emotional one, Dr. Pittman says. "It's when a man can't talk to his wife about his feelings or what's bothering him that he's likely to reach out to another woman," he says.

▶SOLUTIONS

Look smart. Men with an experienced wandering eye don't stare, leer, or ogle; they know that's the surest way to catch hell from an irate spouse or girlfriend. It's also a sure method for making the women around you uncomfortable, flustered, or even angry. This is a very bad thing, particularly in the workplace. Don't embarrass women with your eyes. Rather, learn how to look without appearing that you're looking, particularly when you're with your wife or a date.

"Make it seem like the woman

MEN'S HEALTH INDEX

So, you're a girl-watcher, eh? Here are five great places to ply your trade, as chosen by John Eagan, author of *How to Pick Up Beautiful Women in Nightclubs or Any Other Place.*

1. Outside the ladies' room at a bar or club
2. Fancy coffee shops (women love their coffee)
3. The library of a local college
4. The makeup department at a fancy department store
5. Readings at bookstores

---

you want to check out came into your line of sight accidentally," advises John Eagan, author of *How to Pick Up Beautiful Women in Nightclubs or Any Other Place.* "As she gets closer, pretend to be fixated on a spot where she'll be in the next few seconds." By the time she's in that spot, you'll have already established your "right to look" in that direction.

Explain yourself. Like salmon must swim upstream to spawn, men must look at women—all women. It's a biological imperative. Believe it or not, Dr. Pittman recommends explaining this to your partner. "Tell her that men look at other women because they're aware of the world around them," he says. "They're just taking in the scenery." What if your partner keeps elbowing you in the ribs when an attractive woman passes by? "Say, 'Good Lord, I thought I married a grown-up,'" says Dr. Pittman. "A man shouldn't let a woman tyrannize him into sacrificing his rights for her fragile ego."

Examine your motives. Of course, it's a different story if you feel you're in danger of violating the look-but-don't-touch rule. In this case, a little introspection can save you from a big-time screwup. "To a certain extent, having a wandering eye is natural," says Stanley Teitelbaum, Ph.D., a clinical psychologist and psychoanalyst in private practice in New York City. "But there might be other things going on—a midlife crisis, a feeling of anger or resentment toward your partner—that may be influencing your feelings and behavior. It always helps to understand where you're coming from."

Get out of there, pal. "Opportunity is the only thing that prevents most men from having an affair," says Willard Harley Jr., Ph.D., a clinical psychologist and expert on marital therapy in Whitebear Lake, Minnesota, and author of several books on marriage, including *Give and Take.* So if you truly don't want to give in to temptation, don't give yourself the chance. Stay out of the diner where that cute waitress who gives you free doughnuts works, or phase out those "friendly" lunches with that attractive temp who (you think) is giving you the green light.

▶ALTERNATIVE APPROACHES

Meet her kneads. Giving your partner a massage can help you appreciate her more fully, says Steven Woolpert, a licensed massage therapist and counselor in Portland, Oregon, who has taught couples massage at the Oregon School of Massage in Portland. You don't need to learn any fancy techniques either. Have a quiet, warm place where your partner will feel comfortable, such as your bed or on pillows. Put massage oil or lotion on your hands as you ask your partner where she would like to be touched. Glide your hands lightly over her body. "As you're doing this, look with loving eyes at your partner and recall intimate times together," says Woolpert. "Appreciate the texture of her skin, the way her arms connect to her shoulders, all the features that attracted you to her."

▶PREVENTIVE MEASURES

Zip it. Never complain about your marriage or relationship to a woman you're attracted to, Dr. Harley advises. "Often, two people embark on an affair after griping to each other about their relationships," says Dr. Harley. "Each decides to help the other one out, and that's how it all starts."

Don't deny yourself. Guilt is like an acid; it eats a hole in your soul and makes you keep secrets from your partner. So don't feel guilty for looking or even for imagining what it would be like with that cute cashier at Kmart. "Most men are faithful, but they sure think about being otherwise," says Dr. Pittman. "To pretend that you don't is a lie, and it's a sin to tell a lie. If you give yourself the freedom to proudly look, you won't feel guilty and turn a normal situation into a conflict."

Warts

▶**PROBLEM**

Warts are rough, raised spots on the skin that appear alone or in clusters. "They're usually white, but there can also be variations on that color," says Robert Schosser, M.D., chief of the division of dermatology at the University of Kentucky A. B. Chandler Medical Center in Lexington. "They are rarely brown or dark. On the feet, they may not be raised but appear as rough areas that may look more like calluses than warts." Although all warts belong to the same virus family, there are 100 different types, ranging from plantar (bottom of the foot) warts to the common warts that children get.

▶**CAUSE**

Warts are benign tumors caused by the human papillomavirus, which most of us are in contact with almost every day. Some people develop warts, while others don't, however. In a sense, warts are to the skin what cold viruses are to the respiratory system. Just as children are prone to more colds than adults, they are also more prone to getting warts. That's probably because they haven't yet developed an immunity to the virus. The most common warts in men are warts on the fingers and plantar warts.

▶**HOW SERIOUS**

On your fingers, warts are not so serious. They may take a long time to go away, and can

---

DO THIS NOW

For warts on your hands and feet, if you are otherwise healthy, use an over-the-counter wart remover that contains salicylic acid and leaves a protective film on your skin when it dries, advises Robert Schosser, M.D., chief of the division of dermatology at the University of Kentucky A. B. Chandler Medical Center in Lexington. "My favorite is Occlusal-HP, which has 17 percent salicylic acid," Dr. Schosser says. "Just follow the directions on the package of whichever medication you choose." If you are diabetic or have circulation problems with your hands and feet, you should see your doctor before attempting to treat warts on your own.

Did You Know?

According to Irish folklore, if you steal a piece of meat and apply it (raw) to a wart, then bury the meat in the ground, your wart will disappear. Or you could take some clay from under the feet of men who are carrying a coffin, apply the dirt to your wart, and wish strongly for the wart to go away. It will, so the legend goes. Sure, and maybe you'll find a pot of gold, too.

be ugly and uncomfortable (and spread to other parts of the body), but they don't generally cause further problems.

Warts on your feet (if they interfere with walking) or on your face should be checked by a doctor. Anything that looks like a wart on your penis should also be checked since penile warts can be readily transmitted to sexual partners.

Something that looks like a wart but doesn't go away on its own or after treatment with an over-the-counter medicine such as Occlusal-HP, should be checked by a doctor, says Dr. Schosser, as should wartlike lesions that grow rapidly.

▶SOLUTIONS

Dry out. After you wash a body part that has warts, towel-dry thoroughly, says Suzanne M. Levine, D.P.M., clinical assistant podiatrist at Cornell Medical Center in New York City. Warts thrive and multiply in a moist environment, so don't give them the satisfaction. If you have a plantar wart, sprinkle on a foot powder containing cornstarch or talc to dry your skin after you finish toweling off, Dr. Levine says.

Go in for the dunk. If you have plantar warts, dunk your feet in a tub of water mixed with a special drying preparation, such as Domeboro, recommends D'Anne Kleinsmith, M.D., a staff dermatologist at William Beaumont Hospital in Royal Oak, Michigan. Domeboro contains aluminum salts, which dry and toughen the skin. Mix the solution, which comes in packets or tablets, into water and soak your feet in it for 15 minutes once a day, Dr. Kleinsmith says. For best results, also file down the warts with an emery board and use with an over-the-counter wart medication until the wart goes away.

Just wait. Warts do eventually go away, and this may be one of the reasons that so many old wives' tales about how to get rid of them have flourished. People assume that whatever remedy they've chosen has somehow made the wart disappear in four months, but the truth is that it would have left on its own anyway. "Eventually, your body will generate an immune response to the virus," says Vail Reese, M.D., a dermatologist with the Dermatology Medical Group of San Francisco.

This doesn't mean, however, that the virus goes away. It simply means that your body has become more adept at controlling outbreaks. Once you develop warts, the virus may continue to be a part of you.

Get stoned. Since warts are raised, they can sometimes make it uncomfortable to use your hands easily. "You can pare them down with a pumice stone," Dr. Reese says. Use a pumice stone, available at drugstores, when your hand is wet (in the shower is good) and vigorously rub it across the wart. Continue to rub until the wart is flush with the skin. You don't want to rip the skin; you're just trying to file down the area.

▶ALTERNATIVE APPROACHES

Tape it. Here's another way to use an over-the-counter wart preparation that contains salicylic acid: After showering, dry off the skin around the wart, apply the preparation to the wet wart, then put some adhesive tape over the wart. "This will help break down the skin cells that contain the virus," says Dr. Reese. Each day, pare down the wart with a pumice stone or emery board and repeat.

▶PREVENTIVE MEASURES

Wear a condom. Genital warts spread easily, but a condom is one of the best ways to protect yourself and your partner. Condoms appear to be relatively effective in preventing the spread of warts. "If your partner has warts and you touch her or have unprotected sex with her, you can catch them," Dr. Schosser says. And, of course, if you're the one with the virus, you can spread it to your partner if you hit the sheets unsheathed.

Protect your feet. To prevent plantar warts, don't go barefoot in health clubs, poolside, or anyplace that is wet and heavily traveled says Dr. Schosser. Instead, wear shower shoes or flip-flops.

Wrinkles

▶PROBLEM

Your face looks older than it used to. There are lines across your forehead and a furrow in your brow. The skin near the outside of your eyes is crinkly, and there are new creases running from your nose to your mouth. Sometimes you think that you look distinguished, almost like Clint Eastwood. But sometimes you think that you just look old, kind of like Mr. Burns on *The Simpsons*.

Along with wrinkles, your face may also look darker than it used to, with pigmented blotches on the skin. These age spots, as they are called, are another sign of aging.

▶CAUSE

"The damage you see in your skin as you get older reflects, for the most part, the time you spent in the sun unprotected as a child," says George J. Hruza, M.D., associate professor of dermatology at Washington University School of Medicine in St. Louis. In fact, most sun damage, or photoaging, occurs in the first 10 to 12 years of your life.

When the sun hits your unprotected skin, it alters the structure of the uppermost layer, or epidermis. The noticeable sign that this has happened is a suntan or sunburn. Over time, your skin manages to do some repair work (tans fade, burns heal), but it isn't able to fully finish the job. Meanwhile, you've gone out and gotten another tan (or worse, burn), so now your skin has more damage to undo. But the fact is that your skin never completely recovered from the first tan or burn.

A few other things can contribute to the occurrence of wrinkles. Smoking constricts the blood vessels in your skin and causes it to become papery and thin. It also creates fine lines around your lips when you inhale. That brings us to another common contributor: facial expressions. Sleeping with your face scrunched up in a pillow every night, frowning, and smiling all can cause wrinkles. And, yes, gravity causes some wrinkles, but not as many as everyone thinks.

▶How Serious

The truth is that you could live with the cosmetic changes in your skin if they didn't mean what you fear they do: that permanent damage has been done to your skin. Men may develop wrinkles later in life than women because their skin is thicker, but the flip side is that they are two to three times more likely than women to develop skin cancer. Hardly a fair trade-off. And in 1997, almost 10,000 Americans died from skin cancer.

By the way, none of the suggested remedies for wrinkles can prevent or cure skin cancer. If you notice any changes in your skin, such as pale, waxlike nodules; red, scaly patches; or unusually shaped moles that are larger than six millimeters or growing fast, you should definitely see a dermatologist, says Dr. Hruza.

▶Solutions

Reach for A derivative. Try an over-the-counter antiwrinkle cream that contains retinoids, Dr. Hruza suggests. Retinoids, which are derived from vitamin A, increase cell turnover speed. The result is that you get newer, fresher skin faster. Healthy Skin, a cream made by Neutrogena, is a good choice, says Dr. Hruza.

"It's best to start using these products once a day, at night, and let your skin get used to them," Dr. Hruza says. "Also, they make you more sensitive to the sun, so this is another reason to use a sunscreen."

Retinoids, however, aren't to be considered weaker versions of Retin-A or Renova, the prescription medications developed from vitamin A that have been shown to actually reduce wrinkles within a few months. In fact, the two products are very different, says Dr. Hruza.

Be an alpha male. Over-the-counter products that contain alpha hydroxy acids are another good bet, Dr. Hruza says. These are natural exfoliators (dead skin cell removers) made from glycolic, lactic, or citric acids. And each of these comes from natural sources such as sugarcane or sour milk.

"Most of these products will make wrinkles look less apparent," says Dr. Hruza. "But you have to be patient, and you have to keep using them."

Look for products that contain 8 percent or more glycolic acid, Dr. Hruza

Did You Know?

The latest wrinkle remedy making the rounds in upscale dermatology offices is botox injections. Botox is shorthand for botulism toxin. A sterilized form of the virus temporarily paralyzes the muscle into which it is injected, relaxing the appearance of the wrinkle above it.

"It's not as bad as it sounds," says Joseph W. Rucker Jr., M.D., a plastic and reconstructive surgeon in private practice in Eau Claire, Wisconsin. "Sometimes a person has deep wrinkles because they consistently use a certain muscle, for example, one in their forehead to express astonishment. There was nothing we could do about something like that until botox injections came along."

Usually, a physician will laser the skin over the muscle, which decreases the depth of the wrinkle. The injection allows the laser process to be effective longer than it would normally be, Dr. Rucker says.

---

says. Two that meet this standard of effectiveness are Alpha Hydrox preparations and Avon's Anew line. Use them once a day.

Rub on vitamin C. The newest topical application to fight wrinkles is vitamin C. "We don't have a lot of long-term conclusive information about Cellex-C and other vitamin C products, but the anecdotal reports are very positive," Dr. Hruza says.

Vitamin C helps your skin in two ways. First, it's needed to make collagen throughout your body, and collagen is what supports the skin. Second, it's a free-radical scavenger. "Vitamin C works as an antioxidant to help your skin fight sun damage," explains Lorraine Faxon Meisner, Ph.D., professor of preventive medicine at the University of Wisconsin Medical School in Madison and co-inventor of Cellex-C, the first antiwrinkle product to use vitamin C.

Still, you can't go squeezing an orange on your face and expect to see results. "You need formulations that will allow these high concentrations of vitamin C to penetrate the skin," Dr. Meisner says. Buy a cheap or poorly made product and the vitamin C will never be absorbed by the cells that need it. Cellex-C, which is sold through dermatologists, plastic surgeons, and licensed skin care professionals, utilizes zinc and tyrosine to help make the vitamin C work, Dr. Meisner says.

▶ALTERNATIVE APPROACHES

Put antioxidants on your face. While vitamin C may be the latest antioxidant to bring excitement to the skin care world, moisturizers with added vitamins A and E without extra added chemicals or alcohol also help prevent wrinkles, says Eugene Zampieron, a doctor of naturopathy in Middlebury, Connecticut, and a professional member of the American Herbalists Guild. Look for facial creams with vitamins A and E listed on their labels, and use as directed.

▶PREVENTIVE MEASURES

Think pale. Although wrinkles are a sign of age, you can easily get older without developing wrinkles. Just stay pale. "Suntans aren't considered a sign of health anymore," says Vail Reese, M.D., a dermatologist with the Dermatology Medical Group of San Francisco. "In fact, if you look at many of the male and female movie stars of today, most of them are downright pale." If you want people to know you're healthy, work out, eat well, and use sunscreen.

Keep shaving. "Men have a higher turnover of dead skin cells because their faces are pushed and pulled when they shave," Dr. Hruza says. "Some people theorize that's one of the reasons that men get wrinkles later in life than women do."

Zipper Dangers

▶PROBLEM

Either when pulling your pants zipper up or—more likely—down, you snag your penis. It's painful, and removing your unhappy organ is a delicate task.

▶CAUSE

It's caused by simple carelessness.

▶HOW SERIOUS

It is potentially serious, especially if it's the penile shaft and not the foreskin that is caught in the zipper, says E. Douglas Whitehead, M.D., associate clinical professor of urology at the Albert Einstein College of Medicine of Yeshiva University and director of the Association for Male Sexual Dysfunction, both in New York City.

"If it's the penile shaft, you ought to see a doctor right away, preferably a urologist," Dr. Whitehead says. The shaft can become infected if not treated properly "and could result in limited sexual activity," he adds.

▶SOLUTIONS

Remain calm. Yeah, we know, that's easy to say when it's someone else's penis being pinched. But you are less apt to make things worse if you stay calm, says Thomas Stillwell, M.D., a urologist in private practice near Minneapolis.

Go slow. Proceed slowly and gently in trying to extricate your foreskin from the zipper, advises Dr. Stillwell. A quick yank of the zipper "would probably tear something"—and he's not talking about your trousers. If that fails, you may have to go to a urologist for assistance. If he is not available to see you that day, go to your local emergency room.

DO THIS NOW

In a pinch, apply some mineral oil or salad oil to your penis, suggests Thomas Stillwell, M.D., a urologist in private practice near Minneapolis. It just might lubricate it enough so that you can extract it painlessly.

History Lesson

What's worse than getting your manly member caught in your zipper? Stuck in a swimming pool suction fitting. At a motel, no less.

That's what happened in Lakeland, Florida, in the wee hours one summer morning. According to an Associated Press news report, a clerk at the motel in question dialed 911 to report that the 33-year-old man was trapped in the motel's pool.

When police and paramedics arrived, they found the guy, pants down, penis stuck in the suction hole serving as part of the filtration system on one wall of the pool. The pool's pump was shut off before help arrived, but the man could not free willy because his penis had become swollen in the small hole.

Paramedics inserted a lubricant around the suction fitting, and about 40 minutes later, their man was unplugged. He was treated at a local hospital and released with bruised genitalia and, one suspects, an acute case of embarrassment.

Break the demon zipper. One way to liberate your penis is to find a tool that will break the zipper. Dr. Stillwell and two colleagues once used a bone cutter. You probably don't have one of these around the house, so a wire snip or pliers may do the job, Dr. Stillwell says.

Stem the flow. "If it's bleeding, you ought to put some pressure on it," Dr. Whitehead says. "And you probably ought to put some local antibiotic cream on it"—such as Bacitracin.

Don't be overly concerned about blood, however. "It's not going to be life-threatening," Dr. Stillwell says.

▶ALTERNATIVE SOLUTIONS

Be a button-fly guy. If you're really worried about mangling your member, switch to a different style of trousers, says Dr. Whitehead. "Throw away all your zippered pants and get pants with buttons," he says.

Snip it; snip it good. Okay, this is an extreme measure, but if you chronically abuse your penis in your zipper and you are uncircumcised and have no religious or other objections to being circumcised, then consider getting snipped. "It would seem that guys who are uncircumcised are more likely to have problems because they have a little more skin hanging there and it's easier to get caught," Dr. Whitehead says.

▶**PREVENTIVE MEASURES**

Take your time. In addition to carelessness, some guys zip more than their pants because they're in a big hurry when they urinate, says Dr. Stillwell. This is even more true of little boys, he adds. Slow down. Your penis will thank you.

Wear underwear. This advice is most appropriate if you have a young son. A little boy's penis pokes straight out in harm's way, while a man's is more vertical, says Dr. Stillwell. Underwear affords some protection.

But it's also good advice for grown men, although the reason has to do with urination, says Dr. Whitehead. "It doesn't matter how much you shake and dance, the last few drops go down your pants," he says.

Part Three

In Case of Emergency

Lifesaving Techniques

Men should be prepared for all of life's emergencies, like opening a beer bottle on a countertop when you can't find an opener. Included in your emergency talent arsenal should be what to do in a life-or-death situation.

All too often, people think that the guy next to them will be able to help, that there will be a doctor in the house. Don't take that chance. You want to be prepared—make that *very* prepared—when the life of a friend, a lover, a child, or even a total stranger is at stake.

One of the most important things that you should know is how to get in touch with your local emergency medical services, says Jedd Roe, M.D., assistant professor of emergency medicine at the University of Colorado School of Medicine in Denver. In most, but not all communities, the emergency number is 911. If this isn't true in your community, check the inside cover of your telephone directory for the emergency number. In a serious situation, calling your local emergency services is your best first step, advises Dr. Roe.

WHAT EVERY MAN SHOULD KNOW

The following are five lifesaving techniques that every man should know how to perform properly. They're kind of like that condom you used to carry in your wallet. Odds are that you're never going to actually use any of these. But it's nice to know that they're safely stored, just in case.

It's not enough just to know what to do. You must know how to do it properly. Skills such as rescue breathing and cardiopulmonary resuscitation (CPR) can't be learned from a book alone. Take a first-aid and CPR class at your local hospital or community center, advises Paul Matera, M.D., an emergency medical technician-paramedic and vice chairman and professor of emergency services at Providence Hospital in Washington, D.C. They'll teach you the right way to do these lifesaving techniques, which will come up repeatedly in the following chapters in this emergency first-aid section. What we offer here is just a short refresher for those of you who have already learned these skills. The information we give is only for adults; children and infants require different procedures.

An important concern while giving first-aid is disease transmission. While chances are that you will be helping a family member or friend, you may be helping a stranger. There are simple ways to reduce the risk of disease. Try not to come in contact with the victim's body fluids, such as blood or saliva. Wear disposable latex gloves, or place layers of clean cloth between you and body fluids. Have the victim use their own hands to stop bleeding. You should have a face mask or face shield for doing rescue breathing and CPR. Protect your eyes as well. If you have glasses or sunglasses wear them, or borrow them from a friend. Wash your hands thoroughly after giving first-aid, even if you wore gloves. If you did come in contact with body fluids, tell your doctor. You can get disposable gloves at drugstores and face masks at medical supply stores.

If there is an emergency in a public place like a restaurant or sports arena, and you decide to assist, ask the manager or security officer for a first-aid kit. Public places are usually required to have first-aid kits that should contain "universal precaution kits" with gloves, eye protection, and face masks, says Dr. Matera.

DO IT RIGHT

In the time it takes you to read a couple of chapters in this book, 2 people will be killed and almost 400 will suffer a disabling injury. And odds are that most of them will be men. Males are 1.3 times more likely than women to visit the emergency room because of an injury, and young men up to age 24 are twice as likely to be hospitalized because of an injury. Deaths from injuries are 4.6 times higher in men ages 20 to 24 than in women in the same age group. So odds are that at some time in your life, you will need first-aid yourself or need to give it to somebody else.

"It should be the obligation of all responsible adults to know first-aid," Dr. Matera says.

The following techniques can help you or someone you love from becoming one of those statistics. Just remember: Whenever possible, call 911 before taking any of these steps.

RESCUE BREATHING

In rescue breathing, you supply the breath for someone who has stopped breathing. You usually need to use it after some type of trauma—a bad fall, a seizure, an accident—when the heart is still beating. "Most times, after a few breaths, they'll wake right up and breathe on their own. You only need to breathe for them until spontaneous respiration is reestablished," says Dr. Matera.

If the victim isn't breathing, roll him gently on his back, keeping his head and back in a straight line. Sometimes all it takes to restore someone's breathing is to reopen his airway with the head-tilt/chin-lift technique. Kneel beside the patient and place the palm of your hand on his forehead and push backward to tilt the head back. Take the fingers of your other hand and hook them under the bony point of the chin and lift the chin upward.

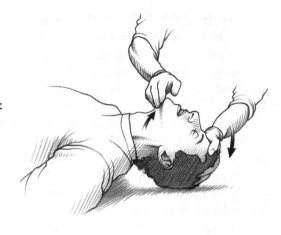

If you suspect a neck or spine injury, use this technique instead. Place your hands on the side of the victim's head, behind the angles of his lower jaw, and move the jaw forward without tilting the head backward.

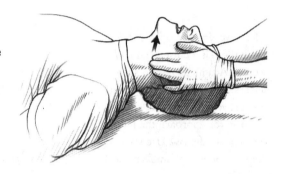

Take three to five seconds to check for breathing. Place your ear over the victim's mouth and nose and listen and feel for breathing. Look at his chest to see if it is rising and falling. If he is breathing, and there are no spinal injuries, place him in the recovery position.

If he is not breathing, start rescue breathing. Keep his head tilted back and pinch his nose shut.

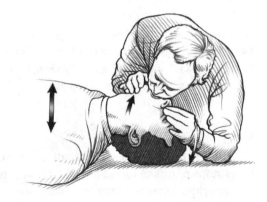

Seal your lips tightly around his mouth. (If you are using a mask or shield, be familiar with how to use them.) Give two slow, deep breaths, each lasting one to two seconds. Check that the chest rises with each breath. If the first breath does not go in, retilt the head and try again.

CHECKING FOR A CAROTID PULSE

To see if you have to move on to CPR, check for a pulse. Many people can easily find the carotid arteries, making it a good place to look for a pulse. But the carotids are also the closest major arteries to the heart muscle. "If you find a carotid pulse, you can be pretty sure that the heart is pumping out some blood," Dr. Matera says. If you locate a pulse, then continue with rescue breathing until the person starts breathing on his own.

If you don't find a pulse, it means that the heart isn't doing its job of pumping blood. Move on to CPR, Dr. Matera says. Don't make the fatal mistake of just listening for a heartbeat in the chest, he warns. You can have a heart beat yet not have a pulse. "In certain shock situations, the heart can be beating, but nothing is being pumped out. The heart can be technically beating and even contracting, but there may be no blood available to pump," he says. Check for a pulse to make sure that blood is pumping through the person's system.

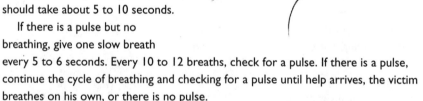

After two deep breaths, check to see if there is a pulse. Find the victim's Adam's apple and slide your fingers down the side of the neck nearest you. You should find the pulse as you approach the level of the angle of the jaw. Use your fingers, not your thumb, to check the carotid artery for a pulse. This should take about 5 to 10 seconds.

If there is a pulse but no breathing, give one slow breath every 5 to 6 seconds. Every 10 to 12 breaths, check for a pulse. If there is a pulse, continue the cycle of breathing and checking for a pulse until help arrives, the victim breathes on his own, or there is no pulse.

CPR

For whatever reason—a heart attack, an accident, loss of blood—the person's heart stops pumping blood and the person stops breathing. CPR gets the heart pumping and lungs working manually. You supply the breaths, and your hands pump the heart. Without this, the major organs, including the heart and brain, will die within minutes because they aren't getting oxygenated, nutritious blood, Dr. Matera says. "When you are giving breaths, you must see the chest rise. When you are giving compressions, a pulse must be detected. Then you know that you are doing your job," Dr. Matera adds.

If there is no pulse, start CPR. Your hands must be positioned properly. Slide the fingers of your hand nearest the victim's feet up his rib cage and find the notch at the bottom of the sternum. Put your middle finger on the notch, and place your index finger next to it. Place the heel of your other hand next to the index finger.

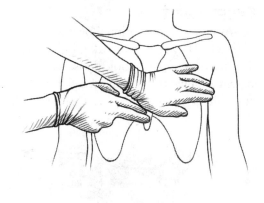

Remove the hand at the notch and place it on top of the hand on the chest. Keep your fingers off the chest. Use the heel of the bottom hand to apply pressure to the chest.

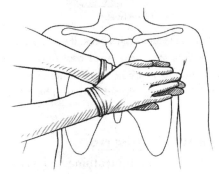

Your shoulders should be directly over your hands. Keep your arms straight and your elbows locked. Push down with your upper body, pivoting from your hips. Don't rock from your knees; instead move straight up and down like a piston. With each compression, the victim's chest should be pushed straight down about two inches. Keep up a steady rhythm and don't stop between compressions. Compress the

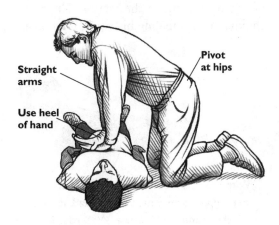

Straight arms

Pivot at hips

Use heel of hand

chest 15 times at the rate of 80 compressions per minute. Then give the victim two deep breaths.

Do three more cycles of 15 compressions and two breaths. Then check the pulse. If there is no pulse, continue doing four cycles of 15 compressions, two breaths, and a pulse check until help arrives, the victim revives, or you are too exhausted to continue. If there is a pulse, return to rescue breathing.

SHOCK POSITION

After a severe emotional or physical trauma, a person may slip into a state of shock. They may be awake, but appear confused, lethargic, or shaky; and they may have pale, cool, moist skin. This happens because the circulatory system is failing to provide enough oxygen-rich blood to the body. Putting them in the shock position helps restore circulation, says Dr. Roe.

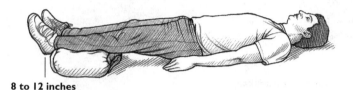

8 to 12 inches

Lay the victim on his back. If you are absolutely certain that there are no head, neck, or spine injuries or broken bones in the legs or hip, raise his feet 8 to 12 inches. If you are not sure if there are head, neck, spine, or leg injuries, keep the victim lying flat. In either case, if he is feeling cool, cover the victim with a blanket.

RECOVERY POSITION

If the victim is breathing and has a pulse but is unresponsive or is vomiting, put him into the left-side recovery position, says Dr. Roe. If you suspect a spine injury, do not move the victim. The recovery position will keep him from choking on or inhaling his vomit if it comes up.

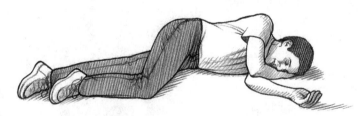

With the victim on his back, kneel at his left side. Bend his left arm at the elbow so his upper arm is next to his head. Place the back of his right hand against his left cheek and hold it there. With your hand behind his right knee, bend the right leg and roll him toward you. In the final position, his right hand supports his head and his bent right leg prevents rolling.

Broken Bones

▶PROBLEM

You have 206 bones in your body, but you also have more than 100 different ways to break them. A sampling includes the greenstick fracture, where one side of the bone breaks and the other side bends. Then there's the impacted kind, where one broken bone fragment drives into the other. Or you can develop the spiral fracture, where the bone twists apart.

▶CAUSE

Any force that applies pressure against a bone could cause it to break: landing wrong on your foot during a pickup basketball game, a bad fall, a feet-first slide into second, you name it. Popular causes for men include motorcycle accidents and sports activity mishaps. To tell if you broke a bone, try to move it, says Paul Matera, M.D., an emergency medical technician-paramedic and vice chairman and professor of emergency services at Providence Hospital in Washington, D.C. "If you can't move it and it hurts, then it's possibly broken. Obviously, if you hear a crunch, then it's probably broken," he says. Just remember that you only move it to find out if it's broken. Once you think it is, stay still.

All broken bones should be seen by a doctor since many are easily treated and will heal nicely. An untreated broken bone may not heal correctly, leaving you with a deformity. If not properly cared for as soon as possible, it may damage surrounding blood vessels and nerves. Internal bleeding can build up around the bone, shutting down blood vessels and causing loss of movement.

DO THIS NOW

Stay still. "You have to keep the bone from moving until you get medical help," says Paul Matera, M.D., an emergency medical technician-paramedic and vice chairman and professor of emergency services at Providence Hospital in Washington, D.C. Moving it around further harms the bone, and it also increases the risk of damaging surrounding blood vessels and nerves, he says. If you suspect a head, neck, or spinal injury, you should absolutely not move the person, he adds. Call for an ambulance right away.

▶SOLUTIONS

Here are some step-by-step tips to follow while waiting for medical help to arrive to care for your broken bone.

Leave the fixin' to the experts. "People should not attempt to put bones back together," says Jedd Roe, M.D., assistant professor of emergency medicine at the University of Colorado School of Medicine in Denver. Moving a broken bone will only cause a lot more pain and further damage. Save the repair work for the doctors at the hospital no matter how bad your break looks.

MEN'S HEALTH INDEX
Here are the different bones that action film star Jackie Chan (*Mr. Nice Guy, Rumble in the Bronx*) reportedly has broken while doing his own stunts.
1. Skull
2. Jaw
3. Shoulder
4. Two fingers
5. Kneecap
6. Nose (three times)
7. Ankle
8. Ribs

Bandage with saline. If the bone breaks through the skin, soak sterile gauze in saline—regular contact lens solution will do, Dr. Roe says. Place the gauze over the bone and the injured skin. "Saline has the same concentration of salt as we have in our body, so it's better for the injured tissues than water," he says. If you don't have saline solution, use dry sterile gauze. Do not use any kind of tape to fasten the gauze to the wound; just lay it on the area. After the wound is covered, sit tight and wait for the ambulance to arrive. Do not move, splint, or elevate a bone that breaks through the skin, Dr. Roe adds.

Be a splendid splinter. If you are out in the woods or are far away from a hospital, you can make a splint to help keep broken bones still until you get medical help, says Dr. Roe. "The splint should cover the areas below and above the break," he says.

Splint the bone the way you found it, no matter how mangled that may be, says Ian Cummings, M.D., director of emergency services at the Day Kimball Hospital in Putnam, Connecticut.

Plenty of common items make a quality splint: cardboard, a ruler, branches, magazines, a pillow, or a thick blanket. When applying a splint, use your hands to support the injured area. You can use cloth ties, neckties, torn clothing, or belts to tie the splint to the injured area. Make sure that any knots are not pressing against the injury. Tie them securely, but not so tightly that circulation is impaired, says Dr. Roe.

If the area beyond the splint becomes pale, numb, or throbs, loosen the ties. You may also need to loosen the ties if the injured area swells after you've applied the splint.

HERE'S HOW TO MAKE AN ANKLE SPLINT

For a broken ankle that has no open wound, place a thick blanket underneath the foot and ankle. Then wrap it lightly with cloth or anything that ties it in place, leaving the toes exposed. After applying the splint, elevate the ankle.

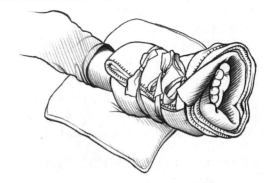

To splint a broken forearm or wrist, you can place a few fairly thick magazines or newspapers rolled into a "U" shape under the lower arm. Make sure that the splint extends from the elbow to the hand. Tie it snugly in place with cloth ties. Make a sling by tying a jacket, shirt, or some other piece of clothing or cloth around the neck.

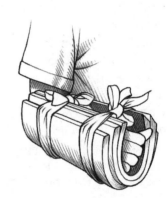

HERE'S HOW TO MAKE A FOREARM SPLINT

If you are alone and have possibly broken your forearm, make a self-splint by holding your broken arm close to your body. Bend the elbow of the broken arm and hold the forearm still against your chest with your opposite hand and arm until you get medical help, says Dr. Cummings.

Put it on ice. After you make the splint, put an ice pack or a cold compress on the break, Dr. Roe says. Keep the ice on for 20 to 30 minutes at a time, and make sure to wrap it in a towel or cloth to prevent the skin from freezing. Ice the area several times in the first 24 hours, says Dr. Roe. The ice keeps down the swelling and lessens some of the pain, he says.

Raise it to the sky. If the bone that you suspect is broken is in your wrist, hand, finger, toe, foot, or ankle, elevate the broken area above your heart, Dr. Roe says. "You can do this lying down if it makes you more comfortable," he says. This slows the blood from pooling in the fractured area and reduces swelling. Do not elevate larger broken bones, particularly the femur or pelvis, Dr. Roe adds.

Treat for shock. When a person breaks a major bone like his femur or pelvis, he may go into shock, says Dr. Roe. For instructions on how to treat for shock, see Lifesaving Techniques on page 579.

Pacify your pain. The homeopathic medicine arnica can accelerate wound healing and relieve the pain, says Michael Carlston, M.D., assistant clinical professor in the department of family and community medicine at the University of California, San Francisco, School of Medicine. Keep an arnica product in your first-aid kit with a potency of 30C. If you suffer a break, take one dose of the 30C arnica every three to four hours for up to five days, Dr. Carlston says.

▶PREVENTIVE MEASURES

Let the pros slide. Sliding into second can take out the second baseman on a double play, but it also can break an ankle. "It's a friendly softball game, yet they slide hard into second. I can't understand why they do that," says Robert McNamara, M.D., professor of emergency medicine and program director of the department of emergency medicine residency at Allegheny University of the Health Sciences–MCP Hahnemann School of Medicine in Philadelphia. Unless the World Series is riding on you, reach the base standing up, he suggests.

Bring protection. Whatever the sport, wear all the necessary protective gear, especially if you're new at it. Dr. McNamara sees a lot of broken-boned men who tried inline skating for the first time—without the pads. "A lot of men are macho and think that they are going to be good at a new activity, so they don't wear the gear. Even professional athletes wear protective gear," Dr. Mc-Namara says.

Put out the light. Every cigarette puff you take steals a bit of strength from your bones. "Smoking does decrease bone density," Dr. Cummings says. Set a quit date and stick to it. Your bones as well as your lungs will thank you later.

Broken Nose

▶PROBLEM

A nose can break in three places: the actual bones found on each side of your nose, and the septum—the ridge of bone and cartilage that divides your nostrils. At first, you might not notice any difference other than a little pain after being popped. But in a few minutes or even a few days, you'll see the telltale signs of swelling, bleeding, difficulty breathing, and the most obvious one—your nose isn't in the same place as it was before.

▶CAUSE

A random elbow during a pickup basketball game, a flying softball, a punch during a barroom brawl, and an accidental head butt from a two-year-old have all been known to break a nose. The possibilities are endless.

DO THIS NOW

Get some ice on your nose. A broken nose will swell up quickly and start to bleed. An ice pack or a cold compress wrapped or covered in a towel to avoid freezing the skin will help reduce the swelling and stop the bleeding, says Sanford Archer, M.D., associate professor of otolaryngology at the University of Kentucky A. B. Chandler Medical Center in Lexington.

An untreated broken nose can obstruct breathing, lose its sense of smell, and leave you open to infections. And unless you're going for that postfight pugilist look, you'll want to get to a doctor soon, especially if you're still having difficulty breathing through your nose a few days after the injury or if the appearance of your nose is not like it should be, says Sanford Archer, M.D., associate professor of otolaryngology at the University of Kentucky A. B. Chandler Medical Center in Lexington.

Most people with broken noses don't need to seek immediate attention, however. As long as they get to a doctor within seven days of suffering the injury, their nose can be reset, if necessary, fairly quickly and easily, Dr. Archer says. Before you head to the doctor's office, dig out a few good photos of yourself so that the doctor can compare your nose before and after the injury. What one doctor might perceive as a crooked, broken schnozzle may just be your nat-

---

Did You Know?

Remember hearing the story that a quick, karate-type shot to the nose could kill a man by pushing the bones into the brain? Sorry to break it to you, but it is a myth perpetuated by too many kung fu movies, says Sanford Archer, M.D., associate professor of otolaryngology at the University of Kentucky A. B. Chandler Medical Center in Lexington.

---

ural nasal disposition. "Some people come in asking if they broke their nose, but it certainly looks the same as it did before to me," Dr. Archer says. Just don't rely on your driver's license photo, he adds. "They usually aren't helpful," he says.

▶SOLUTIONS

Here are some tips to try until you get to a doctor that may help control the bleeding, lessen the pain, and decrease congestion.

Stop the bleeding. Treat blood from a broken nose the same way you would your basic nosebleed. Sit up straight and tilt your head slightly forward so that the blood flows out of your nose and not down your throat, Dr. Archer says. Then apply pressure by pinching the nostrils closed for a few minutes, he says.

Reach for a painkiller. Your everyday over-the-counter pain medicine will help you deal with the pain, Dr. Archer says. But stick with acetaminophen-containing products such as Tylenol, he advises. Nonsteroidal anti-inflammatories such as ibuprofen and aspirin open blood vessels and will actually increase the bleeding.

Grab a decongestant, too. A decongestant nasal spray will help any congestion that may develop after you break your nose. Pills or nasal sprays work fine, although Dr. Archer advises not to use the sprays for more than a few days or else you may become addicted.

Be a gotu guy. The herb gotu kola is an alternative remedy that can get your nose back on track. "It is a wonderful healer of cartilage, tendons, and connective tissue," says Kathleen Maier, director of the Dreamtime Center for Herbal Studies in Flint Hill, Virginia, and a professional member of the American Herbalists Guild. You can take it as a tea or a tincture—a solution of the herb steeped in drinkable alcohol or a similar substance. Steep one tablespoon of the dried herb in a cup of boiling water. You can drink two to three cups of gotu kola tea a day for several weeks, Maier says. If you're using the tincture, put 20 to 30 drops in water and drink two to three times a day for several weeks. You can find gotu kola in health food stores.

Apply some arnica. The arnica plant is used in homeopathic medicine to treat broken bones. "It reduces swelling, bruising, and pain," says Andrea D. Sullivan, Ph.D., a doctor of naturopathy; president of Sullivan and Associates Center for Natural Healing in Washington, D.C.; and author of *A Path to Healing*. You can take two or three pellets of arnica 30C internally as soon as you break your nose, and then again after two hours, Dr. Sullivan says. Then apply an arnica cream or gel to the nose area. But only use the cream or gel if you have no open wound. Continue taking the arnica 30C two times a day for five days and applying the cream or gel as needed for five days, says Dr. Sullivan. Arnica is available at most health food stores and homeopathic stores.

▶PREVENTIVE MEASURES

Fasten your seat belt. Although broken noses are often the result of freak mishaps, there is one way you can lessen your chances. Many a broken nose has been caused by a car accident when a person wasn't wearing a seat belt, Dr. Archer says. Even the slightest bump can send your face flying into the dashboard. Strap yourself in for this and many other reasons.

Wear your headgear. Whatever your choice of sport may be, wearing some protective headgear (if warranted) can help deflect a shot to the nose, says Dr. Archer.

Burns

▶PROBLEM

Even though most burns suffered by people in United States are minor, they still hurt—and for a long time. Just a split second of carelessness when your finger touches a hot plate can keep you in pain anywhere from 7 to 20 days and possibly leave you with a scar.

▶CAUSE

Fire and a hot stove aren't the only things that can char your skin. Exposure to electricity, chemicals, and radiation can all burn you. Even tap water can reach 140°F at times, causing a third-degree burn within five seconds.

Although about two million people are burned in the United States every year, only 5 percent of them need hospital treatment. Small heat burns caused by flames or hot items usually don't go beyond first-degree burns (which look red) or mild second-degree burns (which have some minor blistering), meaning that you can treat them at home, says Jedd Roe, M.D., assistant professor of emergency medicine at the University of Colorado School of Medicine in Denver. But severe second-degree or third-degree burns—usually marked by the skin being white with red spots, wet or waxy looking, severely blistered or charred—should be seen immediately by a doctor. You also should get medical treatment for burns if the burn covers more than 10 to 20 percent of the body; if the face, hands, or genital area has been burned; if you have suffered chemical or electrical burns; or if the burn becomes infected or you start to develop chills and a fever, says Dr. Roe. Signs of infection usually occur two or three days later and include increased redness or pain, swelling, pus, and red streaks spreading from the burn up the extremities.

If you or someone else has suffered a severe second- or third-degree burn,

DO THIS NOW

Place your burn under cool water for at least 15 minutes, says Jedd Roe, M.D., assistant professor of emergency medicine at the University of Colorado School of Medicine in Denver. Don't use the old standby home remedy of ice, he warns. "Ice can cause tissue damage. It essentially freezes the outside layer of the skin," he says.

THE RULE OF NINES

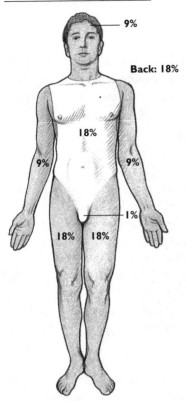

9%

Back: 18%

18%

9%　　　9%

1%

18%　18%

The Rule of Nines is a way to figure out how much of the body is burned. It divides the body into sections and assigns a percentage value to each section. For example, in an adult, the head and arms each equal 9 percent of the body's total surface area. The front and back of the torso and the legs are each worth 18 percent.

you should elevate the burned area and put the victim in the shock position while waiting for medical help to arrive, says Dr. Roe. (For illustrated instructions on how to put someone into this position, see page 584.) Do not disturb any blisters or remove any dead skin, he cautions.

▶SOLUTIONS

The following home remedies can help promote healing of minor burns.

Leave blisters intact. Blisters provide a natural protective layer for the burned tissue. "You should leave blisters alone because they function as a nice, sterile dressing. As long as that skin is intact, there's no avenue for bacteria to get in," Dr. Roe says.

Change and clean daily. If your burn is blistered or open, you should apply an ointment such as Polysporin and bandage it with dry, sterile gauze. Take off the gauze bandage at least once a day, and gently clean the burn area with antibacterial soap and water, says Karl Kramer, M.D., clinical professor of dermatology at the University of Miami School of Medicine. Reapply ointment, and cover the wound with fresh gauze. "As long as it looks better every day, then you are probably doing all right," Dr. Kramer says. You may use the ointment over a small blistered area, but burns with blistering over an area larger than a silver dollar need to be seen by a doctor, he adds.

Buy an aloe plant. "Every kitchen ought to have an aloe vera plant," says Michael Carlston, M.D., assistant clinical professor in the department of family and community medicine at the University of California, San Francisco, School of Medicine. Aloe cools the burn and helps the healing process. If you have an aloe plant, break off a leaf and rub the gel found inside it on the burn. Or use an over-the-counter aloe vera cream found in most drugstores. Just avoid using creams that contain alcohol, as they will irritate the skin, adds Dr. Carlston.

History Lesson

Burns didn't seem to be a problem for early-nineteenth-century performer Signora Girardelli. She entertained audiences by cooking eggs in boiling oil in her palm, running a red-hot poker over her limbs, and attending to baked goods while inside a blazing oven.

Now *that's* one hot babe.

Help the healing along. The mineral zinc aids wound-healing, says Kenneth Singleton, M.D., a physician in private practice in Bethesda, Maryland. Extra zinc helps speed up tissue repair. Take 30 milligrams of zinc supplement twice a day for 10 days, he suggests. But you need to check with your doctor first. Doses above 15 milligrams require medical supervision.

Drink plenty of water. "Blistering sunburns and excessive burns drain the body of fluid," says Don W. Printz, M.D., president of the American Society of Dermatology and a dermatologist in Atlanta. Drink at least eight, eight-ounce glasses of water each day to keep yourself well-hydrated.

▶PREVENTIVE MEASURES

Walk away from the grill. When your propane grill doesn't light right away, shut off the gas and take a walk before you try again, says Ian Cummings, M.D., director of emergency services at the Day Kimball Hospital in Putnam, Connecticut. The gas is heavier than air, so it sits at the bottom of the grill. If it doesn't light right away, and you keep the gas on, the gas collects to the point of a minor explosion when you finally get it to light. "A lot of guys try to light up a propane grill and it blows up in their face," Dr. Cummings says.

Use lighter fluid, not gasoline. Getting charcoal to fire up can be a frustrating experience, but don't get carried away in your quest for a fast barbecue. Only use lighter fluid to light the grill, Dr. Cummings says. Gasoline might give you a quick light, but it will also probably give you a good burn and a trip to a hospital.

Buy a grease fire extinguisher. Many men burn themselves trying to put out grease and oil fires in the kitchen. "Don't put water on it for God's sake," Dr. Cummings pleads. Buy a fire extinguisher made especially for grease fires, and place it in an easy-to-reach location in the kitchen. They're available at hardware and home supply stores. You should also have a fire extinguisher in your workshop area, in your garage, and near wood-burning stoves, adds Dr. Cummings.

Choking

▶PROBLEM

Without even thinking about it, the average person breathes 5,000 gallons of air per day at a rate of about 12 times per minute. But the importance of breathing becomes apparent really quickly when a piece of food goes down the wrong pipe, cutting off your air supply. If you don't unblock that airway, you'll likely be dead within eight minutes.

▶CAUSE

A piece of food, a small object, or even your own tongue lodges in your throat, blocking your ability to breathe in and out through your lungs. It's as if someone has completely cut off your air supply. If you do not remove whatever is blocking your breathing, you will suffocate. The first thing that you or anyone else should do is call for help. Even if you are alone and cannot speak, still dial 911, says Jedd Roe, M.D., assistant professor of emergency medicine at the University of Colorado School of Medicine in Denver. The town you live in may have enhanced 911, where they can trace the call and get help to you even if you can't make a sound. If you have been choking for a few minutes but dislodge the item, you may still want to see a doctor, Dr. Roe says. You could have damaged your larynx or the esophagus.

DO THIS NOW

Try to talk. "If you can speak or even make any sound, then you have a partial airway obstruction and aren't completely choking yet," says Jedd Roe, M.D., assistant professor of emergency medicine at the University of Colorado School of Medicine in Denver. But even a partial airway obstruction can be life-threatening, so regardless of whether you can make any noise, dial 911 or have somebody else call for help and start the suggested solutions right away.

If you can make a noise, try to dislodge the piece of food by coughing. "Someone who can make a noise should be left to try and cough the object up on their own," Dr. Roe adds.

▶SOLUTIONS

The following tips are some things that you can do if you or someone else is choking. Remember to always call for emergency help first.

Keep your hands to yourself. Fight the natural urge to thrust your hand into the mouth, whether it's yours or someone else's, to dig out whatever is stuck. "One thing that you do not want to do is stick your fingers down the back of a conscious person's throat. You end up pushing it deeper down into the airway, making it even harder to get out," Dr. Roe says.

Learn the Heimlich maneuver. Every man should know how to perform the Heimlich maneuver, both on himself and on someone else, Dr. Roe says. For step-by-step instructions on how to do it correctly, see the following illustrations.

PERFORMING THE HEIMLICH MANEUVER ON SOMEONE ELSE

If someone else is choking, stand in back of him and wrap your arms around his waist. Then make a fist with one hand and position the thumb side of your fist just above his belly button. Grab hold of your fist with your other hand.

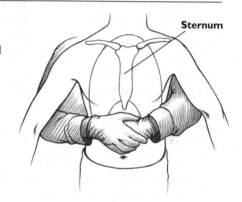

Sternum

Pull in and then up as hard as you can. You may need to do this four or five times to dislodge the object.

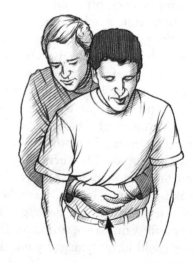

PERFORMING THE HEIMLICH MANEUVER ON YOURSELF

If you're alone and choking, stand at the back of a chair. Lean over the chair so that the top is positioned just above your belly button. Supporting yourself by holding on to the sides with your hands, pull yourself down onto the back of the chair. You may need to do this four or five times until the item comes out.

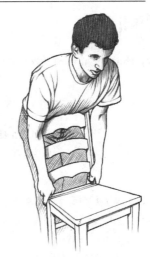

Improvise. If you can't find a chair to perform the Heimlich manuever on yourself, throw a large object on the ground, says Robert McNamara, M.D., professor of emergency medicine and program director of the department of emergency medicine residency at Allegheny University of the Health Sciences–MCP Hahnemann School of Medicine in Philadelphia. "Any object that provides a thrust to the abdominals will do. Just lay something down and flop yourself on top of it," he says.

Save a life. If another person is choking and becomes unconscious, lay him on the floor on his back and check his pulse, Dr. Roe says. If he has a pulse, begin rescue breathing, which is explained and illustrated on pages 580 and 581. Give him two full breaths.

If the breaths won't go in, begin abdominal thrusts, which is similar to the Heimlich maneuver. To do this, straddle the unconscious victim with your legs, placing one hand on top of the other with your palms positioned just above the person's belly button. Your fingers should be pointing toward the person's head. Push upward toward the person's face with 6 to 10 good thrusts, says Dr. Roe.

Then do a finger sweep to see if you have dislodged the object. With your two fingers in a hooked position, place them at one side of the mouth. Using a sweeping motion, move the fingers to the other side. Having your fingers in a hook position pulls the item out toward you instead of pushing it farther down into the airway, Dr. Roe says.

If the object has not been dislodged, recheck the victim's pulse and repeat the steps, beginning with two rescue breaths, Dr. Roe says. If the person has no pulse, begin cardiopulmonary resuscitation, which is explained and illus-

Did You Know?

Dr. Henry Heimlich, who developed the famed Heimlich maneuver in the early 1970s, has never used the technique on a real choking person.

trated on pages 582 and 583. In the event that the person regains consciousness at any time, put him in the recovery position (illustrated on page 584) until medical help arrives.

▶PREVENTIVE MEASURES

Don't drink and eat. "A lot of guys choke on a big chunk of meat after a couple of martinis," says Paul Matera, M.D., an emergency medical technician-paramedic and vice chairman and professor of emergency services at Providence Hospital in Washington, D.C. "As your alcohol level increases, so does your risk of choking," he adds. After a few too many, your motor skills and attention level plummet. "You're drinking and eating, and the next thing you know you're not paying attention and start to laugh. You suck that piece of meat right down your trachea," Dr. Matera says.

Chew thoroughly. There are times that you can get so hungry or so rushed that you practically swallow your food whole. If you don't take the time to chew each piece of food, you increase your chances of getting something stuck and choking on it, Dr. Roe says. Eat slowly and chew each piece completely.

Use your knives. Many people chow down on a piece of food that's too big, Dr. Roe says. Cut up your food into small pieces so that even if it goes down unchewed, it won't lodge in the airway.

Drowning

▶PROBLEM

Some 4,500 people drown each year, making it the fourth most common cause of death from unintentional injury in the United States. And men account for 83 percent of all drowning deaths in the country. But for every one death by drowning, there are four near drownings that result in hospitalization. Those who survive a near drowning can suffer medical complications. Anyone found unconscious in water should receive emergency medical treatment right away, says Jedd Roe, M.D., assistant professor of emergency medicine at the University of Colorado School of Medicine in Denver.

▶CAUSE

There are three main ways that people die by drowning. The vast majority are wet drownings, so named because water, vomit, or some other substance is inhaled into the lungs, causing the victim to suffocate. Dry drownings are those in which the vocal cords snap shut in response to water touching them. While this effectively keeps water out of the lungs, it also keeps out oxygen and may trigger a seizure and death. The third type of drowning, called a secondary drowning, happens when someone who is resuscitated dies within 96 hours.

▶SOLUTIONS

The following tips from the American Red Cross and the National Safety Council may help you or someone else who is in danger of drowning.

Tread and think. Slowly tread water without exerting too much energy, says Michael Espino, senior associate of new prodcuts and services development

DO THIS NOW
Stay calm. Panicking and flailing about in the water will only wear you down, making you more likely to drown. "You want to conserve energy. The more energy you use panicking, the more tired you will become, and you won't be able to help yourself," says Michael Espino, senior associate of new prodcuts and services development for the American Red Cross in Falls Church, Virginia.

SURVIVAL FLOATING

Survival floating in warm water helps you conserve energy while waiting for help. First, hold your breath with your face in the water, letting your arms and legs dangle. Rest in this position for several seconds.

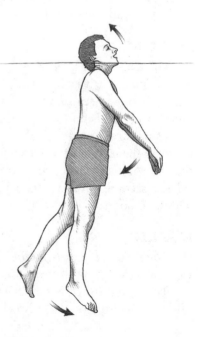

When you need to breathe, slowly lift your arms to about shoulder height and separate your legs with one leg forward and one leg back.

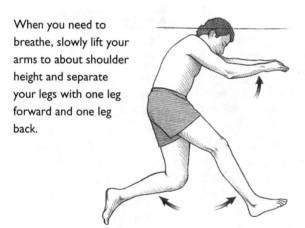

Gently press down with your arms, and bring your legs together at the same time. This helps bring your mouth above water while you take another breath. Then return to the resting position and start all over again.

for the American Red Cross in Falls Church, Virginia. Look around and find your bearings—how far you are from land, how you can get help, how many people are around. Figure out the best way to get out of your situation.

Inflate your clothes. Your clothes make for great floatation devices if you aren't wearing a life jacket, Espino says. While treading water, tuck in your shirt or jacket or tie the shirttail ends together. Unbutton the collar button and take a deep breath. Then bend your head forward into the water, pull the shirt or jacket up to your face, and blow into the shirt. Both your face and your shirt should be in the water when you're blowing the air into your shirt. After inflating your shirt, keep the front of the shirt or jacket underwater and hold the collar closed. The air trapped in the shirt will keep you afloat. With time, the air may seep out of your shirt. If that happens, just repeat the process. "You'll look like the Incredible Hulk," Espino says.

Keep winter clothes on. If it's cold out, don't make the mistake of thinking that heavy winter clothes will weigh you down. Winter clothes may actually help you float and delay hypothermia in cold water, according to the American Red Cross. Lie back, spread your arms and legs, and use a winging motion with your arms to move toward safety, says Espino. The air in the clothes will keep you on top of the water.

Take easy strokes. If you are in cold water, start to swim toward shore. In cold water, you have the added threat of hypothermia. But use easy, gentle strokes to get there. "Swim forward but conserve your energy by doing a breaststroke or a sidestroke. Once you get tired, float for awhile," Espino says.

Go with the flow. If caught up in a strong current, go with it, Espino says. "Don't fight it. People don't realize how strong those currents are," he adds. If the current pushes you farther away from land, swim in a diagonal direction across the current, but not into it.

Be a hero. So what do you do if you happen upon someone else who's drowning? Remember these four words, in order, from the National Safety Council: reach, throw, row, and go. The first option is to find a nearby object—a lightweight pole or long stick—and use it to reach for the victim. If someone else is around, have that person grab your belt or pants and hold you for stability. And make sure that your feet are firmly planted. If you can't find something to reach out with, throw something in the water that floats. An empty picnic jug, life jacket, cushion, piece of wood—anything you can find. If there's a rope handy, tie it to the object so that you can pull it back in or retrieve it to try, try again.

If there's no pole or object to throw, but there's a rowboat, canoe, boogie board, or some other water-worthy craft nearby, then row to the victim, suggests the National Safety Council. Two cautions if you try this: Wear a life jacket. And to avoid capsizing, pull the victim in over the rear of the boat (the stern), not over the side. Jumping in and swimming to save the victim yourself should be your last option if the other three techniques are impossible. But you

History Lesson

On July 3, 1969, London's two evening papers ran the headline "Brian Jones Dead in Pool Tragedy." Jones, a founding member of the Rolling Stones, was found lying facedown at the bottom of his pool in his Cotchford Farm estate. The estate was the former home of A. A. Milne and the place where the author wrote his famous tales of Winnie-the-Pooh and friends.

There's no question that Jones drowned that night. But was it due, in part, to a deadly mix of alcohol and drugs as the coroner ruled? Or was it, as a friend of Jones claims, a murder? Nicholas Fitzgerald, an heir to the Guinness beer fortune, claims that he saw men holding someone down in the pool that night. He said that Jones told him earlier that people were out to get him. Fitzgerald later wrote that one of the men at the farm that night told him, "Get the hell out of here, Fitzgerald, or you'll be next." When he finally published his bizarre tale 16 years later, Fitzgerald claimed that Jones was on the verge of forming a new supergroup with Jimi Hendrix and John Lennon at the time of his untimely demise. (Of course, Jones, Hendrix, and Lennon were already jamming together in Rock 'n' Roll Heaven at the time the claim was made public, so they weren't exactly able to confirm what happened.)

Yet even Rolling Stone Keith Richards has expressed doubts about what happened the night that Jones died. "Some very weird things happened that night," he told *Rolling Stone* magazine in 1972. "It's the same feeling with who killed Kennedy. You never get to the bottom of it."

Paging Oliver Stone.

---

should only try this if you are a capable swimmer trained in water lifesaving procedures. If you are untrained in these procedures; have improper equipment to reach, throw, or row to the victim; or would be putting yourself in danger, go get help instead, Espino says.

Take action. If you have saved someone from a near drowning, you may need to start emergency measures such as rescue breathing and cardiopulmonary resuscitation, says Espino. (Look in Lifesaving Techniques on pages 580 to 583 for step-by-step, illustrated instructions.) If the person was rescued from cold water, you should remove their wet clothing and cover them with a dry blanket, adds Espino.

▶PREVENTIVE MEASURES

Learn to swim. "You'd be surprised how many adults have not learned to swim," Espino says. Many people think that they can swim but really can't, especially if faced with a dangerous situation, he adds. If you can't swim, or never learned how to swim properly, take an adult swimming class at a local pool or call your local American Red Cross chapter for a referral to a pool that offers swimming classes. Many places have adult-only classes so that you don't have to worry about splashing, noisy kids.

Stay dry near water. "When it comes to men, alcohol has a lot to do with water accidents, especially with boating and fishing," Espino says. Alcohol affects your balance and judgment, slows your movements, and reduces your swimming skills, even if you're an excellent swimmer. If you are going to be near water, lay off the booze.

Wear protection. Always wear a life jacket whenever you're in or around water, Espino says. Even if you are just fishing and have no intention of getting wet, put a jacket on, he urges. "That's how a lot of accidents happen. It's people who never thought they would be in the water in the first place," Espino says.

Bring your buddies. Whether boating, fishing, or swimming, always bring a friend along to help if something goes wrong. "The best bet is to never be alone when around water. That way the other person can assist you or at least get help immediately," Espino says.

Electrical Shock

▶PROBLEM

It doesn't take a high-voltage power line to give you a deadly electrical shock. The typical household current of 110 volts can kill.

▶CAUSE

When electricity enters your body, it travels along the path of least resistance, which happens to be your nerves and blood vessels. The electricity injures the nerves, blood vessels, and muscles as it zips along. The current can then work its way toward the heart, where it disturbs the heart cells. This disruption may send your heart into an abnormal rhythm, causing it to stop pumping blood. The electrical shock can also disrupt the nerves that control breathing.

Because most of the damage is internal, you should seek medical attention immediately after a severe shock. "You can look deceptively normal after a shock but actually have a great deal of nerve and vascular damage as well as damage to the muscles. This releases a protein called myoglobin that can clog the kidneys and cause kidney problems," says Ian Cummings, M.D., director of emergency services at the Day Kimball Hospital in Putnam, Connecticut.

▶SOLUTIONS

If you find someone getting an electrical shock, here are the first things you should do.

Turn off the power. To cut off the source

DO THIS NOW

A jolt of electricity may not always be strong enough to render you unconscious, but it can be strong enough to make your muscles involuntarily contract. If this happens, you may find yourself actually gripping the power source with your hand even though you want to let go.

If you have a free hand, grab a wood object or a magazine or any nonconductive material and try to pry or slap your other hand from the wire, says Paul Matera, M.D., an emergency medical technician-paramedic and vice chairman and professor of emergency services at Providence Hospital in Washington, D.C. Or throw your body back so that you pull away from the source, he adds.

of the electricity, unplug the appliance, says Paul Matera, M.D., an emergency medical technician-paramedic and vice chairman and professor of emergency services at Providence Hospital in Washington, D.C. If that can't be done, then turn off a circuit breaker or a fuse box. If you have difficulty cutting off the source to an outside line, call the power company or 911 to see if they can shut it down.

Get help. After you have cut off the power, call 911, says Jedd Roe, M.D., assistant professor of emergency medicine at the University of Colorado School of Medicine in Denver.

Don't rush in. Before jumping in to save someone who has had an electrical shock, make sure that the power is cut off or else you could soon be a victim as well. If someone is trapped in a car that has a power line on top of it, tell them to stay put until the power has been shut off. If you feel your legs tingle as you get near a victim, stop, says Dr. Roe The sensation means that you are on energized ground and that an electrical current is entering your body. Raise one foot off the ground, turn around and hop on one foot to a safe place.

Leave the wires alone. Don't try to move live wires, even with wood objects such as poles, wood handles, or tree branches, according to the National Safety Council. If the voltage is high enough, even these wood objects can conduct electricity and the rescuer will be electrocuted. Definitely don't push wires with metal objects. Wait for properly trained personnel to arrive to deal with the wires.

Go into emergency mode. As soon as you can safely reach the victim, check his breathing and pulse. If he isn't breathing, start emergency breathing procedures, Dr. Roe says. If he isn't breathing and doesn't have a pulse, start cardiopulmonary resuscitation, he adds. (Look in Lifesaving Techniques on pages 580 to 583 for step-by-step, illustrated instructions.)

Leave him lie. Someone who has experienced an electrical shock may also have a spinal injury. Don't move the victim unless absolutely necessary to open his airway or give rescue breathing. Keep him in the position where you found him, and cover the person with a jacket or blanket to keep him warm until medical help arrives, suggests Dr. Roe.

▶PREVENTIVE MEASURES

Pamper your tools. The better you treat your electrical tools, the less of a chance they'll shock you, Dr. Roe says. Store them properly in cabinets away from the elements so that they don't rust and the cords don't fray. Keep them away from water, which could damage them and harm you as well. And throw out any old, damaged power tools instead of taking a chance by using them, he adds.

Look out for power lines. Anyone working outside with a ladder should be vigilant about power lines. "That's a classic—working with a ladder and coming into contact with overhead power lines," says Robert McNamara,

History Lesson

The idea for the electric chair came at the expense of an elderly drunk. One day in 1881, Dr. Alfred Southwick, a dentist and former steamboat engineer, witnessed an old drunken man mistakenly touch the terminals of a live electrical generator in Buffalo. Dr. Southwick was amazed at the quickness and ease of the old man's passing and recounted the story to his friend, New York state senator Daniel H. McMillan.

Sen. McMillan, in turn, was so thrilled with the story that he passed it on to the governor of New York, David B. Hill. Gov. Hill took the idea to the state legislature and asked lawmakers to consider how "the science of the present day" might replace hanging as a form of execution. After years of study, the world's first "Electrical Execution Law" went into effect on January 1, 1889.

Just three months later, William Kemmler killed his lover, Matilda, in Buffalo and consequently became the electric chair's first human guinea pig (although many dogs lost their lives as test subjects in the years leading up to the passage of the law). Unfortunately for Kemmler, he didn't leave this world as easily as the drunk who started it all. It seems that the prison officials who operated the chair never thought about how long to administer the electricity until minutes before the execution. Doctors on the scene theorized that 10 to 15 seconds would do the trick, but they guessed wrong. As the warden began unstrapping the body, doctors realized that Kemmler was still alive. So the chair was fired up again for a much longer period of time to finish the deed.

M.D., professor of emergency medicine and program director of the department of emergency medicine residency at Allegheny University of the Health Sciences–MCP Hahnemann School of Medicine in Philadelphia. The best way to avoid this problem is simply to avoid working near power lines, Dr. McNamara says. If work must be done near power lines, hire an expert to do it, he recommends.

Dig it—carefully. "Digging with power tools over underground cables is a big problem with men and electric shock," Dr. Cummings says. If you have some heavy digging to do, you might be better off handing the job to a professional, Dr. Cummings advises.

Or look in the phone book for the number of your local power company, and call them to find out if there are hidden electrical cables where you want to dig. Some power companies even have special numbers set up to dispense such information, Dr. Cummings says.

Let go of the jumper cables. When you need to jump your car battery, make sure that you don't jump yourself in the process. Let go of the handles before someone starts the engine. "There's a reason that there is insulation on the handles of jumper cables; it's insulating you from the electrical current," Dr. Matera says.

Use batteries in the bathroom. No matter how careful you are with electrical appliances in the bathroom, you are still increasing your chances for electrical shock, Dr. McNamara says. "Having radios and such in the bathroom can kill you," he adds. Use battery operated radios or shavers and keep plugged appliances out of the bathroom.

Fainting

▶PROBLEM

In the movies, it's usually a slender woman being told bad news who faints. But in real life, as opposed to reel life, men can be just as squeamish and prone to fainting. "I had this burly construction worker who came in with a cut on his hand. As soon as I touched him with the needle, he went out cold. All 300 pounds of him," says Paul Matera, M.D., an emergency medical technician-paramedic and vice chairman and professor of emergency services at Providence Hospital in Washington, D.C.

▶CAUSE

Perhaps you can't stand the sight of blood. Or your own blood sugar is low because you've been too busy to eat. Or you just got some bad news. Or maybe you've just been standing in the heat too long. Any of these things and many more can cause you to faint. That's because the two main things that brain cells need are oxygen and glucose.

If you haven't eaten all day, your brain may not be getting enough glucose and you could pass out. If you've been in the heat for a few hours or just got some bad news, your blood pressure could plummet without warning. That temporarily interrupts the blood flow—and, therefore, the oxygen supply—to your brain, which renders you unconscious.

A random fainting incident isn't anything to worry about, Dr. Matera says. As long as you were healthy before you fainted, and you're just as healthy after you come to, it was probably just a freak occurrence. You should seek medical attention if the fainting spell comes with other symptoms such as stomach pain,

Did You Know?

In the early 1880s, a farm worker appeared in Tennessee with three nanny goats and one billy goat that all "fainted," thus forever branding them the Fainting Goats breed. There's even an International Fainting Goat Association (whose symbol is a goat lying on its back with its feet up in the air). The goats don't actually faint, but they have a condition called myatonia, which causes them to lock up and fall over when startled. The stiffness only lasts for about 10 to 15 seconds, after which the goat just gets up and walks off.

fever, pains, or shortness of breath, says Dr. Matera. And you should see a doctor if you start to faint repeatedly.

▶SOLUTIONS

The following step-by-step tips are some things you can do if you or someone else has fainted.

Lie down. If you can't sit down to put your head between your knees when you feel faint, just lie down and elevate your legs 8 to 12 inches, according to the National Safety Council. This jump-starts your blood flow back to the heart, which then pumps it up to the brain.

Assess the situation. If someone has fainted, check his breathing and heart rate to be sure that it is not *more* than a fainting spell. If he isn't breathing, start emergency breathing procedures, Dr. Matera says. If he isn't breathing and doesn't have a pulse, start cardiopulmonary resuscitation, he adds. For illustrated, step-by-step instructions on taking a pulse, rescue breathing, and cardiopulmonary resuscitation, see Lifesaving Techniques, beginning on page 579. If the person who fainted has fallen, or if you didn't witness the fainting and aren't sure whether he fell, check for injury and see Falling on page 611.

Put him on his side. If someone who has fainted is breathing and has a pulse, roll him onto his side, Dr. Matera says. This is in case the person starts to vomit after he passes out. When placed on his side, he will have less chance of choking. (For an illustration showing the proper unconscious recovery position, see page 584.)

Forget the film version. Doubtless you've seen in the movies where someone throws ice-cold water on a fainting victim or slaps the person silly. Don't, Dr. Matera says. If it is a simple fainting spell, the person will be up and around shortly, so there's no need to injure him by slapping him in the face. Cold water can be an additional shock to a system that has already been under some stress. You can use a cool, wet cloth on the person's face instead, Dr. Matera says.

▶PREVENTIVE MEASURES

Beat the heat. Standing or sitting still for a long time in the heat can cause your blood to pool in dilated blood vessels. The pooling decreases your circulation, causing a drop in blood pressure. The drop in pressure slows the flow of blood to your brain, according to the National Safety Council.

If you have to sit still in the heat for some reason—maybe you're at your nephew's college graduation—then flex and extend your lower legs as if you're putting each foot on and off the gas pedal, Dr. Matera says. Do this three to five times every few minutes to squeeze the blood out of your legs and put it back into your body's central circulation, he says.

Watch your triggers. Certain people will always faint in specific situations, says Michael I. Weintraub, M.D., clinical professor of neurology at New York Medical College in Valhalla and chief of neurology at Phelps Memorial Hospital in Sleepy Hollow, New York. Some lose it at the sight of blood, some faint if they keep their neck in a certain position, and some pass out while straining to go to the bathroom while constipated (called micturition syncope).

If you have a factor or situation that often causes you to faint, then take steps to keep away from it, Dr. Weintraub says. Staying away from blood is relatively simple. Holding your neck in certain positions—especially hyperextending your neck during shampooing in a hair salon, for example—can cause a person to faint. So can keeping your neck in the same position for a long time, like maintaining your head in a posture while painting or doing yoga. So try to keep your neck and head in a relatively neutral position, recommends Dr. Weintraub. And for those who strain too hard on the toilet, get some more fiber in your diet or use a stool softener, he suggests.

Falling

▶ PROBLEM

Your stepladder is a little short to reach the eaves, so you back the pickup against the house and set the ladder up in the bed. If your wife's lucky, you'll fall right into the bed. Then she won't have to move you for the drive to the emergency room.

▶ CAUSE

Falls are the number one cause of deaths in the home, accounting for more than 10 times as many home fatalities as firearms. But most are avoidable with a little common sense, says Michael Taylor, manager of the community safety division at the National Safety Council in Itasca, Illinois. Like using a ladder, not a chair, to reach high places.

"I think that a lot of falls by men are guys trying to do the Bob Vila thing, and they just aren't being careful," says Taylor.

As you age, falls are more of a concern. Even small tumbles can cause broken bones such as hip fractures and sometimes even death. In 1996, 350 people between age 25 and 44 died after falling in their homes. That same year, 1,300 people age 65 to 74 died in home falls.

▶ SOLUTIONS

The following step-by-step tips can help you handle a fall.

Take the fall. Your natural inclination is to

DO THIS NOW

Don't move. After a hard fall, resist the temptation to jump up and deny that the accident occurred. Temporary numbness or pain can mask or exaggerate the severity of an injury, cautions **Warren Bowman, M.D.**, medical director for the **National Ski Patrol** who lives in **Cooke City, Montana**, just outside **Yellowstone National Park**.

It is usually safe to wait a few moments to see if pain persists or dies down unless it is clear that you are severely hurt—which means that the pain is intense, you're unable to move, or some part of your body is immovable. Only after a little time passes can you accurately gauge the severity of the injury.

History Lesson

In 1944, a desperate British pilot named Nicholas Alkemade jumped without a parachute from his flaming bomber 18,000 feet above Germany. He hit a fir tree, caromed into a snowbank, and walked away unscathed.

break a fall by putting out your arms or grabbing at something. That may not be advisable because the inertial force can snap a wrist or wrench an arm, says Jay Caputo, a Hollywood stuntman and former world-class gymnast.

It's better to tuck and roll, advises Caputo. "If you roll with your momentum, you can shrug off some of the speed, and then it's safer to stop yourself," he says.

To practice the tuck position, lie down on a mat or rug, grasp your knees to your chest, bring your chin forward, and then rock yourself back and forth until you reach the seated position. This is to help you get used to rolling. "You want to be like a ball that rolls," says Caputo. "It's a position that protects your head and neck."

Stay still. There are times when you absolutely should not move after a fall, says Warren Bowman, M.D., medical director for the National Ski Patrol who lives in Cooke City, Montana, just outside Yellowstone National Park. If you have significant pain in the neck or back; if you experience weakness, numbness, tingling, or paralysis of your arm or leg; if you're unable to use an arm or leg; or if you have a deformity of an arm or leg, let the paramedics be the ones to move you. "The only exceptions to this are if you're alone in a remote area with no chance of getting help or if you're in danger," Dr. Bowman says.

Determine how badly you're hurt. Once you've fallen, ask yourself the following questions, advises Dr. Bowman. You may have to open your clothing to determine how bad your injuries are, he adds.

- Is your pain moderate or severe?
- Are you bleeding?
- Can you move the area below the pain, meaning can you wiggle your toes and fingers?
- Do you have normal sensation below the injured area?
- Is there any deformity? Compare the injured area with the opposite area if necessary (for example, compare an injured arm to your uninjured arm).
- Did you lose consciousness, even for only a moment?
- Did you or are you experiencing any of the following: confusion, dizziness, severe headache, vomiting, weakness, or visual changes such as double vision?

Choose a course of action. From those answers should come the answer to the next question: Do I need to see a doctor, or can I handle this myself? Bloody scrapes you can handle. "But if you can't move the area or there's numbness, you may have a broken bone, a dislocation, or a nerve injury," says Dr. Bowman. Likewise, if your ankle slumps to one side or a finger points the wrong way, you'll definitely need a doctor. And if you've smacked a vital area, like your head, you'd better be safe and see a doctor, says Dr. Bowman. If you believe that you are seriously injured, call 911, he says.

Be wary with the elderly. If you see an elderly person fall, you should assess the person carefully since fractures (especially of the spine and hip) are more common in seniors, says Dr. Bowman. Consult a doctor or take the person to the emergency room if there is any deformity, loss of use, marked swelling, or bruising, or if there is not significant recovery within 24 hours, he says. "I have seen an elderly patient with a hip fracture who was able to limp around for several days before being brought to the doctor," Dr. Bowman says.

▶PREVENTIVE MEASURES

Get a grip. The most likely place to fall in the home is the bathroom, Taylor says. In the tub, always have a rubber mat underfoot or put down those sandpaper-like stick-ons, he recommends. He also advises installing grab bars securely fastened into wall studs at chest level in the shower and tub stall.

"You need something to hold on to when you're getting in or out, or when you're standing on one leg, scrubbing your other foot," Taylor says. And when you get out of the tub, step onto a rubber-backed rug or bath mat rather than a slick, steamy, tiled floor, he says.

Rail against style. Who hasn't slipped and taken a fall down the stairs? All stairs should have a handrail and a back to each step. Steps also should be covered with some type of tractionlike carpeting or rubber grips, says Taylor.

"In new homes, you see these open staircases that start in the middle of the room and go up to a loft. They don't have rails, and even the steps are open," Taylor says. "It sacrifices safety for style."

Sturdy your stepladder. When you're setting up a ladder, make sure that it's on solid ground, not perched on six inches of fresh mulch or the side of a hill. And never stand on the top two rungs of the ladder (even though they're there) because it makes you top-heavy, Taylor says.

If you're using an extension ladder, set it at a 45- to 55-degree angle against the house. "You'll know it's right because it will feel sturdy under you," Taylor says. And, finally, don't reach up once you're on the ladder. Your work—the window or the gutter—should be right in front of you, within easy arm's reach. If not, take time to move the ladder, says Taylor.

Take up tai chi. Elderly people who practice tai chi—the Chinese discipline of moving meditation—improve their sense of balance and have fewer falls, says Robert Whipple, a physical therapist and assistant professor of neurology at the

University of Connecticut Health Center in Farmington. "This is corroborated by research findings at the Pepper Foundation in Tallahassee, Florida. They found significant improvement in the strength and balance of seniors participating in Taoist tai chi training," he says.

But you don't have to be a senior to benefit from tai chi. Just two, 15-minute home practice sessions per day will make anyone more sure on their feet, says Whipple. "Foremost among the many factors affecting balance are body awareness and a consciousness of where your body is in space as you move. Tai chi can definitely improve that," he says.

Whipple recommends learning tai chi from an instructor rather than a video or book. The instructor can critique and correct your movements, and working under group supervision is a powerful learning and motivational tool, he says. To find a tai chi instructor in your area, you can contact the Taoist Tai Chi Society of America, 1310 North Monroe Street, Tallahassee, FL 32303. Or you can check in the Yellow Pages or at your local YMCA or senior health center.

Frostbite

▶PROBLEM

If you've ever wondered what your hands, feet, ears, or other extremities would look like with frostbite, check out the frozen meat section of your local supermarket. "It would look white and waxy just like a frozen chicken leg. That's what it would feel like, too—a frozen chicken leg," says Eric A. Weiss, M.D., assistant professor of emergency medicine at Stanford University Medical Center and author of *Wilderness 911.*

▶CAUSE

Frostbite occurs during cold and windy weather. It usually strikes when people spend 6 to 12 hours in temperatures of –4° to 10°F. But it doesn't have to be that cold for it to happen. "Even if it isn't very cold, high winds can reduce the temperatures to dangerously low levels. It could be 20°F out, but with a 40-mile-per-hour wind, it's just as dangerous as being –20°F," says Dr. Weiss. Getting wet or touching metal objects can also speed up the frostbite process. Once your skin freezes, small, icy crystals form and destroy the skin cells. This causes the blood to clot, cutting off circulation to the area. The flesh hardens, the skin becomes waxy and white, and you lose all feeling in the affected area.

Severe frostbite requires hospitalization and possibly amputation, Dr. Weiss says. Less severe cases can still lead to discolored skin, burning

DO THIS NOW

If you are deep in the frozen tundra and can't get inside immediately, cozy up with a friend to keep your extremities warm, says Eric A. Weiss, M.D., assistant professor of emergency medicine at Stanford University Medical Center and author of *Wilderness 911.* Put your feet or hands inside your partner's clothing. "Take your feet out of your boots and place them against the warm skin of your partner's stomach. Their body heat will help prevent frostnip, where your skin is numb and cold but not frozen, from becoming frostbite," Dr. Weiss says. If you're alone, tuck your hands under your armpits to get them warm or windmill them around to increase blood flow to your fingers, he advises.

pain, numbness, and joint problems. Anyone who develops frostbite should see a doctor, Dr. Weiss says. "You can't tell by looking at skin tissue how serious the damage is. Even terrible looking limbs recover when treated well," he says.

▶SOLUTIONS

If you find yourself in danger of frostbite, follow these steps in this order.

Join the in crowd. Seek shelter as soon as possible. If you notice your skin turning waxy white, get inside before additional frostbite develops in other areas, Dr. Weiss says.

Loosen up. As soon as you get somewhere warm, take off your rings and any other constricting jewelry and clothing, says Dr. Weiss. As your skin begins to thaw, it will swell, making it almost impossible to do this later. If you don't take off a ring, it could act as a tourniquet and cause further damage, he says.

Save the massage for later. Rubbing the frostbitten skin will only cause more damage, Dr. Weiss says. Don't massage or even touch it.

Don't refreeze it. The actual damage that occurs in frostbite happens during the freezing and thawing process, Dr. Weiss says. The more times you freeze and thaw, the more harm you're doing to your body. "If you thaw it out prematurely, and then it refreezes, you are doing three times as much damage as you would if you kept it frozen," Dr. Weiss says. Don't thaw out your skin unless you know that you won't be back out in the cold, he advises.

Make like Frankenstein. The big guy was afraid of fire. You should be, too, if you have frostbite. Your frozen nerve endings can't warn you if your skin starts to cook, so don't try to warm yourself over a flame. Don't heat your hands or feet over a stove either, Dr. Weiss says.

Heat some water. If there is no risk of refreezing the frostbitten area, gradually immerse it in a tub or saucepan of warm (102° to 105°F) water. Circulate the water to help keep the frozen part in contact with the warm water. Since the frozen part is acting like an ice cube, you may need to add more warm water. Rewarming frostbitten fingers and toes is very painful, so you may want to take a painkiller before you start, Dr. Weiss says.

Beet it. After you have seen a doctor, try beets to deal with post-frostbite tenderness. She's not sure why it works, but Andrea D. Sullivan, Ph.D., a doctor of naturopathy; president of Sullivan and Associates Center for Natural Healing in Washington, D.C.; and author of *A Path to Healing*, recommends bandaging fresh beets on the frostbitten area to quell the pain. Keep the sliced beets on the area until the beets dry. Replace them when they are dry, up to several times a day until the tenderness is gone. The beets take the pain out of the thawing process, she says.

▶PREVENTIVE MEASURES

Adapt with Adaptrin. Adaptrin is a combination of 24 herbs used in the ancient Indian practice of Ayurvedic medicine. The concoction opens up blood

History Lesson

You don't even have to set foot outside to get frostbite. One man developed frostbite in his left cheek while enjoying the high-inducing effects of nitrous oxide—a sweet-smelling anesthetic (better known as laughing gas) used in dentistry and surgery.

In another incident, a passenger on a commercial airline flight needed a cold compress. A flight attendant gave the passenger a cold pack made up of a section of dry ice used for cooling in the galley. The passenger developed third-degree frostbite in the lower left side of his back.

---

vessels, expediting blood flow to the extremities, says Jean D. Miller, D.O., holistic medical director of BodyCentered in New York City. Skiers often take Adaptrin to keep warm while hitting the slopes, she adds. You can find it in health food or herbal stores, or they can order it for you.

Two weeks before you expect to be out in the cold, start taking two tablets per day, says Curtis Jacquot, president of Pacific BioLogic, the makers of Adaptrin, in Clayton, California. But, he warns, taking herbal preparations to increase blood flow is no substitute for common sense and dressing properly.

Get hot, hot, hot. Take cayenne pepper capsules before you go out in the cold. They will warm you up as well as stimulate blood flow to your hands and feet, says Kathleen Maier, director of the Dreamtime Center for Herbal Studies in Flint Hill, Virginia, and a professional member of the American Herbalists Guild. She suggests taking two capsules every three hours while you are exposed to the cold.

You can also use an already-made cayenne pepper tincture, which, like the capsules, can be found at health food or herb stores. Use 10 drops of the tincture three times a day as a preventive measure, suggests Dr. Sullivan.

Watch for warning signs. After a few hours in the cold, your skin starts to turn red and you lose sensation in your fingers and toes. That's called frostnip, and it's a warning sign that frostbite is on its way. "If you stop whatever you are doing and warm the skin, you can prevent frostbite and permanent injury," Dr. Weiss says.

Wear a hat. So what if it musses up your hair. A good deal of body heat escapes through an uncapped head in cold weather, says David C. Novicki, D.P.M., president of New Haven Foot Surgeons in New Haven, Connecticut, and past president of the American College of Foot and Ankle Surgeons in Chicago. Wearing a hat keeps your other body parts warm and decreases your vulnerability to frostbite.

Layer it on. With each piece of clothing you wear, air gets trapped between the layers. The air then heats up, creating a self-sufficient insulation system. Wear liners underneath gloves and socks, long underwear under pants, and layers of shirts around your torso, Dr. Novicki says.

Skip the rum punch. Sure, it makes you feel all toasty and warm when it goes down, but alcohol actually lowers the body temperature and is counterproductive in very cold weather, Dr. Novicki says. Chugging down hot toddies won't help your perception skills or reaction time during an emergency either.

But do drink a lot of water and other beverages, adds Dr. Weiss. Dehydration speeds up frostbite. "When you are dehydrated, the blood isn't going to the skin," he says.

Heat Exhaustion and Heatstroke

▶PROBLEM

You've been working hard in hot, humid weather and your body can't shed the heat gained from the environment and activity fast enough. Heat illness can be relatively minor, such as heat exhaustion, or it can be deadly, such as heatstroke. They are two points on a continuum, says Warren Bowman, M.D., medical director for the National Ski Patrol who lives in Cooke City, Montana, just outside Yellowstone National Park. And if not cared for, heat exhaustion may lead to heatstroke.

▶CAUSE

Heat exhaustion is a form of hypovolemic shock, says Dr. Bowman. That means that your vital organs—your brain, heart, lungs—are not getting enough blood. In hot weather, you can lose up to three quarts of fluids and salts an hour through perspiration. If you aren't replacing those fluids and salts, your blood volume decreases. At the same time, more blood has been diverted to your skin to help cool you off. After awhile, says Dr. Bowman, your circu-

---

DO THIS NOW

If you see someone with heatstroke, call 911. Then strip him down to his underwear, pour water over him, and fan him. Place him in a stream, lake, or bathtub full of cool water. If you have ice or a cold pack, wrap it in a thin cloth and place it in his armpits, groin, around the neck and head, or anywhere there are large blood vessels, recommends Warren Bowman, M.D., medical director for the National Ski Patrol who lives in Cooke City, Montana, just outside Yellowstone National Park.

latory system no longer works as efficiently. And with less blood available to your vital organs, you begin to feel light headed and weak. Other symptoms of heat exhaustion include cool, pale, clammy skin; thirst; headache; nausea; a fast, weak pulse; and anxiety.

Heatstroke develops when your body is overwhelmed by the heat and loses its ability to regulate internal temperature, causing it to rise to dangerous levels, says Dr. Bowman. A person with heatstroke almost always has some kind of altered mental state, he says, which can range from confusion to unconsciousness. Other symptoms include very hot, flushed skin; a rapid pulse; and headache. A heatstroke victim's temperature will usually read above 105°F.

As your body temperature climbs uncontrollably, you may become delirious, irrational, and unable to help yourself, warns Dr. Bowman.

With heatstroke, every minute counts. Getting medical attention quickly is essential. Once your body temperature climbs above 105°F, brain damage occurs and death isn't far off, warns Mark Rosoff, an emergency medical technician and director of the Front Range Institute of Safety in Fort Collins, Colorado.

You don't have to have heat exhaustion before heatstroke, says Rosoff. Heatstroke can occur rapidly, most often in healthy people working strenuously in a hot climate. Elderly or chronically ill people who have been exposed to high temperatures for a long time or who can't shed heat effectively because of the medications they are taking are also at risk for heatstroke.

▶SOLUTIONS

Do the following when you first start feeling ill. Preventing heat illness in the first place is your best course of action.

Cool down. Getting woozy in the heat is your body's strong hint to stop what you're doing and get in the shade with a cool drink. If the humidity is less than 75 percent, you can get cool by frequently dousing your clothes in water— even warm water, says Rosoff. As the clothes dry, they'll wick away heat. In a more humid climate, you need to move to a shaded area and sponge with cool water, he says.

Get comfortable. Lie down, prop up your feet 8 to 12 inches, and stay down until you feel better, says Dr. Bowman. Loosen any tight clothing and remove any heavy clothing.

Grab a sports drink. Slowly drink a sports drink like Gatorade, suggests Dr. Bowman. It should be at room temperature, and you can drink up to a quart of it. If you don't have any sports drink on hand, just add a half-teaspoon of salt to a quart of plain water.

Keep track of how you feel. "You should feel better after about 20 minutes. If not, your body may have lost its ability to regulate its temperature," explains Rosoff. In that case, you could be developing heatstroke. This is a medical emergency, says Rosoff, and you need to call 911 immediately.

History Lesson

It was scorching and humid when President Zachary Taylor presided over the laying of the Washington Monument cornerstone on July 4, 1850. He spent the day eating cherries and milk. Clad in a stately high-neck collar and black suit, the Mexican War hero perspired terribly, turned flush, and nearly fainted during the ceremony before he drank a pitcher of water that had also been under the sun for several hours.

Back at the White House, Taylor broke out in chills and sweats and declared that he was "very hungry," before collapsing with stomach cramps. He died five days later, after just 16 months in office.

Historians are not sure exactly what killed Taylor, the 12th president. Some believe that he got sick from the heat. Others think that he may have picked up some sort of bug in the fruit or water and died from "bilious" or typhoid fever.

▶PREVENTIVE MEASURES

Slake your thirst. Never heed the advice of your old football coach who ordered you during August preseason practice not to drink water because then you'd be thirsty all day.

In hot weather, you should be downing an eight-ounce glass of fluid every 20 minutes, and more if you are really exerting yourself and sweating, says Dr. Bowman.

"Unless you drink lots of liquids in hot weather, you won't be able to radiate heat from your body," Dr. Bowman says. Your best choices are plain old water or sports drinks.

Put down the pop. The sugar in many sodas actually slows down absorption of liquid, Dr. Bowman says. So guzzling a giant cola on a hot day isn't quite as refreshing as the multimillion-dollar ad campaigns make it seem.

Delete diuretics. Drinks with caffeine or alcohol—sorry, but yes, that does include ice-cold beer—act as diuretics, which means that they make the fluid loss problem even worse, Dr. Bowman says. So not only don't they count as fluids but they may actually subtract from your daily total. Meanwhile, back at Moe's Tavern, Homer Simpson is sobbing in his beer.

Use your head. Heat illness often occurs when you push yourself too hard or just aren't accustomed to hot outdoor temperatures. In February, you fly to Palm Springs from Poughkeepsie, go for a run, and the paramedics find you prone amongst the Joshua trees with the coyotes circling.

"If you're working hard in the heat, you can bypass heat exhaustion and go straight into heatstroke," Dr. Bowman says. "Most people know when they are overheating; they just need to pay attention to the signals."

Dress for the heat. Sun and wind suck away moisture, bake your body, and just make you feel hotter. It's better to wear a hat, long-sleeve shirt, and loose, cotton clothing. "Cotton is light and porous and does a good job of wicking away the heat," Rosoff says.

Acclimate yourself. If you live in a seasonally cool climate, your body needs time to adjust to the heat. "As the weather gets warmer, you should try to work in the heat a little bit, and then increase it daily," suggests Rosoff. "The other alternative is to exercise year-round, periodically raising your body's core temperature through exertion."

When you acclimate to the heat, your heart pumps out more blood, you start sweating sooner, the amount you sweat may double, and the salt content in your perspiration decreases.

"People who consistently work in hot climates respond to heat more efficiently," Rosoff says.

Know before you go. If you have had trouble with the heat in the past, says Rosoff, you are more likely to have trouble in the future, unless you plan ahead by rehydrating and having plenty of water on hand.

Open Wounds

▶PROBLEM

Open wounds occur as abrasions, lacerations, cuts, or punctures. An abrasion is when the surface of the skin is scraped off. A laceration is a tearing of tissue with jagged and irregular edges. Cuts are smooth slices in the flesh. Puncture wounds are deep and narrow wounds caused by an object such as a nail piercing the skin.

▶CAUSE

You're peeling an apple, skinning a deer, or cutting a slice of quiche and—whoops! The length of the open wound isn't so much a concern as depth. A wound deeper than a half-inch or one that gapes open (such as a wound over the knee or elbow) probably needs stitches to heal properly, says Warren Bowman, M.D., medical director for the National Ski Patrol who lives in Cooke City, Montana, just outside Yellowstone National Park.

In addition to depth, you can judge the severity of an open wound by the type of bleeding. Veins and capillaries near the surface tend to seep blood, but an artery spurts bright red blood with each heartbeat, explains Carl Weil, an emergency medical technician and director of Wilderness Medicine Outfitters in Elizabeth, Colorado. If you have this type of bleeding, or any severe bleeding at all, you should go to the emergency room immediately, says Weil.

Another concern is contamination. If you've fallen off your bike and skidded down the trail or cut your thumb while cleaning a chicken, get a tetanus shot within 72 hours if you haven't had one within 5 years, advises Dr. Bowman. "The tetanus bacterium is found mostly in soil or manure," he says.

"So if you have a wound chock-full of dirt and debris, it's better to play it safe and get a booster shot." If your wound is fairly clean, you may still need a booster if you haven't had one in 10 years. If you're not sure whether you should get a shot, your best bet is to ask your doctor, says Dr. Bowman.

If infection sets in, the wound will swell, become red, hurt worse, and drain pus, in which case you should see a doctor, advises Dr. Bowman.

If you see red streaks radiating from the wound—likely in the direction of the heart—then get to a doctor immediately. You have septicemia, otherwise known as blood poisoning, Weil says. "Blood poisoning can happen fast, within just a day depending on the strength of your immune system. And it can kill you if not treated immediately," he says.

▶SOLUTIONS

Follow these steps in the order they are presented to treat an open wound.

Put on the gloves. If you're treating someone else's open wound, always put on disposable rubber gloves—the latex or vinyl kind used by doctors or food handlers—to protect yourself from any disease-carrying organisms in their blood. The risk is not just from HIV (although that is certainly a concern) but also from hepatitis, Dr. Bowman says.

"I stuff one pair of gloves into a 35-millimeter film canister and then carry them in my car and in my pack when I'm out in the back country," Dr. Bowman says. Just be sure to keep the glove-filled canister out of direct sunlight and extreme heat, as high temperatures for prolonged periods can damage the gloves. You should also inspect the contents of any first-aid kit periodically to make sure that the items have not deteriorated, Dr. Bowman adds.

Get a raise. You can stop most any bleeding with strong direct pressure and by elevating the wound above the heart to lower the pressure on the cut. If your arm is cut, hold it over your head. If it's your leg, lie down and put up your feet, Weil says.

"When blood flow stops, clotting starts," explains Dr. Bowman. "With pressure and elevation, you're giving the body time to do its work."

Clean the junk out. If there is significant bleeding or the wound is a half-inch deep or more (and so probably requires stitches), leave the cleaning to the experts. Apply direct pressure and a sterile gauze compress held in place by adhesive tape, elevate the area, and get to an emergency room, says Dr. Bowman.

If your wound is minor and probably does not require stitches, remove any dirt and debris with tweezers once the bleeding has stopped, Dr. Bowman says. Use sterile tweezers, such as those in a Swiss Army knife flamed in a match or cleaned with an alcohol swab. If bleeding starts up again, just apply direct pressure.

Scrub it. Once the debris is out, cleanse the wound with hydrogen peroxide, pHisoHex soap (an antibacterial skin cleanser), a povidone-iodine solution (a

History Lesson

When Simon and Schuster published *Doctor Dan the Bandage Man*, a children's Little Golden Book, publisher Richard Simon decided, at the last minute, to put a half-dozen adhesive bandages in each book as a gimmick. He wired a friend at Johnson & Johnson, saying, "Please ship two million Band-Aids immediately." The reply the next day said, "Band-Aids on their way. What the hell happened to you?"

topical antiseptic microbicide), or just plain soap and water, which works about as well as anything, Weil says.

"Don't scrub just the wound but also the skin for four inches around the cut," Weil says. "Germs can crawl across skin surfaces."

Rinse it. After you've scrubbed, flush the soap or cleanser out of the wound with clean water. Do not use water from a lake or running stream, no matter how clean it looks, says Weil. "Use only the cleanest of drinking water," he advises.

Cover it. Let the skin surface dry thoroughly, and, if you have it, apply a small bead of triple antibiotic ointment (bacitracin, neomycin, and polymyxin B) such as Neosporin or Mycitracin Plus to the cut, says Weil.

For shallow wounds, cover with a commercial bandage strip. If the wound gapes, but isn't deep enough for stitches, use adhesive tape or butterfly bandages to pull it closed from each side.

Check it. Once the wound is clean and bandaged, you should check it every two days and reapply a clean bandage, Dr. Bowman says. Check the wound sooner if there are any signs of infection. If the bandage gets wet from showering, replace it. To prevent it from getting wet, tape plastic wrap over the bandage before showering—or take a bath, Dr. Bowman adds.

▶PREVENTIVE MEASURES

Stay sharp. Keep your kitchen knives properly honed, recommends Dr. Bowman. Although it may not seem obvious at first, a sharp knife is actually a safer knife because you don't need to exert as much pressure to cut through food. It's when you're exerting too much pressure on the knife that it's most likely to slip and slice you instead of whatever you're trying to cut, he says.

Cut away. Always cut in the direction away from your body, not toward it. This decreases the odds of slicing yourself if the knife slips. For example, many a man has found himself in the emergency room when all he really wanted was a bagel for breakfast. So here's how to slice a bagel safely, according to Mark Smith, M.D., chairman of the department of emergency medicine at

Washington Hospital Center and clinical professor of emergency medicine at the George Washington University School of Medicine and Health Sciences, both in Washington, D.C.: With your thumb and index finger, hold the bagel perpendicular to the table. Your thumb and index finger should be shaped like an upside-down "U." Put the knife edge in the space between the thumb and index finger and cut down.

Clean it quick. We know that this goes against our basic genetic programming as guys but do not just drop a knife into a sinkful of pots and dishes, says Dr. Bowman. It may dent or nick the knife, making it more likely to injure you the next time you use it. Leaving knives in the sink also poses a threat to you or the person who eventually reaches his hand in to start cleaning the mess, he says. Grab the knife by the blade, and you can go back to the top this chapter and start reading again.

Poisoning

▶PROBLEM

This isn't just a problem of kids getting into the Drano. More than 25 percent of emergency calls to the nation's poison control centers deal with adults. You don't have to ingest a dangerous substance to suffer the effects of poisoning. Just coming into contact with some chemicals, or inhaling the fumes, can hurt you.

▶CAUSE

For men, mishaps with prescription medications and household chemicals bring about the most cases, says Rose Ann Soloway, R.N., administrator of the American Association of Poison Control Centers in Washington, D.C.

Some poisons are potentially fatal, while others cause skin problems, respiratory ailments such as pneumonia, and even permanent conditions such as blindness or kidney failure. But most problems can be taken care without a trip to the hospital. In fact, 75 percent of calls to national poison control centers are taken care of over the phone, Soloway says.

▶SOLUTIONS

Follow these first aid tips for poisoning, then immediately call the Poison Control Center.

Jump in the shower. If the problem is a chemical that you've come in contact with, you need to get it off your body or out of your eyes as soon as possible. If it is a dry chemical, brush if off before getting wet. If you have quick ac-

DO THIS NOW

If you have swallowed a poisonous substance, drink a half-glass (four ounces) of milk or water. The drink will flush the chemicals out of your mouth and esophagus, where it can do the most damage, and send it to your stomach. But don't drink much more than a half-glass, warns Rose Ann Soloway, R.N., administrator of the American Association of Poison Control Centers in Washington, D.C. If you flood your stomach with too much liquid, it will distend, exposing an even larger surface area to the poison. Once you've downed the milk or water, call the poison control center immediately.

cess to a shower, hop in and stay under lukewarm water for 15 to 20 minutes, Soloway says. It's easier and more effective to wash off the substance in the shower than washing at a sink or with a cloth. If you are near a hose or a sprinkler, you can use water from those instead. If the chemical is in your eye, look straight into the shower head and blink your eyes under the water for 15 to 20 minutes as well, she says.

Take it all off. Shed every piece of clothing you have on if you've come in contact with a poisonous chemical, even if you don't think it was contaminated, Soloway says. Wash it immediately, and don't mix it with other clothes.

Get some fresh air. Inhaling poisonous fumes can be just as dangerous as ingesting a chemical. If you've inhaled fumes, get to fresh air immediately, Soloway says.

Don't automatically throw up. Many people mistakenly believe that they have to force themselves to vomit if they've ingested poison. Don't, says Bruce Anderson, Pharm.D., director of the Maryland Poison Center at the University of Maryland School of Pharmacy in Baltimore. "Always contact your poison control center first for their treatment recommendations. If certain substances get into your stomach in a small amount, it's not that bad. But if it goes down the wrong pipe and gets into your airways, it can be dangerous. Making yourself throw up increases the likelihood that it will go down the wrong pipe," Dr. Anderson says.

Call the local poison control center. As soon as you have taken these immediate measures—to dilute the poison, rinse your skin or eyes, or get fresh air—call your local poison control center. You can find the number on the inside cover or first page of the phone book. When you call, have the container of the poisonous substance on hand, says Kathy Ray, educator of the Poison Prevention Program of Lehigh Valley Hospital in Allentown, Pennsylvania. They will either tell you how to handle the situation at home or advise you to call the proper authorities if you need medical attention. Then they will alert the facility where you are going and let them know that you are on the way and what the nature of the problem is. They'll also advise you whether you should induce vomiting.

Be prepared. When you call the poison control center, you may be instructed to use either syrup of ipecac or activated charcoal. So it's a good idea to keep them on hand in case of emergency. Use them only as instructed.

Comfort with comfrey and calendula. After you have done what the poison control center suggests, you could try this: Make a poultice of either calendula flowers or comfrey leaves, suggests Kathleen Maier, director of the Dreamtime Center for Herbal Studies in Flint Hill, Virginia, and a professional member of the American Herbalists Guild. Both are available at health food stores. Take a handful of dry or fresh flowers or leaves and just cover them with boiling water. Let them sit for 10 to 15 minutes and then gently squeeze out the excess water. Take a layer of sterile gauze bandaging and lay it on your skin. Put

History Lesson

Bank robbers have used all sorts of weaponry during the years to perpetrate their crimes. But one especially creative criminal actually used poison to carry out his heist. In 1948, a thin, distinguished-looking man wearing a white coat and an armband with the word *Sanitation* on it walked into the Teikoku Bank in Tokyo just as the bank was closing. He claimed to be a civilian doctor with General Douglas MacArthur's staff sent to immunize the bank's employees against dysentery, which was going around at the time. The doctor ordered the entire staff to drink a medicine he gave them. As the workers drank, they fell down in excruciating pain. Only 4 of the 16 survived. The fake doctor left the bank with 181,805 yen—about $500 American.

After the murders, Tokyo police learned that the bogus doctor had conducted "rehearsals" at two other banks but that the intended victims did not fall sick after drinking the "medicine." But at one of the two test runs, the impostor gave a bank employee a business card stating that he was Dr. Shigeru Matsui. Police tracked down the real Dr. Matsui and found that he had given out 96 of his business cards to patients and businessmen.

Police interviewed every person who received a card, and focused on 56-year-old Sadamichi Hirasawa. The struggling artist was in desperate need of money yet somehow managed to deposit 44,500 yen a few days after the robbery. Hirasawa cracked under interrogation and admitted that he used potassium cyanide to kill the bank workers. (He also admitted that the two previous attempts failed because his poisonous concoction was too weak.) Hirasawa was found guilty and sentenced to death, but various appeals dragged the case out until he died of pneumonia on May 10, 1987, at the age of 95, making him the oldest person on death row in the world.

---

the flowers or leaves on the gauze and top it with another layer of gauze. Bandage it in place and leave it on for up to a half-hour. Calendula combats infections, and comfrey is a "supreme wound healer" when used externally as a poultice, Maier says. Reapply as needed, up to three times a day, until your skin heals.

▶PREVENTIVE MEASURES

Read the label. This simple deed will practically guarantee that you'll never have to call the poison control center. Chemicals and medications have directions and warnings for a reason, Soloway says. "Companies want to make using their products as easy as possible. They are not going to put a warning there or give detailed directions for use if they are not really necessary," she says.

Be a marked man. Here's a common male poisoning mistake: Guy puts antifreeze in a soda bottle to save space in the garage; guy forgets he did that; guy drinks antifreeze. "Keep all chemical products and medications in their original containers," Ray says.

Never, ever siphon gas. Okay, a lot of us did this when we were young and foolish—especially those of us who lived through the Arab oil embargo and gas lines of the 1970s. It may have seemed like a good idea at the time, but so did disco and leisure suits. Enough said. This idea literally sucks, and you can wind up with a mouthful of gasoline. "If you cough or choke and so get gasoline into your lungs, you could develop pneumonia," Soloway says. Do yourself a favor and don't even try it, she says.

Leave it to the scientists. You think that you're creating the supercleaning agent of all time by mixing ammonia and chlorine bleach: What you are really getting is a dangerous mixture that emits a poisonous gas, Ray says. Never mix chemicals and chemical products unless you're absolutely sure what you're doing.

Removing a Fishhook

▶ PROBLEM

You were angling for a big old bass but instead buried your lure deep into your own flesh. You're hooked good, too, because the barb—the angular part of the hook extending from the point—goes in easy but comes out hard.

▶ CAUSE

Perhaps a sudden gust of wind sent your perfect back cast awry, and that Size 12 Beadhead Nymph pierced your earlobe like some kind of New Age jewelry.

Actually, most fishermen hook themselves while removing the hook from a fish's mouth, says Joe Healy, avid fisherman and editor of *Saltwater Fly Fishing* magazine in Bennington, Vermont.

"You get a fish up to the boat, you're excited, and you're trying to remove the hook. The fish thrashes around, and the hook gets imbedded in your hand," Healy explains.

If you can get the hook out and minimize the chance of infection, you'll probably have nothing worse than a small puncture wound, says Warren Bowman, M.D., medical director for the National Ski Patrol who lives in Cooke City, Montana, just outside Yellowstone National Park.

If you're hooked deeply, pierced with more than one hook (a treble hook) or snagged around the eye and face, however, you better head straight to the emergency room, Dr. Bowman says.

DO THIS NOW

Immediately cut the line so that the hook or lure is hanging freely, suggests Joe Healy, avid fisherman and editor of *Saltwater Fly Fishing* magazine in Bennington, Vermont.

That way, if the rod falls over, it won't jerk the line and embed the hook deeper. You can also avoid embedding the hook deeper if you stay calm and don't jerk away when you hook yourself.

If your partner hooked you, let him know so that he doesn't jerk back on the rod or start reeling in the lure.

▶SOLUTIONS

Follow these steps—in order—to remove and treat a fishhook injury.

FISHING LINE METHOD

Tie a loop using a two-foot length of 20- to 30-pound test fishing line. (If you only have the lighter, more common 10- to 12-pound test, make a double loop.) Slip one end of the loop around your wrist and grip firmly. Loop the other end around the curve of the embedded hook.

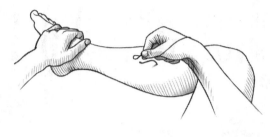

Next, determine the location of the hook's barb and the direction of penetration by gently rocking and rotating the hook between your thumb and forefinger. You're looking to position the hook in the path of least resistance. You are trying to back it out of the same hole it entered.

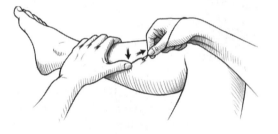

With the thumb of your opposite hand, apply firm, downward pressure on the shank, or straight end, of the hook. This should disengage the barb from the flesh and open the wound enough so that the hook can come out backward.

Finally, while maintaining pressure on the hook, give the fishing line a quick jerk by pulling horizontally on the line or at a slight, upward angle. The hook should come out fast. Be sure that no one is standing in the line of fire, or else they'll be nailed by the hook.

Push it out. If the barb is through the skin or lodged just beneath, you can opt to push it on through, says Howard Backer, M.D., a physician who practices emergency sports and wilderness medicine for Kaiser Permanente Medical Centers in the San Francisco Bay area and teaches wilderness medicine through the Wilderness Medical Society. Once the barb is through, snip it off with wire cutters or pliers and then back the rest of the hook out of the wound. Pushing a hook through should only be an option if the line-and-jerk method fails, Dr. Backer says.

"It's a painful, sort of bite-the-bullet cure. But it works," says Dr. Backer.

Purify the puncture. Once the hook's out, clean the wound thoroughly

History Lesson

Before the advent of metals, people made fishhooks from thorn bushes, stone, shells, wood, horns, and animal bone. On Easter Island in the Pacific, there were no large mammals to provide bone for hooks. Instead, after destruction of the island's small animals and the beginning of cannibalism, the Easter Islanders used human bones.

with soap, preferably a germicidal soap like Dial. Get rid of any dirt, fish flesh, or worm slime. Then put on an adhesive bandage. If you've had a tetanus shot or booster within the last five years, you're probably in no danger of a tetanus infection. But if you are uncertain about how long it has been since you had a shot, you should get one within 72 hours, says Dr. Bowman. "Tetanus is nasty, so it's always better to err on the conservative side," he adds. Antibiotics are usually not necessary, but if an infection develops, go see your doctor, he says. The signs of infection are increasing pain, redness, swelling, fever, discharge of pus from the wound, and red streaks running up your arm.

▶PREVENTIVE MEASURES

Shield the skin. Always wear glasses and a hat. Fly fisherman, who typically whip the line back and forth a few times before setting the fly on the water, sometimes hook themselves in an ear, back, or neck, Healy says. "Sometimes, they hook their buddies who are standing behind them," he adds.

Boat and bait fishermen do somewhat less casting than fly fishers, but they're fishing in a small space surrounded by lots of gear and hooks. "In a boat, you should always wear shoes so that you don't step on a hook," Healy advises. "And I've heard of people sitting on hooks, so look behind you before you plop down in your seat."

Seizures

▶PROBLEM

They last for as little as 30 seconds or up to several minutes, but seizures can be a frightening experience—for both the person having the seizure and those around them. Someone in the midst of a seizure loses consciousness, and their muscles involuntarily contract. They may also lose control of their bladder and suffer from mental confusion after the attack.

▶CAUSE

On a normal day, your brain circuits take turns firing off messages. But when a seizure comes on, the circuitry gets out of sync and launches a rapid-fire assault. Your brain goes into overload, and you react by losing consciousness and muscle control. "Seizures are an explosion of electricity in the brain," says Michael I. Weintraub, M.D., clinical professor of neurology at New York Medical College in Valhalla and chief of neurology at Phelps Memorial Hospital in Sleepy Hollow, New York.

If you have never experienced a seizure before, get medical help right away. While not normally dangerous in their own right, seizures usually signal more serious medical problems, including brain tumors, brain injuries, or strokes, says Paul Matera, M.D., an emergency medical technician-paramedic and vice chairman and professor of emergency services at Providence Hospital in Washington, D.C. People with epilepsy or a history of seizures do not necessarily need medical attention after an episode, as long as they are under the care of a doctor for

Did You Know?

Some special dogs can sense when a person is about to have a seizure, even if the person himself can't feel one coming. Seizure alert dogs warn their master about the oncoming seizure so that the person can prepare and get to a safe area. How the dogs know about the seizure is unknown, although scientists theorize that the dogs sense or smell a body chemistry change that may come right before the episode.

their condition, Dr. Matera says. People with epilepsy should, however, discuss their antiseizure medication and other measures of seizure prevention and control with their doctor if the seizures become more frequent.

▶SOLUTIONS

If you see someone having a seizure, do these in the following order.

Clear the decks. If you feel a seizure coming on, or are around someone who's having a seizure, quickly move any furniture, sharp objects, or other potentially harmful items out of the way. "Move anything near them that could cause injuries," says Georg Weber, M.D., Ph.D., assistant professor of medicine and a researcher at the Dana-Farber Cancer Institute at Harvard Medical School.

Cushion the head. Put a pillow or something else soft under your head and lie down if you feel a seizure coming. The same goes when you see that someone else going into a seizure. "Don't let them bang their head on anything," Dr. Matera says. The cushion protects them from head injuries during the seizure.

Put your money where your mouth is. A man's wallet is a perfect-size tool to keep a seizure victim from biting or swallowing his tongue, says Dr. Weber. If you sense a seizure coming, insert your wallet—take the change out first—between your teeth and chomp down on it. The same technique obviously can be used if you're around someone else who's going into a seizure.

If you don't have a wallet, use something that's not sharp and is big enough that you won't swallow it. Take care not to obstruct the airways, says Dr. Weber. Put the wallet in the side of the mouth. Don't stuff the whole thing into the mouth. Remove dentures if applicable, he adds. But if a person's in the midst of a full-blown seizure, don't try to force anything in his mouth, Dr. Matera adds. You could hurt them and yourself.

Let them be. Seizures can seem like they last forever. In reality, they usually last anywhere from 30 seconds to five minutes, Dr. Matera says. During that time, be patient and don't panic. People who try to hold the victim down usually only end up hurting themselves and the person having the seizure. "Don't try to shake them or wake them up. Let the seizure abate itself," he says.

During the seizure, put them in the left-side recovery position, if you can do this without injury to the victim or yourself. If not, wait until after the seizure is over to put them in the recovery position. Check to make sure that they are breathing and have a pulse. If not, call 911 and give rescue breathing or cardiopulmonary resuscitation as needed. If they do, monitor them until they fully recover. (For step-by-step information on the recovery position, rescue breathing, and cardiopulmonary resuscitation, see Lifesaving Techniques, beginning on page 579.)

Don't be alarmed. After a seizure, the victim may appear dazed, disoriented, even combative, says Dr. Matera. Don't worry, he says. This is normal, and it lasts from a few seconds to a few minutes. Just stay with him until he recovers.

▶PREVENTIVE MEASURES

Keep the water flowing. For some people, dehydration is a stepping-stone to a seizure, Dr. Weber says. Drink at least eight, eight-ounce glasses of water a day to prevent your body from drying out on the inside.

Get a good night's rest. Sleep shouldn't be what you sacrifice to keep your hectic life on schedule. "Sleep deprivation is a known trigger for seizures," Dr. Weber says. Go to bed and wake up the same time each day, which forces your internal clock to stay in line with your daily schedule. Don't spend too many nights staying up late to get things done, Dr. Weber cautions.

Go easy on the booze. Drinking heavily can destroy your body and your life. And once you're hooked on alcohol, even taking the steps to go on the wagon can have physical repercussions. Alcohol abusers and people with alcoholism often have seizures during withdrawal, Dr. Weber says. By taking it easy on alcohol, you reduce your chances of becoming dependent in the first place. "You can develop a lifestyle that will effectively reduce the risk of seizures," Dr. Weber says.

Check your medications. Certain drugs, combinations of drugs, or withdrawal from drugs may increase the likelihood of a seizure. If you are on medications, check with your doctor about their possible risks, says Dr. Weber.

Severed Appendages

▶ PROBLEM

Of the approximately 156,000 people who lose a limb each year, accidents are responsible for 75 percent of lost arms and 20 percent of lost legs. And these numbers only represent people who lost entire arms or legs. There are even more who lose smaller parts of the body, such as a fingers or toes.

▶ CAUSE

Blades of all kinds are the most common way of severing an appendage. Lawn mowers, saws, even plain old kitchen knives can cut through skin, muscle, and bone.

Other possible causes include freak mishaps while playing sports and machinery accidents.

▶ SOLUTIONS

While you are waiting for emergency assistance, do these in this order.

Hold on tight. Apply direct pressure to the wound using the cleanest object around, such as a shirt or a towel. Keep direct pressure on the stump until you get to the hospital. This will help stop the bleeding without the use of tourniquets and clamps, which often do more damage and are unnecessary if medical help is on the way, says Jedd Roe, M.D., assistant professor of emergency medicine at the University of Colorado School of Medicine in Denver. (For more tips on how to treat slice wounds, see Open Wounds on page 623.)

Elevate the body part. If you can, elevate the injured appendage above

DO THIS NOW

Whether you cut off your foot or just the tip of your finger, you should call 911 immediately, says Jedd Roe, M.D., assistant professor of emergency medicine at the University of Colorado School of Medicine in Denver.

You can bleed to death in five minutes if a cut has severed a major artery. Even less-severe amputations like the tip of your finger can cause complications and be very painful.

And the quicker you get to a hospital, the more likely doctors will be able to reunite you and your severed body part, he says.

Did You Know?

Take a second and try to pick up something, or do anything for that matter, without using your thumb. It can be very difficult. As humans, we need the thumb to function, and losing a thumb can be devastating. But doctors have found that if you lose a thumb, your big toe makes a great replacement.

Because you need your thumb more than you need your big toe, surgeons have started to perform big-toe transplants on patients who have severed a thumb. Toe transplants are considered better than finger or thumb reconstruction because the big toe looks a lot like a thumb and the toe is flexible. The transplant hasn't caught on in the Far East, though, because people wear zori-type sandals, which require a big toe to stay on the foot.

heart level, Dr. Roe says. Blood flows down with the help of gravity. By raising the body part above heart level, you'll slow down the blood loss.

Keep it attached. If the appendage is hanging off or is only partly amputated, leave it alone, Dr. Roe says. Removing a hanging piece of tissue will do more damage and make it harder to reattach. Apply direct pressure to the stump and support the other piece as best you can.

Make contact. Soak a sterile gauze with saline solution—the kind regularly used for contact lenses—and wrap the detached body part, Dr. Roe says. "It keeps the tissue moist and healthier," Dr. Roe says. Saline is the best choice because it has the same salt content as human tissue, so it keeps the proper balance between salt and water in the cells.

If you don't have saline solution, place the detached body part on dry, sterile gauze and cover it with the gauze. Try to avoid contact with regular water since it could be absorbed by the tissue, causing swelling and complications.

Put it on ice. Once you've wrapped the severed part in sterile gauze soaked in saline solution, place it in a watertight container. Put the part in a cooler filled with ice, says Ian Cummings, M.D., director of emergency services at the Day Kimball Hospital in Putnam, Connecticut. You want to keep it cool, but don't freeze it. Ice could damage the tissue.

Also, don't allow water to get into the container, Dr. Cummings warns. Soaking the appendage in water could also damage tissue and make it harder to reattach.

Bring it along. Even if you think that it is impossible to reattach, bring the severed part to the hospital. "You'd rather bring something with you that can't be attached than not bring something that could be," Dr. Roe says.

Lie down. If you feel light-headed, lie down with the stump elevated and wait for the ambulance, says Dr. Roe.

▶PREVENTIVE MEASURES

Go unplugged. Before sticking your hand into a fax machine, a printer, a copier, or any piece of machinery, unplug it, Dr. Roe says. That simple step may save you a few fingers.

Beware of the lawn mower, man. There were 74,582 injuries caused by lawn mowers in 1995. "For some reason, people don't get the message that you shouldn't fool with the workings of the lawn mower when it is still on," says Robert McNamara, M.D., professor of emergency medicine and program director of the department of emergency medicine residency at Allegheny University of the Health Sciences–MCP Hahnemann School of Medicine in Philadelphia. Shut off the lawn mower before you tinker with it. And keep your feet out from under it. It sounds obvious, but tell that to the guys walking around with nine toes or less. And you don't get a break in the winter: The same rules apply to snowblowers.

Use a push stick. Men who glide wood into a saw blade using their hands often end up gliding their hands in as well, says Dr. Cummings To save your hands, don't take off the saw guard that comes with your table saw. You can also make a push stick out of a piece of scrap lumber a couple of feet long, he suggests. Use the stick to maneuver the wood in and out of the blade's pathway. Be extra careful with any kind of saw, he adds. Chain saws caused 31,356 injuries in 1995. They are notorious for injuries to the foot, knee, thigh, and hand. What's worse, he says, is that they make messy wounds. They remove tissue, damage tendons, and with all the ground-in dirt, chain saw wounds are likely to become infected.

Watch what you wear. When you work around power tools or industrial equipment, dress properly, suggests Dr. Cummings. Don't wear rings, jewelry, or ties. They can get caught and you could get dragged into the machinery. Also, wear steel-tipped shoes to avoid severed toes, he says.

Sport flashy moves, not jewelry. Take off all your jewelry before taking to the basketball court or any sports venue, says Paul Matera, M.D., an emergency medical technician-paramedic and vice chairman and professor of emergency services at Providence Hospital in Washington, D.C. Dr. Matera knows of a man who went up for a slam dunk. His ring and finger got caught on the net—but the rest of his body still came down. "Never, never, never, never wear a ring when you are playing sports. I don't care what your wife says," Dr. Matera says.

Struck by Lightning

▶PROBLEM

Lightning kills about 100 people and injures another 400 each year, more than hurricanes and tornadoes combined. "Lightning is the most dangerous natural phenomenon that people encounter," says Ron Holle, research meteorologist at the National Severe Storms Laboratory in Norman, Oklahoma. "Nearly everyone has lightning strike near them each year."

Studies over the past century have consistently shown that 85 to 90 percent of those injured by lightning are men. That's because men do more outdoor work and sports and are exposed to lightning more than women. And younger men, teens through their thirties, seem to be the more frequent victims, says Holle. "They feel invincible and take more risks than older men," he adds.

A little rain won't stop many golfers, but standing on a treeless fairway, wearing shoes with spikes, and wielding a long, thin, metallic club makes you a superb conduit for the billion volts of energy produced by the average one- to two-inch-wide lightning bolt.

▶CAUSE

Take a direct hit and you're probably history. Most folks get it from side flashes coming off trees or charges surging through the ground. Ground strikes can blow you right out of your shoes, says Holle.

DO THIS NOW

If someone near you is struck by lightning, is knocked unconscious, and has no pulse, start cardiopulmonary resuscitation immediately, says Mary Ann Cooper, M.D., director of the Lightning Injury Research Program at the University of Illinois in Chicago. Lightning acts like a defibrillator and stops the heart.

Depending on the youth and health of its owner, the heart usually starts beating again by itself, Dr. Cooper says. If the person is not breathing, administer mouth-to-mouth resuscitation. The respiratory arrest lasts longer than the cardiac arrest, so the beating heart can eventually stop from lack of oxygen. In either case, seek emergency care immediately.

History Lesson

Being a guy, Ben Franklin was a little cavalier about lightning's lethality, even though he once jolted himself senseless while electrocuting a turkey with glass batteries. To prove that lightning contained electricity, Franklin proposed an experiment where a man would sit in a tower beneath a long iron rod so that "when such clouds are passing low [the man] might become electrified and afford sparks." Franklin never did the tower bit himself but used a kite instead. After reading of Franklin's electrical experiments, a Swedish physicist put up just such an experimental rod , succeeded in drawing "electrical fire" from clouds . . . and died.

Up to 80 to 90 percent of people hit by lightning survive, but that doesn't mean that they come away unscathed, says Mary Ann Cooper, M.D., director of the Lightning Injury Research Program at the University of Illinois in Chicago. "It's like when you pass a charge through a computer. The box on the outside may look okay, but the software inside is a little scrambled," she says. So anyone who has been struck by lightning should see a doctor.

Sometimes the concussive boom of the strike breaks your eardrums, and causes some type of hearing loss. You may be temporarily blinded and have a small chance to develop cataracts in the coming months. Or you could be crippled by the voltage surging through your brain or spinal cord. Neurological problems may be subtle and only show up later as memory or learning problems, says Dr. Cooper.

In fatal strikes, most people die from cardiac arrest. Lightning stops their heart and paralyzes their chest muscles. Burns tend to be superficial since lightning usually travels on the outside of the body, leaving a characteristic fernlike pattern on the skin that disappears after a few hours.

▶SOLUTIONS

Here are some tips to help someone who has been hit by lightning until medical help arrives.

Calm the nerves. There is little first-aid to give conscious lightning victims except comfort, says Dr. Cooper. They'll be dazed and unable to remember what happened. Make sure that they don't wander off a cliff, fall in the water, or hurt themselves, she says.

Balm the burns. Check for burns, which can be deep when the lightning vaporizes metal jewelry or turns a person's sweat into steam, Dr. Cooper adds. "If there are any burns, wash them with soap and water, remove any debris, and cover with bandages," she says. (See Burns on page 592 for more tips.)

Soothe your cells. If you survive the hit, Dr. Cooper suggests that you take a nonsteroidal anti-inflammatory such as ibuprofen (Advil or Motrin IB) for few days. The sooner you start taking them, the better. Lightning damages cell structure and the anti-inflammatory agent may prevent additional damage. The dosage for the average-size person should be about 100 milligrams per hour or about two tablets every four hours.

"It's a little like being punched in the nose or twisting an ankle. For a few days afterward, the damaged cells will leak out some nasty chemicals and cause swelling," Dr. Cooper says.

▶ PREVENTIVE MEASURES

Go undercover. The best protection is in a permanent building with plumbing, electrical wiring, a lightning rod, or some metal component that can ground the charge, says Dr. Cooper. Stay away from isolated trees, ridges, hill-tops, and sheds on the golf course. "Those sheds just make you a taller target," she adds. The safest place to be if you are golfing is the clubhouse, says Michael Cherington, M.D., a neurologist at the Lightning Data Center at Centura Health Saint Anthony's Hospital in Denver.

Cars are safe, but not because of the rubber tires. When lightning hits a car, the electrical charge stays on the outside metal skin. If you take shelter in a hardtop (not a convertible), keep the windows up and don't touch anything metal, Dr. Cooper says.

Be cautious. If a storm is in the area, don't plan on outdoor activities, says Holle. If you are already outside, don't wait until the storm gets close to seek safe shelter.

Know the warning signs of impending storms, such as ominous clouds and thunder. If a storm is approaching and you are in the water, get out and seek safe shelter. Stay away from metal objects such as golf clubs and bicycles. Don't go back out too soon either. "Most people are struck at the beginning or end of the storm when they thought it was safe to be outside," Dr. Cherington says.

Power down. You're not necessarily safe in a house if you ride out the storm by gabbing on the telephone, surfing the Internet, or soaking in a hot tub. When lightning hits a home, the current usually travels along the plumbing and electrical lines. Better to pull the plugs on all your electronic devices when you hear the first thunder, delay the bath, take a seat in the living room, and watch the light show outside, says Holle.

Get down with your bad self. If you're in the woods, find shelter in a thick grove of small trees. In an open field, go to the lowest point. If your skin tingles or hair stands up, squat, grab your legs, and lower your head. Don't lie down. Balance on the balls of your feet to limit ground contact, says Holle.

"Of all the places in your life to be, this is one of the worst," says Holle. "The cloud overhead is electrified and ready to put down a flash in a small area. You never want to put yourself into this position."

Index

Underscored page references indicate boxed text. **Boldface** page references indicate illustrations.